ENSURING GLOBAL FOOD SAFETY

EXPLORING GLOBAL HARMONIZATION

Ensuring Global Food Safety

Exploring Global Harmonization

Christine E. Boisrobert
Air Liquide, Houston, Texas, USA

Åleksandra Stjepanovic
Norwegian University of Life Sciences, As, Norway

Sangsuk Oh
Ewha Womans University, Seoul, Korea

Huub L.M. Lelieveld
Formerly Unilever R&D, Vlaardingen, The Netherlands

ELSEVIER

AMSTERDAM • BOSTON • HEIDELBERG • LONDON • NEW YORK • OXFORD • PARIS
SAN DIEGO • SAN FRANCISCO • SINGAPORE • SYDNEY • TOKYO
Academic Press is an imprint of Elsevier

Academic Press is an imprint of Elsevier
32 Jamestown Road, London, NW1 7BY, UK
30 Corporate Drive, Suite 400, Burlington, MA 01803, USA
525 B Street, Suite 1900, San Diego, CA 92101-4495, USA

First edition 2010

Library of Congress Cataloging in Publication Data
A catalog record for this book is available from the Library of Congress

British Library Cataloguing in Publication Data
A catalogue record for this book is available from the British Library

ISBN: 978-0-12-374845-4

For information on all Academic Press publications
visit our website at www.elsevierdirect.com

Printed and bound in United States of America
Transferred to Digital Printing, 2011

Contents

Foreword

The production, processing, distribution, retail, packaging and labeling of foodstuffs are governed by a vast number of laws, regulations, codes of practice and guidance. Most food safety legislation and regulations were devised in the first decades after the Second World War, at times when analytical methods were much less advanced than today. More recent legislation and regulations often have been developed in response of media scares. Today's reality is that there are differences in regulations between countries that force the food community to check the safety over and over again, depending on where the products are produced, from where they or their ingredients originate, or to where they are exported. In addition to wasting time and money, this also too often leads to severe measures such as the destruction of huge quantities of food, despite lacking any scientific justification, to protect consumers, while a large part of the human population suffers from undernourishment. This book provides examples and discusses possible means of improvement of the current situation in the field of food regulations. It strongly supports the idea of the necessity to establish an integral system of globally accepted food safety protocols. Actually, this idea was launched by the Global Harmonization Initiative (GHI), a network of scientific organizations and individual scientists that was initiated to help eliminate differences in regulations and legislation. This book represents a step forward towards the harmonization of food safety regulations and legislation worldwide.

The intention of this book is to bundle the extensive information on food regulations through history and over all continents into a comprehensive reference; and it presents, complete, up-to-date information on contemporary food safety issues related to the global food supply chain. Various questions and issues relating to food production frequently raised in the supply chain from farming to retail are covered, including control of microbiological risks, approaches to managing low level contaminants in foods, processing issues, applications of antibiotics in food, traditional and organic foods in the scope of safety and nutrition, carcinogenicity and toxicity issues, and finally, the issue of balance between benefits and safety risk. Possibilities for global harmonization of test protocols and analytical methods are also discussed, while the interest in further research into novel methods and ingredients and novel food processing technologies against regulatory hurdles is argued.

Combining scientific, technological, and legal aspects, over 30 carefully selected scientists and food safety professionals from academia, industry, and government across the world have contributed unique expertise and knowledge ensuring the safety and quality of the food supply for consumers.

Prof. Dr. Viktor Nedović

Assistant Minister for International Scientific and Technological Cooperation Ministry of Science and Technological Development Government of the Republic of Serbia

Ass. Prof. at Dept. of Food Technology and Biochemistry, Faculty of Agriculture, University of Belgrade, Belgrade, Serbia

Member of the Executive Committee of the European Federation of Food Science & Technology (EFFoST)

Preface

Food safety is generally recognized as the biological, chemical or physical status of a food that will permit its consumption without incurring excessive risk of injury, morbidity or mortality. It is also true that assessing food safety risk is frequently steeped in either or both political and normative considerations. National governments promote and promulgate food safety laws, regulations and legislation that can be in sharp contrast to those of other countries. These disparities frequently give rise to onerous trade barriers that masquerade as public health protection. Science and certainly scientific consensus on the status of the food, from a food safety perspective, may be overlooked during the rule-making process.

International differences in food safety regulations are disruptive to trade and frequently cause confusion among consumers as to the public health status of a food. Food deemed safe by an exporting nation may be regarded as unsafe by an importing nation. This debate often results in the seizure and destruction of food without a clear scientific basis or justification. Likewise novel food processing and preservation technologies or novel food ingredients are scrutinized for safety using protocols, procedures and standards that differ by country. These measures are taken to protect consumers from exposure to food that may adversely affect their health.

It is difficult to conceive, generally, that a food considered safe for one population would be unsafe for another. Yet and because of differences in food use and preparation among countries, food safety regulations frequently have a basis in the local history and tradition rather than science. Harmonization of food safety regulations would potentially reduce the legal, but scientifically unjustified, destruction of food. Likewise harmonization of legislation and standards may result in eliminating the duplication in the need to prove the safety of novel foods and food ingredients, and consequently the high costs, to satisfy local authorities.

The Global Harmonization Initiative (GHI) is a non-governmental organization that seeks to obtain consensus among individual scientists, globally, on those contentious issues that require resolution. Consensus documents and white papers developed by GHI may be used as powerful tools in the discussions between stakeholders and are intended to promote the development of regulations based on sound science. The authors that have contributed to this work have described many of the reasons why regulations differ and what difficulties must be overcome to resolve such differences. The book provides a detailed insight into food safety regulations around the world and discusses methods to determine the safety of foods, ingredients and food-contact materials. It also addresses food contaminants, including the impact and implications for food safety of those that may be present in very low levels. Furthermore, it provides abstracts of additional reading materials accessible through the publisher's website about integrating risk assessment and cost benefit analysis, food additives and other substances added to foods, and benefits and risks of organic food in relation to harmonization of food safety regulations.

Considering the abundance of pre-existing literature on the topic and the complexity of the subject, this book does not cover genetically modified food.

The editors are immensely grateful to the authors who contributed tremendous effort and time to create this volume. In addition, we thank Nancy Maragioglio and Carrie Bolger of Elsevier for their support and patience with us, the editors, during the development of this book.

Christine Boisrobert, Åleksandra Stjepanovic, Sangsuk Oh and Huub Lelieveld, August 2009.

Acronyms and Abbreviations

2-AAF: 2-acetylaminofluorene.

25(OH)D: 25-hydroxyvitamin D.

3-MC: 3-methylcholantene.

4-AAF: 4-acetylaminofluorene.

AB: Alamar Blue.

AB: Appellate Body.

ACFCR: ASEAN Common Food Control Requirements.

ADA: American Dietetic Association.

ADFCA: Abu Dhabi Food Control Authority.

ADI: Acceptable Daily Intake.

ADME: Absorption, Distribution, Metabolism and Excretion.

AFB_1: Aflatoxin B_1.

AFM: Atomic Force Microscope.

AFNOR: Association Française de Normalisation (*French*).

AFSC: Australian Food Standards Code.

AIDS: Acquired Immune Deficiency Syndrome.

AK: Adenylate Kinase.

ALARA: As Low As Reasonably Achievable.

ALOP: Appropriate Level of Protection.

ALS: Amyotrophic Lateral Sclerosis.

AMA: American Medical Association.

AMPA: α-amino-3-hydroxy-5-methyl-4-isoxazole propionate.

ANSI: American National Standards Institute.

ANZCERTA: Australia New Zealand Closer Economic Relations Trade Agreement.

ANZFA: Australia New Zealand Food Authority (*renamed* FSANZ).

AOAC: Association of Analytical Communities (*formerly* Association of Official Analytical Chemists).

APEC: Asia-Pacific Economic Cooperation.

AQIS: Australian Quarantine and Inspection Service.

AQSIQ: General Administration of Quality Supervision, Inspection and Quarantine of PRC.

ARfD: Acute Reference Dose.

ARLs: ASEAN Reference Laboratories.

ASEAN: Association of Southeast Asian Nations.

ATP: Adenosine Triphosphate.

AU: African Union.

B(a)P: Benzo(a)pyrene.

B(e)P: Benzo(e)pyrene.

BHA: Butylated Hydroxyanisole.

BHT: Butylated Hydroxytoluene.

BIS: Bureau of Indian Standards.

BLEB: Buffered Listeria Enrichment Broth.

BMC: Bone Mineral Content.

BMD: Bone Mineral Density.

BMELV: Federal Ministry of Food, Agriculture and Consumer Protection (Bundesministerium für Ernährung, Landwirtschaft und Verbraucherschutz, *German*).

BNF: British Nutrition Foundation.

bp: base pair.

BRC: British Retail Consortium.

BSE: Bovine Spongiform Encephalopathy.

BSI: British Standards Institution.

BVL: Federal Office of Consumer Protection and Food Safety (Bundesamt für Verbraucherschutz und Lebensmittelsicherheit, *German*).

bw: body weight.

CAC: Codex Alimentarius Commission.

CACCLA: Codex Alimentarius Coordinating Committee for Latin America.

CACM: Central American Common Market.

CAFTA: Council of Food Technology Associations.

CAP: Chloramphenicol.

CARICOM: Caribbean Community and Common Market.

CASCO: Committee on Conformity Assessment.

CAST: Council for Agricultural Science and Technology.

CBA: Cost-Benefit Analysis.

CBOs: Community-Based Organizations.

CCFAC: Codex Committee on Food Additives and Contaminants.

CCFH: Codex Committee on Food Hygiene.

CCFL: Codex Committee on Food Labelling.

CCFNSDU: Codex Committee on Nutrition and Foods for Special Dietary Uses.

CCP: Critical Control Point.

CDC: Centers for Disease Control and Prevention.

CEDI: Cumulative Estimated Daily Intake.

CEDR: European Council for Agricultural Law (Comité Européen de Droit Rural, *French*).

CEF: EFSA Panel on food contact materials, enzymes, flavourings and processing aids.

CEN: European Committee for Standardization (Comité Européen de Normalisation, *French*).

CEO: Chief Executive Officer.

CEPI: Confederation of European Paper Industries.

CETEA-ITAL: Packaging Technology Center – Institute of Food Technology.

CF: Consumption Factor.

CFIA: Canadian Food Inspection Agency.

CFR: Code of Federal Regulations.

CFSAN: Center for Food Safety and Applied Nutrition.

CFSI: Caribbean Food Safety Initiative.

CFTRI: Central Food Technological Research Institute.

CFU: Colony-Forming Unit.

CHO: Chinese Hamster Ovary.

CIA: Central Intelligence Agency.

CIAA: Confederation of the Food and Drink Industries of the EU (Confédération des Industries Agro-Alimentaires de l' UE, *French*).

CIES: The Food Business Forum (Comité International d'Entreprises à Succursales, *French*)

CMC: Common Market Council (Consejo del Mercado Común, *Spanish*).

COAG: Council of Australian Governments.

CoE: Council of Europe.

COPAIA: Pan American Commission for Food Safety (Comisión Panamericana de Inocuidad de los Alimentos, *Spanish*).

CP: Cyclophosphamide.

CRS: Chinese Restaurant Syndrome.

CSREES: Cooperative State Research, Education, and Extension Service.

CUT: Come-Up Time.

CYP: Cytochrome P450

CytK: Cytotoxin K.

DAFF: Department of Agriculture, Fisheries and Forestry.

DC: Dietary Concentration.

D-E: Deficiency-Excess.

DEFT: Direct Epifluorescent Filter Technique.

DEH: Department of Environment and Heritage.

DG: Directorate General (Directorat Général, *French*)

DG SANCO: Directorate General for Health and Consumers (Directorat Général de Santé et Protection des Consommateurs, *French*).

DIG: Digoxigenin.

DM: Dry Matter.

DMN: Dimethylnitrosamine.

DMSO: Dimethyl Sulfoxide.

DNA: Deoxyribonucleic Acid.

DON: Deoxynivalenol.

DP: Degree of Polymerization.

DRF: Simulant D Reduction Factor.

DSB: Dispute Settlement Body.

dsDNA: Double-stranded DNA.

DSHEA: Dietary Supplement Health and Education Act.

DV: Daily Value.

EAR: Estimated Average Requirement.

EC: European Commission.

EC Treaty: European (Economic) Community Treaty (of 1957)

ECCS: Electrolytic Chromium Coated Steel *also see* TFS.

EDI: Estimated Daily Intake.

EDTA: Ethylenediaminetetraacetic acid.

EEC: European Economic Community.

EFFoST: European Federation of Food Science and Technology.

EFLA: European Food Law Association.

EFSA: European Food Safety Authority.

EFTA: European Free Trade Association.

EHEDG: European Hygienic Engineering and Design Group.

EIA: Enzyme Immunoassay.

ELIFA: Enzyme-Linked Immunofiltration Assay.

ELISA: Enzyme-Linked Immunosorbent Assay.

ELOSA: Enzyme-Linked Oligosorbent Assay.

ENM: Engineered Nano Materials.

EPA: Environmental Protection Agency.

EPHX1: Epoxide Hydrolase 1.

ERIC: Enterobacterial Repetitive Intergenic Consensus.

ERP: Expert Review Panel.

ERS: Economic Research Service.

EtOH: Ethanol.

EU: European Union.

EuCheMS-FCD: European Association for Chemical and Molecular Sciences-Food Chemistry Division.

EVM: Expert Group on Vitamins and Minerals.

FAO: Food and Agriculture Organization.

FASEB: Federation of American Societies for Experimental Biology.

FCCP: Carbonyl cyanide 4-(trifluoromethoxy) phenylhydrazone.

FCD Act: Foodstuffs, Cosmetics and Disinfectants Act.

FCM: Food Contact Material.

FCN: Food Contact Notification.

FCS: Food Contact Substance.

FCS: Food Control System.

FDA: Food and Drug Administration.

FDAMA: Food and Drug Administration Modernization Act.

FD&C Act: Federal Food, Drug and Cosmetic Act (*also* FFDCA, FDCA).

FFDCA: Federal Food, Drug and Cosmetic Act (*also* FDCA, FD&C).

FFR: Food Fortification Regulation.

FLAG: Food Legislation Advisory Group.

FMC: Food Microbiology Subcommittee.

FNB: Food and Nutrition Board.

FRF: Fat Reduction Factor.

FSANZ: Food Standards Australia New Zealand (*formerly* ANZFA).

FSC: Food Standards Committee.

FSD: Food Supplements Directive.

FSIS: Food Safety and Inspection Service.

FSO: Food Safety Objective.

FSSAI: Food Safety and Standards Authority of India.

f_T: Food-type distribution factor.

FT-IR: Fourier Transform Infrared.

FVO: Food and Veterinary Office.

GA: Glutamic Acid.

GABA: Gamma-Aminobutyric Acid.

GAPs: Good Agricultural Practices.

GATT: General Agreement on Tariffs and Trade.

GC: Gas Chromatography.

GCC: Gulf Cooperation Council.

GC/MS: Gas Chromatography/Mass Spectrometry.

GCS: g-glutamylcysteine synthetase.

GDP: Gross Domestic Product.

GFL: General Food Law.

GFSI: Global Food Safety Initiative.

GHI: Global Harmonization Initiative.

GHPs: Good Hygienic Practices (*also* Good Hygiene Practices).

GI: Gastrointestinal.

GLPs: Good Laboratory Practices.

GM: Genetically Modified.

GMO: Genetically Modified Organism.
GMC: Common Market Group (Grupo Mercado Común, *Spanish*).
GMP: Disodium 5'-Guanosine Monophosphate.
GMPs: Good Manufacturing Practices.
GRAS: Generally Recognized As Safe.
GSFA: General Standard for Food Additives.
GSH: Glutathione.
HAA: Heterocyclic Aromatic Amine.
HACCP: Hazard Analysis Critical Control Point.
HBL: Hemolysin BL.
HCN: Hydrogen cyanide (hydrocyanic acid).
HDL: High-Density Lipoprotein.
HEATOX: Heat-generated food toxicants, identification, characterization and risk minimization.
HFFA: Health/Functional Food Act.
HFFs: Health/Functional Foods.
HHP: High Hydrostatic Pressure.
HHS: Department of Health and Human Services.
HMPA: Hexamethylphosphoramide.
HPP: High Pressure Processing.
HPP: Hydrolyzed Protein Product.
HPRT: Hypoxanthine Phosphoribosyltransferase
HPS: Health Physics Society.
HT-2: HT-2 toxin.
IARC: International Agency for Research on Cancer.
ICC: International Association for Cereal Science and Technology (*formerly* International Association for Cereal Chemistry).
ICMSF: International Commission on Microbiological Specifications for Foods.
IDB: Inter-American Development Bank.
IDF: International Dairy Federation.
IEC: International Electrotechnical Commission.
IFIC: International Food Information Council.
IFS: International Food Standard.
IFT: Institute of Food Technologists.
Ig: Immunoglobulin.
IHR: International Health Regulations.

IMACE: International Margarine Association of the Countries of Europe.
IMF: International Monetary Fund.
IMP: Disodium 5'-Inosine Monophosphate.
INFOSAN: International Food Safety Authorities Network.
INTI: National Institute of Industrial Technology.
INTN: National Institute of Technology and Standardization.
INU: Intended Normal Use.
IOM: Institute of Medicine.
IPCC: Intergovernmental Panel on Climate Change.
IPCS: International Programme on Chemical Safety.
IQ: 2-amino-3-methylimidazo[4,5-*f*]quinoline.
IPPC: International Plant Protection Convention.
IRAM: Argentine Standardization Institute (Instituto Argentino de Normalización y Certificación, *formerly* Instituto Argentino de Racionalización de Materiales, *Spanish*).
ISI: Indian Standards Institution.
ISO: International Organization for Standardization.
ISR: International Sanitary Regulations.
ITU: International Telecommunication Union.
IUFoST: International Union of Food Science and Technology.
IVO: Iran Veterinary Organization.
JECFA: Joint FAO/WHO Expert Committee on Food Additives.
JEMRA: Joint FAO/WHO Expert Meetings on Microbiological Risk Assessment.
JETRO: Japan External Trade Organization.
JFDA: Jordan Food and Drug Administration.
JHAVC: Japan Hygienic Association of Vinylidene Chloride.
JHOSPA: Japan Hygienic Olefin and Styrene Plastics Association.
JMPR: Joint FAO/WHO Meetings on Pesticide Residues.
JRC: Joint Research Centre.
KFDA: Korea Food and Drug Administration.
KFT: Karl Fischer Titration.

LATU: Technological Laboratory of Uruguay (Laboratorio Tecnológico del Uruguay, *Spanish*).

LbL: Layer-by-Layer

LC-MS-MS: Liquid Chromatography-Mass Spectrometry-Mass Spectrometry.

LDL: Low-Density Lipoprotein.

LEB: Listeria Enrichment Broth.

L-GA: L-Glutamic Acid.

LNT: Linear Non-Threshold.

LOAEL: Lowest-Observed-Adverse-Effect-Level.

LOD: Limit of Detection.

LOQ: Limit of Quantitation.

LPM: Lithium Chloride-Phenylethanol-Moxalactam.

LT: Linear Threshold.

M/S: ratio (mass of food stuff contained/ contact surface area of FCM)

MALDI-MS: Matrix-Assisted Laser Desorption/ Ionization Mass Spectrometry.

MC: Microbiological Criteria.

MeIQ: 2-amino-3,4-dimethylimidazo[4,5-*f*] quinoline.

MeIQX: 2-amino-3,8-dimethylimidazo[4,5-*f*] quinoline.

MERCOUSUL: Common Market of the South (Mercado Commum do Sul, *Portuguese*).

MERCOSUR: Common Market of the South (Mercado Común del Sur, *Spanish*).

MDG: Millennium Development Goal.

MED.: Minimum Effective Dose.

mGST-1: microsomal Glutathione-S-Transferase.

MHLW: Ministry of Health, Labour and Welfare.

ML: Maximum Level.

MLA: McBride Listeria Agar.

MN: Micronuclei.

MoA: Ministry of Agriculture (India).

MOA: Ministry of Agriculture (Japan).

MoC: Ministry of Commerce.

MoCA: Ministry of Consumer Affairs.

MoFPI: Ministry of Food Processing Industries.

MoHFW: Ministry of Health and Family Welfare.

MOHWF: Ministry of Health, Welfare and Family Affairs.

MOU: Memorandum of Understanding.

MOXA: Modified Oxford Agar.

MPA: Medroxyprogesterone acetate.

MPN: Most Probable Number.

MPPO: Modified Polyphenylene Oxide.

MRC: Medical Research Council.

MRL: Maximum Residue Limit.

MRPL: Minimum Required Performance Limit.

mRNA: Messenger Ribonucleic Acid.

MRSA: Methicillin-resistant *Staphylococcus aureus*.

M/S: ratio (mass of foodstuff contained/contact surface area of FCM).

MSG: Mono-Sodium Glutamate.

MTR: Maximum Tolerable Risk.

NAFTA: North American Free Trade Agreement.

NASA: National Aeronautics and Space Administration.

NAT: *N*-acetyl transferase.

NAT 1: *N*-acetyl transferase 1.

NCFST: National Center for Food Safety and Technology.

NCTR: National Center for Toxicological Research.

ND: Not Detected/Not Detectable.

NEPA: National Environmental Policy Act.

NFA: National Food Authority.

NFP: Nutrition Facts Panel.

NGFIS: Netherlands Government Food Inspection Service.

NGOs: Non-Governmental Organizations.

NHE: Non-Hemolytic Enterotoxin.

NHMRC: National Health and Medical Research Council.

NIAS: Non-Intentionally Added Substances.

NIOSH: National Institute for Occupational Safety and Health.

NIP: Nutrition Information Panel.

NIR: Near Infrared.

NLEA: Nutrition Labeling and Education Act.

NMDA: N-methyl-D-aspartate.

NMSP: Nanoscale Materials Stewardship Program.

NNI: National Nanotechnology Initiative.

NOAEL: No-Observed-Adverse-Effect-Level.

NOEL: No-Observed-Effect-Level.

NordVal: Nordic System for Validation of Alternative Microbiological Method.

NRC: National Research Council.

NRCS: National Regulator for Compulsory Specifications.

nRDA: New Recommended Daily Allowance.

NRV: Nutrient Reference Value.

NSW: New South Wales.

NTP: National Toxicology Program.

OAS: Organization of American States.

OD: Oven Drying.

OECD: Organisation for Economic Co-operation and Development.

OIE: World Organisation for Animal Health (*formerly* Office International des Epizooties, *French*).

OLF: Other Legitimate Factor.

OMA: Official Methods of Analysis.

OML: Overall Migration Limit (expressed in mg/kg or mg/dm^2) (EU and MERCOSUR (=LMT, Límite de Migración Total, *Spanish*)).

OSHA: Occupational Safety and Health Administration.

OTA: Ochratoxin A.

OWCs: Organic Wastewater Contaminants.

OXA: Oxford Agar.

PA: Polyamide.

PAHO: Pan American Health Organization.

PALCAM: Polymyxin Acriflavine Lithium chloride Ceftazidime Aesculin Mannitol.

PAS: Publicly Available Specification.

PATP: Pressure Assisted Thermal Processing.

PC: Polycarbonate.

PCBs: Polychlorinated biphenyls.

PCDDs: Polychlorinated dibenzodioxins.

PCDFs: Polychlorinated dibenzofurans.

PCR: Polymerase Chain Reaction.

PE: Polyethylene.

PEF: Pulsed Electric Fields.

PEMBA: Polymyxin pyruvate egg-yolk mannitol bromothymol blue agar.

PEN: Project on Emerging Nanotechnologies.

PET: Polyethylene Terephthalate.

PFA: Prevention of Food Adulteration Act.

PFAC: Pure Food Advisory Committee.

PFGE: Pulsed Field Gel Electrophoresis.

PhIP: 2-amino-1-methyl-6-phenylimidazo [4,5-*b*]pyridine.

PLA: Polylactic Acid.

PMMA: Polymethyl Metracrylate.

PMP: Poly(4-methyl-1-pentene).

PO: Performance Objective.

POPs: Persistent Organic Pollutants.

PP: Polypropylene.

ppb: parts per billion (1 in 10^9).

PPCPs: Pharmaceuticals and Personal Care Products.

ppm: parts per million (1 in 10^6).

ppt: parts per trillion (1 in 10^{12}).

PRC: People's Republic of China.

PRPs: Prerequisite Programs.

PS: Polystyrene.

PTDI: Provisional Tolerable Daily Intake.

PTH: Parathyroid Hormone.

PTI: Provisional Tolerable Intake.

PTMI: Provisional Tolerable Monthly Intake.

PTWI: Provisional Tolerable Weekly Intake.

PVA: Polyvinyl Alcohol.

PVC: Polyvinyl Chloride.

PVDC: Polyvinylidene Chloride.

QM: Quantity in Material (limit on the residual quantity of a substance left in the finished material expressed in mg/kg) (EU and MERCOSUR (=LC, Límite de Composición, *Spanish*)).

QMA: Quantity in Material per surface Area (limit on the residual quantity of a substance left in the finished material expressed as mg per 6 dm^2 of the surface in contact with the food) (EU and MERCOSUR (=LCA, Límite de Composición por Area de superficie de contacto, *Spanish*)).

QMA(T): group concentration limit (limit on the residual quantity left in the finished material expressed as mg of total of moiety or substance(s) indicated per 6 dm^2 of the surface in contact with the food) (EU and MERCOSUR (=LCA(T), Límite de

Composición grupal por Area de superficie de contacto, *Spanish*)).

QM(T): group concentration limit (limit on the residual quantity left in the finished material expressed as total of moiety or substance(s) indicated, in mg/kg) (EU and MERCOSUR (=LC(T), Límite de Composición grupal, *Spanish*)).

QMRA: Quantitative Microbiological Risk Assessment.

RAPD: Randomly Amplified Polymorphic DNA.

RASFF: Rapid Alert System for Food and Feed.

RD: Reference Drying.

R&D: Research and Development.

RDAs: Recommended Daily Allowances (*also* Recommended Dietary Allowances).

RDIs: Reference Daily Intakes (*also* Recommended Daily Intakes).

RF: Russian Federation.

RFLP: Restriction Fragment Length Polymorphism.

RIA: Radioimmunoassay.

RIVM: National Institute for Public Health and the Environment (Rijksinstituut voor Volksgezondheid en Milieu, *Dutch*).

RNA: Ribonucleic Acid.

ROS: Reactive Oxygen Species.

RPHA: Reverse Passive Haemagglutination.

RPLA: Reverse Passive Latex Agglutination.

rRNA: Ribosomal Ribonucleic Acid.

RTE: Ready-To-Eat.

RTQ: Real-Time Quantitative.

S/M: ratio (contact surface area of FCM/mass of foodstuff or simulant

SABS: South African Bureau of Standards.

SAIC: State Administration for Industry and Commerce.

SAIF: Surface Adhesion Immunofluorescence.

SARS: Severe Acute Respiratory Syndrome

SCENIHR: Scientific Committee on Emerging and Newly Identified Health Risks.

SCGE: Single Cell Gel Electrophoresis.

SEM: Semicarbazide.

SF: Sampling Frequency.

SFDA: Saudi Food and Drug Authority.

SFDA: State Food and Drug Administration.

SGT 3: MERCOSUR Working Sub-Group 3 (Sub-Grupo de Trabajo 3, *Spanish*)

SIG: Special Interest Group.

S/M: ratio (contact surface area of FCM/mass of foodstuff or simulant).

SML: Specific Migration Limit (expressed in mg/kg) (EU and MERCOSUR (=LME, Límite de Migración Especifica, *Spanish*)).

SML(T): Group Migration Limit (expressed as total of moiety or substance(s) indicated, in mg/kg) (EU and MERCOSUR (=LME(T), Límite de Migración grupal, *Spanish*)).

SPC: Standard Plate Count.

SPM: Scanning Probe Microscopy.

S-PMF: Soft Palm Mid-Fraction.

SPS: Sanitary and Phytosanitary Measures.

SULs: Safe Upper Limits.

SULT: Sulfotransferase.

SVRs: Surface-to-Volume Ratios.

T-2: T-2 toxin.

TAA: Total Antioxidant Activity.

TB: Tuberculosis.

TBS: Tanzania Bureau of Standards.

TBT: Technical Barriers to Trade.

TC: Technical Committee.

TCDD: 2,3,7,8-tetrachlorodibenzo-para-dioxin.

TDI: Tolerable Daily Intake.

TD-NMR: Time-Domain Nuclear Magnetic Resonance.

TEQ: Toxic Equivalent.

TFA: *Trans* Fatty Acids.

TFDA: Tanzania Food and Drugs Authority.

TFS: Tin-Free Steel *also see* ECCS.

TIE: Toxicologically Insignificant Exposure.

TMI: Tolerable Monthly Intake.

TNase: Thermostable (heat-resistant) nuclease.

TNC: Transnational Corporation.

TOR: Threshold of Regulation.

TP: Total Polyphenol.

TRF: Total Reduction Factor.

Trp-P-1: 3-amino-1,4-dimethyl-5H-pyrido [4,3-*b*]indole.

Trp-P-2: 3-amino-1-methyl-5H-pyrido [4,3-b]indole.

TRIPS: Trade-Related Aspects of Intellectual Property Rights.

TTC: Threshold of Toxicological Concern.

TTMRA: Trans-Tasman Mutual Recognition Arrangement.

UAE: United Arab Emirates.

UBSL: Universally Banned Substances List.

UDPGT: UDP-glucuronosyl transferase.

UF: Uncertainty Factor.

UGT: Glucuronosyltransferase.

UK: United Kingdom.

UN: United Nations.

UNECA: United Nations Economic Commission for Africa.

UNFPA: United Nations Population Fund (*formerly* United Nations Fund for Population Activities).

UNIDO: United Nations Industrial Development Organization.

UNWTO: United Nations World Tourism Organization.

URAA: Uruguay Round Agreement on Agriculture.

US/USA: United States (of America).

USC: United States Code.

USDA: United States Department of Agriculture.

US RDAs: US Recommended Daily Allowances.

UV: Ultraviolet.

UVB: Ultraviolet B.

UVM: University of Vermont.

VCM: Vinyl Chloride Monomer.

WC: Water Content.

WEF: World Economic Forum.

WFS: World Food Summit.

WG: Working Group.

WHO: World Health Organization.

WTO: World Trade Organization.

Contributors

Fadwa Al-Taher Illinois Institute of Technology National Center for Food Safety and Technology, Summit-Argo, IL, USA

Lucia E. Anelich Consumer Goods Council of South Africa, Craighall, South Africa

Kalapanda M. Appaiah Retired Head, Food Safety and Analytical Quality Control Laboratory, Central Food Technological Research Institute, Mysore, India

Alejandro Ariosti INTI (National Institute of Industrial Technology), Plastics Center, Buenos Aires, Argentina

Janis Baines Food Standards Australia New Zealand, Canberra BC ACT, Australia

Gustavo V. Barbosa-Canovas Center for Nonthermal Processing of Food, Washington State University, Pullman, WA, USA

Daniela Bermúdez-Aguirre Center for Nonthermal Processing of Food, Washington State University, Pullman, WA, USA

Christine E. Boisrobert Air Liquide, Houston, TX USA

Hans Bouwmeester RIKILT - Institute of Food Safety, Wageningen UR, Wageningen, The Netherlands

Adelia C. Bovell-Benjamin Department of Food and Nutritional Sciences, Tuskegee University, Tuskegee, AL, USA

Paul Brent Food Standards Australia New Zealand, Canberra BC ACT, Australia

Julie Larson Bricher National Center for Food Safety and Technology, Illinois Institute of Technology, International Commission on Microbiological Specifications for Foods, Summit-Argo, IL, USA

Elaine Bromfield Department of Food and Nutritional Sciences, Tuskegee University, Tuskegee, AL, USA

Frank F. Busta University of Minnesota, St. Paul, MN, USA

Martin Cole[*] National Center for Food Safety and Technology, Illinois Institute of Technology, Summit-Argo, IL, USA

[*]On behalf of The International Commission on Microbiological Specifications for Foods (www.icmsf.org)

Pamela L. Coleman Silliker, Inc., Homewood, IL, USA

Firouz Darroudi Department of Toxicogenetics, Leiden University Medical Centre, Leiden, The Netherlands

Thibaut Dubois Department of Toxicogenetics, Leiden University Medical Centre, Leiden, The Netherlands

Veronika Ehrlich Institute of Cancer Research, Department of Medicine I, Medical University of Vienna, Vienna, Austria

Anthony J. Fontana Silliker, Inc., Homewood, IL, USA

Neal D. Fortin Institute for Food Laws & Regulations, Michigan State University, East Lansing, MI, USA

Tracy Hambridge Food Standards Australia New Zealand, Canberra BC ACT, Australia

Jaap C. Hanekamp Roosevelt Academy, Middelburg, HAN-Research, Zoetermeer, The Netherlands

Vincent Hegarty Institute for Food Laws & Regulations, Michigan State University, East Lansing, MI, USA

Heinz-Dieter Isengard University of Hohenheim, Institute of Food Science and Biotechnology, Stuttgart, Germany

Lauren S. Jackson US Food and Drug Administration, National Center for Food Safety and Technology, Summit-Argo, IL

Edward Jansson The New South Wales Food Authority, Silverwater NSW, Australia

Frans W.H. Kampers Wageningen UR, Wageningen, The Netherlands

Larry Keener International Product Safety Consultants, Seattle, WA, USA

Ji Yeon Kim Division of Nutrition and Functional Food, Bureau of Nutrition and Functional Food, Korea Food & Drug Administration, Seoul, Korea

Siegfried Knasmüller Institute of Cancer Research, Department of Medicine I, Medical University of Vienna, Vienna, Austria

Gisela Kopper University of Costa Rica, San José, Costa Rica

Jan H.J.M. Kwakman President-Seafood Importers and Processors Alliance

Oran Kwon Department of Nutritional Science and Food Management, Ewha Womans University, Seoul, Korea

Huub L.M. Lelieveld Formerly Unilever R & D, Vlaardingen, The Netherlands

Rebeca López-García Logre International Food Science Consulting, México, DF, México

Volker Mersch-Sundermann Department of Environmental Health Sciences, Freiburg University Medical Centre, Freiburg, Germany

David Miles The New South Wales Food Authority, Silverwater NSW, Australia

Carmen Moraru Department of Food Science, Cornell University, Ithaca, NY, USA

Sangsuk Oh Department of Food Science and Technology, Ewha Womans University, Seoul, Korea

William R. Porter New South Wales Food Authority, Newington, NSW, Australia

Margherita Poto University of Torino, Italy; Wageningen University, The Netherlands; and the African Institute for Comparative and International Law, Songea, Tanzania

V. Prakash Director, Central Food Technological Research Institute, Mysore, India

Keith C. Richardson Food Science Australia, North Ryde, NSW, Australia

Syed S.H. Rizvi Department of Food Science, Cornell University, Ithaca, NY, USA

Vijay D. Sattigeri Central Food Technological Research Institute, Mysore, India

Bert Schwitters International Nutrition Company, Loosdrecht, The Netherlands

Mun-Gi Sohn Korea Food & Drug Administration, Seoul, Republic of Korea

Glenn Stanley Food Standards Australia New Zealand, Canberra BC ACT, Australia

Cynthia M. Stewart Silliker, Food Science Center, South Holland, IL, USA

Juanjuan Sun Law School at Shantou University and future PhD student of Law School at Nantes University

John G. Surak Surak and Associates, Clemson, SC, USA

Elizabeth A. Szabo The New South Wales Food Authority, Silverwater NSW, Australia

Martinus AJS (Tiny) van Boekel Wageningen University & Research Centre, Product Design & Quality Management Group, Wageningen, The Netherlands

Bernd van der Meulen Wageningen University and European Institute for Food Law, Wageningen, The Netherlands

Mandyam C. Varadaraj Department of Human Resource Development, Central Food Technological Research Institute, Mysore, India

Yuriy Vasilyev Director of the Stavropol Branch of the North Caucasus Civil Service Academy; and Head of the Law department at the Stavropol Stage Agricultural University, Russian Federation

Axelle Wuillot Department of Toxicogenetics, Leiden University Medical Centre, Leiden, The Netherlands

Ensuring Global Food Safety—A Public Health Priority and a Global Responsibility

Julie Larson Bricher

National Center for Food Safety and Technology, Illinois Institute of Technology,
International Commission on Microbiological Specifications for Foods,
Summit-Argo, IL, USA

'Only if we act together can we respond effectively to international food safety problems and ensure safer food for everyone.'

—Dr. Margaret Chan, Director-General, World Health Organization

The march toward globalization appears inexorable, even as the trend remains politically controversial on the world stage. The International Monetary Fund defines globalization as 'the process through which an increasingly free flow of ideas, people, goods, services, and capital leads to the integration of economies and societies' (IMF, 2006). At its core, globalization is a process driven by free trade economics and an ideal driven by the promise of greater societal benefits for all peoples of the world. Proponents put forward that an economy without borders spurs greater market competition and therefore economic freedom, driving down prices and increasing availability and variety of affordable goods and services for a greater number of people. In turn, globalization promises further benefits, such as increases in productivity, access to new technologies and information streams, and higher living, environmental and labor standards for those in both developed and developing countries. Critics charge that inherent economic and infrastructure inequalities that exist between developed and developing nations preclude less developed and poorer nations from fully realizing these benefits.

Some socioeconomic benefits of an interconnected world market have been realized in countries such as China, India and Vietnam, where poverty rates have substantially declined in concert with more liberalized international trade policies. However, whatever the measurable positive benefits experienced by some countries over the years, there are also tangible challenges brought on by the rapid acceleration of globalization in the world economy. The agro-food production and distribution supply chain is a key case in point. Nearly a decade into the twenty-first century, the challenges of ensuring food security, food safety and nutrition on a global scale continue to grow in complexity. Recent statistics show that the levels of world hunger, malnutrition, and food and waterborne disease are among the most critical global public health issues facing the international community. For example:

- According to a 2008 report on international food security by the Food and Agriculture Organization (FAO) of the United Nations, 963 million people are undernourished, up from 923 million in 2007 (FAO, 2008).
- Although world food prices have stabilized, FAO officials report that lower prices have not ended the food crisis in developing countries, raising concerns about the feasibility of reaching the World Food Summit goal to reduce the number of world's hungry by 50% by 2015 (FAO, 2008; World Food Summit, 1996).
- The World Health Organization (WHO) reports that foodborne diarrhoeal disease is one of the most common illnesses worldwide, estimated at between 2.2 and 4 million cases per year (WHO, 2004; Schlundt, 2008).
- Each day, thousands of people die from preventable foodborne disease. In developing countries, 1.8 million children under the age of five die each year because of diarrhoeal diseases. Up to 70% of these cases may be caused by foodborne pathogens (WHO, 2004; Schlundt, 2008).
- In developed countries, one in three consumers gets a foodborne disease associated with microbes or their toxins every year. This does not include other foodborne diseases associated with naturally-occurring or man-made chemical contaminants, such as aflatoxin, acrylamide, furan or dioxin (Schlundt, 2008).

The WHO Initiative to Estimate the Global Burden of Foodborne Diseases identifies the rapid globalization of food trade as a worldwide trend that has introduced an increased potential for contaminated food to adversely affect greater numbers of people (WHO, 2004). As the food supply chain becomes more integrated, the potential for massive foodborne illness outbreaks caused by pathogens, chemicals, viruses and parasites increases—as do the difficulties in controlling foodborne infections, morbidity, disability and mortality. Rapid globalization also has exposed critical gaps in national and international capabilities to assure adequate levels of food safety and quality. Disparities related to national infrastructural and technological capacities and international food production, distribution and handling standards and law have become more visible as global commerce becomes more interconnected. As a result, WHO and other food-related international public health, development and standard-setting bodies have targeted these gaps as priority items and are working together to reinforce the need to use an integrated international food safety regulatory system in the era of 'one global market.' To be effective, these organizations agree that such a system must include: 1) advancing the use of risk analysis and management to better direct resources towards areas of high risk; 2) providing a scientific basis for international food safety action; 3) moving from conventional 'vertical' legislation within nations to more 'horizontal' rulings among nations to attain harmonization of standards and reduce barriers to trade; and 4) building capacity to promote the availability and use of new food safety technologies, testing and prevention strategies that will reduce the public health risks of foodborne disease around the globe.

In this book, members of the Global Harmonization Initiative (GHI) contribute to the world dialogue, discussing tools for promoting harmonization of scientific methods, standards and regulations. Launched in 2004, GHI is a network of international scientific organizations and individual scientists that aims to achieve objective consensus on the science of food regulations and legislation to ensure the global availability of safe and wholesome food products for all consumers. With support and participation of its individual members and member organizations, GHI has conducted a series of meetings at which members have formulated approaches to critically (re-)evaluate the scientific evidence used to underpin existing global regulations in the areas of product composition, processing operations, and technologies or measures designed to prevent foodborne illness. The chapters in this book address the differences between existing regulations and illustrate why they need to be aligned in concert with efforts from international public health and food safety authorities, including WHO, FAO, and the Codex Alimentarius Commission (CAC).

GHI's overarching objective is to provide regulators, policymakers and public health authorities with a foundation for sound, sensible, science-based international regulations in order to eliminate hurdles to scientific advancement in food safety technology. For example, there is no question that, the more avenues of global trade narrow, the higher the probability of traffic jams in worldwide commerce. Barriers to trade in the form of differing—and sometimes conflicting—country-by-country import/export rules and requirements, can and do make it difficult for food businesses to get traction in overseas markets. Food safety concerns are frequently cited by individual nations as underpinning the justification for their legislative acts and rulemaking—and for erecting trade barriers and other measures that have the impact of curtailing free trade. Unfortunately, in some cases, the science used to inform and bolster food safety policymaking is insufficient, inconsistent or contradictory, creating a roadblock to the promulgation of laws that have a clear and evident benefit to protecting public health. National differences in food safety regulations and laws also trigger a red light to the advances offered by science and technology. Though many food companies throughout the world have invested significant monies in food safety and nutrition technology research and

development efforts, industry is understandably hesitant to apply newly-developed capabilities on an international scale in an uncertain, maze-like regulatory environment.

By streamlining international regulations, laws and standards, GHI expects that the private sector will find it increasingly beneficial to invest in food safety and nutrition research and development, making individual nations' food industries more competitive in the world market. Legislative harmonization will also spur the adoption and use of innovative technologies, which in turn will raise industry's confidence in investing corporate funds and other resources in technologies that will further ensure the safety, quality and security of the global food supply.

Ultimately, 'globalizing' food safety regulations and laws based on sound science can only serve to help bridge public health gaps and create opportunities for all stakeholders to realize the big-picture benefits promised by economic globalization, including measurable global reductions in morbidity and mortality associated with foodborne disease; increases in food availability to combat malnutrition and enhance food security for consumers worldwide; and decreases in poverty rates among less-developed or impoverished nations through capacity building that enables full participation in the global economy. For public health agencies responsible for overseeing the safety of the international food supply, harmonization of food safety and quality standards and regulations will bring a higher level of confidence that risk-reduction strategies and food safety measures are effective, that decisions taken are based on science and not on underlying political agendas that may be in conflict with public health goals, and that available resources are allocated where they have the highest impact on the most pressing food disease-related problems.

To paraphrase WHO Director-General Chan, only if we act together can we fully embrace our global responsibility to respond effectively to the challenges of ensuring food security, food safety and nutrition for everyone. As the authors in this book attest, meeting that global responsibility requires co-operation, collaboration and consensus-building if we are to achieve harmonization of food regulations and standards, and thereby accomplish even greater gains in ensuring global public health.

References

Food and Agriculture Organization. (2008). *The state of food insecurity in the world 2008.* www.fao.org/docrep/011/i0291e/i0291e00.htm

International Monetary Fund. (2006). *Glossary of selected financial terms.* http://www.imf.org/external/np/exr/glossary/showTerm.asp#91

Schlundt, J. (2008). *Food safety: A joint responsibility.* 14th World Congress of Food Science and Technology, Shanghai, China. 20 October 2008.

World Food Summit. (1996). www.fao.org/WFS/ index_en.htm.

World Health Organization. (2004). *Global burden of disease: 2004 update.* http://www.who.int/healthinfo/global_burden_disease/2004_report_update/en/index.html

Development of Food Legislation Around the World[1]

[1]Bernd van der Meulen is professor of Law and Governance at Wageningen University (The Netherlands). See <www.law.wur.nl>. He took responsibility for integrating the contributions to this chapter and wrote the sections on international food law and on the EU. These sections elaborate on his contributions to the European Food Law Handbook. Comments are welcome at: <Bernd.vanderMeulen@wur.nl>.

2.1 INTRODUCTION

Bernd M.J. van der Meulen
Wageningen University, The Netherlands

2.1.1 We Always Eat

Eating and drinking are among the few things that, without a single exception, everyone does. A custom we share with all our contemporaries and ancestors. It is obvious that where a concept of law is developed it will quickly lead to rules related to the acquiring and distributing of food. German introductory literature (for example, Lips & Beutner, 2000) on food law likes to refer to the discovery of a Phoenician inscription that dates back to 1000 BC. Some believe this the oldest food regulation still in our possession.[2] It reads: 'Thou shall not cast a spell on thy neighbor's wine'.

There is, however, much more law than just statutory regulations. Echoes of food law resound from an even more distant past. The oldest pieces of writing, for instance, that remain of Pharaonic Egypt are food labels (Seidlmayer, 1998). They date back to the first dynasty, i.e. 3000 BC. Archaeologists are very fond of labels as they provide a wealth of information on many different aspects of a culture. They contain at least three types of texts: names of products,[3] specifications of quantities[4] and dates.[5] For lawyers it is just a small step to suspect a general rule behind the label stipulating that the product, quantity and date stated must be correct. It does not matter whether that general rule has been issued by a ruler, has a religious origin or is rooted in the conviction of the parties concerned that this is as it should be. All constitute a source of law and thus a rule of law. Of course we do not know what the consequences were of violation of that rule of law. Were there sanctions? Could a buyer return an improperly labeled product?

The role of the authorities in ancient Egyptian food law is also unknown. The Bible-book of Genesis[6] shows that a vice-pharaoh who in times of plenty had stores laid up to feed his people in the years of famine was regarded as extremely wise. It seems that concern for his people, although appreciated, was not one of the standard responsibilities of a ruler.

2.1.2 Food and Values

In modern time food is recognized as a human right. The right to adequate food is mentioned in the Universal Declaration on Human Rights (Article 25) and laid down in several international treaties of which the International Covenant on Economic, Social and Cultural Rights (Article 11) is probably the most important. International organizations such as the Food and Agriculture Organization (FAO) and the UN Committee on Economic, Social and Cultural Rights have further elaborated this right.[7] The right to adequate food is realized if people have access to food that:

- provides sufficient nutritional value and micronutrients for a person to lead a healthy and active life;
- is free of hazardous substances;
- is acceptable within a given culture.

---

[2]This is debatable, however. The famous Babylonian Code of Hammurabi is about a millennium older and also holds provisions that may be understood to relate to the adulteration of food.

[3]They provide information on language.

[4]They provide information on measurements and weights.

[5]They provide information on chronology—crucial to archaeologists.

[6]Genesis 41: 37–57.

[7]See for example the Voluntary Guidelines to support the progressive realisation of the right to adequate food in the context of national food security: <http://www.fao.org/docrep/meeting/009/y9825e/y9825e00.htm>.

Rights always go hand in hand with obligations. Human rights go hand in hand with state obligations. Regarding the right to food three types of obligations are distinguished:

1. The obligation *to respect*. In general people are able to care for themselves and their families. This ability may not be curbed without sound legal justification; this is in line with other fundamental rights such as the freedom of expression for instance.
2. The obligation *to protect*. If the ability of citizens to provide for themselves is threatened by other citizens the government must do its best to protect these citizens from the others.
3. The obligation *to fulfill*. This obligation is composed of a policy obligation and a relief obligation. On the one hand a prudent government is expected to adopt policy geared towards supporting and promoting the ability of the population to provide for itself, on the other hand it must do its best to provide assistance if people find themselves in a situation in which they cannot provide for themselves through no fault of their own.

Here below we will see that it is mainly the second aspect of adequate food (safety) and the second state obligation (to protect) that is taken up in the food regulatory systems as we find them today in all over the world.

2.1.3 This Chapter

Legislation on food is not only widely distributed in time, but also in space. We may expect to find law relating to food in all corners of the globe. This book is not a place to attempt a systematic overview. In this chapter a variety of systems are presented (International, India, South Africa, Eastern Africa, Australia and New Zealand, United States of America, Canada, Latin America, the EU, the Near East, Northeast Asia, China and the Russian Federation) in the perspective of their development to give an impression of the features found in food law and the reasons why they have taken certain forms. Each section has its own separate author or authors, indicated at its beginning. The authors have based their contributions on an open question to present highlights in development, not on strict guidelines. Personal differences in style and approach of the subject matter have been respected.

In the systems presented we repeatedly find a complex situation due in part to the distribution of the subject matter over different competent authorities. We find product specific provisions alongside legislation of a more general nature. In all systems presented here, safety is an important consideration for the legislators concerned who increasingly rely on science. Repeatedly reference is made to international developments and standards such as the *Codex Alimentarius*. For this reason this chapter opens with a section introducing international food law as a background to the national and regional systems discussed thereafter.

2.2 INTERNATIONAL FOOD LAW

Bernd M.J. van der Meulen
Wageningen University, The Netherlands

2.2.1 *Codex Alimentarius*

In 1961 the Food and Agriculture Organization (FAO) and the World Health Organization (WHO) established the Codex Alimentarius Commission (CAC). Over the years the CAC has established specialized committees. These committees are hosted by member states all over the world. Some 175 countries, representing about 98% of the world's population, participate in the work of *Codex Alimentarius*.

Food standards are established through an elaborate procedure of international negotiations (FAO/WHO, 2006). All standards taken together are called '*Codex Alimentarius*'. In Latin this means 'food code'. It can be seen as a virtual book filled with food standards. The food standards represent models for national legislation on food.

Beside the food standards, *Codex Alimentarius* includes advisory provisions called codes of practice or guidelines. These codes of practice and guidelines mainly address food businesses.

At present the Codex comprises more than 200 standards, close to 50 food hygiene and technological codes of practice, some 60 guidelines, over 1,000 food additives and contaminants evaluations and over 3,200 maximum residue limits for pesticides and veterinary drugs. Finally, the *Codex Alimentarius* includes requirements of a horizontal nature on labeling and presentation and on methods of analysis and sampling (FAO/WHO, 2002, 2006; Masson-Matthee, 2007).

2.2.2 Procedural Manual

The 'constitution' of the *Codex Alimentarius* is the Procedural Manual. The Procedural Manual not only gives the procedures and format for setting Codex Standards and Guidelines, but also some general principles and definitions (Table 2.1). The principles relate among other things to the scientific substantiation of the work of *Codex Alimentarius* and the use of risk analysis for food safety (Table 2.2).

2.2.3 Standards

The work of the CAC has resulted in a vast collection of internationally agreed food standards that are presented in a uniform format. Most of these standards are of a vertical (product specific) nature. They address all principal foods, whether processed, semi-processed or

TABLE 2.1   Some definitions in the *Codex Alimentarius* Procedural Manual

Food means any substance, whether processed, semi-processed or raw, which is intended for human consumption, and includes drink, chewing gum and any substance which has been used in the manufacture, preparation or treatment of "food" but does not include cosmetics or tobacco or substances used only as drugs.

Food hygiene comprises conditions and measures necessary for the production, processing, storage and distribution of food designed to ensure a safe, sound, wholesome product fit for human consumption.

TABLE 2.2   Some principles in the *Codex Alimentarius* Procedural Manual

Statements of Principle concerning the role of science in the Codex decision-making process and the extent to which other factors are taken into account

1. The food standards, guidelines and other recommendations of *Codex Alimentarius* shall be based on the principle of sound scientific analysis and evidence, involving a thorough review of all relevant information, in order that the standards assure the quality and safety of the food supply.

2. When elaborating and deciding upon food standards *Codex Alimentarius* will have regard, where appropriate, to other legitimate factors relevant for the health protection of consumers and for the promotion of fair practices in food trade.

3. In this regard it is noted that food labelling plays an important role in furthering both of these objectives.

4. When the situation arises that members of Codex agree on the necessary level of protection of public health but hold differing views about other considerations, members may abstain from acceptance of the relevant standard without necessarily preventing the decision by Codex.

raw. Standards of a horizontal nature are often called 'general standards', like the General Standard for the Labeling of Pre-packaged Foods.[8]

---

[8]CODEX STAN 1-1985 (Rev. 1-1991).

According to this general standard, the following information shall appear on the labeling of pre-packaged foods:

- the name of the food; this name shall indicate the true nature of the food;
- list of ingredients (in particular if one of a list of 8 allergens is present);
- net contents;
- name and address of the business;
- country of origin where omission could mislead the consumer;
- lot identification;
- date marking and storage instructions;
- instructions for use.

2.2.4 Codes

In addition to the formally accepted standards the Codex includes recommended provisions called codes of practice or guidelines. There is, for example, a 'Code of Ethics for International Trade in Food',[9] and a set of hygiene codes like the 'Recommended International Code of Practice General Principles of Food Hygiene' and the 'Hazard Analysis and Critical Control Point (HACCP) System and Guidelines for its Application' (Table 2.3).

2.2.5 Legal Force

The Codex standards do not represent legally binding norms. They present models for national legislation. Member states undertake to transform the Codex standards into national legislation. However, no sanctions apply if they do not honor this undertaking.

By agreeing on non-binding standards, the participating states develop a common language. All states and other subjects of international law will mean the same thing; for example, when they meet to negotiate about food, they mean 'food'

TABLE 2.3   The principles of HACCP according to *Codex Alimentarius*

Principle 1	Conduct a hazard analysis.
Principle 2	Determine the Critical Control Points (CCPs).
Principle 3	Establish critical limit(s).
Principle 4	Establish a system to monitor control of the CCP.
Principle 5	Establish the corrective action to be taken when monitoring indicates that a particular CCP is not under control.
Principle 6	Establish procedures for verification to confirm that the HACCP system is working effectively.
Principle 7	Establish documentation concerning all procedures and records appropriate to these principles and their application.

as defined in the Codex. The same holds true for 'milk' and 'honey' and all the standards that have been agreed upon. The notion of HACCP has been developed—and is understood—within the framework of *Codex Alimentarius*.[10] In this way the *Codex Alimentarius* provides a common frame of reference, but there is more.

The mere fact that national specialists on food law enter into discussion on these standards will influence them in their work at home. A civil servant drafting a piece of legislation will look for examples. As regards food s/he will find examples in abundance in the Codex. In these subtle ways the *Codex Alimentarius* is likely to have a major impact on the development of food law in many countries even without a strict legal obligation to implement.

It turns out more than once that soft law has a tendency to solidify. Once agreements are reached, parties tend to put more weight on them than was initially intended. This is true for Codex standards as well. Due to several

---

[9]CAC/RCP 20-1979 (Rev. 1-1985).

[10]Recommended International Code Of Practice General Principles Of Food Hygiene CAC/RCP 1-1969, Rev. 3-1997, Amd. (1999).

developments they are well on their way to acquiring at least a quasi-binding force.

2.2.6 World Trade Organization/Sanitary and Phytosanitary Agreement

The World Trade Organization[11] (WTO) tries to remove barriers to trade. To achieve this, several measures have been taken. Tariff barriers were reduced and to the extent that this was successful non-tariff barriers became more of a concern. The basic treaty addressing trade in goods is the General Agreement on Tariffs and Trade (GATT). The GATT recognizes that certain exceptions to free trade can be necessary to protect higher values like health and (food) safety.

In the food trade, differences in technical standards like packaging requirements may cause problems. However, it is mostly concerns about food safety, human health, animal and plant health that induce national authorities to take measures which may frustrate the free flow of trade. To address these concerns two WTO treaties were concluded: the Agreement on Technical Barriers to Trade (the TBT Agreement) and the Agreement on the Application of Sanitary and Phytosanitary Measures (the SPS Agreement).

The SPS Agreement was drawn up to ensure that countries only apply measures to protect human and animal health (sanitary measures) and plant health (phytosanitary measures) based on the assessment of risk, or in other words, based on science. The SPS Agreement incorporates, therefore, safety aspects of foods in trade. The TBT Agreement covers all technical requirements and standards (applied to all commodities), such as labeling, that are not covered by the SPS Agreement. Therefore, the SPS and TBT Agreements can be seen as complementing each other.

To a certain extent the WTO is a supranational organization. The treaties concluded between its members are binding. There is the Dispute Settlement Understanding, providing an arbitration procedure to resolve conflicts. If a party wants to present a conflict, a Dispute Settlement Body (DSB) is formed to arbitrate on the basis of WTO law. If a party does not agree with the decision of the DSB, it can take the case to an Appellate Body (AB). The WTO does not have powers to enforce decisions taken in this arbitration procedure. It can condone, however, that if the decision reached is not implemented by the party found at fault, the winning party may implement economic sanctions. These sanctions usually take the form of additional import levies on goods from the state found at fault. If the levies are condoned by the DSB (or the AB), setting them does not in itself constitute an infringement of WTO obligations.

As follows from the above, the SPS Agreement is very important from a food safety point of view. The SPS Agreement recognizes and further elaborates on the right of the parties to this agreement to take sanitary and phytosanitary measures necessary for the protection of human, animal or plant life or health. The measures must be scientifically justified and they may not be discriminating, nor constitute disguised barriers to international trade.

If the measures are in conformity with international standards, no scientific proof of their necessity is required. These measures are by definition considered to be necessary. The most important international standards regarding SPS are set by the so-called three sisters of the SPS Agreement: the Codex Alimentarius Commission, the International Office of Epizootics (OIE[12]) and the Secretariat of the International Plant Protection

---

[11]Established 1 January 1995 by the Agreement Establishing the World Trade Organization as the result of the so-called Uruguay round of trade negotiations and signed in Marrakesh on 15 April 1994 (WTO Agreement). The WTO is the institutional continuation of the General Agreement on Tariffs and Trade 1947 (GATT).

[12]The abbreviation follows the French spelling. In 2003, the International Office of Epizootics became the World Organisation for Animal Health, but kept its historical acronym.

Convention (IPPC). The standards on food and on food safety are mainly to be found in the *Codex Alimentarius*.[13]

2.2.7 Conclusion

The inclusion of the *Codex Alimentarius* in the SPS Agreement, greatly enhances its significance. WTO members who follow Codex standards are liberated from the burden to prove the necessity of the sanitary and phytosanitary measures they take. If they cannot base their measures on Codex, they have to prove that their measures are science-based.

2.3 INDIA

Vijay D. Sattigeri and Kalapanda M. Appaiah
Central Food Technological Research Institute, Mysore, India

2.3.1 Introduction

Adequate, nutritious and safe food is essential to human survival and it is the duty of the government to see that the consumers are provided with such safe food. The assurance of safe food production is a multidisciplinary task involving food producers, processors, food scientists, technologists, toxicologists and food regulators. The general public may consider that 'safe food' means food with zero risk. But from a regulatory point of view, safe food means food that has an appropriate level of protection (ALOP). Today, globalization of food trade and increasing problems worldwide with emerging and re-emerging foodborne pathogens have increased the risk of cross-border transmission of infectious diseases. The standards, guidelines of hygienic practices and recommendations established by the Codex Alimentarius Commission

are recognized as the basis for harmonization by the World Trade Organization. India, being a signatory to WTO agreements, has taken adequate steps to harmonize the laws based on risk analysis. Furthermore, food safety is not limited to concerns related to foodborne pathogens, physical hazards or toxicity due to contaminants—in today's context it is extended to include nutrition, food quality, labeling and awareness. The food control system in India is geared to meet these additional requirements.

In this context, it is fascinating to see the evolution of Indian Food Legislation which has evolved over the last fifty years or so with a paradigm shift from gross adulteration to subtle contamination in foods. This has reflected a blend of social, economical, political and scientific factors, which is sometimes marked by little coherence in its development resulting into over-complexity with fragmented measures, contradictions and sometimes lack of consistency. However, these shortcomings are being addressed in the New Food Safety and Standards Act 2006.

2.3.2 Food Legislation in India

Food laws and regulations existed in some forms in most ancient cultures to deal with food safety and consumer concerns. In Charak Samhita, there are references about the quality of food articles for maintaining a good health. The great economist Chanakya in his 'Arthashastra' written in 375 BC, was mentioning food adulteration and punishments to be given to traders indulging in such anti-social activities. People in pre-historic times knew about the benefits and safety of various foods and the sale of adulterated food was dealt with by Criminal Acts that existed during those periods.

It is possible that Food Legislation in India dates back to 1860 with certain sections of the Indian Penal Code dealing with food adulteration. However, the exclusive food laws were enacted

---

[13] The Agreement on Technical Barriers To Trade (TBT Treaty) has similar articles.

only early in the twentieth century. Before independence in 1947, Indian provinces under British rule, had their own acts and rules to deal with prevention of food adulteration (e.g., The Bengal Food Adulteration Act 1919, The Bombay Prevention of Food Adulteration Act 1925, The Calcutta Municipal Act 1923, The Madras Prevention of Food Adulteration Act 1918, The Punjab Pure Food Act, 1929, etc.).

These laws were based largely on the British Food and Drug Act, 1872 and generally dealt with gross adulteration of cereals and pulses with extraneous matter, spices with colors, milk with water etc. These laws had the provisions for seizure of such foods followed by prosecution in the courts of law. In 1943, a Central Advisory Committee was appointed, which recommended establishment of Central Legislation to bring about uniformity in food legislation throughout the country.

Consequently, the national food law, namely the Prevention of Food Adulteration Act (PFA Act), was enacted in 1954 (Act 37), which came into force from 1 June 1955, vide Notification No. SRO 1085, dated 10 May 1955, Gazette of India (MoHFW, 1954). The objective of the PFA Act is to protect the consumers against impure, unsafe and fraudulently labeled foods. The PFA covers food production, processing, formulation, packaging, labeling and distribution. Furthermore, limits for additives and contaminants in foods have been specified. These standards and regulations apply to both domestic and imported foods.

The Directorate General of Health Services, through the Central Committee for Food Standards, under the Ministry of Health and Family Welfare, Government of India, lays down food standards and has the power to amend the rules as and when necessary. The implementation of the rules goes through the State governments and local bodies. Till this day, the rules have been amended more than 200 times to meet the current requirements of safety as enunciated in SPS, TBT and other agreements of WTO. Some of the major amendments till this date are listed in Table 2.4.

2.3.3 Aspects of India's Food Legislation

The evolution of Indian Food Legislation involves three aspects, namely: 1) legislation; 2) administration; and 3) participation of stakeholders. These are briefly discussed here.

2.3.3.1 *Legislation Aspects*

Apart from amendments in PFA, the following important statutory quality legislation and orders have been promulgated to regulate different categories of processed foods such as processed fruit and vegetable products, meat and meat products, milk and milk products, vegetable oils etc. Some of the important acts/

TABLE 2.4 Highlights of the development of food legislation in India

1976	Minimum of six month jail for the persons indulged in food adulteration.
1986	Introduction of Consumer Protection Act under which the consumer is eligible to submit a food product for testing to the state laboratory.
1998	Vegetable oils to be sold only in packed conditions to avoid adulteration.
2004	Harmonization of food laws with reference to food additives such as Synthetic sweeteners, bulk sweeteners, preservatives antioxidants, etc. in traditional sweets, snacks, instant mixes, confectionery products, etc. Limits for pesticide residues, antibiotic residues, toxic metals and aflatoxins have been laid down for various products based on risk analysis.
2004 & 2006	Microbiological requirements for sea foods, fruit and vegetable products and milk products have been introduced.
2008	Nutritional labeling covering nutrients such as protein, fat, carbohydrates, calories, added vitamins and minerals and trans-fats (for products containing hydrogenated vegetable oil) for the prepackaged foods is made compulsory; health claims are permitted.

orders and the year in which they were promulgated are given below:

(a) Essential Commodities Act, 1955 A number of Orders have been formulated under the provisions of the Essential Commodities Act in 1955 with the objectives to regulate the production, supply, distribution and trade and commerce of essential commodities, including foods.

These orders include:

(i) *Fruit Product Order, 1955* The order is administered by the Ministry of Food Processing Industries. It lays down standards for processed fruit and vegetable products, hygienic and sanitary requirements, food additives and contaminants (MoFPI, 1955).

(ii) *Meat Food Products Order, 1973* This order, laying down conditions for licensing and hygienic requirements, is implemented by the Directorate of Marketing and Inspection, Ministry of Agriculture (MoA, 1973).

(iii) *Solvent Extracted Oil, De-oiled Meal and Edible Flour (control) Order, 1967* Standards, packing and labeling requirements for the solvent extracted products have been laid down in this order, which is regulated by the Department of Consumer Affairs, Ministry of Consumer Affairs (MoCA, 1967).

(iv) *Vegetable Oil Products (Regulation) Order, 1998* This order is implemented by the Directorate of Vanaspati, Vegetable Oils and Fats under the Ministry of Consumer Affairs. It provides for compulsory licensing for manufacturing units and lays down standards for these products (MoCA, 1998).

(v) *Milk and Milk Products Order 1992* The order is implemented by the Ministry of Agriculture. It provides for compulsory registration of the units and lays down hygienic and sanitary requirements (MoA, 1992).

(b) Export (Quality Control and Inspection) Act, 1963 (Amended in 1984) The government has established the Export Inspection Council under the Ministry of Commerce to ensure the safety and quality of foods meant for export through consignment testing, premise inspection and implementation of Quality Assurance systems such as GMP,[14] GHP[15] and/or HACCP in the processing units (MoC, 1963).

(c) Standard of Weights and Measures Act, 1976 Under this act, rules were laid down in 1977 for prepackaged products to regulate interstate trade. It is regulated by the Ministry of Consumer Affairs. As per the act every package shall have: (a) Name of the product, (b) Net quantity in standard units of weight and measures, (c) Unit sale price and (d) Name of Manufacturer, packer or distributor (MoCA, 1976).

(d) Voluntary Based Product Certifications

(i) *Bureau of Indian Standards Act, 1986* In 1947, the government, recognizing the role of standardization in the industry to promote competitive efficiency and quality production, set up the "Indian Standards Institution (ISI)", as a registered society. In 1986 the government gave ISI a Statutory status through the Bureau of Indian Standards (BIS) Act 1986. The organization runs a voluntary certification scheme known as the "ISI" Mark for certification of consumer goods, including processed food products (BIS, 1986). Under the provisions of the PFA Act, it is compulsory to have BIS certification for food additives, condensed milk, milk powder, Infant Milk substitutes and packaged drinking/mineral water.

(ii) *Agmark Grading and Marking Act and Rules,1937* Under the Directorate of Marketing and Inspection under the

[14] Good Manufacturing Practices.
[15] Good Hygiene Practices.

Ministry of Agriculture, operates a voluntary scheme of certification of raw and processed agricultural commodities (AGMARK, 1937).

2.3.3.2 *Administrative Aspects*

A closer look at the PFA Act and rules reveals that the enforcement of the act rests with the Food (Health) Authority of the States. Norms have been laid down by the authority for the appointment of qualified Food Safety Officers (Food Inspectors) with requirements of adequate training and awareness and provision for accreditation of the central /state testing laboratories to establish competence of the analysts/chemists.

2.3.3.3 *Participation of Stakeholders*

As food safety involves major stakeholders such as government, food industry and consumers, provisions have been made for adequately representing these stakeholders in various scientific panels /committees.

2.3.4 Development of Integrated Food Laws

It is evident from the above evolution of Indian Food Laws that India has a multiplicity of food laws, that are implemented through different ministries and departments. To avoid inter-ministerial confusions and contradictions, a Task Force was appointed in 2002 to review the Food and Agro Industries Management Policy (TASK FORCE, 2002).

One of the major recommendations was the consolidation of various food laws under one umbrella so that a single authority could formulate laws and supervise effective implementation of various food laws. The Ministry of Food

Processing Industries (MoFPI) drafted a new Food Bill in 2002. The government constituted a group of Ministers to formalize the new legislation. The group drafted the Food Safety and Standards Bill 2005. On further review by the Parliamentary Standing Committee on Agriculture, the Bill was passed by the parliament and the Food Safety and Standards Act 2006 came into effect from 24 August 2006. Once the rules are framed under this Act, the PFA Act and orders under Essential Commodities Act will stand repealed.

Under the new act, the Central Government has constituted the Food Safety and Standards Authority of India (FSSAI) headed by a chairman with twenty-two members drawn from ministries, foods industry and food technologists. Scientific Panels for Food Additives, Contaminants, Labeling, GM Foods, Nutraceuticals, etc. are being constituted. The act is expected to boost the food processing sector by providing a single window for all regulatory issues as it is considered to be industry friendly, transparent, and science based (FSSAI, 2006).

2.4 SOUTH AFRICA

Lucia E. Anelich[16]
Food Safety Initiative at the Consumer Goods Council of South Africa.

2.4.1 Introduction

South Africa had its own Public Health Act in 1919, followed by the Food, Drugs and Disinfectants Act in 1929. These Acts have since been replaced with others as indicated below. Since democracy in 1994, South Africa became a member of the *Codex Alimentarius*, the IPPC[17] (plant health) and the OIE[18] (animal health). In

---

[16]Sincere acknowledgement goes to Dr Theo van de Venter, former Director: Food Control, Department of Health, and to Mr Andries Pretorius, current Director: Food Control, Department of Health.
[17]International Plant Protection Convention.
[18]World Organisation for Animal Health (formerly Office International des Epizooties).

1995, South Africa became a signatory to the WTO as well.

In South Africa the control over foodstuffs is fragmented between a number of authorities and components at national, provincial and local level. Typically, national government departments governing food safety, are responsible for writing policies and regulations, whilst local authorities are responsible for enforcement. Foodstuffs are not always regulated as foodstuffs but also as animals, animal products, plants, plant products or reproductive material. The objectives of such control relate to human health concerns such as food safety and nutrition, as well as to quality and to animal and plant health. Economic and environmental considerations also play a role. The relevant South African legislation and the authorities that are involved in the administration and enforcement of such legislation are discussed here below.

2.4.2 Foodstuffs, Cosmetics and Disinfectants Act

The Foodstuffs, Cosmetics and Disinfectants Act, 1972 (Act 54 of 1972) (FCD Act) is the most important set of legislation related to foodstuffs within the health sector in South Africa. Those aspects of this Act that relate to foodstuffs are administered by the Directorate: Food Control of the Department of Health and are enforced by local authorities in their areas of jurisdiction. Food imports are controlled by the provincial health departments on behalf of the national Department.

According to its long title, the Act is there "to control the sale manufacture and importation of foodstuffs, cosmetics and disinfectants; and to provide for incidental matters". Its objectives can however be summarized more clearly as follows:

1. It forbids the sale of foodstuffs, cosmetics and disinfectants that may be detrimental or harmful to human health.
2. It endeavors to protect the consumer from exploitation by false or misleading claims.

3. It attempts to provide the consumer with such information as is necessary to make informed choices according to individual needs and wishes.

The second and third objectives obviously refer to labeling.

The philosophy of the Act is that it is reactive as well as prohibitive:

- *Reactive* because no provision is made for the registration or approval of foodstuffs, or for the labels on such commodities. The onus also rests on the law enforcer to establish whether the product being manufactured, imported or sold, does in fact comply with the legal requirements. The law enforcer therefore reacts to a particular situation and cannot take recourse to any registration or approval to ensure the safety of a product. The Act does, however, make provision for approval by means of regulation for the use of certain *ingredients* in these commodities. A good example is the listing of permissible food additives, as well as the stipulation of the maximum permissible levels of specific substances that a foodstuff may contain.
- *Prohibitive* because nothing may be added to or removed from a foodstuff unless permitted by regulation or unless necessary for the manufacture of such foodstuff, or unavoidably present as a result of the process of its collection or manufacture.

Table 2.5 lists some regulations that, among others, have been published in terms of the Act by the Minister of Health.

The FCD Act (as for other Acts) is amended from time to time to include any significant changes as required.

2.4.3 Other Legislation on Food

2.4.3.1 *Health Act*

The Health Act, 1977 (Act 63 of 1977). Regulations under this Act govern the hygiene

TABLE 2.5   South African regulations on food under the FCD Act (Act 54 of 1972)

Anti-caking agents—Amounts that may be used in foodstuff

Baking powder and chemical leavening substances

Preservatives and antioxidants

Irradiated foodstuffs

Emulsifiers, stabilizers and thickeners and the amounts that foodstuffs may contain

Labelling and advertising of foodstuffs

Guar Gum—Prohibiting as a foodstuff

Colourants—Food

Soft drinks

Herbs and spices

Milk and dairy products

Metals in foodstuffs

Food fortification

Microbiological standards for foodstuffs and related matters

Mineral hydrocarbons in foodstuffs

Pesticide residues that may be present—Maximum levels in foodstuffs

Radio activity in foodstuffs

Marine food

Certain seeds in certain agricultural products—Tolerances for

Certain food additives in certain wheaten and rye products—Use of

Salt

Substances in wine, other fermented beverages and spirits—Additives, amounts, tolerances

Acids bases and salts—The amounts thereof that foodstuffs may contain

Fungus-produced toxins in foodstuffs—Tolerances for

Food additives containing nitrite and/or nitrate and other substances

Sweeteners in foodstuffs—Relating to the use of

Veterinary medicine and stock remedy residues—Regulations governing the maximum limits

Fats and oils—Edible

Foodstuffs for infants, young children and children

Certain solvents

Articles imported in transit and addressed to or intended for transmission to Botswana, Lesotho and Swaziland

Perishable foodstuffs

Inspectors and analysts—Duties of

Jam, conserve, marmalade and jelly

Mayonnaise and other salad dressings

Raw boerewors (a unique type of South African sausage), raw species sausage and raw mixed species sausage—Composition and labeling of

Manufactured or processed foodstuffs

Hazard Analysis and Critical Control Point

Labeling of foods produced by certain techniques of genetic modification.

aspects of food premises (including milking sheds) and the transport of food. These are also administered by the Directorate: Food Control of the Department of Health and enforced by local authorities in their areas of jurisdiction.

2.4.3.2 IHR

The International Health Regulations (IHR). These regulations of the World Health Organization, as adopted by South Africa, have certain provisions that relate to the provision and handling of food, as well as the control of foodborne diseases of global concern. The Department of Health is responsible for the approval of the source of food for consumption on the premises of ports and airports as well as on vessels and aircraft. Currently the provincial health authorities are conducting these approvals on behalf of the national Department. The Act also tasks local authorities to inspect the premises and to take food samples for analysis.

2.4.3.3 Agricultural Product Standards Act

The Agricultural Product Standards Act, 1990 (Act 119 of 1990). This Act controls and promotes specific product standards (e.g. meat, dairy products, cereals, certain canned products, fruit and vegetables) for local and for export purposes. It is administered and enforced by the Division: Food Safety and Quality Assurance of the Department of Agriculture.* Various assignees such as the Perishable Products Export Control Board are appointed and authorized as assignees to do physical inspections under the Act.

2.4.3.4 The Liquor Products Act

The Liquor Products Act, 1989 (Act 60 of 1989). Addresses requirements for wines and spirits. It is also administered and enforced by the Division: Food Safety and Quality Assurance of the Department of Agriculture, Forestry and Fisheries.

2.4.3.5 The Liquor Act

The Liquor Act, 1989 (Act 27 of 1989). This Act is administered by the Department of Justice and controls aspects such as liquor licenses and selling hours.

2.4.3.6 The Meat Safety Act

The Meat Safety Act, 2000 (Act 40 of 2000). Administered by the Division: Food and Veterinary Services of the Department of Agriculture, Forestry and Fisheries. It addresses food safety and hygiene standards in abattoirs. These regulations are enforced mainly by the provincial agriculture departments. The import and export of unprocessed meat is also controlled by this Act. This aspect is enforced by the national Department.

2.4.3.7 The Animal Diseases Act

The Animal Diseases Act, 1984 (Act 35 of 1984). Administered by the Division: Food and Veterinary Services of the Department of Agriculture, Forestry and Fisheries and enforced by the provincial components, except for import control which is a national responsibility. The Act controls animals as well as animal products, including meat, eggs and their products from an animal disease point of view.

2.4.3.8 The Genetically Modified Organisms Act

The Genetically Modified Organisms Act, 1997 (Act 15 of 1997). Administered and enforced by the Division: Biosafety of the Department of Agriculture, Forestry and Fisheries. This Act controls issues such as the licensing and importation of live genetically modified organisms. These may currently include foods such as maize, soy beans and tomatoes.

*Department of Agriculture, Forestry and Fisheries (www.daff.gov.za).

2.4.3.9 The National Regulator for Compulsory Specifications Act

The National Regulator for Compulsory Specifications Act, 2008 (Act 5 of 2008). Administered by the National Regulator for Compulsory Specifications (NRCS) (www.nrcs.org.za), (formerly known as the regulatory division of the South African Bureau of Standards). The NRCS is a public entity within the Department of Trade and Industry and is responsible for the administration of technical regulations, including compulsory specifications based on standards that protect human health and safety, and the environment. The NRCS was launched as recently as October 2008. It typically administers compulsory specifications for:

1. Canned meat and canned meat products;
2. Canned fish, marine mollusks and crustaceans;
3. Frozen fish and marine mollusks;
4. Frozen rock lobster;
5. Frozen shrimp, langoustines and crab;
6. Smoked snoek.

The NRCS exercises import and export control over these products, and is recognized by the European Union and other countries as the competent authority for certifying exports of fish and fishery products.

2.4.3.10 The Fertilizers, Farm Feeds, Agricultural Remedies and Stock Remedies Act

The Fertilizers, Farm Feeds, Agricultural Remedies and Stock Remedies Act, 1947 (Act 36 of 1947). Administered by the Division: Feeds, Stock Remedies, Pesticides and Fertilizers of the Department of Agriculture, Forestry and Fisheries. Animal feeds, stock remedies and agricultural remedies are registered in terms of this Act, which therefore has indirect implications for food safety.

2.4.3.11 The Medicines and Related Substances Act

The Medicines and Related Substances Act, 1965 (Act 101 of 1965). Administered and enforced by the Chief Directorate: Medicines Administration of the Department of Health. This Act *inter alia* provides for the registration of veterinary drugs as well as for the registration of foodstuffs and food supplements with medicinal effects or in respect of which medicinal claims are made.

2.4.3.12 Agricultural Legislation

The Plant Breeders Rights Act, 1976 (Act 15 of 1976), the Plant Improvement Act, 1976 (Act 53 of 1976), and the Agricultural Pests Act, 1983 (Act 36 of 1983), are all administered by various divisions in the Department of Agriculture, Forestry and Fisheries. The regulations made in terms of these Acts have implications for certain foodstuffs. The Agricultural Pests Act, 1983, for example regulates the importation of certain controlled goods such as plants, plant products, honey, used apiary equipment, exotic animals, etc.

2.4.3.13 Industrial Legislation

The Trade Metrology Act, 1973 (Act 77 of 1973), and the Trade Marks Act, 1963 (Act 62 of 1963). Both have certain implications for food labeling. The Trade Metrology Act is administered by the NRCS whilst the Trade Marks Act is administered by the South African Bureau of Standards (SABS).

2.4.4 Food Legislation Advisory Group (FLAG)

The Director: Food Control created the Food Legislation Advisory Group (FLAG) some years ago by inviting a number of stakeholders to nominate persons to advise him on matters that relate to his regulatory responsibilities. FLAG is non-statutory by nature, and members attend meetings (biannually) in their own time and

TABLE 2.6 Members of the Food Legislation Advisory Group in South Africa

Government:	Department of Health (various national and provincial components)
	Department of Agriculture (Food Safety and Quality Assurance)
	Department of Trade and Industry
Statutory:	South African Bureau of Standards
	Council for Scientific and Industrial Research
	Agricultural Research Council
	National Regulator for Compulsory Specifications
Other:	Allergy Society of South Africa
	Association for Dietetics in Southern Africa
	Consumer Goods Council of South Africa
	South African Association for Food Science and Technology
	South African Association for Flavor and Fragrance Manufacturers
	South African Milk Chamber of Milling/Chamber of Baking
	South African Soft Drinks Federation
	University of Stellenbosch
	Botswana Ministry of Health
	National Consumer Forum
	International Life Sciences Institute of South Africa

at own cost. In spite of being only an advisory body, most of its members are experts in the various fields of food control, and play an important role in the preparation and revision of regulations. The objective is to obtain as much consensus as possible on draft regulations even before they are published for comment. Table 2.6 lists the organizations that are represented on FLAG.

2.5 EASTERN AFRICA

Margherita Poto
African Institute for Comparative and International Law, Songea, Tanzania

2.5.1 Introduction

The global regulation of food safety has a great impact on developing countries, such as those in Africa. Food supplies in many African countries are inadequate in quantity and quality. This contributes to widespread malnutrition on the continent. It has been found that at least 60% of the food supply is imported to supplement the local production.[19] With such a trend, there is the need for a local food safety system that ensures food for better health and agricultural trade opportunities.

Many African countries do not currently have effective food safety regimes and hence the safety of imported food cannot be assured, thus adding the risk of widespread contamination of

[19]See <http://www.fao.orgnewsroom/en/news/2005/2005/107908/index.html>. See also FAO/WHO Regional Conference on Food Safety for Africa Harare, Zimbabwe, 3–6 October 2005, final report, p 121.
[20]<http://www.fao.org/newsroom/en/news/2005/107908/index.html>.

food.[20] In this section, the situation in Tanzania is presented as an example.

In Tanzania and other African countries to achieve high food safety standards, a need is recognized to revise legislation relating to food safety in order to harmonize it with international standards such as the SPS Agreement, *Codex Alimentarius*, IPPC and importing country or regional regulations such as EU legislation.[21]

The importance of food safety does not lie in health and international trade alone. Firstly, Food *safety* is a critical element of food *security*. Secondly, lack of food safety has a high cost. Each outbreak of foodborne illness causes not only human suffering, but also direct and indirect costs. Thirdly, improving food safety has the added advantage of helping reduce food losses or even avoid them. In short, the improved safety of food can contribute to increased availability of food.[22] To meet all these, African countries are challenged to improve the food safety situation by improving their basic infrastructures such as regular access to electricity, safe water, transportation and storage.[23] These countries also need capacity building in food safety planning. Donors should provide technical assistance and traffic through national borders should also be monitored to prevent the importation of sub-standard foodstuff.[24]

So far, African food safety does not progress at the required pace, in its socio-economic and political aspects, as the failure of many African produced food products to meet international food safety and quality standards hampers the continent's efforts to increase agricultural trade both intra-regionally and internationally. The repercussion is that many African farmers miss out on another chance to improve their economic well-being.[25]

After discussing Tanzania, this section will turn its attention to the African Union.

2.5.2 Tanzania

2.5.2.1 *Situation*

The economy of Tanzania is based on agriculture (including animal production and fisheries) which accounts for more than 60% of the GDP. More than 80% of the population is rural based and depends entirely on agriculture for food and cash earnings.

The food safety situation in Tanzania as in many African countries is problematic. Illustrations from the press are disturbing. In 2008, there were people in Dar es Salaam (Tabata Dampo) whose houses were demolished owing to a court decree. These people have been provided with some foodstuff, some of which has been discovered to be unfit for human consumption.[26] Imported foods in Tanzania seem to have difficulties in meeting the standard food safety qualities. For instance, Zanzibar's Pharmaceutical and Cosmetics Board declared 70 tons of rice and wheat flour imported into the Isles from Dubai unfit for human consumption and to be destroyed.[27] This is evidenced by the Government act of destroying foodstuff

---

[21]United Nations Conference on Trade and Development, Geneva: Costs of Agri-Food Safety and SPS Compliance: United Republic of Tanzania, Mozambique and Guinea: Tropical Fruits Selected Commodity Issues, in the Context of Trade and Development, Unctad/Ditc/Com/2005/2, at 9.

[22]FAO/WHO Regional Conference on Food Safety for Africa: Harare, Zimbabwe, 3–6 October 2005 Final Report, p 34.

[23]*Ibid*, Challenges of food Safety, 35.

[24]*Ibid*.

[25]<http://www.fao.org/newsroom/en/news/2005/107908/index.html>.

[26]Makamba Atoa Msaada Wa Mchele Mbovu Kwa Waliobomolewa Nyumba Tabata, www.jamboforums.comshow-thread.phpt=11173KwaWaliobomolewaNyumbaTabata-JamboForums_com.htm (visited on 24 March 2008).

[27]Tanzania Standard NewspapersHome www.dailynews.habarileo.co.tzsportsindex.phpid=2950.htm (visited on 24 March 2008).

that was found to be unfit for human consumption.[28] Such acts of destruction have been made several times while the food concerned was already on the market.[29] Such foodstuffs are imported through the Tanzanian harbors. This brings more questions than answers. That is: how did such food pass through the port? Are the legally established agencies not working? Is the foodstuff destroyed tantamount to the whole food imported? If this foodstuff was discovered to be unfit for human consumption how many times has it passed through the ports thereby affecting the health of the citizens?

Unfortunately, it was also revealed that in the case of the rice and wheat flour imported from Dubai, both products were covered with green fungus and the consignments lacked indications for both the expiry and manufacturing dates. This apart from being dangerous to health, infringes the public/consumer right to know important information about the product before making the decision whether to buy or not.[30] This right is irrespective of the health situation of the food. According to FAO, Tanzania should indulge in building an effective food safety regime as an urgent necessity to save lives and create economic opportunity across the continent.[31]

All these examples show that it is a necessity to create the conditions for a "bottom up" democracy, where the citizens raise their awareness in considering Food Safety as another way to give their needs the right voice.[32]

In the Annual Report of the Commission on the Social Dimensions of Globalization T. Halonen, President of Finland and B.W. Mkapa, former President of the United Republic of Tanzania, expressed this opinion with the following words:

> "[t]here is a wide international agreement on the essentials which we must urgently strive for: […] a vibrant civil society, empowered by freedom of association and expression, that reflects and voices the full diversity of views and interests. Organizations representing public interest, the poor and other disadvantaged groups are also essentials for ensuring participatory and socially just governance."

This idea is linked to the recognition of two sources for the challenges facing developing countries, Africa in particular, in the global system.

> "One is domestic; the other one is systemic. […] [S]olutions to the difficulties will have to come from these two sources. African countries will hardly make any impact in global trade negotiations if they fail to take trade issues and trade rules seriously at home. It is becoming crystal that participation and strategic and clever moves at International negotiations can make a difference to what a country gets from such negotiations."

This discourse referred to global trade law, but it can easily apply to food safety law. The idea is that the problem has to be faced both at an international and national level, through an aware participation with the intention at least to temper the abuse of the stronger interlocutor.

---

[28] *Ibid.*

[29] *Ibid.*

[30] Pacific Law Journal, 1988–1989, 969.

[31] <http://www.fao.org/newsroom/en/news/2005/107908/index.html>.

[32] It is worth noting that, despite the mentioned remarkable attempts, public opinion still underestimates the importance of reaching high standards in food safety as part of the protection of human health. See the key points summed up in the report of The African Food Safety and Traceability Conference. The African Food Safety and Traceability conference 2007 that took place from 11th to 13th April 2007 welcomed more than 120 participants. The conference was organized by GS1 Kenya and Insysnc Ltd. under the auspices of the Ministry of Trade and Industry and sponsored by Syngenta. Speakers included policymakers, academics industry leaders and solution providers.

For the last two decades, Tanzania has been carrying out micro- and macro-economic adjustments in line with globalization and market liberalization forces in the world. Such adjustments have recognized food safety as a prerequisite for national food security and for both regional and international trade in food. It is in view of this recognition that food function in the country is in the process of re-organization to ensure food safety and food security.[33]

2.5.2.2 Law

In line with the idea of food safety as a prerequisite of food security, and considering the two regimes deeply interconnected, the Ministries of Health, Agriculture and Food Security, Natural Resources and Tourism, and Ministry of Industries and Trade carry out food safety and quality control functions in Tanzania. Laws empowering these ministries had been considered to be adequate for the monitoring and control of transboundary safety emergencies. Among these laws are notably the Tanzania Food, Drugs and Cosmetics Act and Food Security Act .

Within this law, there is also a provision concerning the necessity for the exchange of information. In particular, Article 12 states that

"(1) [f]or the purposes of securing the proper performance of its functions under this Act, the Department may require in writing any department, organization, authority or body of persons, to furnish it with such information required for the purpose of food security planning and operations as the Board or the Director may deem necessary; (2) [a]ny person who

is required to furnish information under subsection (1) of this section shall comply with that requirement and any person who refuses or fails to comply with that requirement shall be guilty of an offence and be liable on conviction to a fine not exceeding ten thousand shillings, or a jail term not exceeding six months, and he shall be ordered by the trial court to furnish the information required."

The mentioned provision seems to be unidirectional, referring to the possibility of information transfer only from the Authority to the citizens and not *vice versa*. The expected goal should be a cross cooperation between authority and citizens, through the provision of an asset of "participatory rights" for the citizens and all the actors belonging to civil society in general (non governmental organizations, international organizations and so on).

The Tanzania Food, Drug and Cosmetics Act establishes the Tanzania Food and Drugs Authority (TFDA). This is the main agency for the control of food safety in Tanzania. To achieve food safety the Act vests the TFDA with the following objective, *inter alia* (a) to regulate all matters relating to quality, and safety of food, drugs, herbal drugs, medical devices, poisons and cosmetics; (b) to regulate the importation, manufacture, labeling, marking or identification, storage promotion, selling and distribution of food, drugs, cosmetics, herbal drugs and medical devices or any materials or substances used in the manufacture of products regulated under the Act.

Actually, the development of the matter seems to be an ongoing process. Even from the

---

[33] In Tanzania, the institutions involved in the regulatory system and standard-setting system are the Tanzania Bureau of Standards (TBS), under the authority of the Ministry of Industry and Trade, the Plant Health Services (PHS) in the Ministry of Agriculture and the Tanzania Food and Drugs Authority (TFDA), under the Ministry of Health. See the Workshop of the United Nations Conference on Trade and Development, *Costs of Agri-Food Safety and SPS Compliance: United Republic of Tanzania, Mozambique and Guinea: Tropical Fruits, Selected Commodity Issues in the Context of Trade and Development*, New York and Geneva, 2005.

point of view of access to information it seems to be a work in progress. Most importantly, the awareness of the need to participate in the same network as the Food Safety agencies is still feeble, if not non-existent. However, the main objective of the Authority is to become the best agency in regulating food, drugs, cosmetics and medical devices by 2015.

2.5.3 African Union and the Harmonization of Food Law

2.5.3.1 African Model Law on Safety in Biotechnology

One of the most remarkable attempts to create a network of interlocutors in food safety is the development of the African Union (AU). The African Union may be considered an example of the desegregation of the barriers between international and national domains. It is an actor of the network, contributing to the building of linkages between international institutions and civil society.

The African Union shall play this role of interlocutor between the International Organizations, the various African States and civil society, cooperating with the WTO and with International Organizations in general.

The AU Assembly of Heads of State and Government in July 2003 in anticipation of the entry into force of the Cartagena Protocol endorsed the draft African Model Law on Safety in Biotechnology, finalized in May 2001. The Model Law is an attempt to harmonize existing and future biosafety legislation in Africa. It provides a comprehensive framework of biosafety regulations designed to protect Africa's biodiversity, environment and health. Deeply connected with the compliance of the African Model Law is the creation of a competent authority.

The African Model Law provides (in Article 3) that the Government shall designate or establish a competent authority to follow up, supervise and control the implementation of this law. The powers and duties of the Competent Authority shall include: prescribing criteria, standards, guidelines and regulations as may be necessary for the fulfillment of the objective of this law; taking into account the policy recommendations and other guidelines of the National Biosafety Committee in making decisions on the import, transit, contained use, release or placing on the market of a genetically modified organism; establishing of Institutional Biosafety Committees at relevant institutions or nominating independent panels or any other body of experts, as appropriate, as technical and scientific advisors on issues of biosafety; keeping genetically modified organisms globally under constant review and when any one of them is suspected of posing a serious risk to human health or to the environment, banning its transit through the country's territories and notify the Clearing-House, the customs and trade officials accordingly; informing the Secretariat of the Cartagena Protocol, if appropriate, that it has no access to the Clearing-House; maintaining and making available to the public on request, a database on genetically modified organisms and products of genetically modified organisms intended for direct use as food or feed, or for processing.

The Law also provides that a National Biosafety Committee comprising of representatives of governmental and non-governmental organizations, and the private sector that are relevant to the issues of biotechnology and biosafety shall be established by the government to provide, as appropriate, policy recommendations and guidelines to the competent authority. The National Biosafety Committee will further develop based on its general responsibility, its terms of reference and may draw up its own rules of procedure.

A member of the National Biosafety committee who finds a conflict of interest in the case at hand must declare it and withdraw from the Committee in so far as that case of conflict of interest is concerned. Institutional Biosafety

Committee Institutions that are involved in the import, export, handling, contained use, release or placing on the market of genetically modified organisms or products of genetically modified organisms will establish Institutional Biosafety Committees to institute and control safety mechanisms and approval procedures at the institution level.

2.5.3.2 Risk Assessment

A workshop was held in Addis Ababa from 23 to 25 August 2007,[34] organized by the African Union Experts Meeting on the revised African Model Law on Safety in Biotechnology. This was the first attempt to comply with international standards concerning the risk assessment settled upon in the mentioned Cartagena Protocol.

The objectives were to enable participants to learn about risk assessment and risk management in the context of the Biosafety Protocol;[35] to review the general concepts, principles and methodologies; to exchange practical experience; to review the existing guidance materials on risk assessment and risk management; to consider the need for further guidance; to review the format and key elements of risk

assessment reports; and to identify mechanisms for promoting cooperation and networking between experts and agencies.

The efforts undertaken by the African Union are likely to be the first achievements in harmonization of food safety regulation in Africa. It is worth mentioning the recent goals reached by the African Union Commission, together with many other actors, with respect to the Capacity building and Exchange of Experiences on Risk Assessment and Risk Management of Living Modified Organisms.

The FAO/WHO Regional Conference on Food Safety for Africa in Harare, Zimbabwe, from 3 to 6 October 2005, is another cooperative attempt in the promotion of food safety situation in Africa. The participants of the meeting were nearly all the African countries, as well as some international organizations in the area of food safety and observer countries such as Italy and the USA.[36]

The important issues discussed were National Food Safety Systems in Africa—A Situation Analysis,[37] Prioritization and Coordination of Capacity Building Activities,[38] Informal Food Distribution Sector in Africa (Street foods): Importance and challenges,[39] Assuring Food

---

[34] The workshop was attended by fifty seven participants from twenty five countries and sixteen organizations involved in risk assessment and risk management. Amongst the organizations represented, there were Addis Ababa University, AfricaBio, African Biodiversity Network, African Union Commission, United Nations Economic Commission for Africa (UNECA) and University of Rome 'La Sapienza'. For the official documents concerning the meeting, see <http://www.cbd.int/doc/meetings/bs/rwcbafr-01/official/rwcbafr-01-02-en.pdf>. The meeting is one of the most recent attempts of the global actors to settle a 'corpus' of standards in Food Safety. For further examples, see the African food safety meeting held on the 6 October 2005 in Geneva/Rome—The first pan-African food safety meeting attended by 147 food regulation officials and experts from some 50 countries, unanimously recommended a Strategic Plan for Food Safety in Africa for adoption by UN food and health agencies and the African Union. See <ftp://ftp.fao.org/es/esn/foodsafetyforum/caf/CAF_foodsafetyclose.pdf>. To consult the list of the main meetings on this topic see: <http://www.who.int/foodsafety/publications/newsletter/18/en/index.html>.

[35] For the text of the Protocol see <http://www.cbd.int/biosafety/>.

[36] FAO/WHO Regional Conference on Food Safety for Africa: Harare, Zimbabwe, 3–6 October 2005 Final Report See the list of participants, at 13–30.

[37] Paper prepared by FAO Regional Office for Africa, Accra, Ghana, *ibid* pp 47–87.

[38] Paper prepared by the FAO/WHO secretariat, *ibid* pp 88–97.

[39] Paper prepared by Zimbabwe *ibid*, 98–107.

Safety And Quality In Small and Medium Size Food Enterprises[40] and International, Regional, Sub-regional and National Cooperation In Food Safety in Africa.[41] This meeting, apart from other things, formulated a resolution to ensure the eradication of problems associated with food safety in Africa.[42]

The increasing globalization of the food trade has notably resulted in shifting food consumption patterns, new production methods and technologies, faster trans-boundary transfer of microbiological and chemical hazards between regions.[43] With this, there can be no successful food safety without dealing holistically with the concerns of the main players in the food industry.[44] This, in fact, underlines the importance of cooperation. Cooperation at national, sub-regional, regional and international levels provides opportunities in synergy and maximized benefits for improved human health and economic development.[45]

These are good examples of cooperation to implement the standards and develop the exchange of information amongst the actors in the global arena. The mentioned examples testify to the progress towards cooperation between authorities to reach the goal of Food Safety in Africa and to assure the respect of a fundamental human right, the right to safe food.

2.5.4 Conclusion

In Eastern Africa developments in food take place both at national and at international level. Tanzania has established a food safety authority. A small step, such as the implementation of the Tanzanian Food Safety legislation with the

provision of participatory rights, can consolidate the edification of a "common core" of global standards. The regulation of a transparent procedure, where citizens can participate in the decision-making processes, helps reach a more efficient distribution of information.

It was further observed that, establishing pan-African food safety standards will not only save lives and improve the health of African people but will also go a long way towards helping Africans to join international trade and raise African living standards. This is particularly true in rural areas where the most poor are subsisting.[46]

The African Union, confronted with the challenges created by biotechnology and the issue of biosafety, has moved to formulate an African Model Law on Safety in Biotechnology. It contributes to establish the concept of risk assessment in African food law.

2.6 AUSTRALIA AND NEW ZEALAND

Keith C. Richardson and William R. Porter
Food Science Australia, North Ryde, New South Wales, Australia
New South Wales Food Authority, Newington, New South Wales, Australia

2.6.1 International Development of Food Law and its Application in Australia

The development of food law internationally is well documented. O'Keefe (1968) identifies six centuries of adulteration in a wide range of

---

[40] Paper prepared by Botswana *ibid*, 108–120.
[41] Prepared by the WHO Regional Office for Africa, BP 06, Brazzaville, Republic of Congo *ibid* ,121–131.
[42] On the resolution see *ibid*, 134–135.
[43] *Ibid*, 45.
[44] *Ibid*.
[45] *Ibid*,121.
[46] *Ibid*.

foodstuffs, the ineffectiveness of officials and the ad hoc statutory provisions to remedy the matter in the UK as significant factors. Add to that the rise of analytical chemistry and the increased awareness of the level of food adulteration and particularly a series of articles published by the Lancet, and the findings of a Select Parliamentary Commission (1855). These resulted in the passage of the UK Adulteration of Food and Drink Act 1860.

At the time of white settlement in Australia, the laws then in place in Britain were considered to apply in the new colony of New South Wales. However, legislation subsequently passed by the British Parliament had no application in the colonies unless expressly provided. Consequently the 1860 UK Act did not apply.

2.6.2 Federal and State Responsibility

Australia is a federation of six States and two Commonwealth Territories. From 1788 there was just the colony of New South Wales; New Zealand was first to split away, then Victoria and Queensland, followed by the proclamation of the other Australian colonies. Prior to federation in 1901, each State was an independent colony of Great Britain with its own legislative system including matters relating to food.

Laws regulating food were first introduced in the State of Victoria in the mid-nineteenth century as a response to concern over adulterated food. The Victorian Public Health Act of 1854 empowered the Board of Health to inspect, seize and destroy unwholesome food (Anon, 1988). Specific legislation followed as analytical techniques developed to permit a closer examination of what was being added to food. In 1838, the New South Wales government passed an Adulteration of Bread Act, and in 1879 the first general legislation, the Adulteration of Food Prevention Act. The Act appears to have had little or no use (Madgwick, unpublished material).

When Australia became a Federation, domestic food legislation was not among the powers

vested in the Commonwealth and each State individually introduced specific legislation to control manufacture and sale of food. This activity was led by Victoria, which introduced its Pure Food Act in 1905 and by 1912 most of the other States had followed with similar, but not identical, legislation aimed primarily at preventing the sale of adulterated food. New Zealand had eliminated its provincial governments in 1876 and as a consequence its Sale of Food and Drugs Act of 1877 applied throughout the country (Farrer, 1983).

Regulations were progressively made under the State Food Acts to set standards for foods, including labeling requirements. In NSW the Pure Food Advisory Committee established by the Act consulted extensively with the food industry and took evidence as part of their regulation-making process (PFAC minutes).

The non-uniformity of food regulations in Australia created real difficulties for the burgeoning interstate trade and a series of Commonwealth/State conferences were held in 1910, 1913, 1922 and 1927 to set uniform standards for foods. Many of these were adopted under State Food Acts and remained unchanged through to the 1950s. Nonetheless the need for uniform adoption of these standards was emphasized. A Royal Commission was held in 1925 to endeavor to overcome the problems but without notable success. In particular the Commission made the following recommendation "That the States transfer to the Commonwealth the Constitutional power to legislate for the control of food and drugs" (Downer, 1995).

In 1936, the National Health and Medical Research Council (NHMRC) was established within the Commonwealth Department of Health with responsibility for advising both Commonwealth and State Governments on matters of public health. Food was considered part of its interest because food was seen as a public health matter.

The initial concern of the NHMRC on food was primarily the nutritional value of the Australian food supply. No reference was made in the NHMRC report to food legislation until November 1952 when the NHMRC adopted recommendations from its Public Health Committee (made up of representatives of the States as well as Commonwealth officers) concerning the need for national uniformity of food and drug regulations. The NHMRC noted the need for closer liaison between the Commonwealth, the State Food Advisory Committees and industry organization, viz., the Chamber of Manufacturers and the Council of Food Technology Associations (CAFTA) to achieve this end. This led to the formation of the Food Standards Committee (FSC) of the NHMRC.

2.6.3 Towards a Model Food Standards Code

The FSC had its first meeting in 1955 when it identified as its purpose to recommend to the NHMRC model food standards that would be adopted without material change in all States so that food legislation might be uniform throughout Australia. It was not concerned with the legal machinery for the policing of these regulations, which remained with the States.

The FSC was made up of senior officers of the State and Federal governments together with an industry representative nominated by CAFTA. A unique feature of this system was that first drafts for any proposed standard or amendment would be supplied by CAFTA, giving the industry body the opportunity to be fully involved in the standard making process. It was the FSC's wish that industry would not communicate with it directly but through CAFTA. This clearly showed that the FSC acknowledged CAFTA's ability to speak for industry in a balanced and ethical manner (Reuter, 1997).

Before the establishment of the FSC, the NHMRC had acted to review existing controls on additives and contaminants in the food supply with particular reference to preservatives and colors. They did this by establishing a

Food Additives Committee in 1953. The early work of this committee is described in detail by Farrer (1990). The terms of reference of the Food Additives Committee as enunciated when it subsequently became a subcommittee of the FSC were to enquire into and advise the FSC on matters concerning food science and technology including:

1. the specifications for purity and identity of food additives;
2. the technological need for and safety of food additives;
3. contaminants in food; and
4. the use of coloring substances in cosmetics, pharmaceuticals and food.

Australia provided a representative at the first meeting of the Joint FAO/WHO Expert Committee on Food Additives (JECFA) in 1956 and has maintained regular representation since that time.

While the major food safety concern of the NHMRC and its reference groups in matters of food law were with chemicals in foods, microbiological standards began to appear in product standards, particularly dairy products, on an ad hoc basis in the mid-1960s. Greater recognition of the importance of microorganisms in food safety led in 1965 to the establishment of the Food Microbiology Subcommittee (FMC) to assist the FSC in the preparation of microbiological standards (Smith, 1978).

Faced with a lack of information on the microbiological status of Australian foods, one of the first initiatives of the FMC was to organize a comprehensive survey of the States of a range of ready-to-eat foods using standard laboratory methodology. The FSC proved reluctant to clutter the regulations with microbiological standards of doubtful value, recommending Codes of Practice whenever possible.

Since a major reason given for States being unable to adopt uniformly the model food standards recommended by the NHMRC system was the inherent differences in the Food Acts, moves were commenced in 1975 to have a uniform Food Act for the States and Commonwealth territories. This so called Model Food Act was eventually adopted at a Health Minister's Conference in 1980. The path to achieving this was by no means straightforward and is described in some detail by the first chairman of the Food Standards Committee (Reuter, 1997). It then took some years for all the States to change their Food Acts so that food standards generated through the NHMRC could be incorporated automatically as regulations under State law.

However this was facilitated by the model food standards being endorsed by all parties and gazetted in whole as the NHMRC's Australian Food Standards Code (AFSC) in 1986.

While some success could be claimed for introducing uniformity between States with regard to food standards this was by no means complete. In addition, the Code and the way it was amended continued to be the subject of criticism by the food industry and by consumer groups who now took a marked interest in food. Industry representatives complained that the Code was overly prescriptive, difficult to have amended and inhibited innovation. Consumer representatives criticized the lack of information on labels.

2.6.4 Winds of Change

In 1989 food standards development was transferred from the NHMRC to the Bureau of Consumer Affairs in the Attorney-General's Department in the Commonwealth Government. While the representation on the former food standards committee was enlarged, the committee system continued to operate with, in the view of the industry, its inherent deficiencies. This view was at least partly shared by three major review committees reporting to the Commonwealth government around this time.

Following further discussion by State Premiers, it was agreed in 1990 that a new body, the National

Food Authority (NFA), which later became the Australia New Zealand Food Authority (ANZFA), responsible to the Minister for Health and Human Services should be established. ANZFA was to undertake a number of functions in re-ordering the food regulatory system of which the principal one was to identify more specific objectives for domestic food standards which would:

- protect public health and safety;
- provide sufficient information on food ingredients to allow consumers to make informed choices;
- promote fair trading practice at the national level; and
- promote domestic uniformity and alignment with international requirements to promote trade and commerce in the food industry.

Recommendations of the NFA were referred to the National Food Standards Council that comprised State Health Ministers and the Commonwealth Minister for Consumer Affairs. The National Food Standards Council was supported by the Uniform Food Law Interpretation Committee made up of Commonwealth and State officers, usually Chief Food Inspectors or their equivalent, which had come into being under the previous system. Health officers from the New Zealand Department of Health started attending meetings of the NFA as they had done prior to that of the AFSC. These officers had observer status and contributed to discussions. Under the Act of the Commonwealth Parliament which established the NFA, it was also responsible for developing food inspection policies for imported food.

Under a 1991 Inter Governmental Agreement between the Commonwealth and State and Territory governments, the States and Territories agreed to adopt, without variation, food standards recommended by the National Food Authority. The purpose of the agreement was to consolidate responsibility for developing food standards in one specialist agency and to ensure the uniformity of food standards across all States and Territories, which continued to have primary responsibility for enforcing food laws.

In 1996 the Australian and New Zealand governments agreed to establish a bi-national regime to develop food standards that were to apply in both countries. This agreement took effect by way of a treaty which outlined four specific aims focused at reducing unnecessary barriers to trade by adopting a joint system for the development of food standards. These were the same as listed above. The treaty applies generally to food standards within the AFSC except for those standards addressing maximum residue limits for agricultural and veterinary chemicals, specifications for food hygiene requirements, which are the responsibility of the New Zealand Food Safety Authority (Winger, 2003) in that country. It also contains provisions that allow New Zealand to opt out of a joint standard for exceptional reasons relating to health, safety, trade, environmental concerns or cultural issues. For example, New Zealand has opted out of the Code's country of origin labeling requirements.

The commitments contained within the treaty were implemented by a new body, the Australia New Zealand Food Authority, which subsequently became Food Standards Australia New Zealand (FSANZ) by virtue of the revised amended Commonwealth, State and Territory Agreement in 2000. The 2000 agreement left standards development as the prime responsibility of FSANZ, but vested policy development as the responsibility of the Food Regulation Ministerial Council, assisted by the Food Regulation Standing Committee. The objectives for developing food standards were reduced to three with the protection of public health and safety retained as the primary objective (Healy, Brooke-Taylor, & Liehne, 2003).

In Australia, additional legislation applies to imported food at the point of entry. Implementation of the Imported Food Control Act of 1992 requires food to be safe and to meet the requirements of the Australian Food Standards Code. In New Zealand, imported food is subject to the New Zealand Customs and Excise Act of

1996. In addition, the Australia/New Zealand treaty does not apply to export requirements relating to third country trade.

There remains another significant area of non-uniformity in the shape of the Trans-Tasman Mutual Recognition Arrangement (TTMRA). This arrangement, which commenced in 1997, allows for the sale in either country of foods which comply with the laws in the other. Thus for example, foods imported from New Zealand can be sold in Australia without country of origin labeling, notwithstanding the application of the Food Standards Code in Australia. New Zealand also has its Dietary Supplements Regulations 1985 which allow the sale in New Zealand of foods and drinks with added vitamins, minerals and other substances not permitted under the Code. Under TTMRA these products may be legally imported from New Zealand and sold in Australia, although it would be an offence to manufacture such products in Australia.

A major review of the Australian Food Standards Code was commenced in 1994 and this review was continued as a vehicle to develop the joint Australia New Zealand Food Standards Code. The basic principle underlying the policy for the review was efficient and effective regulation. The reform of food product standards aimed to reduce the level of prescription and to construct standards that apply across all foods or a range of foods (Healy et al., 2003). The first general or horizontal standard to be completed was the joint standard for food additives and this was also the first standard to be adopted as a joint Australian and New Zealand standard. The process of reviewing food additive regulation at a fundamental level enabled the development of a standard that recognizes the principles of the Codex General Standard for Food Additives (Codex Alimentarius Commission, 1995) as well as the food additive regulations of the major trading partners (Brooke-Taylor, Baines, Goodchap, Gruber, & Hambridge, 2003).

The most notable reforms have occurred in food hygiene requirements. Within Australia, hygiene requirements for food, with the exception of a small number of microbiological standards, had traditionally been specified within the legislation of each State or Territory with some local municipal councils (the third tier of government in Australia) introducing additional requirements. This resulted in a lack of national consistency and also many prescriptive requirements which were of little or no relevance to food safety. The policy guiding the reform required that food safety standards represent international best practice and particular note was taken of the guidelines for the use of hazard analysis critical control point (HACCP) systems as defined by the Codex Alimentarius Commission (1997),[47] which had already been partially introduced in New Zealand by the New Zealand Food Safety Authority and by State and Territory Primary Production Authorities.

Basic hygienic requirements for food in the Food Standards Code are now in four food safety standards. Three of the four were approved in 2000 as mandatory standards. These are Standard 3.1.1, Interpretation and Application; Standard 3.2.2, Food Safety Practices and General Requirements; and Standard 3.2.3, Food Premises and Equipment. The fourth Standard, 3.2.1, Food Safety Programs, which specifies requirements for HACCP based food safety plans was originally approved as a voluntary standard to provide a model set of requirements for those States and Territories wishing to introduce such requirements. The introduction has to date not been uniform but significant progress has been made. In addition the Food Standards Code now includes a mandatory standard for Food Safety Programs for Food Service to Vulnerable Persons. Standard 3.3.1, which calls up Standard 3.2.1.

2.6.5 Model Food Act, Part 2

Uniformity across State and Territory Food Acts remains the holy grail of food regulators.

The 1980 Model Food Act was adopted in a desultory fashion at best by the States and Territories. The second "Model Food Bill" was finalized in October 2000. On 3 November 2000, the Council of Australian Governments (COAG) signed an Inter-Government Agreement agreeing to a new food regulatory system. The Commonwealth of Australia and all the Australian States and Territories are signatories to the Agreement. The new arrangements required a renegotiation of the Treaty with New Zealand prior to full implementation. This Inter-Governmental Agreement is also known as the Food Regulation Agreement.

The Agreement states in part that States and Territories will use their best endeavors to submit to their respective Parliaments, within twelve months of the date of signing this Agreement, legislation which gives effect to the provisions listed at Annex A and Annex B of this Agreement which provide for the effective and consistent administration and enforcement of the Food Standards Code (including the Food Safety Standards). Annex A was to be adopted without change, except in respect of separate legislation governing safe primary food production. Annex B was completely optional.

Some States and Territories honored the agreement without delay. New South Wales fell across the line in 2003. At the time of writing West Australia has yet to enact the model food provisions.

2.6.6 Where To From Here?

At the time of writing, FSANZ is in the process of developing standards for primary production and processing paving the way for a complete food chain approach to food safety. Standards for the seafood and dairy industries have been completed with work being undertaken on the egg, poultry, meat, and dairy (raw

[47]See section 2.2 above.

milk products) industries. Administration of "paddock to plate" standards continues to be problematic with only New Zealand and New South Wales having through chain agencies.

The October 2008 meeting of the Food Regulation Ministerial Council agreed in principle to commission an independent, comprehensive review of food labeling law and policy. The review would be undertaken by an independent expert panel. The expert panel is to comprise prominent individuals appointed by the Ministerial Council who collectively possess knowledge and expertise in the fields of public health, regulatory, economics/public policy, law and consumer behavior and business. The review is to be chaired by an independent public policy expert.

The Australian Government has been active in progressing food regulation reform. Much of the drive for reform has come from the Commonwealth Productivity Commission. In October 2008 the COAG Business Regulation and Competition Working Group agreed that the Commission should benchmark food safety regulation in 2009, "and report by December 2009. In November 2008, the Council of Australian Governments (COAG) agreed to consider options to improve national consistency in the monitoring and enforcement of food standards and options to improve food labeling law and policy in early 2009 (COAG). This could be seen as a move toward the Commonwealth assuming administrative responsibility for certain aspects of food regulation. As mooted in 1925 and many times since.

2.7 THE UNITED STATES AND CANADA

Neal D. Fortin
Institute for Food Laws and Regulations, Michigan State University, East Lansing, MI, USA

2.7.1 Introduction

As food trade expands and food processing increases, so does the opportunity and the scope of adulteration. Legislatures have followed rather than led food safety reform. Scientists and analytical methods have played a critical role in increasing awareness of food safety risks. Public outrage has also played a role. The food industry also plays an important leadership role out of enlightened self-interest in improved food safety. However, rarely have any of these factors alone been enough. Major food law revision occurs when all—scientists, the public, and food industry leadership—are galvanized, too often by outrageous tragedy.

2.7.2 The Early Years

And chalk, and alum and plaster are sold to the poor for bread.
   —Alfred Lord Tennyson, *Maud* (1886)

The history of adulteration of food is as old as the trade in food (Hart, 1952). The corresponding history of food law and the efforts to detect adulteration similarly run as far back as commerce itself (*Ibid.*). The earliest adulteration was comparatively simple, in large part because food was mostly unprocessed. Whole coffee beans, for instance, provide less opportunity for adulteration than ground coffee. The more processing, the greater the opportunities for adulteration. Grinding grain into flour provides one opportunity, and the mixing and baking of the flour into bread provides additional opportunities. Therefore, it is no coincidence that the earliest food laws covered the earliest processed foods: bread, wine, and beer (*Ibid.*).

In these earliest years, consumers served as their own food inspectors. They sniffed fish and meat for freshness, squeezed fruit and vegetables to check for soundness, and examined grain for mold (Janssen, 1975). Lack of analytical techniques limited the ability to detect adulteration.

However, most food trade was local, so consumers assessed the reputation of the purveyors of food.

In their colonial years, before the founding of the United States and the confederation of Canada, the British common law applied the earliest food safety law. The essence of the common law was plain and direct: 1) Do not poison food, and 2) Do not cheat (Hutt, 1960). "Adulterated food" in the common law consisted of food that was unfit for human consumption or contained some deleterious substance, whereby rendering it dangerous to health (*Ibid.*). Packaged food with labels was rare, so there was no common-law offense of mislabeling. However, our basic concept of mislabeling existed as the common law offense of falsely representing merchandise for sale (*Ibid.*).

The sixteenth, seventeenth, and eighteenth centuries were an era of colonial expansion in the United States and Canada. This expansion coincided with increased trade in agricultural goods from the New World (Hart, 1952). As demand and value of exported goods rose, so did incentive and the opportunity to adulterate (*Ibid.*). During this same period, food production began shifting from the home to manufacturers. As people moved to the cities, consumers bought more processed and manufactured foods. Reputation weakened as a means of control. Laws were enacted to prohibit adulteration, but without analytical methods of detection, the laws provided only minimal protection (*Ibid.*).

The legislative food laws of this era were largely ones that protected commerce rather than food safety. For instance, seventeenth century colonial bread laws penalized short weight and the failure to identify the maker of the bread (Janssen, 1975). Merchants pushed for the establishment of food inspection laws because they recognized the marketing problems created by inferior goods, and they wished to create a level playing field (*Ibid.*). Honest dealings were important in creating and preserving the export markets, so the colonies created laws on food export.

2.7.3 The State and Local Legislative Era in the United States

The first food safety law in North America is thought to be the Massachusetts "Act against selling unwholesome Provisions" passed on 8 March, 1785 (Hart, 1952; Janssen, 1975). However, not until the latter half of the nineteenth century were major food safety laws enacted. Rapid development of analytical methods began in the early 1800's, and these tools identified adulteration of shocking scope. In 1820 Frederick Accum documented adulteration so widespread that he found it difficult to find a single type of food that was not adulterated; and some foods he scarcely ever found genuine (Accum, 1820; Hutt & Hutt, 1984).

The public was shocked and dismayed, but legislative reform was slow in coming. The early nineteenth century was the height of *laissez faire* capitalism. This economic philosophy called for deregulation of business, not food protection.[48] At the same time, however, the exodus from farms to the cities continued. The development of large cities by the middle of the nineteenth century required increased national commerce in food. More people purchased processed food, and adulteration increased. This degradation of the food supply was increasingly documented as scientists found new ways to detect adulteration[49] (Batrershall, 1887; Beck, 1846; Byrn, 1852; Felker, 1880; Hoskins, 1861; Richards, 1886).

---

[48]This was not called the era of the "robber barons" for nothing.

[49]For example, in the period around 1880, over 73% of the milk in Buffalo, New York, was watered; 41% of the samples of ground coffee in New York were adulterated; and 71% of the olive oil in New York and Massachusetts were adulterated (Hart, 1952).

The period from 1865 to 1900 was one of increased state legislative activity. The Georgian Code of 1867 provided fines, imprisonment, and whipping up to 39 strokes, or chain gang for up to one year for knowing sale of unwholesome food or drink (Hart, 1952). Massachusetts, New York, Michigan, New Jersey, Rhode Island, and others jurisdictions passed food laws in this period (*Ibid.*).

2.7.4 The Federal Era

Both Canada and the United States are federations. Some powers are assigned to the federal or national government, but other powers are reserved to the individual provinces or states. This division of power from time to time has created questions of the proper role of the federal government in regulating food. However, increasing national and international commerce along with growing magnitude of the problem made national regulation inevitable.

Both federal governments hold authority over commerce. However, unlike the United States, the Canadian Constitution Act, 1867, assigns criminal law power and presumably power over health and safety concerns to the federal government. Therefore, food safety legislation falls naturally under federal authority in the Canadian system.

2.7.4.1 *Canada*

Canada confederated in 1867. Canada's first federal food law was the Inland Revenue Act of 1875, enacted just seven years after confederation.[50] The act prohibited the adulteration of food and drink and covered alcohol and drugs. The definition of adulterated was nearly the same as in the common law and similar to English statutes of that era (Hutt & Hutt, 1984). Adulterated meant, "all articles of food or drink with which there has been mixed any deleterious ingredient or any material or ingredient of less value than is understood or implied by the name under which the article is offered for sale" (Blakney, 2009).

Adulterated liquor apparently was a great cause of concern and adulterants included ferrous sulfate, opium, hemp, strychnine, and tobacco (Gnirss, 2008). According to a report by the Commissioner of the Inland Revenue Act, 50% of all foods sold in Canada at the time were adulterated (*Ibid.*) Similar to the United States, nearly all coffee and pepper were adulterated, milk was diluted with water, and other high value items, such as tea and chocolate were often adulterated (*Ibid.*).

The Inspection Law, 1874, established a system of quality and grade inspections for staple food commodities, such as butter, flour, and meal (Blakney, 2009). Although the grading was voluntary for domestic product, some grades were mandatory for export goods (*Ibid.*) In 1884, the Inland Revenue Act of 1875 was amended and renamed by the Adulteration Act of 1884. Standards of identity began with a standard for tea in 1894, but standards soon followed for milk, milk products, honey, maple products, and foods (Gnirss, 2008). These standards served as important tools to prevent adulteration and as food safety controls.

2.7.4.2 *United States*

We face a new situation in history. Ingenuity, striking hands with cunning trickery, compounds a substance to counterfeit an article of food. It is made to look like something it is not; to taste and smell like something it is not; to sell like something it is not, and so deceive the purchaser.

—US Congressional Record,
49 Congress I Session 1886

---

[50]37 Vict. c. 8.

Through the late 1800s, nearly all of the early food laws in the United States were state and local. The limited federal activity was largely to regulate imports and exports. For instance, in 1883 the United States Congress enacted a law to prevent the importation of adulterated tea. The oleomargarine statute followed in 1896, which was passed because of the dairy industry's objections to the sale of fats colored to look like butter.[51] In 1890, Congress passed a meat inspection act to facilitate the export sale of meat (Hutt & Hutt, 1984). A live cattle inspection law followed in 1891 (*Ibid.*). In 1899, Congress authorized the Secretary of Agriculture to inspect and analyze any imported food, drug, or liquor when there was reason to believe there was a danger (*Ibid.*).

From the beginning of federal regulation, analytical chemistry played an important role. When the United States Department of Agriculture (USDA) was created in 1862, Congress authorized the agency to employ chemists. This Chemical Division eventually became the US. Food and Drug Administration (FDA) in 1930 (Hutt, 1990). The FDA was transferred from USDA in 1940. In 1883, Dr. Harvey Wiley became the chief chemist of the USDA Bureau of Chemistry. Dr. Wiley expanded research and testing of food and documented the widespread adulteration (FDA, 2002). He helped spur public indignation by his dramatic and highly publicized "Poison Squad." The volunteers in the Poison Squad consumed questionable food additives, such as boric acid and formaldehyde. Observation and documentation of the ill effects and symptoms of the volunteers provided a crude gauge of food additive safety.[52]

2.7.4.3 The 1906 Pure Food and Drug Act

Public support for passage of a federal food and drug law grew as muckraking journalists exposed in shocking detail the frauds and dangers of the food industry, such as the use of poisonous preservatives and dyes in food. A final catalyst for change was the 1905 publication of Upton Sinclair's *The Jungle* (Sinclair, 1905). Sinclair's portrayal of nauseating practices and unsanitary conditions in the meatpacking industry captured the public's attention. On 30 June 1906, President Theodore Roosevelt signed both the Pure Food and Drug Act[53] and the Meat Inspection Act[54] into law.

2.7.4.4 Evolution of the Food Statutes

Not long after passage of the Pure Food and Drug Act, legislative battles began to expand and strengthen the law. For example, leaders in the food industry called for more stringent product quality standards to create a level playing field. Consumers wanted stronger safety standards and fair dealing. However, major revision of the 1906 Act stalled until a precipitous tragedy occurred. The agonizing deaths of more than 100 children from sulfanilamide spurred the passage of the Federal Food, Drug, and Cosmetic Act of 1938.

This pattern for major revision of the national food law repeats itself. A tragedy alone is not enough. Concerns of a few interested parties are not enough. Typically, scientists, the food industry, and the public must all be interested in addressing the issue of the day.

The food laws continued to evolve based upon the concerns and issues of the times. In the 1950s, concerns over synthetic food additives,

---

[51]Margarine was patented in 1869 (Hutt & Hutt, 1984).
[52]The data is collected in the USDA, Bureau of Chemistry, bulletin no. 84 (1902–1908).
[53]21 U.S.C. § 1 *et seq.*
[54]21 U.S.C. § 601 *et seq.*

pesticides, and cancer were high. Consequently, in 1958, the Food Additives Amendment was enacted, requiring the evaluation of food additives to establish safety. The Delaney Clause forbade the use of any substance in food that was found to cause cancer in laboratory animals.

In 1920, the Canadian Adulteration Act was repealed and replaced with the Food and Drug Act of 1920. While the predecessor acts were significantly influenced by British law, this new statute looked more like the US Pure Food and Drug Act of 1906 (Gnirss, 2008). The Canadian Food and Drug Act of 1920 was revised in 1952-53 to cover cosmetics and therapeutic devices and to increase the regulation over labeling, packaging, and advertising (Blakney, 2009).

2.7.5 Conclusion

Food law is again at a crossroads. Rapid improvement in analysis and technology combines with rising global trade and more processing of food before reaching consumers. These conditions set the stage for increased adulteration, public outrage, unstable markets, and need for greater food safety oversight.

The past decade has been an American experiment with food safety deregulation. The results have left Americans with a growing sense of the failure of their government to ensure food safety. A series of foodborne disease outbreaks—melamine in pet food and then in human food, *E. coli* in spinach, lettuce, *Salmonella* recalls on tomatoes, peppers, and peanut butter—have left the public feeling vulnerable and intensified calls for reform of the food safety system. Firms have lost hundreds of millions of dollars in recalls and lost market share.

The history of adulteration in food reveals that increased processing and globalization will magnify the challenges to ensure pure and safe food. History instructs that the legislatures will follow rather than lead food safety reforms. Scientists play a critical role in increasing

awareness of food safety risks. Public outrage also plays a role. The food industry must play a leadership role. Enlightened self-interest points to stringent but fair food safety regulation as necessary to preserve and grow food trade.

Major food law reform usually occurs only when all—scientists, the public, and food industry leadership—are galvanized by current events. Sadly, all too often this has been outrageous tragedy.

2.8 LATIN AMERICA

Rebeca López-García
Logre International Food Science Consulting, Mexico, DF, Mexico

2.8.1 Introduction

Latin America is a very complex region that faces diverse challenges due to a disparity of social, economic and cultural conditions. Each country and even each sub-region has its own strengths, weaknesses and challenges, so it is difficult to portray the whole region in just a few pages without making generalizations. Latin American countries are most definitely not strangers to the "globalization processes" and have been quickly gaining a position in global markets with unique products. In addition, Latin America represents a huge market that is very attractive for companies around the world and commercial activities within the region have increased through the participation in several free trade agreements. These new market opportunities have helped shape the region's industry and food regulations and have sparked the interest in actively participating in International Organizations such as the *Codex Alimentarius*.

Latin American countries have only recently sought to promote a policy shift from protecting national industries through openly protectionist policies towards an open market, free commerce system that seeks to foster competition within the "global market" framework. The shift to free markets has not come without opposition. Of course, there is the responsibility of the state to defend the health and safety of its national consumers. However, most Latin American countries are subject to private sector pressures and are struggling to find the balance between encouraging more open commerce while making sure the products being imported are safe. In primary production, the shift from subsistence agriculture to competitive productive systems has faced a lot of cultural resistance and in many countries land reform has fractionated land to a point where it is almost impossible to compete without proper cooperation. How can small Central American producers compete with the economies of scale? How will they make the transition when the Central American Free Trade Agreement is fully operational? What are their options and their real competitive strengths?

2.8.2 First Steps Towards Harmonization

Harmonization is not new to the region. In fact, long before other regions of the world began to imagine a framework of food standards beyond their national borders, in 1924, in Buenos Aires, at the first Latin American Congress of Chemistry, a Commission composed of two delegates from each country represented in the Congress proposed the development of a *Codex Alimentarius Sudamericanus*. This Commission accomplished their objective and in 1930 at the following Congress in Montevideo they presented a Code that had 154 articles and was considered for adoption by all countries in Latin America. The Code contained definitions of food products and general dispositions. Unfortunately, then, as now, turning a proposal into a reality was not easy. Although many countries in Latin America have adopted "modern" and well thought out food legislation, as a region Latin America did not achieve an early effective regional regulation of food. In the following Latin American Congresses of Chemistry, there was much discussion on the

same topic always with the vision of developing a Latin American Code. During the sixth Congress in Caracas in 1955, after much discussion, there was a vote for a new commission that was composed of official representatives of each country. In addition, a group of specialists in Bromatology was formed. This group was charged with the project and after working for three years the Commission presented a new document that was unanimously approved. The Revised Latin American Food Code was published in Spanish in 1960. This document is highly relevant since it represents the regional efforts towards harmonization. In addition, its value is that in combination with European Legislation, it served as a source for the *Codex Alimentarius* (Acosta & Marrero, 1985; Nader & Vitale, 1998). Despite these very valuable efforts, with so much diversity in the region and with the problems Latin America has had to face, it is not surprising that food regulation has also been challenging.

The Codex Alimentarius Coordinating Committee for Latin America (CACCLA) was created in 1976 with the mandate to define the region's challenges and needs for food regulations as well as inspection systems, to strengthen the inspection infrastructure and to recommend the establishment of international standards for products of interest to the region; particularly products that in the Committee's judgment could have commercial potential in international markets; to establish regional regulations for products that are traded almost exclusively in regional markets; to identify important challenges unique to the region; and to promote the coordination of all food regulatory activities promoted by international organizations, local government and non-governmental organizations (Acosta & Marrero, 1985).

2.8.3 Challenges of Regional Food Regulation

A 1988 study of food regulation in Latin America sponsored by the Pan-American Health

Organization (2008) and the Food and Agriculture Organization noted the following deficiencies common in the region:

- Insufficient commitment on a national level to protect food.
- Lack of coordination between responsible agencies.
- Deficiencies in the laws and regulations.
- Problems in the infrastructure of agencies enforcing the laws and regulations.
- Lack of information.
- Insufficient participation in the preparation of international norms and a subsequent difficulty in accepting and applying them.
- Investigation.
- Inadequate sanitation education.

Since 1988 the region has made strides to overcome some of these deficiencies, but there is still a long way to go. According to Pineiro (2004), there are several key problems in the region. These can be grouped into three major areas: 1) inadequate food control systems (FCS); 2) lack of prevention and control policies and strategies coordinated into integrated national plans of action; and 3) insufficient awareness and funding. All these alone or in combination have important health and economic effects. From these issues, the first and foremost problem in the region is a weak FCS. Pineiro defines a FCS as a system of voluntary and mandatory activities carried out by food producers, processors, marketers and national or local authorities to provide consumer protection and ensure that all foods, domestically produced or imported, conform to national requirements of quality and safety. An adequate FCS has several major components that include Food Legislation, Quality Assurance, Food Inspection and Analysis (including infrastructure and human resources), Food Control Management and Information and Cooperation. From a weak FCS the other two major areas of concern inevitably follow and this, obviously complicates any regional efforts.

Harmonization is also complicated by the diversity of food control systems since these are at very different stages of development and are not always organized, developed, comprehensive or effective. In most Latin American countries, the systems are heavily challenged by problems of growing population and lack of resources. In many cases, there are sufficient food regulations but the enforcement capabilities are missing so the control is not always translated into better availability of a safe food supply. Even if there have been many efforts, in many cases, the regulatory framework is not harmonized with international standards.

2.8.4 Regional Intentions for Improvement: The Pan-American Commission for Food Safety (COPAIA 5)

Harmonizing regulatory requirements to assure safe and good quality foods and promote trade is of increasing interest to all countries in the Americas. In general, in the region, there are no structures and processes to achieve these objectives in a harmonized manner. Work towards regional structures and processes in the Americas has been strengthened and promoted via the activities of the Pan American Health Organization (PAHO), which is one of six regional organizations of the World Health Organization, and the Food and Agriculture Organization of the United Nations.

For example, PAHO plans and executes many training activities in the Americas. Recently, PAHO has supported establishment of a hemispheric Commission for Food Safety (COPAIA). Training and research links between the COPAIA and academic institutions in the Americas may be especially useful to promote collaborations and leverage resources (FAO, 2002).

Almost 20 years after the original PAHO study, it seems that, in reality, although the framework has improved and there are now commercial blocks trying to harmonize their regulatory systems, the challenges remain very much the same. During the Fifth Meeting of the Pan-American Commission for Food Safety (COPAIA-5) celebrated in Rio de Janeiro, on 10 June 2008, the members of the Commission that consisted of delegates from the ministries of health and agriculture and representatives of the consumers and producer sectors of the sub-regions of the Andean Area, the British Caribbean, Central America, the Latin Caribbean, the Southern Cone and North America made the following statement:

'Recognizing that access to safe food and nutritionally adequate diet is a right of each individual, and convinced that:
- Food safety is an essential public health function, which protects consumers against health risks posed by biological, chemical and physical hazards associated with food;
- If uncontrolled, the risks associated with food may become a major cause of diseases and premature death, as well as entailing losses owed to diminished productivity and serious economic damage to the agricultural, livestock and tourist sectors including agri-food industry, food processors, food distribution and retailers;
- Effective risk management and communication requires surveillance systems that can link disease outbreaks and illness to specific food supply chains;
- Appropriate implementation of food safety measures among and within countries can improve food safety on both a regional and a global scale;
- Integrated food safety systems can make possible the management of potential risks throughout the food chain from production to consumption;
- Measures aimed at food safety should be based on scientific evidence and on risk analysis principle, and avoid raising unnecessary barriers to food trade;
- The production of safe food is a primary responsibility of the food industry;
- Consumer education is an essential factor in promoting appropriate measures for ensuring food safety at home; and the sale of foods in general;
- Interactive communication with consumers is important for ensuring that society's values

and expectations are taken into consideration in decision-making.

Now therefore, the COPAIA 5 delegates recommend the:
- Designation of competent food safety authorities as independent entities under a comprehensive legal framework encompassing the entire food chain from production to consumption;
- Adoption of regulations and other measures based on risk analysis to ensure food safety along the entire food chain from production to consumption, consistently with the guidelines and norms of the Codex Alimentarius Commission and other relevant organizations that work on the definition of norms and standards;
- Ensuring the food legislation's effective enforcement through methodologies based on risk analysis, such as the Hazard Analysis and Critical Control Points (HACCP) whenever possible;
- Adoption of programs for the monitoring of food, total diet studies and disease surveillance systems, so as to obtain prompt, reliable information about the prevalence and emergence of food transmitted diseases and biological and chemical hazards in food sources;
- Establishment of procedures, such as traceability and alert systems throughout the food industry, to allow the prompt identification and investigation of incidents related to contaminated food, and report to the WHO incidents contemplated in the International Health Regulation (WHO, 2005) through the International Food Safety Authorities Network-INFOSAN and the IHR focal points;
- Promotion of communication and effective consultation with consumers, the food industry, and other relevant sectors with a view to the formulation, implementation and review of food safety policies and priorities, including education with a systematic focus along the entire food chain from production to consumption;
- Proceeding further with the strengthening of capabilities in respect of food safety by means of effective cooperation between developed and developing countries, as well as among

developing countries, so as to promote the access to food safety for all; and

- *Establishment of cooperation programs among international and regional technical cooperation organizations involved in food safety in areas of common interests and pursuant to the Member States mandates.'*

This declaration seems to cover the challenges faced by the region. However, the greatest challenge is in the actual implementation of the actions and promotion of true regional harmonization.

2.8.5 General Regulatory Structure

There are many general strategies to group different Latin American countries in blocks. These divisions are made based on geographical location, cultural background, language spoken, level of development, etc. The following statements are based on an informal division based in part on a geographical division as well as common typical regulatory structure. This division is by no means formal. In general, Caribbean countries have individual laws and regulations for consumer products. Some of the islands are associated with the European Union or the US and follow their regulatory structure while others have decided to adopt Codex standards as their own. Central American countries have individual laws and regulations and, again, in many cases have opted for the adoption of Codex standards. Most countries in South America have individual laws and regulations for products. However, five have entered a common market arrangement known as MERCOSUR. In addition, even when countries such as Bolivia, Chile, Colombia, Ecuador, the Falkland Islands, French Guiana, Guyana, Paraguay, Peru, Suriname have existing trade agreements, they maintain individual laws and standards for products. Chile, for example has very specific unprecedented laws for toluene limits in children's products.

2.8.6 Trade Agreements

There are several associations and trade agreements within the region. Each of these agreements varies widely in terms of their scope and the degree of harmonization.

2.8.7 The North American Free Trade Agreement

The North American Free Trade Agreement (NAFTA) between Mexico, the United States and Canada has had a profound effect in Mexican regulations. So, even when technically speaking this is not a Latin American Agreement, it is still of extreme importance to the region. NAFTA includes text on sanitary and phytosanitary measures, modeled after the Uruguay Round Agreement on sanitary and phytosanitary measures. Article 756 of NAFTA recommends that the three countries 'pursue equivalence of their respective sanitary and phytosanitary standards.' This article was drafted to assist in avoiding trade disputes among the three regarding the preparation and processing of food products that are traded. The idea is that the countries pledge to harmonize food production processes to 'the extent feasible' and that measures do not become disguised trade restrictions.

To avoid barriers to trade, the NAFTA agreement encourages countries to use relevant international standards, if existent, when developing their SPS measures. However, each country is permitted to adopt a standard more stringent than international standards to achieve an appropriate level of desired protection of human, animal or plant health if the standard is based upon scientific principles. The NAFTA signatories have agreed to work toward 'equivalent' SPS measures without reducing national levels of desired, appropriate protection. Equivalency recognizes that different methods may be used to reach the same level of protection. Each country agreed to accept the others' SPS measures as equivalent, provided the exporter shows that its SPS measures meet the importer's desired level of protection as long as it is based on risk assessment techniques (Looney, 1995).

Mexico's inclusion in the NAFTA agreement has permitted it to reach a level of parity with the US that other Latin American trade partners may not reach for several years. But before this could occur, officials in Mexico, the US and Canada, spent years comparing standards in food regulation and making changes that would permit this trade partnership to go forward on a common basis. No other countries in Latin America have attempted, much less achieved, what Mexico has done up to this moment in time to warrant inclusion in a regional trade agreement with the US.

2.8.8 Andean Community

The Andean Community (Peru, Ecuador, Colombia, and Bolivia) is a South American organization that was founded to encourage industrial, agricultural, social and trade cooperation. In 2005, this organization signed an agreement with MERCOSUR. Through this, the Andean Community gained four new associate members, Argentina, Brazil, Paraguay and Uruguay. Among the objectives of this association is to facilitate the participation in the regional integration process, with a view to the gradual formation of a Latin American common market. At the time of writing, the Technical Committees have been able to finalize a few common (harmonized) Andean standards, with several more in the project stage. The Andean Group Member Countries are also working on the harmonization of health and consumer safety requirements for processed foods, pharmaceutical products and cosmetics. Members are considering the creation of Ad Hoc Committees to consider standards-related aspects of security, health, consumer protection, the environment and national defense of Andean Group members. The Andean countries have adopted the

ISO/IEC guidelines related to standardization and conformity assessment procedures. With respect to the adoption and/or development of Andean standards, Decision 376 sets out an order of preference from which these should be drawn, proceeding from international standards, to regional standards, to national standards of Member Countries, followed by those of non-member countries and lastly, to those of private standards organizations (OAS, 1998).

2.8.9 Caribbean Community and Common Market

The Caribbean Community and Common Market (CARICOM) is an organization that aims at the eventual integration of its members and economies and the creation of a common market. Its members include: Antigua and Barbuda, Belize, Grenada, Montserrat, St. Vincent and the Grenadines, Turks and Caicos Islands, The Bahamas, British Virgin Islands, Guyana, St. Kitts and Nevis, Suriname, Barbados, Dominica, Jamaica, Saint Lucia, and Trinidad and Tobago. As signatories to the WTO, CARICOM countries are expected to harmonize national and regional food safety standards with Codex standards in the import and export of food products, and to adopt the WTO approach to food safety.

The Caribbean Food Safety Initiative (CFSI) was designed by the CARICOM Secretariat, the US Department of Agriculture (USDA), the Food and Drug Administration (FDA) and the Interamerican Development Bank (IDB). The purpose of this initiative was to develop a model approach to assist countries in meeting their WTO Sanitary and Phytosanitary obligations. The outcome of the first mission of specialists was used by the CARICOM Members to achieve greater harmony among national and regional food safety policies and infrastructures; promote technical cooperation among developing countries, and leverage financial support from international donor groups (FAO, 2002).

2.8.10 Central American Common Market

The Central American Common Market (CACM), is a well integrated group of five Central American economies (Guatemala, Honduras, El Salvador, Nicaragua and Costa Rica). The progress in this regional integration has been the consequence of forty years under the CACM, this is a far-reaching trade agreement that, among other things, ensures tariff-free exchange for 99.9% of the native products within the region. The CACM also provides common regulation in many areas from services to product registry to dispute resolution. The region has now been working for a few years in upgrading the common market into a Central American Customs Union. This means extending the integration process to a point in which internal customs procedures for trade within the isthmus become redundant and are eliminated, while customs procedures for trade with non-regional partners are homogenized and administrated jointly. However, at the time of writing, although Central American Countries have adopted Codex Standards as their own, in practice, each country still follows their own individual rules.

2.8.11 MERCOSUR

Argentina, Brazil, Paraguay, and Uruguay created MERCOSUR in March 1991 with the signing of the Treaty of Asuncion. MERCOSUR was originally created with the ambitious goal of creating a common market similar to the European Union. Venezuela became a full member in 2006. Similar to the EU, MERCOSUR has different legislative and technical organizations that create legislation and standards that are voted on and if passed are supposed to be adopted into national law. Although many hundreds of standards have been created and adopted by MERCOSUR, individual country adoption is still lagging. Food law harmonization has been conducted by the SGT-3 (Technical Regulations Work Subgroup) under the responsibilities of the Food Committee. Originally, the objective was to have all food law harmonized in time for the start of the single market. However, not only were few MERCOSUR resolutions adopted by 1 January 1995, but of those, very few were actually implemented by the member countries at that time. In general, the process as followed before the adoption of a MERCOSUR initiative by the member countries is (De Figuereido Toledo, 2000):

1. Elaboration of the proposals to be discussed jointly by governmental and private institutions.
2. Submission of the proposals to all member countries during an ordinary meeting of the SGT-3 Food Commission.
3. Discussion of the proposal by the specific ad hoc group.
4. Approval of the proposal by consensus.
5. Elaboration of a MERCOSUR project of technical regulation.
6. Internal discussion of the project within each member state by all interested parties
7. Approval of the project by the SGT-3
8. Submission of the harmonized project to the GMC for approval as a resolution.

In order to supplement the scientific knowledge required to set food standards, *Codex Alimentarius* standards, guidelines and recommendations as well as EU directives and the US FDA regulations are consulted. The process is well established. However, with the participation of four (now five) countries with different laws, habits, idiosyncrasies and interests, harmonization has not progressed as originally planned.

2.8.12 Conclusion

Although food law harmonization is highly desirable to set a level playing field for global food trade, its implementation, in reality, may be hampered by many challenges. In the Latin

American region, these challenges are further complicated by the diverse level of development of national food control systems. Each country must first face the challenges of their own internal system before participating in a more regional approach. This development could be facilitated by the adoption of already internationally recognized standards such as the *Codex Alimentarius*. However, it is important to consider that each country has its own idiosyncrasies and needs and thus, the level of adoption and the activities for implementation may still be very different. The process of regional harmonization will still take some time and will depend on technical assistance and the use of sound risk assessment activities that are already available through international organizations. In some cases, harmonization activities may already be well-defined on paper. However, the challenge still resides in making them a reality.

2.9 EUROPEAN UNION

Bernd M.J. van der Meulen
Wageningen University, The Netherlands

2.9.1 Introduction

From its beginning in 1958 the European Economic Community devoted much of its attention to agriculture. Initial motivators where the desire to gain self sufficiency and to support the rural areas and their agricultural population. Almost immediately legislation started to develop addressing food as a commodity in its own

right.[55] At first this legislation originated from the directorate general (DG) responsible for agriculture, but emphasis shifted to the DGs responsible for industry, enterprises and the internal market.

From the early 1960s until the eruption of the BSE crisis in the mid-1990s, European food law was principally directed at the creation of an internal market for food products in the EU.

This market-oriented phase can be divided into two stages. During the first, emphasis was on harmonization through vertical directives. This stage ended with the 'Cassis de Dijon' case law. During the second stage emphasis shifted to harmonization through horizontal directives.[56]

The BSE crisis and other food scares in the 1990s brought to light many serious shortcomings in the existing body of European food law. It became evident that fundamental reforms would be needed. In January 2000 the European Commission announced its vision for the future development of European food law in a "White Paper on Food Safety".[57]

The "White Paper on Food Safety" emphasized the Commission's intent to change its focus in the area of food law from the development of a common market to assuring high levels of food safety. In the years since its publication, a complete overhaul of European food legislation has taken place.

2.9.2 Creating an Internal Market for Food in Europe

When the six original members of what is today the European Union signed the Treaty of Rome in 1957, they created a community with an economic character. This was reflected

---

[55] It took some decades, however, before food law developed as an academic specialization. The European Council for Agricultural Law (CEDR: Comité Europeèn de Droit Rural: <www.cedr.org>) for example was established in 1957. The European Food Law Association (EFLA: <www.efla-aeda.org>) in 1973.

[56] The distinction between horizontal and vertical directives will be discussed hereafter.

[57] COM(1999) 719 def. Commission White Papers traditionally contain numerous proposals for Community action in specific areas, and are developed in order to launch consultation processes at the European level. If White Papers are favorably received by the Council, they often form the basis of later "Action Programs" to implement their recommendations.

not only in its original name—the European Economic Community—but also in the original objective to create a common market.

At the heart of the instruments to achieve this objective are the so-called four freedoms of the European Union: the free movement of labor, the free movement of services, the free movement of capital and the free movement of goods. The free movement of goods[58] has been vital to the development of food law.

During the first years of implementing the ambitious idea of trade without frontiers, Community legislation aimed primarily at facilitating the internal market through the harmonization of national standards. Agreement about the quality and identity of food products was considered necessary. To reach such agreement directives were issued on the composition of certain specific food products. This is called vertical (recipe, compositional or technical standards) legislation. Vertical legislation resembles the product standards of the *Codex Alimentarius*.

Early attempts to establish a common market for food products in Europe by prescribing harmonized product compositions faced two substantial obstacles. Firstly, at that time all legislation required unanimity in the Council, which gave each member state a virtual right of veto over new legislation. Secondly, there was the sheer scale of the task. Browse through a supermarket in any EU member state and consider the variety of products on the shelves. There are, as the Community institutions soon realized, simply too many food products to deal with. Creating compositional standards for each product would have been a mission impossible, and

the Commission wisely chose to seek alternatives. Nevertheless quite a few products remain subject to European rules on compositional standards.[59] These compositional standards form the legacy of the first phase of EU food law. They are being updated or replaced when necessary but no new products are being added.

2.9.3 Advancement Through Case Law

It was the Court of Justice of the European Communities that showed the way out of the deadlock through new, broad, interpretations of the key provision on the free movement of goods in the common market: Article 28 of the EC Treaty.[60] This Article prohibits quantitative restrictions on imports and all measures having equivalent effect.[61]

This article should be read in connection with Article 30 of the EC Treaty which lists possible exceptions to the free movement of goods, such as the protection of health and life of humans, animals or plants.

The landmark decision in this context was Cassis de Dijon.[62] A German chain of supermarkets sought to import Cassis de Dijon, a fruit liqueur, from France. The German authorities, however, refused to authorize the import because the alcohol content was lower than allowed by German national law, which stipulated that such liqueurs should contain at least 25% alcohol. Cassis de Dijon contained just 20% alcohol.

The German authorities acknowledged that this was a restriction on trade, but sought to justify it on the basis that beverages with too little alcohol pose several risks. The German

---

[58] Now Article 3 (1)(c) and Article 23–31 EC Treaty.

[59] E.g. sugar, honey, fruit juices, milk, spreadable fats, jams, jellies, marmalade, chestnut puree, coffee, chocolate, natural mineral waters, minced meat, eggs, fish. Wine legislation is a body of law in itself. For legislation on fresh fruit and vegetables. Compositional standards still figure prominently in the *Codex Alimentarius*.

[60] At that time numbered Article 30.

[61] On the relevance of Article 25 EC Treaty banning customs duties and charges having equivalent effect, see Broberg (2008), sections 2.3 and 2.4.

[62] EC Court of Justice 20 February 1979, Case 120/78 (Cassis de Dijon), ECR 1979, page 649.

authorities argued that alcoholic beverages with low alcohol content could induce people to develop tolerances for alcohol more quickly than beverages with higher alcohol content, and that consumers trusting the (German) law might feel cheated if they purchased such products with the expectation of higher alcohol content. Finally, Germany submitted that in the absence of such a law, beverages with low alcohol content would benefit from an unfair competitive advantage because taxes on alcohol are high, and beverages with lower alcoholic content would be saleable at significantly lower prices than products produced in Germany according to German law.

The Court held that the *type* of arguments presented by the German authorities would be relevant, even where they did not come under the specific exceptions contained in the EC Treaty, provided that those arguments met an urgent need. This is known as the rule of reason.

The Court found that Germany's public health argument did not meet this standard of urgency. The Court specifically cited the availability of a wide range of alcoholic beverages on the German market with alcohol content of less than 25%. As to the risk of consumers feeling cheated by lower than expected alcohol content, the Court suggested that such a risk could be eliminated with less effect on the common market by displaying the alcohol content on the beverages label.

For cases such as this one, in which there are no specific justifications for restrictions on the trade between Member States, the Court introduced a general rule: products that have been lawfully produced and marketed in one of the member states, may not be kept out of other member states on the grounds that they do not comply with the national rules. This is called the *principle of mutual recognition*.

With its ruling the Court in Luxemburg laid the legal foundation for a well-functioning common market. Food products that comply with the statutory requirements of the member state where they are brought on the market must, in principle,[63] be admitted to the markets of all other member states.

Several commentators expressed concern that the Cassis de Dijon decision would lead to product standards based on the lowest common denominator. It is clear that manufacturers established in member states with the most lenient safety or technical requirements or legal procedures do gain a competitive advantage.

The limitations and drawbacks of the principle of mutual recognition highlighted the need for further harmonization of food requirements at the European level. For member states with more stringent national standards, European-level legislation became the best hope for raising neighbors' standards. The Cassis de Dijon ruling marked a significant change in the perception of the benefits of harmonization. Before Cassis, harmonization was seen merely as a condition for the functioning of the internal market. Afterwards, emphasis shifted to the need to alleviate the consequences of the internal market. In legal terms, too, the wave of harmonization that followed Cassis differed from earlier efforts. Emphasis shifted from product-specific legislation, to horizontal legislation, meaning general rules addressing common aspects for a broad range of foodstuffs.

Mutual recognition remains the rule up to this day. Food products that have legally come to the market in any member state, may in principle be sold without restrictions across the whole territory of the European Union.

2.9.4 Breakdown

The heyday of market-oriented food law based on mutual recognition ended in tears. The food and agricultural sectors in the European Union emerged deeply traumatized from the

---

[63] Exceptions can be based only on Article 30 of the EC Treaty or the rule of reason.

1990s. A series of crises resulted in a breakdown of consumer confidence in public authorities, industry and science. The current third phase of EU food law can only be truly fathomed if the trauma to which it responds is understood.

Although the bovine spongiform encephalopathy (BSE) crisis was not the first and, in terms of death toll, not the worst[64] food safety crisis in the EU it caused an earthquake in the legal and regulatory landscape of Europe. Subsequent food safety scares,[65] outbreaks of animal diseases[66] and scandals over fraudulent practices, added to a sense of urgency to take protective measures. These fraudulent practices included the discharge of waste in animal feed[67] and the underworld involvement in the supply and employment of growth hormones[68] mounting to the murder of the veterinarian who brought the use of these illegal substances to the attention of the authorities and the public (Butler, 2002).

Public awareness of the BSE-epidemic, and the time it had taken British and European authorities to address it, presented a major challenge to European cooperation in the area of food safety. When the extent of the crisis became public, the European Union issued a blanket ban on British beef exports. In response, Britain adopted a policy of non-cooperation with the European institutions, and sought to deny the extent and seriousness of the BSE problem.[69]

The European Parliament played a crucial role in defusing this crisis. A temporary Enquiry Committee was instituted to investigate the actions of the national and European agencies involved in the crisis.[70] The Enquiry Committee presented its report in early 1997 (Ortega Medina Report, 1997). The report strongly criticized the British government as well as the European Commission. The Commission was accused of wrongly putting industry interests ahead of public health and consumer safety, science had been biased and transparency had been lacking.

Paradoxically, this reproachful report followed by a motion of censure proposed to the

[64] *See* Abaitua Borda *et al.* (1998); Gelpí *et al.* (2002) (finding that the toxic oil syndrome (TOS) epidemic that occurred in Spain in the spring of 1981 caused approximately 20,000 cases of a new illness. Researchers identified 1,663 deaths between 1 May 1981 and 31 December 1994 among 19,754 TOS cohort members. Mortality was highest during 1981). The poisoning was caused by fraud consisting of mixing vehicle oil with consumption oil.

[65] One example is the Belgian dioxin crises. It was caused by industry oil that had found its way into animal feed and subsequently into the food chain (Whitney, 1999). Another example is the introduction of medroxyprogesterone acetate (MPA) into pig feed in 2002 (Graff, 2002). Sugar discharges from the production of MPA, a hormone used in contraceptive and hormone replacement pills, were used in pigs feed and by that route MPA entered the food chain. In 2004 a dioxin crisis broke out in the Netherlands.

[66] Like Food and Mouth Disease, SARS and Avian Influenza.

[67] Probably the cause of the first dioxin crisis (Whitney, 1999).

[68] Community and national legislatures in the EU have been battling the use of artificial hormones—DES (diethylstilbestrol) in particular—for years. When it turned out to be impossible to separate their use from body-proper hormones and to get them under control, finally all hormones were banned. The legislation on the use and application of hormones started with Directive 81/602 (prohibiting certain matters with hormonal effects and of stuffs with thyrostatic effects). Directive 81/602 has been supplemented by Directive 85/358/EEC and replaced by Directive 88/146/EEC (prohibition of applications of certain stuffs with hormonal effect in the cattle breeding sector). A next one, Directive 88/299 is aiming at the trade in animals and meat treated with stuffs with hormonal effect referred to in Directive 88/146.

[69] A symbolic event was shown on TV where the responsible Secretary of State, John Gummer is shown feeding his little daughter a hamburger, to convince the public that nothing was wrong with British beef (16 May 1990, BBC). Text, picture and video available at BBC (16 May 1990).

[70] OJ 1996 C 261/132.

European Parliament provided the Commission with the impetus it had hitherto lacked; indeed with a window of opportunity, to take the initiative for restructuring European food law in a way that considerably strengthened its own powers. The Commission undertook far-reaching commitments to implement the Committee's recommendations.

Progress was made along institutional lines as well as policy lines. The Directorate General (DG) XXIV "Consumer Policy" created two years earlier, was reinforced and renamed "Consumer and Health Protection Policy" and included the scientific advisory committees from the DGs for Industry and Agriculture.[71] A Scientific Steering Committee was created to bring wider scientific experience and overview to consumer health questions. The internal market "product warning system" was also transferred from DGIII (Agriculture) to DGXXIV. As of 1997, the centre of gravity in food legislation moved from DG Agriculture to DGXXIV, now called "SANCO."

As early as May 1997, the Commission[72] published a Green Paper on the general principles of food law in the EU.[73] It set out the structure of a legal system capable of getting a firm grip on food production. Consumer protection was made the main priority. The Commission committed to strengthening its food safety control function. This led directly to the establishment of the Food and Veterinary Office (FVO) in Dublin in 1997.[74] The FVO was charged with carrying out the Commission's control responsibilities in the food safety sector, to include controlling animal health and welfare and auditing third countries that wish to export to the EU. Furthermore, the Commission announced the establishment of an independent food safety authority.[75]

The Commission kept the pressure on beyond 1997, eventually gaining the support of the European Court of Justice for the measures that had been taken against Great Britain at the climax of the crisis.[76]

On 12 January 2000 the Commission published its famous White Paper on Food Safety.[77]

2.9.5 The White Paper: A New Vision on Food Law

The Commission's vision on the future shape of EU food law, its blueprint so to speak, was laid down in the White Paper on Food Safety. Before the BSE crisis, European food safety law was subordinated to the development of the internal market. The shortcomings in the handling of the crisis clearly revealed a need for a new, integrated approach to food safety.

The Commission aimed to restore and maintain consumer confidence.

The White Paper focused on a review of food legislation in order to make it more coherent, comprehensive and up-to-date, and to strengthen enforcement.

---

[71]Knudsen & Matikainen-Kallström (1999); European Parliament Fact Sheets 4.10.1. Consumer Policy: principles and instruments, chapter 3 Reform in the wake of the BSE crisis, Green Paper on general principles of food law.

[72]Interestingly, DG Industry was the instigator.

[73]*Commission Green Paper on the General Principles of Food Law in the European Union*, COM(1997) 176.

[74]*See generally* DG Sanco (2002 and 2007).

[75]Communication of the European Commission, Consumer Health and Food Safety COM(97) 183 fin. of 30 April 1997. See also: James, Kemper, & Pascal (1999).

[76]*See* Case C-157/96, The Queen v. Ministry of Agric., Fisheries and Food, 1998 ECR I-02211; Case C-180/96, United Kingdom of Great Britain and Northern Ireland v. Commission, 1996 ECR I-03903; Case C-209/96 UK vs. Commission.

[77]COM(1999) 719 final. Unlike a Green Paper that is intended mostly as a basis for public discussion, a White Paper contains concrete policy intentions.

Furthermore, the Commission backed the establishment of a new European Food Safety[78] Authority, to serve as the scientific point of reference for the whole Union, and thereby contribute to a high level of consumer health protection.

2.9.6 Implementing the Vision

The Annex to the aforementioned White Paper is the Action Plan on Food Safety, a list of 84 legislative steps that the Commission deemed necessary to create a regulatory framework capable of ensuring a high level of protection of consumers and public health.

The turn of the millennium saw the beginning of the planned overhaul of European food law. The first new regulation took effect in 2002 and at the time of writing most of the 84 steps have been taken.[79] The new regulatory framework is based on regulations rather than directives.

Only two years after the White Paper was published, the cornerstone of new European food law was laid: 'Regulation 178/2002 of the European Parliament and of the Council of 28 January 2002 laying down the general principles and requirements of food law, establishing the European Food Safety Authority and laying down procedures in matters of food safety'.[80] This regulation is often referred to in English as the 'General Food Law' ('GFL'). The Germans speak of it as a 'Basisverordnung'—perhaps a more precise phrase given that the regulation is in fact the basis upon which European and national food laws are now being reconstructed.[81] The main objective of the General Food Law is to secure a high level of protection of public health and consumer interests with regard to food products. It does so by stating general principles, establishing the European Food Safety Authority and giving procedures to deal with emergencies.

After the General Food Law, whole packages of new legislation followed (Table 2.7).

It is next to impossible to predict how long we will remain in the third phase of EU food law and what will come afterwards.

The window of opportunity for large-scale legislative projects on food that opened after the animal health and food safety scares of the 1990s seems to be closing. Some finalising proposals are underway. If no major crisis sparks new

TABLE 2.7   Highlights in the overhaul of EU food law

2002	Regulation 178/2002 (GFL)
2003	Regulations 1829/2003 and 1830/2003 GMO package
2004/2005	Regulations 852-854/2004 Hygiene package
	Regulation 882/2004 Official controls
	Regulation 1935/2004 Food contact materials
2006/2007	Regulation 1924/2006 nutrition & health claims
2007	White Paper A Strategy for Europe on Nutrition, Overweight and Obesity related health issues
Ongoing	Obesity policy
	Modernization pesticides legislation
	Modernization legislation on additives, flavorings, enzymes and novel foods
	Modernization of labeling legislation

---

[78]In the White Paper the Commission speaks of a European Food Authority. The word 'safety' was inserted later.

[79]See Knipschild (2003), Nöhle (2005), and Berends & Carreno (2005).

[80]OJ 1.2.2002 L 31/1.

[81]New European food law displays several characteristics in which it is different from its predecessor: more emphasis on horizontal regulations (than on vertical legislation), more emphasis on regulations that formulate the goals that have to be achieved, so-called objective regulations, than on means regulations; increased use of regulations (rather than directives) and thus increasing centralization.

action, it seems unlikely that more legislation of fundamental nature will be undertaken in the near future. The EU legislator will probably feel prompted to make an attempt at simplification and reduction of burdens for the food sector.

The most pressing issue on the agenda for the years to come is probably overweight and obesity. So far the EU legislator has not found suitable instruments to deal with this problem. Measures are currently limited to providing consumers with information directly and on food product labels.

2.9.7 Analysis

The quantity of European legislation regarding food is overwhelming. The food sector has become the third most regulated sector in the EU (after automobiles and chemicals). At closer look, however, the structure turns out to be rather straightforward. There are public powers of law enforcement[82] and incident management and legislation addressing food businesses.

Legislation addressing food businesses usually can be grouped in one of three categories: legislation on the product, legislation on the process and legislation on presentation.

The whole structure is embedded in general principles.

2.9.7.1 *Principles of EU Food Law*

The General Food Law provides some general concepts, obligations, requirements and principles of food law. Food law should aim at the protection of human life and health and (other) consumers' interests (Article 5). In protecting life and health it should be science based, that is to say based on risk analysis (Article 6). When scientific risk assessment is inconclusive the precautionary principle justifies temporary measures to be taken to protect from possible risks (Article 7). The authority responsible for risk assessment is the European Food Safety Authority—EFSA (Article 22).

Where international standards—like the *Codex Alimentarius* exist—or their completion is imminent, they shall in general be taken into consideration in the development or adaptation of food law (Article 5(3) GFL). The definition of food for example is tailored to the Codex and also the principle of HACCP as elaborated in the Codex is incorporated in EU food law (see hereafter). The legion of product standards that is available in the Codex has less influence on EU legislation as product specific legislation has been largely abandoned in the EU (see above).

Food businesses are responsible for ensuring compliance. Member states are responsible for enforcement (Article 17).

2.9.7.2 *Product*

Legislation addressing the product can be further subdivided in three categories: 1) compositional standards, 2) market access requirements, 3) restrictions.

Above we have encountered (vertical) legislation about the composition or quality of products. This type loses in relevance.

The general rule is that producers are free in their choice of ingredients. Increasingly exceptions to this rule are made in the sense that approval is required of certain products. Approved products are included in so-called positive lists (lists of products that may be used).

The most important categories for which approval is required are food additives,[83] genetically modified foods[84] and novel foods.[85] Food additives are synthetic substances that are not foods by themselves but are added to foods for

---

[82]Regulation 882/2004.

[83] *See* Additives Framework Directive 89/107; Sweeteners Directive 94/35; Colours Directive 94/36 and Miscellaneous Additives Directive 95/2. A proposal for a modernization of this legislation is currently in procedure.

[84] Regulations 1829/2003 and 1830/2003.

[85] Regulation 258/97. A proposal for a modernization of this legislation is currently in procedure.

technological reasons like preservatives, gelling agents and colors. Genetically modified foods are foods consisting of, made from or made with organisms to which gene technology has been applied. Novel foods are all (other) foods that have not been consumed to a significant degree in the EU prior to 1997.

The most important criterion for approval is scientific risk assessment.

Finally, there is legislation setting limits to the presence of undesirable substances (contaminants) or organisms in food.[86] The limits are set on the basis of scientific risk assessment. To products that have not been approved or for which no lowest safety level can be established, a zero tolerance may apply.

2.9.7.3 Process

It has been recognized that in order to ensure food safety processes must be under control in production as well as in trade. Practices aimed at the prevention of food safety risks are known as 'hygiene'. At the heart of EU legislation on food hygiene is the so-called HACCP-system: Hazard Analysis and Critical Control Points.[87] This system requires food businesses to make such an analysis of their processes that they know where hazards may occur, how to recognize them and how to deal with them in order to maintain food safety. Application of the system must be well documented.

In trade a requirement of traceability applies (Article 18 GFL). Food businesses must record where their inputs come from and where their products go. If a food safety incident occurs this information must enable the authorities to swiftly identify the origin of the problem and

its dispersal in order to eliminate the cause and take care of the consequences.

Finally, businesses that have reason to believe that a food they have brought to the market may not be in conformity with food safety requirements, are under obligation to withdraw it from the food chain and recall it from consumers (Article 19 GFL).

2.9.7.4 Presentation

A large part of food legislation addresses the information food businesses provide to consumers regarding their product through advertising and—mainly—labeling. The most important codification of these rules is to be found in Directive 2000/13 of the European Parliament and of the Council of 20 March 2000 on the approximation of the laws of the Member States relating to the labeling, presentation and advertising of foodstuffs: the so-called 'Labeling directive'.[88] Labeling means 'any words, particulars, trade marks, brand name, pictorial matter or symbol relating to a foodstuff and placed on any packaging, document, notice, label, ring or collar accompanying or referring to such foodstuff'. Labeling may not be misleading.

All pre-packaged food products must be labeled in a language that is easily understood. Usually this means in the national language of the member state. Other information is mandatory, restricted or forbidden.

There are about twelve required (mandatory) pieces of information, the most important of which are: the name under which the product is sold; the list of ingredients; the quantity of certain ingredients or categories of ingredients; the presence of allergens; in the case of pre-packaged

---

[86] See Framework regulation 315/93; Regulation 1881/2006 on mycotoxins and chemicals; Regulation 2073/2005 on microbiological criteria; Regulation 396/2005 on pesticide residues; Regulation 2377/90 on veterinary drugs and Directive 96/22 on hormones.

[87] See Regulation 852/2004.

[88] OJ 6.5.2000 L 109/29. A proposal for a modernization of this legislation is currently in procedure.

foodstuffs, the net quantity; the date of minimum durability or, in the case of foodstuffs which, from the microbiological point of view, are highly perishable, the 'use by' date; the name or business name and address of the manufacturer or packager, or of a seller established within the Community.

Specific labeling requirements demand that the presence of additives, novel ingredients and GMOs be mentioned on the label.

In 2006 a new Regulation on nutrition and health claims was published.[89] Nutrition claims must conform to the annex to this regulation. The annex states among other things that the expression 'light' may be only used in case of a reduction of at least 30% of certain nutrients or energy. Health claims e.g. claims about the effects of a certain food on health must be approved and science based. Foods bearing health claims are sometimes called 'functional foods'.

At present nutrition labeling, e.g. mentioning the nutrients and energy present in the food product, is voluntary except when a claim is made.[90] Legislation is in preparation to make it mandatory.

2.9.8 Science in EU Food Law

The general principle that food law in the EU is science based mainly means that authorities need scientific advice—for which the European Food Safety Authority is responsible at the community level—when they take decisions on requests for approval of certain foods or health claims and when they set maximum levels for contaminants.

2.10 NEAR EAST

P. Vincent Hegarty
Institute for Food Laws and Regulations, Michigan State University, East Lansing, MI, USA

[89]Regulation 1924/2006.
[90]Directive 90/496.

2.10.1 Geography

When dealing with food safety issues in this part of the world care must be taken to use the correct geo-political terminology. "Near East" is the term used by *Codex Alimentarius*. The Near East countries listed by Codex are the ones discussed in this section. They are: Algeria, Bahrain, Egypt, Iran (Islamic Republic of), Iraq, Jordan, Kuwait, Lebanon, Libyan Arab Jamahiriya, Oman, Qatar, Saudi Arabia, Sudan, Syrian Arab Republic, Tunisia, United Arab Emirates and Yemen. It is important to draw a distinction between this list and the equivalent regional grouping of countries used by the World Health Organization and by various national governments. In a food safety context the countries in the "Near East" listed above do not always equate with the countries in the various geo-political definitions of the term "Middle East."

2.10.2 History

The history of food safety in the Near East is short. One reason is some of the countries became independent in recent times. So, it has taken time to develop a national food safety system. A second reason is countries in the Near East are net importers of food. There was a tendency until recently to sometimes rely on the safety measures taken by the authorities in the food exporting country to ensure that the food entering the region was safe. This is no longer the situation. National emphasis is now placed on the safety of both imported *and* exported food, resulting in a streamlining of food safety programs. Furthermore, food safety was assessed by multiple agencies in most countries. This resulted frequently in unnecessary duplication and breakdowns in communication between agencies. Adding to the problem was the application of different safety criteria to a food depending on whether it was produced locally or was imported; higher food safety requirements usually applied to the imported food. A significant impetus to food safety in the region is the rapid growth of tourism. This has produced increased efforts to ensure a safe food supply nationally and regionally.

Countries in the Near East who have made significant progress recently in modernizing and streamlining their food safety programs include Jordan, Saudi Arabia, United Arab Emirates, Egypt and Lebanon.

2.10.3 Jordan

Jordan established the Jordan Food and Drug Administration (JFDA) on 16 April 2003. It was established under the JFDA Act, 2003. The basic legislation regulating food control in Jordan is Food Law no. 79/2001. This law makes JFDA the responsible official agency entrusted to regulate and supervise food control activities in Jordan. Considerable resources were committed recently to ensuring that food laws were consistent with WTO rules and international standards. Laboratory facilities were improved significantly.

2.10.4 Saudi Arabia

Saudi Arabia established the Saudi Food and Drug Authority (SFDA) on 10 March 2003. This consolidated into one government authority all agencies previously involved with food and drug safety. The Saudi FDA was given a 5-year period to develop its structure, hire staff and establish laboratories. It was then required to submit a food safety law to ensure that all imported and indigenous food conforms to national and to internationally recognized standards.

2.10.5 United Arab Emirates

United Arab Emirates (UAE) has the Emirates Authority for Standardization and Metrology to regulate standards. Municipalities have the responsibility for ensuring food safety within each of the seven emirates in the UAE. The largest of these are in Dubai (Food Control Department under Public Health Services) and Abu Dhabi (Abu Dhabi Food Control Authority, ADFCA). Each emirate has its own food inspection system and food safety laboratories. Dubai has an annual food safety conference which is a forum for regional and international issues in food safety.

2.10.6 Egypt

Egypt has food laws dating back to the 1940s. The laws, inspection service and food safety laboratories have now been considered as inadequate by both the public and private sectors.

Much activity is taking place to improve the entire system by creating a single, unified food safety authority in Egypt. At the time of writing, a draft food safety law is being prepared for presentation to the Egyptian parliament.

2.10.7 Lebanon

Lebanon has made access to safe and healthy food a priority. It is modernizing its food safety legislation and strengthening public administration concerned with quality control and safety along the entire food chain. The Minister of Economy and Trade mandated the Lebanese Food Safety Panel to draft the new Lebanese Food Law by May 2003 to comply with international requirements. This is a work in progress still.

2.10.8 Other Countries

Algeria, Bahrain, Iran (Islamic Republic of), Iraq, Kuwait, Libyan Arab Jamahiriya, Oman, Qatar, Sudan, Syrian Arab Republic, Tunisia and Yemen are engaged also, to varying degrees, in modernization and streamlining their national food safety programs. In this group the Islamic Republic of Iran has the longest history in food safety. Its Ministries of Agriculture, Health, Hygiene and Medical Education and the Iran Veterinary Organization (IVO) are engaged in food safety work. The Institute of Standards and Industrial Research of Iran was established in 1960.

2.10.9 Harmonization

There are encouraging signs of increased harmonization of food safety regulations between countries in the Near East. There is also a growing awareness of the importance of harmonization with internationally accepted food safety regulations. Examples of harmonization at the national level include the 2005 Memorandum of Understanding (MOU) signed between Dubai and Abu Dhabi on food control and veterinary services. This was done to better coordinate food safety and public health issues between the two authorities within the UAE.

The countries of the Gulf Cooperation Council (GCC) have a coordinated system of food control which they are improving further. The GCC countries are: Bahrain, Kuwait, Oman, Qatar, Saudi Arabia and the United Arab Emirates.

An example of interest in harmonization at the regional level was the discussion paper on mutual recognition agreements between Near East countries on import/export accreditation. This was presented in 2005 by Jordan at the 3rd Session, Joint FAO/WHO Food Standards Program, FAO/WHO Coordinating Committee for the Near East. It describes a conceptual framework of a harmonized and cooperative regional approach towards the application of mutual recognition agreement(s) on a bilateral and/or multilateral basis between countries in the region. The paper highlighted the importance of accreditation of imports/exports and for the need to establish mechanisms for food import and export control based on equivalency systems.

Some recent examples of regional harmonization efforts are the drafting of a Code of Practice for Street Vended Foods, a regional Code of Practice for the Packaging and Transport of Fresh Fish, nutritional labeling in the region, and regional standards for harissa, doogh, pomegranate and for halawa with tehena. All of these were to be discussed at the January 2009 meeting of the FAO/WHO Coordinating Committee for the Near East.

In summary, there are efforts by all countries in the Near East region to improve and streamline their food safety systems. This is being done with attention to coordination with international standards and procedures.

2.11 NORTHEAST ASIA

Mun-Gi Sohn
Korea Food and Drug Administration, Seoul, Republic of Korea

2.11.1 Introduction

Public concern regarding the safety of food is increasing due to the frequent food safety incidents such as BSE, dioxin, and melamine contamination of food that occurred over the past few years. In order to protect the health of the public, significant advances in food regulations and regulatory systems have been made to modify and upgrade the existing regulations and control systems in the Northeast Asia.

The food regulations in the region used to focus on the traditional food safety control measures such as necessary legal powers, relevant government bodies, regulatory enforcement actions, criminal investigations, import controls, business licenses, inspection and certification systems, quality and safety standards of foods, prohibition of unapproved/illegal uses of drugs and chemicals, and penalties/punishments for adulterated/misbranded foods or fraudulent health claims.

In recent years, however, more emphasis has been made on harmonized approaches with the international standards, science-based risk analysis, enhanced risk communication, better coordination among different authorities, and emergency response systems. The recently adopted "Food Safety Basic Law" in Japan and Korea provides a legal basis for consolidated efforts for coordinated regulatory framework and policy implementation among different agencies involved.

2.11.2 Development

The food regulations in most countries used to focus mainly on the traditional food safety control measures such as the designation of authorities with necessary legal powers for regulatory actions and criminal investigations, enforcement schemes, import controls, inspection and certification systems, business licenses, quality and safety standards of foods, prohibition of unapproved/illegal uses of drugs and chemicals, penalties and punishments for adulterated/misbranded foods or fraudulent health claims. Due to the diversity and complex nature of numerous food products ranging from agricultural, fisheries, meat and poultry products to processed foods, various ministries and local authorities were involved in the food control schemes by sharing the responsibilities of the safety and quality of the foods at different stages of the food supply chain; production, manufacturing, distribution, and sales of foods.

For the past few decades, China, Japan, and Korea had a Food Hygiene Law that played an important role in their national food safety control systems in covering the basic rules of hygienic practices and requirements for safe food to protect the public health. Each country has its own texts of the Food Hygiene Law, which was first enacted in Japan in 1947, followed by the Republic of Korea (South Korea) in 1962, and by the People's Republic of China in 1965.

Since the establishment of the World Trade Organization (WTO) in 1995, increasing volumes of international food trade have emerged. Because of growing concerns over food safety due to continuous occurrences of food safety incidents such as BSE, dioxin, and melamine contamination, there is an urgent need for significant changes in updating and upgrading food regulations and food safety control systems.

In an attempt to restore public confidence and consumer assurance, new legislation by the name of Food Safety Basic Law was introduced covering new control measures for prompt responses in emergency situations, securing science based risk analysis approach, better coordination and cooperation among different ministries to minimize any loopholes in the control system by establishing the Food Safety Commission or Food Safety Council.

Japan enacted the Food Safety Basic Law in 2003, and South Korea enacted its Food Safety Basic Law in 2008. China enacted its Food Safety Law on 28 February 2009 with the concept of organizing the Food Safety Council under the State Council to control and coordinate the works done by different ministries/authorities more efficiently. The Food Safety Council in Korea oversees the overall activities of the relevant authorities for policy directions and coordination, while the Food Safety Commission in Japan performs the risk assessment activities independently from other government agencies responsible for risk management decisions. At the time of writing, it has not yet been determined what role the Food Safety Council to be established in China will play; however, the Food Safety Law of China came into effect on 1 June 2009 and it replaces the Food Hygiene Law entirely.

The Food Safety Basic Law generally reflects the current interests and demands of the consumers in each country for better public assurance and emphasizes the importance of transparency, public information, traceability, nationwide food safety education, prompt response and preparedness for emergency situations. In addition, harmonization with the international standards based on sound scientific evidence, responsibilities of governments and business operators, and role of consumers are emphasized to ensure the safety of foods.

2.11.3 Food Regulations in Japan

Japanese food regulations and administration are currently based on the Food Safety Basic Law enacted in May 2003, the Food Sanitation Law, the Abattoir Law, the Poultry Slaughtering Business Control and Poultry Inspection Law, and other related laws.[91] The Food Safety Basic Law was introduced to solve the various challenges faced by the relevant authorities, triggered by the occurrence of BSE (Bovine Spongiform Encephalopathy, so called Mad Cow's Disease) in 2001. An internationally harmonized risk analysis approach was broadly applied to the food safety policy of Japan by establishing the Food Safety Commission under the Cabinet Office mainly responsible for science based risk assessment, independent from the risk management roles carried out by the Ministry of Health, Labour and Welfare (MHLW) and the Ministry of Agriculture (MOA).

The Food Safety Commission is composed of seven Members, 16 Expert Committees, and the Secretariat. The Committees such as 'Planning Expert Committee', 'Risk Communication Committee', and the 'Emergency Response Committee' with 11 other Expert Committees review technical information for the risk assessment of potential hazards in foods.

The Food Sanitation Law (11 Chapters, 79 Articles) enacted in 1947, has been revised more than 30 times. It covers various responsibilities of the hygiene requirements of the manufacture and sale of food, business licenses, and standards/specifications for food, food additives, and food packages. The Abattoir Law

and the Poultry Slaughtering Business Control and Poultry Inspection Law cover the hygiene requirements for livestock meat products for processing and sales. The Ministry of Health, Labor and Welfare is mainly responsible for the safe processing and sales of the food, while the Ministry of Agriculture is responsible for the safe production of agriculture, fisheries, and meat and poultry products under the Agricultural Products Quality Control Law and other related regulations such as the Plant Protection Law and the Quarantine Law.

2.11.4 Food Regulations in Korea

Food regulations and administration in Korea are currently based on the Food Safety Basic Law enacted in June 2008, the Food Sanitation Law, the Meat and Poultry Products Processing Law, the Health Functional Food Law, the Agricultural Products Quality Control Law, along with other related quarantine regulations.

The 2008 Food Safety Basic Law emphasized enhanced coordination and cooperation of different authorities dealing with various food safety issues more efficiently and effectively. The Food Safety Council was established under the Prime Minister's Office to oversee and coordinate the overall aspects of food safety activities and issues with an emphasis on risk management, risk assessment, and risk communication approaches for enhanced cooperation activities among relevant authorities. The emergency response system, promotion of public information, traceability, expert committees, and harmonization efforts with the international standards and norms are also emphasized.

The Food Sanitation Law (13 Chapters, 102 Articles) revised in full in 2009 covers the basic responsibilities and the hygiene requirements of the manufacture, process, distribution and sale of food, standards/specifications for food,

[91]Japanese Laws and Regulations, Cabinet Secretariat, Japan

food additives, and food packaging materials, The Ministry of Health, Welfare and Family Affairs (MOHWF) and Korea Food and Drug Administration (KFDA) are responsible for policy directions and enforcement of the overall food safety control systems.

The most recent revision of the Food Sanitation Law reinforced government's responsibility for emergency preparedness and prompt response, foodborne disease surveillance, inspection, certification of official laboratories, immediate recalls and prohibition of sale of contaminated food, extensive monitoring for risk assessment, establishment of the food safety information center, enhanced consumer participation to promote consumer assurance on various food safety issues.

The Meat and Poultry Product Processing and Handling Law enacted in 1962 highlighted the hygiene requirements and conditions for the processing and handling of meat and poultry products for distribution and sale and currently managed by the Ministry of Agriculture.

2.11.5 Food Regulations in China

The People's Republic of China Food Safety Law[92] was recently enacted on 28 February 2009, fully revising and replacing the existing Food Hygiene Act of 1995, and came into effect on 1 June 2009. Food hygiene regulations implemented and authorized by the State Council in 1965 have been revised and updated in various forms of regulations such as the Food Hygiene Act, the Product Quality Act, Animal Quarantine Act, and other related regulations.

The Food Safety Law enacted in 2009 (10 Chapters, 104 Articles) includes the fundamental hygiene requirements for the manufacture, processing, distribution and sale of food, mandatory safety assessment requirements for food additives and novel foods, legal requirements for standards, specifications for food, food additives, reporting of foodborne disease incidents, record keeping, risk assessment, and import and export inspection and certification systems, and the role and responsibilities of relevant authorities.

The Food Safety Law also authorizes the State Council to establish a Food Safety Council in order to enhance efficient coordination and cooperation among relevant authorities. The Ministry of Health is responsible for overall coordination and comprehensive management[93], investigation of major food related incidents, while the Ministry of Agriculture focuses on the production sector along with other relevant authorities. The General Administration of Quality Supervision, Inspection and Quarantine (AQSIQ) is responsible for import, export and quarantine of the products and inspection of the food manufactures. The State Food and Drug Administration (SFDA) supervises hygiene requirements of restaurants, and drugs. State Administration for Industry and Commerce (SAIC) regulates market activities and trade for consumer products including food products on sale.

The next section of this chapter discusses the situation in China more in detail.

2.11.6 Conclusion

The food regulations and food control systems in China, Japan, and Korea share some similarities and differences based on their social, political, and cultural backgrounds. In order to promote public confidence and consumer assurances for food safety, Japan and Korea have adopted new legislation, the Food Safety Basic Law, for complementary cooperation and better coordination among competent authorities. They have also reinforced the provisions of Food Hygiene Laws for prompt responses and

[92]China Food Safety Web, the People's Republic of China.
[93]Food Laws and Regulations, China Light Industry Press 2006.

management of the increasing number of food safety incidents.

China recently enacted the Food Safety Law complementing and replacing existing Food Hygiene Law to minimize the occurrence of food safety incidents and strengthen the coordination of multiple authorities involved in the food safety control system. The Food Safety Commission of Japan carries out the role for science based risk assessment activities, while the Food Safety Council of Korea mainly carries out the consultative role for decision making by coordinating all aspects of food safety activities of the ministries involved. China's Food Safety Council will be expected to carry out a similar role as the Food Safety Council of Korea to strengthen and streamline inter-agency coordination of food safety management system.

Due to recent advances in telecommunications including internet and cellular phones and increased international food trade, food safety in one country is no longer just a national issue. More transparent efforts should be made to enhance the food safety control systems and their capabilities to protect the health of consumers and to ensure fair practices in the international food trade.

2.12 CHINA

Juanjuan Sun
Shantou University and Nantes University

2.12.1 Introduction

Having the largest population in the world, China always had a tough mission to ensure food security for its people. Meanwhile, with economic and social developments, especially the improvement of people's living standards,

people have increasingly higher requirements and expectations on food safety, health and nutrition. However, the repeatedly emerging food safety issues within and outside China have triggered the public's great concerns and injured their confidence in food safety. The melamine incident in 2008 was a case in point. Given the importance of food safety regulation both for consumer protection and for food trade, the current food safety regulation in China is submitted to a reform for which the implementation of the Chinese Food Safety Law will be a catalyst. In this context several special issues on Chinese food safety regulation are worth mentioning to better understand the necessity of its reform. These can be analyzed as follows.

2.12.1.1 *Gaps in the Current Food Legal Framework*

The overall legal framework of China has changed significantly after implementation of the policy of reform and opening up in the late 1970s. Though China is a unified country, its legislative structure is multi-level, including the state laws (Constitution and basic laws) made by the National People's Congress and its Standing Committee, administrative laws and regulations by the State Council and its relevant departments respectively, and local regulations formulated by the relevant administrative organs of ordinary localities and governments etc.[94] With regard to food regulation, the total number of the food related laws, regulations and regulatory documents drafted by government departments at the ministerial level or above amounted to 832, but more than 40 have been invalidated since December 1978 (Zhang, 2008). Among the existing laws regarding food, the Food Hygiene Act and Product Quality Act are relatively important. The purpose of the Food Hygiene Act is to regulate the food activities such as the food

[94]For more information about the legislative structure in China, see <http://www.china.org.cn/english/kuaixun/76212.htm>.

production, processing, distribution, storage, purchasing, marketing and displaying, etc. The Product Quality Act is aimed at regulating the production and marketing of processed food. Although several stages of the food chains have been covered by these two acts, and the regulatory tasks based on sectors have been assigned to different competent authorities, not every stage of the food chain from farm to fork was being regulated in accordance with these laws. For example, the coverage of the Food Hygiene Act did not include plant agriculture and animal husbandry, and one contributing factor to the contaminated milk powder incident of 2008 was a lack of regulation on milk collection from individual farmers. Thus, a systematic and complete legal framework in the field of food safety regulation did not exist yet. This was partly because law making was done on an ad hoc basis and legislative power had been delegated to various agencies with different functions and at different levels. As a result, duplications and gaps, as well as regulatory conflicts between the different specialized laws made law enforcement difficult. Besides, the existing Food Hygiene Act was not sufficient to provide a legal basis for the whole food safety regulatory activities in the mainland. In this situation, the eagerly awaited first Chinese Food Safety Law has been promulgated and came into force on 1 June 2009.

2.12.1.2 Outdated Food Technological Standards

With the development of science and technology, technological standards concerning food safety have become obsolete, and to make matters worse, most of China's food technological standards were established back in the 1960s when the issue of food safety had not yet been well recognized. Generally speaking, the issues with the current food technological standards can be grouped into six key points. First of all, the high number of standard setting bodies has given rise to conflicting standards, for example between

hygiene standards and quality standards. Secondly, some standards are inconsistent with the associated laws. Thirdly, the standards set by food companies are conflicting with government standards. Fourthly, there are no hygiene standards for certain foods which are already in production and being marketed on a large scale. Fifthly, the threshold for the same food products can differ from standard to standard. Sixthly, a large number of the food standards are out of date (Du Gangjian, 2008).

2.12.1.3 The Complicated Food Regulatory System

A typical issue in the multi-agency food regulatory system, is the ambiguity of the functions and responsibilities of the various competent authorities. These involve the Ministry of Health, the Ministry of Agriculture, the State Administration for Industry and Commerce, the General Administration of Quality Supervision, Inspection and Quarantine (AQSIQ), etc. Previously, great efforts have been made to try to solve this issue. Pursuant to article 3 of the Food Hygiene Law of 1995, the Ministry of Health, which is the administrative department of public health under the State Council, is in charge of supervision and control of food hygiene throughout the country while other relevant departments under the State Council shall, within the scope of their respective functions and duties, be responsible for control of food hygiene. However, lack of clarity in the delineation of the functions and responsibilities in this area has led to the system being dubbed as 'over eight departments that cannot figure out how to regulate one pig coordinately'. In this context, there have been administrative rules set up for clarifying the functions and responsibilities of the concerned departments like the Decision of the State Council on Further Strengthening Food Safety issued in 2004. Up until 2007, the attribution of the functions and responsibilities was sector based: the production of primary agricultural products is supervised by the agriculture department; the quality and daily hygiene supervision of food processing is overseen by the quality supervision and inspection department; supervision of food circulation and distribution is done by the department of industry and commerce; and that of the catering industry and canteens is taken care of by the health department. The integrated foodsafety supervision and coordination as well as investigation of and penalties imposed for major incidents in this regard are the responsibility of the department of Food and Drug Administration, while imported and exported agricultural products and other foodstuffs are supervised by the quality supervision and inspection department.[95] Unfortunately, during the new round of administrative reform early in 2008 the Ministry of Health was reorganized; the State Food and Drug Administration (SFDA) was incorporated in that ministry. Several functions and responsibilities have been redistributed. The previous functions of the SFDA to supervise and coordinate activities with regard to food safety as well as to investigate major food safety incidents have been transferred to the newly established "Super Ministry of Health" while the SFDA is only responsible for the new tasks such as the supervision of food circulation and distribution. So far, the newly established 'Super Ministry of Health' did not succeed in preventing criminal acts such as the melamine incident.

2.12.2 The Chinese Food Safety Law

2.12.2.1 Introduction

The Chinese Food Safety Law was passed during its fourth review at the seventh session of the Eleventh National People's Congress Standing Committee in early 2009 and will come into force quickly. After several revisions, this law puts greater emphasis on the accountability of both the central government (relevant competent authorities) and local governments and the responsibility of food operators. The significance of the Chinese Food Safety Law, is analyzed here below.

2.12.2.2 The Authority of the Food Safety Law

Although food safety regulation is only one kind of administrative activity undertaken by the government to ensure food safety and to promote the food economy, the enactment of the Food Safety Law should still be in the form of basic law, given its important role serving as the legal basis in the food safety regulatory framework. As a basic law, it should be enacted and amended by the National People's Congress in China and all of the administrative regulations issued by the departments of government should be subjected to it. In other words, both law enforcement activities and law-making activities of the relevant competent authorities responsible for food safety regulation should conform to the Food Safety Law once it is in force.

2.12.2.3 The Main Elements of the Food Safety Law

As mentioned above, the Food Safety Law is a basic law. Its main concerns are the general principles and requirements. The Chinese legislators have taken inspiration from the principles and requirements as enacted elsewhere even though they may differ from country to country. Generally speaking, the following points have been embodied in the existing basic food laws in some countries/regions or recommended by international organizations such as FAO and WHO.

---

[95]State Council Information Office. 2007. White Paper on Food Quality and Safety. For more detailed information, see: The State Council, The Decision of the State Council on Further Strengthening Food Safety in 2004.

2.12.2.4 The Role of Science in Terms of Risk Analysis

It is universally recognized that food safety regulation should be based on scientific grounds as there are a growing number of risks that are becoming threats to human health. Against this background, a risk based measure, risk analysis, has been widely applied by developed countries. Risk analysis is composed of risk assessment, risk management and risk communication. However, the application of risk analysis in reality still varies from country to country and in China, only risk assessment has been put into place up till now. In this regard, the Chinese Food Safety Law has set up the provisions on risk assessment in order to base the whole food safety regulation on science. Several issues have been emphasized, including the monitoring system on risk, the circulation of the information about risks, the organization of risk assessment and its application, etc.[96]

2.12.2.5 The Food Standards

Chinese food standards consist of state standards, local standards, industry standards and enterprise standards. The multi level standards sometimes conflict with each other, and most of those standards are outdated or lower than the international ones. To systematize those food standards, China has committed to unify national food safety standards by conferring standard making powers on the Ministry of Health.[97] Furthermore, given situations such as the production and marketing of substandard food and food products, the conflicting standards set by different bodies, the regulation based on outdated standards or without established standards, it is also necessary to set up the general principles and requirements with regard to the standard setting procedures in order to ensure uniformity and consistence. To this end, Article 23 has provided that the national food safety standards should be approved by the national committee on standard review which consists of experts with food related background and government officials. In addition to this, before decisions are taken, the committee should consider the comments of different stakeholders and the results of risk assessment as a basis for setting standards.[98]

2.12.2.6 The Regulatory System

As mentioned above, after the latest round of administrative reform in early 2008, the food regulatory system still failed to realize its commitment to ensure the food safety. In light of the seriousness of this issue, this has been readdressed in the Chinese Food Safety Law which clarifies the functions and responsibilities of the different competent authorities with the Ministry of Health taking the leading role. Also, a new national food safety committee will be established to take charge of the cooperative and coordinated work in the field of food safety. Given the unknown structure of the newly created national food safety committee and the potential conflicts between the functions and responsibilities of the committee and the Ministry of Health (since both have been mentioned to have the function to coordinate work in regulation), it is still too early to conclude if the Food Safety Law will play out its role as designed.

2.12.3 Conclusion

Admittedly, there are high expectations for the Chinese Food Safety Law since it intends to introduce a new paradigm in the field of food safety regulation with its role serving as the sound legal foundation. Nonetheless, the formulation of a new food safety law is not a panacea

[96]Articles 11-17, Chinese Food Safety Law, 2009
[97]Articles 21 and 22, Chinese Food Safety Law, 2009.
[98]Article 23, Chinese Food Safety Law, 2009.

to solve existing food safety issues, as this also depends on law enforcement and compliance, let alone that there is still much room for improvement of the new food safety law in its current state. But it goes without saying that the enactment and implementation of the food safety law is still an essential step to improve food safety regulation in China, since as a 'constitution' in this field, the Food Safety Law will provide a legal basis for people to ensure their right to adequate food and for the regulators and regulatees to fulfill their obligation respectively.

2.13 THE RUSSIAN FEDERATION

Yuriy V. Vasilyev
Stavropol Branch of the North Caucasus Civil Service Academy, Russia

2.13.1 Introduction

Food law is not officially considered to be a separate branch of law in the Russian Federation. Politicians and scientists identify food quality and safety as a separate area of a more complicated sphere of social relations which is defined as food security. In its turn, food security is a part of an even more complex system determining the degree of social stability, and is included into the general notion of national security (Figure 2.1).

Food Law proper includes rules of constitutional, civil, administrative, criminal, customs law and some other items out of different spheres of Federal legislation as well as numerous by-laws (governmental decrees, departmental instructions, regulations, orders, etc.).

Food Law is considered an important element of consumer safety and even national security. The most important factors determining this attitude are the following:

1. Numerous counterfeit food items produced both domestically and abroad increasingly threaten consumers' lives and health. According to the National Fund of Protection of Consumers' Rights 50–85% (Chernova, 2008) of food items and 95% (Khurshudyan, 2008) of bioactive supplements at wholesale markets in the Russian Federation are forged in toto or partially, alcoholic beverages topping the list.

2. Poor quality food items both home made and imported do not meet normative requirements. 10-13% of the tested food items are reported as not corresponding to standards (Platishkin, 2007). Sanitary control authorities check more than 3,000,000 food items annually. In 2007 alone, 20% of imported fish and seafood, 14% of canned food, 66% of cereals and 60% of margarine were rejected as defective (APK, 2008). Every year around 1,000,000 people in Russia die prematurely of unnatural causes, one of the main reasons being diseases of the digestive system.

3. Increased use of genetically modified organisms in food items, among them such popular products as sausage, sweets, yogurts, chocolates, pastry and bread, corn, potatoes, tobacco and so on. Although the consequences of consuming genetically modified products are not yet sufficiently studied, scientists are extremely alerted as according to some oncological research, liver, blood, kidney diseases, alongside obesity

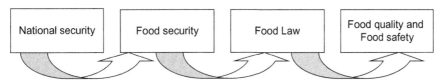

FIGURE 2.1   The hierarchy of food security in the general notion of national security in Russia.

and allergies, may be caused by such kinds of food. Sanitary authorities annually report around 2,000 non-registered transgenic food items (Platishkin, 2007). Unfortunately, consumers are not always necessarily informed about food composition, thus their subjective right of choice is violated.

4. Other Factors. Poor quality of food can be responsible as an indirect cause of a large number of demographic, medical, social and other federal problems.

It is a common truth that 17–20% of imported foods in the domestic market are considered crucial, and it is well-known that the developed countries are planning to decrease the share of imported food items down to zero. On the other hand, over 40% of food items in Russia are imported, the quantity increasing up to 70% in bigger cities. These and some other factors become a serious threat to lives and health of practically all the citizens of the Russian Federation. This is the reason why establishing a national food security system has become a matter of vital importance for the government and for the nation. In terms of its formation and efficient functioning the role of normative and legal regulations in the sphere of Food Law cannot be overestimated. It can significantly diminish the risks and improve the current situation.

2.13.2 The Current Condition of Legislation

It might seem while analyzing the Russian Federation Food Law that Russia is the most advanced country in terms of the quantity of current laws and by-laws defining the quality of food and its safety. But the truth is that Russia suffers more from the abundance of laws and their low quality rather than from their insufficiency. The multitude of by-laws hinders their implementation, as departments and controlling authorities (numbering more than

ten at present) result in overlapping functions and activities. Therefore, the whole food chain has become inefficient. This directly causes the growth of the bureaucratic apparatus, thus encouraging corruption and massive violations of the law.

Apart from this the definitive part of the Russian legislation is of the reference nature and has some declarative elements. To implement the law, many ministries and departments have to elaborate regulations and instructions of their own, besides the above mentioned regulations. These are not necessarily well coordinated with each other. This factor also facilitates corruption and hinders the establishment of efficient control and supervision system.

One can see quite a clear-cut formally established legislation vertical in the sphere of food safety and subjective rights of the Russian Federation citizens who are the rightful participants of food legal relationship. In the number of its articles (Article 7, 17, 41, etc.), the Russian Federation Constitution of 1993 corroborates that the state assumes the functions of social protection and health care of its citizens, and that the appropriate provision of food supplies is considered to be one of the conditions for adequate life and free development of a person.

The main normative basis for providing the home market of the Russian Federation with food items all the way through the food chain are the following main Federal laws:

- No. 52-Ф3 'On sanitary and epidemiologic well-being of population,' dated 30 March 1999, edited in 2007;
- No. 29-Ф3 'On quality and safety of food items,' dated 2 January 2000, edited in 2008;
- No. 86-Ф3 'On the state regulation of genetic engineering,' dated 5 July 1996, edited in 2000;
- No. 184-Ф3 'On technical regulation,' dated 12 December 2002;
- No. 2300-1 'On protection of consumers' rights,' dated 1 February 1992, edited in 2008.

Alongside the above-mentioned, there are several fundamental normative legal acts being elaborated on in the Parliament (Duma) and in the government of the Russian Federation. They are as follows:

- Doctrine of food safety of the Russian Federation;
- Federal law 'On food security of the Russian Federation';
- A number of standards, technical regulations and Federal programs of the food market.

Presently there exist over 7,000 specifying hygienic regulations of food safety, among them 1,024 on sanitary chemical indicators; 1,432 on sanitary microbiological indicators; 2,890 on pesticides; 917 on substances and materials contacting food items, and 797 on biologically active supplements (Tutelyan, 2008). Basic notions of *'counterfeit food items'* and *'identification of food items'* are defined in the above mentioned Federal law 'On quality and safety of food items'. The term *'counterfeit product'* is defined in the Civil Code, although the Criminal Code of the Russian Federation and the Administrative Violations Code lack quite a number of principal notions from the sphere of substantive and procedural law which prevents the efficient and successful counteraction to the corresponding violations of law.

Current realities are such that the existing system of federal control and supervision over the quality and safety of food items cannot adequately cope with the recent changes in agricultural production and turnover. No proper attention is paid to control of the raw agricultural product.

Contemporary systems of quality management are based on thorough studies of the whole technological production process. Control and supervision over the manufactured items cannot be efficient at all. Another significant shortcoming is that legislators are especially interested only in a couple of parameters of control and supervision, for example, in obligatory testing of standard safety criteria evaluation. Other quality indicators are thus ignored by producers and this cannot be considered a positive tendency of the food law development.

2.13.3 Nearest Prospects

The forthcoming membership of the Russian Federation to the WTO involves multiple legal and organizational issues. Actual markets convergence requires coordination of national legal and technical normatives with international ones. Special committees are working on including provisions of *Codex Alimentarius* into many national standards and regulations.

A major joint project of the European Union and the RF Ministry of Agriculture was launched in Russia in February 2007. The Federal Service of Veterinarian and Herbal Supervision participates in the Project with the purpose of coordinating normative regulations in the sphere of sanitation and herbal sanitation in Russia. The Project was timed to function for 30 month with a budget of € 4,000,000.

Summing it all up, one can say that the Russian Federation is fully aware of the positive reaction on global integration and is working hard in that direction even though reckless convergence into the world market is fraught with economic dependence and loss of national identity.

2.14 CONCLUDING OBSERVATIONS

Bernd M.J. van der Meulen
Wageningen University, The Netherlands

2.14.1 Introduction

This chapter may well be unique in the development of food law as an international academic discipline. It may be the first time that such a wide variety of jurisdictions has been addressed in a single publication.

The materials on the worldwide development of food legislation that have been brought together in this chapter are of an explorative nature. They do not allow to draw hard conclusions, nevertheless some interesting observations can be made.

2.14.2 Current Situation

2.14.2.1 Rights Based?

In all the countries and regions presented in this chapter, the subject matter of food law clearly overlaps with the scope of the human right to food as recognized in the International Covenant on Economic, Social and Cultural Rights and similar international documents. Ensuring people access to safe and wholesome food and protection against risks to their life and health are key issues. Nevertheless, only in a few sections specific reference is made to this human right (e.g. Eastern Africa, Latin America, China and Russia). Probably food law is not usually perceived as human rights based.

2.14.2.2 Incident Driven

The sections in this chapter show that food legislation has developed worldwide since the dawn of time, but most rapidly during the last century. In most of the examples presented (with the exception of East Africa and the Near East), we see that legislation on food has a long history (current forms are often based on Nineteenth Century legislation in the UK as is the case with India, South Africa, Australia, New Zealand, USA and Canada). Food law's development over a longer period of time has given rise to a complicated structure (India, South Africa, Australia, New Zealand). Development has been prompted by incidents that occurred more or less spontaneously (animal health incidents, BSE in particular, EU, Japan) and by fraudulent adulteration (South Africa, Australia, New Zealand, USA, China, Russia). The latter was dealt with under criminal law (India, USA).

We have seen similar occurrences taking place in times and places far apart. An observation in the section on the Russian Federation for example ('50–85% of food items and 95% of bioactive supplements at wholesale markets in the Russian Federation are in toto or partially forged') sounds like an almost word perfect repetition of information given in the section on the USA ('Frederick Accum documented adulteration so widespread that he found it difficult to find a single type of food that was not adulterated; and some foods he scarcely ever found genuine') and Canada ('50% of all foods sold in Canada at the time were adulterated. Similar to the United States, nearly all coffee and pepper were adulterated, milk was diluted with water, and other high value items, such as tea and chocolate were often adulterated'). The Russian section refers to the situation as it stands today. The section on the USA and Canada on the other hand, is about a distant past (almost two over one century ago, respectively). Apparently, the battle against adulteration is a timeless feature of food law. In the Russian Federation, food safety is even considered a matter of national security.

Some authors observe a relationship between the occurrence of incidents and technological development. New ways of processing food bring new opportunities for fraud and new risks (USA, Canada). Genetic modification in particular is mentioned as a concern (in the contributions on Eastern Africa, EU and Russia). On the other hand, new technologies increase the possibilities to identify problems (USA, Canada).

A factor partly related to the protection against risks and incidents and partly a value in itself that stimulated development of food law, is the desire to facilitate interstate trade in federal societies (India, Australia, USA), international trade (WTO, Codex, Eastern Africa, Latin America, EU, Russia) and globalization more in general (Eastern Africa) sometimes expressed in terms of telecommunications (Northeast Asia). Even tourism is mentioned as a factor stimulating the development of food law (Near East).

2.14.3 The Way Forward

2.14.3.1 *Quality of Food Law*

Problems encountered within food legislation are expressed in terms of complexity, fragmentation, lack of cooperation, coordination (Latin America), coherence and consistency (India, Russia, China), conflicting provisions (China), scattered responsibility (South Africa, Near East, Northeast Asia), overlapping competences (India, Russia, China), bureaucracy and corruption (Russia). Implementation, supervision and enforcement are problematic issues as well (Australia, New Zealand, Eastern Africa, Latin America, China, Russia).

Developments like increase in national and international trade, globalisation more in general, increased processing of food accompanied by increased adulteration (USA, Canada, Russia), have contributed to a sense of urgency to take measures to reduce barriers (Australia, New Zealand, EU) to trade but also to protect public health and food safety (Australia, New Zealand). This issue is at the forefront in all countries discussed, but in particular in those that have been struck by food safety crises resulting in public outrage (sulphanilamide-USA, BSE-EU, melamine-China).

2.14.3.2 *General Legislation*

Recognition of food law as a branch of law in its own right seems to be a relatively new development in most countries and is only about to start in some other countries (Russian Federation). This development is expressed in attempts at chain integration (from farm to fork and from paddock to plate) (Australia, New Zealand, Latin America, EU, China) and the enactment of basic or general laws holding principles (EU: General Food Law, 2002, Japan: Food Safety Basic Law, 2003; India: Food Safety and Standards Act, 2006; Korea: Food Safety Basic Law, 2008; China: Food Safety Law, 2009). Maybe also the African Model Law on Safety in Biotechnology (AU) can be mentioned in this context.

Recurring expressions are harmonization (Latin America, EU, Near East, Russia) (or even uniformity—Australia) and mutual recognition (Australia, New Zealand, Latin America, EU, Near East).

2.14.3.3 *Food Safety Authorities*

Many countries have instituted a specialized body or central authority to consolidate food safety issues under 'one umbrella'. The roles of these authorities greatly vary from advice (FLAG-South Africa), coordination (Food Safety Council-Korea; Food Safety Council-China), risk assessment (EFSA-EU; Food Safety Commission-Japan), to regulation/legislation (Food and Drug Administration-USA; FSANZ-Australia and New Zealand; Tanzania Food, Drug Authority), and enforcement (Food and Drug Administration-Korea; State Food and Drug Administration-China), or combinations (Food Safety and Standards Authority of India; Jordan Food and Drug Administration). In some situations importance of independence is underscored (Eastern Africa, EU, Japan).

2.14.4 Outlook

Generally the contributions in this chapter are optimistic in tone. Food legislation is seen as progressing and improving. There are some concerns regarding its capability to ensure food safety (China, Russia). Hardly any side effects are mentioned except for the risk that too tight legislation may inhibit innovation (Australia). Deregulation is not mentioned as a way to go, but was once a part of the cause of problems (USA).

2.14.5 Features of Future Food Law

2.14.5.1 *Common Aspects Worldwide*

In twenty-first century food law, we seem to encounter similar features worldwide like the pre-market approval of food additives (South Africa,

USA, EU, China) and sometimes other foods like food supplements and GMOs (South Africa, EU, China), an emphasis on health protection through food hygiene (including HACCP) (Codex, India, South Africa, Australia, New Zealand, Latin America, EU) and powers of incident management, sometimes on traceability (EU, Japan, Korea) and on labeling requirements (Codex, India, South Africa, Australia, New Zealand, EU) including protection of consumers from misleading practices (South Africa, EU) and empowering them to make informed choices (Australia, New Zealand, Eastern Africa, EU, Russia). Stakeholder involvement seems to be a feature increasing in relevance in the creation of food legislation (India, South Africa, Eastern Africa, Australia, New Zealand, Latin America, Japan, Korea, China). Still the aim of reducing barriers to trade is present in virtually all systems.

2.14.5.2 Science Based

More markedly we see a worldwide influence of the WTO and increasing reliance on international standards—the *Codex Alimentarius* in particular—(India, South Africa, Eastern Africa, Australia, Russia, Northeast Asia) and on natural science through the risk analysis methodology for the protection of public health (Codex, SPS Agreement, India, Eastern Africa, Australia, New Zealand, Latin America, EU, Near East, Northeast Asia, China). By consequence science holds an increasing responsibility. It is precisely this responsibility that is at the heart of the Global Harmonization Initiative.

References

Abaitua Borda, I., Philen, R. M., Posada de la Paz, M., de la Cámara, A. G., Ruiz-Navarro, M. D., Ribota, O. G., et al. (1998). Toxic oil syndrome mortality: The first thirteen years. *International Journal of Epidemiology*, 27, 1057–1063. Available from http://ije.oxfordjournals.org/cgi/content/abstract/27/6/1057.

Accum, F. (1820). *A treatise on adulterations of food and culinary poisons*. Longman.

Acosta, A., & Marrero, T. (1985). Normalización de alimentos y salud para América Latina y el Caribe. 4. Labor del Comité Coordinador Regional de la Comisión del Codex Alimentarius. *Bol of SanPPanmn*, 99(6), 642–652.

AGMARK. (1937). Directorate of Marketing and Inspection, Ministry of Agriculture, *Agricultural Produce (Grading and Marking) Act*; www.agmarknet.nic.in.

Agro-Industrial Complex (APK). (2008). *Economics and Management*, 8, 9 (АПК: экономика, управление. 08.2008., с. 9).

Anon. (1988). Report of an inquiry into food regulations in Australia. Part 1—National issue. Business Regulation Review Unit, Commonwealth of Australia.

Batrershall, J. P. (1887). *Food adulteration and its detection*. London.

Beck, L. C. (1846). *Adulteration of various substances use in medicine and the arts.*

Berends, G., & Carreno, I. (2005). Safeguards in food law—ensuring food scares are scarce. *European Law Review*, 30, 386–405.

BIS. (1986). Bureau of Indian Standards, Ministry of Commerce, New Delhi. Available from www.bis.org.in.

Blakney, J. (2009). Lecture: The Regulatory Framework, Food Regulation in Canada (on file with the Institute for Food Laws & Regulations, Michigan State University).

Broberg, M. P. (2008). *Transforming the European Community's Regulation of Food Safety*, SIEPS, 5. http://www.sieps.se/publikationer/rapporter/transforming-the-european-communitys-regulation-of-food-safety.html.

Brooke-Taylor, S., Baines, J., Goodchap, J., Gruber, J., & Hambridge, T. (2003). *Food Control*, 14, 375–382.

Butler, K. (2002, June 5). *Four men found guilty of contract hit on vet.* p. 11. Independent (London), Available from http://findarticles.com/p/articles/mi_qn4158/is_20020605/ai_n12618881.

Byrn, M. L. (1852). *Detection of fraud and protection of health: A treatise on the adulteration of food and drink.*

Chernova, E. V. (2008). Food safety in Russia: Current condition and provision tendencies. *Economics and Management*, 2, 39 (Е.В. Чернова Продовольственная безопасность в России: современное состояние и тенденции обеспечения. // Экономика и управление № 2. 2008. с. 39).

Codex Alimentarius Commission. (1995). *General standard for food additives*. Rome: Food and Agriculture Organization.

Codex Alimentarius Commission. (1997). Hazard analysis and critical control point (HACCP) system and guidelines for its application. In: *Food hygiene basic texts*. Rome: Food and Agriculture Organization.

Du Gangjian. (2008). Several issues on the Legislation of Food Safety Law. *Pacific Journal*, 3, 55.

FAO. (2002). New approaches to consider in capacity build-
ing and technical assistance—building alliances. In *FAO/
WHO global forum of food safety regulators*, Marrakech,
Morocco, 28–30 January.

FAO/WHO. (2002). *Report of the evaluation of the Codex
Alimentarius and other FAO and WHO food standards
work*. Available from http://www.who.int/foodsafety/
codex/eval_report/en/index.html.

FAO/WHO. (2006). *Understanding the Codex Alimentarius*,
(3rd ed.). Rome. Available from ftp://ftp.fao.org/
codex/Publications/understanding/Understanding_
EN.pdf.

Farrer, K. T. H. (1983). *Fancy eating that* (p. 156). Melbourne,
Australia: Melbourne University Press.

Farrer, K. T. H. (1990). *Food Australia, 42*, 146–152.

FDA (United States Food and Drug Administration). (2002).
*FDA Backgrounder: Milestones in U.S. Food and Drug Law
History*. Available from http://www.fda.gov/opacom/
backgrounders/miles.html (last accessed August 5,
2002).

Felker, P. H. (1880). *What the grocers sell us: A manual for buyers.*

De Figueireido Toledo, M. C. (2000). Southern common
market standards. In N. Rees & D. Watson (Eds.),
International standards for food safety (pp. 79–94). US:
Springer.

FSSAI. (2006). *Food safety and standards authority of India*.
New Delhi: Ministry of Health and Family Welfare
Available from www.fssai.gov.

Gelpí, E., Posada de la Paz, M., Terracini, B., Abaitua, I.,
de la Cámara, A. G., Kilbourne, E. M., et al. (2002).
The Spanish toxic oil syndrome twenty years after its
onset: A multidisciplinary review of scientific knowledge. *Environmental Health Perspectives, 110*, 457–464.
Available from http://www.pubmedcentral.nih.gov/
articlerender.fcgi?artid = 1240833.

Gnirss, G. (2008). A history of food law in Canada. *Food in
Canada, 38*.

Graff, J. (2002, July 21). One sweet mess. *Time*. Available from
www.time.com/time/nation/article/0,8599,322596,00.
htm.

Hart, F. L. (1952). A history of the adulteration of food before
1906. *Food, Drug, Cosmetic Law Journal, 7*, 5–22.

Healy, M., Brooke-Taylor, S., & Liehne, P. (2003). *Food
Control, 14*, 357–365.

Hoskins, T. H. (1861). *What we eat: An account of the most common adulterations of food and drink.*

Hutt, P. B. (1960). Criminal prosecution for adulteration
and misbranding of food at common law. *Food, Drug,
Cosmetic Law Journal, 15*, 382–398.

Hutt, P. B. (1990). Symposium on the history of fifty years of
food regulation under the federal food, drug, and cosmetic act: A historical introduction. *Food, Drug, Cosmetic
Law Journal, 45*, 17–20.

Hutt, P. B., & Hutt, P. B., II. (1984). A history of government
regulation of adulteration and misbranding of food.
Food, Drug, Cosmetic Law Journal, 39, 2–72.

James, P., Kemper, F., & Pascal, G. (1999). *A European
food and public health authority. The future of scientific
advice in the EU*. Available from http://ec.europa.
eu/food/fs/sc/future_food_en.pdf.

Janssen, W. F. (1975). America's first food and drug laws.
Food Drug Cosmetic Law Journal, 30, 665–672.

Khurshudyan, S. A. (2008). Counterfeited food
items: Scientific, methodological and normative legal foundations for counteraction. *Economics and Management, 9*, 56C (A.
Хуршудян Фальсификация пищевых продуктов:
научные, методологические и нормативно-
правовые основы противодействия. // Пищевая
промышленность № 9. 2008. c. 56).

Knipschild, K. (2003). *Lebensmittelsicherheit als Aufgabe
des Veterinär- und Lebensmittelrechts* (diss.). Germany:
Nomos Verlagsgesellschaft Baden-Baden.

Knudsen, G., & Matikainen-Kallström, M. (1999) *Joint
parliamentary committee report on food safety in the
EEA*. Available from secretariat.efta.int/Web/
EuropeanEconomicArea/eea_jpc_resolutions/
1999FoodSafety.doc.

Lips, P., & Beutner, G. (2000). *Ratgeber Lebensmittelrecht* (5th
ed.). München.

Looney, J. W. (1995). The effect of NAFTA (and GATT) on
animal health laws and regulations, Oklahoma. *Law
Review, 48*(2), 367–382.

Madgwick, W. J. (unpublished). *History of food law in new
South Wales.*

Masson-Matthee, M. D. (2007). *The Codex Alimentarius
Commission and its standards. An examination of the
legal aspects of the Codex Alimentarius Commission*. The
Netherlands: Asser Press.

van der Meulen, B., & van der Velde, M. (2008). *European
food law handbook*. Wageningen Academic Publishers.
Available from http://www.wageningenacademic.
com/foodlaw.

MoA. (1973). *Meat food products order*. New Delhi: Directorate
of Marketing and Inspection, Ministry of Agriculture.
Available from www.agmarknet.nic.in/mfpo1973.htm.

MoC. (1963). *Export (Quality Control and Inspection) Act*, 1963.
Ministry of Commerce. Available from www.eicindia.org.

MoCA. (1967). *Solvent extracted oil, de-oiled meal and edible flour (control) order*. New Delhi: Department of
Consumer Affairs, Ministry of Food and Consumer
Affairs. Available from http://www.fcamin.nic.inwww.
fcamin.nic.in.

MoCA. (1998). *Vegetable oil products (regulation) order*. New
Delhi: Directorate of Vanaspati, Vegetable Oils and Fats,
Ministry of Food and Consumer Affairs. Available from
www.fcamin.nic.in.

MoFPI. (1955). *The fruit products order*. New Delhi: Ministry of Food Processing Industries. Available from www.mofpi.nic.in.

MoHFW. (1954). *The Prevention of Food Adulteration Act 1954, and Rules*. New Delhi: Directorate General of Health Services, Ministry of Health and Family Welfare. Available from www.mohfw.nic.in/pfa.htm.

Nader, A., & Vitale, G. (1998). Legislación alimentaria—al alcance de la mano. Revista Alimentos Argentinos No. 8. S.A.G.P. y A.—Dirección de Promoción de la Calidad Alimentaria, Buenos Aires, Argentina, September, 1998. Available from http://www.alimentosargentinos.gov.ar/0-3/revistas/r_08/08_06_codex.htm (accessed March 20, 2009).

Nöhle, U. (2005). Risikokommunication und Risikomanagement in der erweiterten EU. *Zeitschrift des gesummten Lembensmittelrechts*, 3, 297–305.

OAS. (1998, February). Standards and the regional integration process in the western hemisphere. Organization of American States. Trade Section. Available from http://www.sedi.oas.org/DTTC/TRADE/PUB/STUDIES/STAND/stand2.asp (accessed March 20, 2009).

O'Keefe, J. A. (1968). *Bell and O'Keefe's sale of food and drugs* (p. 8). London: Butterworth & Co.

Ortega Medina Report. (1997). Report of the Temporary Committee of Inquiry into BSE, set up by the Parliament in July 1996, on the alleged contraventions or maladministration in the implementation of community law in relation to BSE, without prejudice to the jurisdiction of the community and the national courts of 7 February 1997, A4-0020/97/A, PE 220.544/fin/A. The report is often referred to by the name of the chairman of the Enquiry Committee, namely the Ortega Medina report. Available from http://www.mad-cow.org/final_EU.html.

Pan American Health Organization. (2008). Agriculture and health: Alliance for equity and rural development in the Americas. In *Fifteenth inter-American meeting at ministerial level on health and agriculture*, Rio de Janeiro, Brazil, 11–12 June.

Pineiro, M. (2004). Mycotoxins: Current issues in South America. In D. Barug, H. P. Van Egmond, R. López-García, W. A. van Osenbruggen, & A. Visconti (Eds.), *Meeting the mycotoxin menace* (pp. 49–68). The Netherlands: Wageningen Academic Publishers.

Platishkin, A. (2007). Russian food basket. *Russian Federation Today*, 9, 22A. (Платишкин Что на столе россиянина. № 9. 2007. c. 22).

Reuter, F. H. (1997). The Australian Model Food Act. Personal reminiscences on the road to uniform food legislation in Australia. *Food Australia* (Suppl.), 49, 3.

Richards, E. H. (1886). *Foods materials and their adulterations*.

Seidlmayer, S. (1998). Van het ontstaan de staat tot de 2e dynastie. In: *Regine Schulz en Matthias Seidel (red.) Egypte. Het land van de farao's*, Köln.

Sinclair, U. (1905). *The jungle*.

Smith, S. W. C. (1978). Food Technology in Australia, 30, 255–259.

TASK FORCE. (2002). *Task force report on India's Food and Agro-industries Management Policy*. Available from www.nic.in/pmecouncils/reports.food/.

Whitney, C. (1999, June 9). Food scandal adds to Belgium's image of disarray. *New York Times*. Available from http://query.nytimes.com/gst/fullpage.html?res = 9F06E0DC1139F93AA35755C0A96F958260.

Winger, R. (2003). *Food Control*, 14, 355.

World Health Organization. (2005). *International health regulations* (2nd ed.). Switzerland: WHO.

Zhang, J. X., & Chen, Z. D. (2006). Food regulations in China. In: *Food Laws and Regulations* (pp. 268–315). Beijing, China: China Light Industry Press.

Zhang, Y. (2008). Objective assessment of the severity of food safety issues and further strengthening the food legislation in China. *Shantou University Law Review*, 2, 9.

Further reading

Butler, K. (1996, March 19). *Why the mafia is into your beef: The EU ban on growth hormones for cows has created a lucrative black market*. Independent (London). Available from http://findarticles.com/p/articles/mi_qn4158/is_19960319/ai_n14035042.

DG Sanco. (2002). European Commission's Health and Consumer Protection DG, FVO at Home and Away, 7 Consumer Voice, September.

DG Sanco. (2007). European Commission's Health and Consumer Protection DG, Safer Food for Europe—over a decade of achievement for the FVO, Health & Consumer Voice, November.

Downer, A. H. (1985). *Food Technology in Australia*, 37, 106–107.

European Commission. (1997). Green Paper on the General Principles of Food Law in the European Union, COM (1997) 176. Available from http://www.foodlaw.rdg.ac.uk/eu/green-97.doc.

European Commission. (2000). White Paper on Food Safety COM (1999) 719 final. Available from http://ec.europa.eu/dgs/health_consumer/library/pub/pub06_en.pdf.

FSANZ Annual Report. (2006/2007). Food Standards Australia New Zealand. Available from http://www.foodstandards.gov.au/newsroom/publications/annual-report/index.cfm.

Goodrich vs People, 3 Park Cr. 630 (1858), 19 NY, 578 (1859).

Hilts, P. J. (2003). *Protecting America's health: The FDA, business, and one hundred years of regulation*. New York: Alfred A. Knopf.

Kwak, N. S., Park, S., Park, E. J., et al. (2008). Current food and drug policies in China. In *Policy review on food and drug safety in foreign countries* (pp. 202–235). KFDA Policy Report 55. Seoul: KFDA.

NSW Pure Food Advisory Committee minutes, 1909–1912.

Squibb, E. R. (1879). Address to the Medical Society of the State of New York, Proposed Legislation on the Adulteration of Food and Medicine.

USDA (United States Department of Agriculture), Bureau of Chemistry (1902–1908). Bulletin no. 84.

Wilson, B. (2008). *Swindled: The dark history of food fraud, from poisoned candy to Counterfeit Coffee*. Princeton University Press.

3

The Global Harmonization Initiative

Christine E. Boisrobert[1], Larry Keener[2] and Huub L.M. Lelieveld[3]

[1]Air Liquide, Houston, TX, USA
[2]International Product Safety Consultants, Seattle, WA, USA
[3]Formerly Unilever R&D, Vlaardingen, The Netherlands

OUTLINE

3.1 INTRODUCTION

The past few decades have witnessed a marked acceleration in the globalization of the food supply. As the world progresses into the twenty-first century, food systems are undergoing changes at an unprecedented rate driven by global economic and social shifts (FAO, 2004). The increased complexity, interdependence and integration of modern food supply systems have been brought into sharp focus in recent years with a number of highly disruptive and widely publicized food scares ranging from mad cow disease (bovine spongiform encephalopathy, BSE) to the latest melamine adulteration incident.

Despite immediate reactions from national governments to tighten legislation to restore diminishing consumer confidence, the far-reaching effect of such food safety crises can have no other result than to point out the critical and urgent need for global harmonization of food safety laws and regulations. As the world grows more tightly connected, so does the impetus for harmonizing food safety regulations and reaching global consensus on their founding principles (Motarjemi, van Schothorst, & Käferstein, 2001).

3.2 DRIVERS FOR GLOBAL HARMONIZATION OF FOOD SAFETY LEGISLATION AND REGULATIONS

3.2.1 Global Food Security—Availability of Safe and Wholesome Food

Contemporary public health debates on food safety are inevitably and intrinsically linked to the longstanding, overarching issue of global food security:

3.2.1.1 The Right to Food

As strongly illustrated in Box 3.1, ensuring the global availability of safe and wholesome foods to feed a fast-growing world population continues to be one of the world's main development challenges. The right to food—and its implicit corollary, the right to safe food—is a fundamental human right and a binding obligation under international law, as recognized in the *Universal Declaration of Human Rights* adopted by the United Nations (UN) in 1948, as well as the 1966 *International Covenant on Economic, Social and Cultural Rights* (Motarjemi *et al.*, 2001; UN, 2006).

3.2.1.2 Defining Food Security

Originated in the mid-1970s, the initial concept of food security focused primarily on the volume and stability of food supply (FAO, 2003). The decades that followed saw numerous attempts at definition, inherently reflecting the broad acknowledgement in public policy of the complex and multi-dimensional nature of this phenomenon. By the mid-1990s, the concept of food security expanded to include food safety as well as nutritional balance. Although food security has no set definition, the latest and most careful consideration to this topic took place during the *World Food Summit* (WFS), held in Rome in 1996. The summit, convened by the Food and Agriculture Organization (FAO) of the United Nations to renew global commitment to the fight against hunger, defined food security as existing *'when all people, at all times, have physical and economic access to sufficient, safe and nutritious food to meet their dietary needs and food preferences for an active and healthy life'* (FAO, 1997).

3.2.1.3 The World Food Summit and Millennium Development Goals

Successful in increasing the international community's awareness of the extent of hunger and malnutrition worldwide, the 1996 World Food Summit led to the adoption by 185 countries and the European Community of the *Rome Declaration on World Food Security* and the *World Food Summit Plan of Action*. These two documents set forth strategies to achieve food security and eradicate hunger in all countries, with a clearly defined and immediate target of reducing the *number* of undernourished people by half by the year 2015 (FAO, 1997). As the new century began, world leaders further committed their nations to a new global partnership to reduce extreme poverty at the historic Millennium Summit in New York in 2000. In adopting the *United Nations Millennium Declaration*, they renewed their pledge to the World Food Summit's time-bound goal, placing

---

BOX 3.1

GLOBAL FOOD SECURITY AND FOOD SAFETY – FACTS AND FIGURES

- New estimates published by the World Bank in August 2008 reveal that 1.4 billion people in developing countries (one in four) were living in extreme poverty* in 2005 (UN, 2008d).
- Higher food prices are expected to result in 1 billion people to go hungry, while another 2 billion will be undernourished (UN, 2008d).
- The proportion of children under 5 who are undernourished decreased from 33% in 1990 to 26% in 2006. However, by 2006, the number of children in developing countries who were underweight still exceeded 140 million (UN, 2008d).
- FAO estimates show that the number of chronically hungry people in the world reached 923 million in 2007, an increase of more than 80 million since the 1990–1992 base period (FAO, 2008a).
- The world population is expected to grow from 6.7 billion in 2006 to 9.2 billion in 2050. This increase will be absorbed mostly by the less developed nations (UN, 2007).

- FAO estimates that global food production must nearly double by 2050 to feed a projected world population of over 9 billion people (FAO, 2008b).
- Food and waterborne diarrheal diseases are leading causes of illness and death in less developed countries, killing an estimated 2.2 million people annually, 1.8 million of whom are children (WHO, 2002).
- In developed countries, up to 30% of the population is affected by foodborne diseases each year (WHO, 2002).
- US studies in 1995 estimated that the annual cost of the 3.3–12 million cases of foodborne illness caused by seven pathogens amounted to US $6.5–35 billion (WHO, 2002).

*Based on the results of the 2005 *International Comparison Program* (ICP), released in 2008, the World Bank has updated its past international poverty line of US$1 a day to US$1.25 in 2005 prices.

---

eradicating hunger and extreme poverty at the top of the list of the UN's eight Millennium Development Goals (MDGs) (UN, 2000).

Despite global focus on the MDGs and remarkable successes in certain areas, results to date show insufficient progress towards the MDG target of reducing by half the *proportion* of people suffering from hunger by 2015 (UN, 2008a). In the latest and most comprehensive global assessment of progress made so far, the United Nations warned that the number of underweight children in developing countries still exceeded 140 million in 2006 and that soaring food prices were now threatening to undo many previous achievements

(UN, 2008a). Looking ahead to 2015, FAO expressed similar concerns over the unlikely prospects of attaining the WFS and MDG hunger reduction targets (FAO, 2008a). In *The State of Food Insecurity in the World 2008*, FAO reported that, for the first time, the number of chronically hungry people in the world had actually surpassed the 1990–1992 baseline to reach an estimated total of 923 million in 2007. FAO further blamed high food prices for the fastest rise in chronic hunger experienced in recent years, citing production shortfalls, changing diets, market volatility, emerging biofuel demand, and trade policies amongst the many underlying factors.

3.2.1.4 *The Right to Safe Food*

With long-term global food security under threat, a safe food supply is all the more critical. As eloquently put during the first *FAO/WHO Regional Conference on Food Safety for Africa* in 2005, scarcity of food places an even stronger emphasis on the importance of ensuring the safety of that food. For example, in Africa, home to 15 of the 16 countries where the prevalence of hunger already exceeds 35% (FAO, 2008a), an outbreak of acute aflatoxicosis due to contaminated maize claimed more than 120 lives in 2004. Adding to the devastating toll was the economic cost and challenge of supplying 166,000 metric tons of safe replacement food to 1.8 million people in the affected zones over a 6-month period (FAO/WHO, 2005).

During the 1992 *International Conference on Nutrition*, the World Health Organization (WHO) of the United Nations first explicitly recognized, along with FAO, that *'access to nutritionally adequate and safe food is a right of each individual'* (FAO/WHO, 1992). Eight years later, increasingly concerned about the threat presented by microbial pathogens, biotoxins and chemical contaminants in food to the health of millions of people, WHO endorsed food safety as an essential public health function in resolution WHA53.15 of the *Fifty-third World Health Assembly* (WHO, 2002). Food and waterborne diarrheal diseases are considered to be leading causes of illness and death in less developed countries, claiming an estimated 2.2 million people annually, mostly children (WHO, 2002). Even in more advanced nations, 30% of the population is affected by foodborne diseases each year. Food safety is a basic human right and a global public health priority. Consequently, to the extent that each individual should be provided the same level of food safety assurance and the same degree of health protection from foodborne hazards, global harmonization of food safety legislation and regulations is a critical step in fulfilling that right (Motarjemi *et al.*, 2001).

To consider the example of Africa once more, an estimated 700,000 deaths occur each year in this region from food and waterborne diseases. Attributing this unbearable public health burden to the lack of efficient food safety systems, experts and officials assembled at the 2005 *FAO/WHO Regional Conference on Food Safety for Africa* drew particular attention to outdated, inadequate and fragmented food legislation in most African countries. Thus, when devising a *Five-year Strategic Plan for Food Safety in Africa*, conference participants were prompt to identify as a key element the harmonization of food safety standards and regulations between the countries of the region as well as with international requirements (FAO/WHO, 2005).

While one could argue that standards aimed at improving food safety will also reduce losses due to food spoilage, and consequently enhance food availability, it should still be noted that harmonization of food safety legislation will not single-handedly ensure all individuals access to safe and wholesome foods (Motarjemi *et al.*, 2001). Proper consumer protection requires additional critical components, including food control management, food inspection, enforcement, laboratory services, foodborne disease surveillance systems and public information, education and communication. This responsibility lies with all stakeholders—governments, food producers, food processors, retailers, consumers, as well as academic and scientific institutions. For a more detailed discussion of capacity and need for capacity building in food safety, refer to Chapter 8 (Capacity Building: Harmonization and Achieving Food Safety) and Chapter 9 (Capacity Building: Building Analytical Capacity for Microbial Food Safety).

3.2.2 Globalization of Food Safety Issues

While the universal right to safe food speaks to the rationale for harmonization of food safety regulations, rapid globalization of the world economy and society in the late twentieth and early twenty-first centuries adds to the undisputable necessity of international food safety standards (Motarjemi *et al.*, 2001). As national borders become more permeable to the flow of goods, capital, people and information, food contaminated in one country is more likely to pose a risk in other countries (Käferstein, Motarjemi, & Bettcher, 1997; Käferstein & Abdussalam, 1999; Motarjemi *et al.*, 2001; WHO, 2002). This *de facto* globalization of food safety problems is a complex result of many, and often interdependent, forces (Motarjemi *et al.*, 2001).

3.2.2.1 Globalization of Agricultural Trade and Food Supply Chain

Over the past decades, multiple technological advances have largely contributed to the globalization of the food supply (Motarjemi *et al.*, 2001). By preserving product quality, reducing shipping costs and shortening delivery times, developments in processing, packaging, logistics and transportation technologies have made it possible to deliver perishable foods to consumers thousands of miles away (Motarjemi *et al.*, 2001; Coyle, Hall, & Ballenger, 2001; Bruinsma, 2003). For instance, airfreight has been a significant factor in the rapid growth in food trade from Africa and Asia to Europe and North America (Saker, Lee, Cannito, Gilmore, & Campbell-Lendrum, 2004).

This process further accelerated in the 1990s through the establishment of various bilateral, regional and global trade agreements, and most notably, the successful completion of the Uruguay Round of Multilateral Trade Negotiations in 1994 and the subsequent creation of the World Trade Organization (WTO) in 1995 (Motarjemi *et al.*, 2001; Saker *et al.*, 2004; Hawkes, Chopra, Friel, Lang, & Thow, 2007). By establishing a framework to reduce barriers and distortions to trade for agricultural products, the Uruguay Round Agreement on Agriculture (URAA) marked a historic point in the reform of the agricultural trade system and laid the foundation for the liberalization of international food trade (Diakosavvas, 2001; Bruinsma, 2003). As a testament to trade liberalization, the nominal value of world agricultural exports is reported to have increased tenfold since the early 1960s, to reach around US$604 billion in 2004 (FAO, 2007). That same year, processed food products accounted for about 65% of the total food trade.

Closely tied to this increase in food trade is the continuing consolidation of agricultural and food companies into large transnational corporations (TNCs) and the overall globalization of the agri-food industry (Chopra, Galbraith, & Darnton-Hill, 2002; Hawkes *et al.*, 2007). Most often vertically integrated and based in the United States or Western Europe, these TNCs dominate today's global market drawing on global brand names and marketing strategies while still adapting to local tastes (Chopra *et al.*, 2002; Bruinsma, 2003; Saker *et al.*, 2004). Again, making use of cheaper transport systems, these companies are able to source ingredients from different parts of the world, manufacture products in less expensive labor markets, and distribute those worldwide (Saker *et al.*, 2004). Similarly, standardized retail and food service outlets, often owned by multinational companies operating in numerous countries, have had an unprecedented expansion in the last decade (Frazão, Meade, & Regmi, 2008). An interesting case in point, the share of supermarket sales in Latin America increased from 15 to 30% of national retail food sales before the 1980s to 50 to 70% in 2001, exhibiting in two decades the level of growth experienced in the US over five decades.

Together with the integration and consolidation of the agri-food industry, the globalization of food trade is changing the patterns of food production and distribution. Increased economies of scale and changes in farming and production practices are creating an environment in which both known and new foodborne diseases can become prevalent (Käferstein et al., 1997; Käferstein & Abdussalam, 1999; WHO, 2002). To cite an example, intensive animal husbandry technologies, which have helped reduce production costs, have also been a factor in the emergence of new zoonotic diseases that affect humans (WHO, 2002). Similarly, complex and extensive distribution systems may lead to widespread dissemination throughout the world of contaminated food and feed, as exemplified by the bovine spongiform encephalopathy variant Creutzfeldt-Jakob disease (BSE/vCJD) crisis in the UK (Motarjemi et al., 2001; WHO, 2002; Saker et al., 2004). Hazards can be introduced or exacerbated at any point in the food chain from the farm to the consumer's plate (WHO, 2002). In one incident, fraudulent addition of melamine, believed to have occurred at milk collection centers in China to boost apparent protein content, triggered multiple recalls due to confirmed contamination of a wide array of products containing milk or milk-derived ingredients. Contaminated products, ranging from infant formula to cookies and candy, found their way to all continents, affecting not only China, but also Singapore, Hong Kong, Japan, South Korea, Thailand, Indonesia, New Zealand, Australia, the United Kingdom, the Netherlands, France, South Africa, Tanzania, the United States of America, and Canada.

As a matter of fact, in its *Global Risks 2008* report, the World Economic Forum (WEF) Global Risk Network pointed to supply chain vulnerability as one of four emerging issues likely to impact the world economy and society in the next ten years (WEF, 2008). The report recognized that advances in technology and global logistics, combined with reduced trade barriers, have resulted in increased efficiency and historic expansion of international trade in the last two decades. However, the report also warned that extended supply chains may concentrate risks and increase vulnerabilities to disruptions.

3.2.2.2 Population Mobility Within and Across National Borders—Migration, Urbanization and Travel

Technological innovations and lower trade barriers have significantly reduced transaction costs for movements of not only goods but also people (Bruinsma, 2003). While population mobility is not a new phenomenon, the current volume, speed, and reach of travel are unprecedented (Saker et al., 2004). Cheaper and faster transportation, easier communication and the advent of the Internet have increased people's awareness and curiosity about the world and allowed them to travel more frequently and to further away places. According to the United Nations World Tourism Organization (UNWTO), the global total of international arrivals worldwide reached a new record figure of over 900 million in 2007, with leisure travel accounting for just over half of that figure (UNWTO, 2008). UNWTO's *Tourism 2020 Vision* further forecasts that international arrivals will grow to nearly 1.6 billion by the year 2020, including 378 million long-haul travelers. In the same manner as short-term travel, long-term migration has grown rapidly. In 2005, international migrants numbered 191 million (UNFPA, 2008), compared with 75 million in 1965 (UNFPA, 2003). On the even larger scale of internal migration, one billion people, representing about one sixth of the world's population, moved within their respective national borders in the mid-1980s (Saker et al., 2004).

Increased population mobility is also intimately linked to the incidence and spread of foodborne diseases, therefore adding to the globalization of food safety problems (Käferstein et al., 1997). International travelers can be exposed to infections they have not encountered before, and consequently are not immune to, such as gastroenteritis caused by *Giardia* (Saker et al., 2004). Furthermore, while incubation periods for diseases have remained the same, the virtual explosion in distance and speed of travel achieved over the past two centuries has made it possible for a traveler to be exposed to a foodborne disease in one country and expose others to that infection thousands of miles away (Käferstein et al., 1997). Depending on travel destination, risk of contracting a foodborne illness can be as high as 50%. As further evidence of the impact of this phenomenon on some countries, 80 to 90% of salmonellosis cases in Scandinavia have been attributed to international travel.

Finally, both international and internal migration combined with population growth have led to an accelerated process of urbanization, particularly in developing countries, where a number of 'megacities' counting more than 10 million inhabitants have emerged since 1945 (Saker et al., 2004). After breaking the 50% mark in 2008, the world's population living in urban areas is actually expected to reach 70% by 2050 (UN, 2008b). Intensified urbanization places heavier demands on transport, storage and preparation of food (WHO, 2002). Income growth and urban lifestyle often result in a larger share of food consumed away from home. In recent years, developing countries have witnessed a shift in food consumption from homemade foods to ready-to-eat foods, often prepared by street vendors (WHO, 2002; FAO/WHO, 2005). Conversely, consumers in developed countries spend up to 50% of their food budget on food prepared outside the home (WHO, 2002). This higher reliance on food away from home increases the potential for consumer exposure to a single source of contamination, with possible global repercussions. Particularly at risk are developing countries, which are further challenged by overcrowding, inadequate sanitation, and insufficient access to safe water and facilities for safe food preparation (WHO, 2002; Saker et al., 2004).

3.2.2.3 Changing Demographics and Globalization of Food Consumption Patterns

Adding to the accelerated urbanization process, the liberalization of international food trade and globalization of the food industry have resulted in a growing convergence of food consumption patterns across various countries and regions (Bruinsma, 2003; Frazão et al., 2008). Diets around the world are becoming increasingly similar over time. For instance, the overlap in the diets of Japan and the United States rose from only 45% in 1961 to about 70% in 1999 (Bruinsma, 2003). Furthermore, worldwide food preferences and dietary habits are mutually influenced by the increasing standardization and expansion of retail and food service chains (Frazão et al., 2008). Between 2000 and 2005, sales of packaged foods worldwide increased from US$1.095 billion to US$1.455 billion, with ready-meals registering a 45% growth in that time period (Hawkes et al., 2007).

In developing countries, rising income levels have resulted in a shift from grain-based diets to livestock-based diets (Bruinsma, 2003). This preference for meat and poultry can increase the potential for foodborne illness (WHO, 2002), especially in the case of insufficient cold chain infrastructure. In affluent economies, consumers have grown accustomed to year-round availability of a large diversity of foods, regardless of growing season or geographical location (Saker et al., 2004). Furthermore, these same consumers are raising food safety stakes by demanding fresh and minimally processed foods, with extended shelf-lives, no chemical preservatives and reduced salt and sugar content (Käferstein & Abdussalam, 1999).

Public concern about foodborne diseases has also stretched beyond national boundaries. Amidst serious food safety outbreaks and their extensive media coverage, consumers in both industrialized and developing societies share growing concerns over the risks posed by pathogens and chemical compounds in the food supply (Motarjemi et al., 2001; WHO, 2002; FAO/WHO, 2005). Rising consumer activism, long a characteristic of developed countries, is now also gaining importance in the developing world (FAO/WHO, 2005).

Compounding these trends are changes in demographic profiles affecting both developed and developing countries. Greater life expectancy, population aging, and growing numbers of immuno-compromised individuals place a higher percentage of the population at risk for foodborne illness (Käferstein & Abdussalam, 1999; WHO, 2002).

3.2.2.4 Environmental Factors—Global Climate Change

In further association with human activities, global food safety is faced with new environmental challenges. Most notably, global climate change is expected to exacerbate the growing pressure from transboundary pests and diseases due to globalization, trade and traffic (FAO, 2008b). According to the *Fourth Assessment Report* of the Intergovernmental Panel on Climate Change, global temperatures are projected to rise by 1.8 to 4°C by the end of the century (IPCC, 2007). Although the scientific evidence is not unambiguous, it may be wise to take into account that possibility may prove correct. In addition to global warming, climate change is also likely to result in more frequent extreme weather events, such as heavy precipitations and droughts (FAO, 2008c). The impact of climatic influences, particularly temperature and humidity, on the prevalence of food and waterborne diseases has already been well-documented and is cause for future concern over an escalating threat of pathogenic infections and mycotoxin contamination. For instance, weeks of elevated ambient temperature often signal increases in reported cases of salmonellosis and campylobacteriosis. Similarly, the climatic event El Niño has been responsible for increases in cholera and diarrheal disease in Peru (Käferstein & Abdussalam, 1999; FAO, 2008c). Pathogens with documented stress tolerance responses, such as enterohemorrhagic *E. coli* and *Salmonella* can also be anticipated to better compete under changing climate conditions (FAO, 2008c).

3.2.2.5 An International Regulatory Framework for the Twenty-First Century

Through the rapid and growing integration of economies and societies, food safety has thus become a transnational challenge and a shared responsibility and, as such, must be addressed on a global scale. This indisputably requires increased international cooperation in setting standards and regulations (Käferstein *et al.*, 1997). While the establishment of global food safety standards will help protect people throughout the world from the risks of foodborne illness, it will also allow them to reap the many benefits brought about by the globalization of the food trade (Motarjemi *et al.*, 2001; WHO, 2002). Access to a diverse and affordable supply of safe and high-quality foods not only contributes to a healthy and nutritionally-balanced diet, it also measurably enriches the consumers' eating experience with a wider variety of flavors and gastronomic options.

Although indirect, but equally important, trade liberalization and globalization create opportunities for developing countries to increase their foreign earned income with food products exports (WHO, 2002; FAO/WHO, 2005). The adoption and enforcement of international harmonized standards would facilitate access of these countries to more lucrative markets, which, in turn, would foster economic development and thus improve population welfare. In absence of such harmonization, export prospects can indeed become severely limited for some countries. To illustrate this point, Otsuki, Wilson, and Sewadeh (2001) analyzed the impact of changes in the EU standards for aflatoxin contamination levels on bilateral trade flows between Africa and Europe. Using trade and regulatory survey data for 15 European countries and 9 African countries between 1989 and 1998, they estimated that, while reducing health risk by about 1.4 deaths per billion a year, the new EU-harmonized standard would decrease African exports of cereals, dried fruits, and nuts to Europe by US$670 million, compared to the implementation of an international standard.[1]

Although many national governments have achieved significant progress in ensuring a safe food supply, they have often done so by developing diverse legislative and regulatory systems in response to very different circumstances which were specific to their respective food markets (Bruinsma, 2003). This long history of independent national policy-making has inevitably resulted in regulatory disparities, and thus, barriers to food trade. As the pace of globalization accelerates, the international community and world trade need a coherent and harmonized legal and regulatory framework that will address common threats and, particularly in the case of developing countries, facilitate welfare-enhancing entry into the global marketplace (Josling, Roberts, & Orden, 2004a).

3.3 ADVANCES AND ACHIEVEMENTS IN HARMONIZING FOOD SAFETY POLICY[2]

If we look back in history, formal efforts in setting international food standards can be observed in the late 1890s with the establishment of the *Codex Alimentarius Austriacus* to help regulate the movement of food in the Austro-Hungarian Empire (FAO/WHO, 2006). The International Dairy Federation, founded in 1903, can also be credited for its early involvement in developing international standards for milk and milk products. It was not until the mid-twentieth century, however, that harmonization of food standards started garnering international interest.

Most important, the Food and Agriculture Organization (FAO) and the World Health Organization (WHO) of the United Nations, formed in 1945 and 1948, respectively, received the mandate to establish international food standards addressing nutrition and human health. Following several regional efforts, such as the Latin American food code *'Código Latino-Americano de Alimentos'* proposed in 1949, and the European Codex Alimentarius *'Codex Alimentarius Europaeus'* created in 1958 under Austrian leadership, FAO and WHO established the Codex Alimentarius Commission (CAC) in 1963 to implement their Joint Food Standards Programme[3] aimed at protecting the health of consumers, ensuring fair trade practices in the food trade and promoting coordination of all food standards work undertaken by governmental and international organizations. Consisting of over 170 member countries representing 99% of the world's population, this intergovernmental standard-setting body, commonly referred to as 'Codex,' gained further prominence with the conclusion of the aforementioned Uruguay Round of Multilateral Trade Negotiations in 1994 and the implementation of the World Trade Organization (WTO), thus becoming the main harmonization instrument for food safety standards worldwide.

---

[1]A recent World Bank report shows that the actual impact of the EU-harmonized aflatoxin regulation on African exports was much lower than the original estimates due to other factors (Diaz Rios & Jaffee, 2008). Chapter 12 (Mycotoxin Management: An International Challenge) provides a more in-depth account of this topic.

[2]For the purpose of this chapter, only harmonization of food safety regulations is considered. Refer to Chapter 20 (Harmonization of International Standards) for a discussion on international harmonization of private-sector standards through the International Organization for Standardization (ISO) and the Global Food Safety Initiative (GFSI).

[3]FAO/WHO Food Standards—*Codex Alimentarius*. Available from URL: http://www.codexalimentarius.net (accessed 31 March 2009).

3.3.1 *Codex Alimentarius* and the World Trade Organization

First to deal with the liberalization of trade in agricultural products, the Uruguay Round of Multilateral Trade Negotiations, which began in Punta del Este, Uruguay in 1986 and concluded in Marrakesh, Morocco in 1994, established the World Trade Organization (WTO) to supersede the General Agreement on Tariffs and Trade (GATT) as the umbrella organization for international trade. While agreeing to reduce tariff barriers for many agricultural commodities in order to encourage free trade, countries participating in the negotiations recognized the potential for national governments to increasingly use non-tariff barriers, such as sanitary, phytosanitary and other technical requirements, as a means of discriminating against imports and disguising barriers to trade (WHO, 1998; FAO/WHO, 2006). This concern resulted in two binding multilateral Agreements relevant to food safety regulations: the Agreement on the Application of Sanitary and Phytosanitary Measures (SPS Agreement) and the Agreement on Technical Barriers to Trade (TBT Agreement).

Specifically addressing food safety and animal and plant health regulations, the SPS Agreement acknowledges that WTO Member governments have the right to take sanitary and phytosanitary measures, provided that such measures are based on scientific principles and applied only to the extent necessary to protect human, animal or plant health. These should also not arbitrarily or unjustifiably discriminate between Members where identical or similar conditions prevail (WHO, 1998). In order to harmonize sanitary and phytosanitary measures on as wide a basis as possible, SPS provisions further encourage governments to base their national requirements on international standards, guidelines and recommendations where such exist. In the case of food safety, Annex A to the SPS Agreement explicitly refers to 'the standards, guidelines and recommendations established by the Codex Alimentarius Commission relating to food additives, veterinary drug and pesticide residues, contaminants, methods of analysis and sampling, and codes and guidelines of hygienic practice.' Therefore, national measures conforming to Codex standards are presumed to be consistent with the provisions of the Agreement. While WTO Members retain the sovereign right to maintain or introduce sanitary measures resulting in stricter standards, the Agreement requires that such measures be justified and based on a scientific risk assessment taking into account risk assessment techniques developed by the relevant international organizations. In addition to setting the rights and obligations of the current 153 WTO Members, the SPS Agreement also establishes information exchange and enforcement mechanisms (Bruinsma, 2003). These include notification procedures for informing trading partners of changes in SPS measures, the establishment of an SPS committee to discuss these issues on a continuing basis, and the use of the WTO dispute settlement system for resolving in a timely manner conflicts between countries over trade-distorting barriers. Through the adoption of Codex standards as the benchmark against which national measures and regulations are evaluated, the SPS Agreement has thus served a critical role in promoting the international harmonization of food safety regulations (WHO, 1998; Motarjemi *et al.*, 2001).

The TBT Agreement, which complements the SPS Agreement by covering all other technical regulations and standards, such as packaging, marking and labeling requirements, similarly encourages countries to use international standards where appropriate. However, it does not require them to change their levels of protection as a result of standardization.[4]

---

[4]WTO. Legal Texts—The WTO Agreements. Available from URL: http://www.wto.org/english/docs_e/legal_e/legal_e.htm (accessed 31 March 2009).

As could be expected, the specific recognition of Codex standards as integral parts of the multilateral legal framework within WTO has generated considerable interest in the activities of the Codex Alimentarius Commission (FAO/WHO, 2006). Accordingly, the Commission has observed a significant increase in attendance, particularly by developing countries. Aware of its critical role in the harmonization of national regulations, Codex acknowledges the importance for each country to take an active role in Codex's standard-setting activities (WHO, 1998; FAO/WHO, 2006).

While the responsibility for developing standards rests with the Codex Alimentarius Commission and its subsidiary bodies, independent expert committees established by FAO and WHO provide the essential scientific basis for the CAC's work by undertaking the function of risk assessment. These groups, which publications act as international references, are the Joint FAO/WHO Expert Committee on Food Additives (JECFA), the Joint FAO/WHO Meetings on Pesticide Residues (JMPR) and the Joint FAO/WHO Expert Meetings on Microbiological Risk Assessment (JEMRA) (FAO/WHO, 2006).

From its inception, the Codex Alimentarius Commission has adhered to the principle of science-based standards, adopting close to 300 standards on commodities and food safety issues, over 3000 maximum limits for pesticide residues and veterinary drugs, over 1000 food additives provisions, dozens of guidelines for contaminants, as well as codes of practice to prevent contamination and various texts on food hygiene which have become global benchmarks (FAO/WHO, 2006; UN, 2008c). Early on during the Uruguay Round negotiations, the Commission realized the increased legal relevance that the SPS Agreement would confer to the Codex standards and consequently set out to examine and define more clearly its standard-setting procedures (Jukes, 2000). After first reconfirming the fundamental role of science in its standardization work at the 1991 FAO/WHO Conference on Food Standards, Codex also came to recognize that other more subjective but legitimate factors, such as consumer concerns, technological need, and ethical and cultural considerations should be integrated into its decision-making processes. This eventually led to Codex's adoption in 2003 of the risk analysis framework encompassing three interrelated components: risk assessment, risk management and risk communication (FAO/WHO, 2006).

European consumer objections to Genetically Modified (GM) foods and hormone-treated beef and their impact on EU food safety regulations give some appreciation for the importance of these other legitimate factors (OLFs) and the challenge of effective risk communication (Motarjemi *et al.*, 2001; Verbeke, Frewer, Scholderer, & De Brabander, 2007). The latter case bears particular significance, as the first WTO dispute involving the SPS Agreement centered on the long-running feud between the EU and the US on growth promoting hormones in beef cattle (Bruinsma, 2003). Soon after their adoption by Codex in 1995, the Maximum Residue Limits (MRLs) for meat hormones served as a reference point in the US challenge to the EU's hormones ban (Jukes, 2000). The dispute was officially resolved through the WTO settlement system in favor of the complainant on the basis of insufficient scientific justification. However, the EU continued to ban hormone-treated beef and consequently suffered retaliatory tariffs. Another approach could have hardly been expected from European governments seeking public reassurance within a context of strong consumer resistance, further exacerbated by the BSE crisis and other food scares (Jukes, 2000; Josling *et al.*, 2004a). This official resolution, which in essence remains unsatisfactory for all parties, implies practical limits to the role of science and scientific consensus in securing regulatory convergence when differences in public perceptions prevail (Josling *et al.*, 2004a). Given that consumer risk perception might differ substantially from that of experts, it also further illustrates the necessity for effective risk communication strategies (Verbeke *et al.*, 2007).

3.3.2 Additional Harmonization Efforts through Regional Economic Integration and Bilateral Agreements

In conjunction with global trade integration under the auspices of WTO, the trend towards regional economic integration has also encouraged harmonization of food safety regulations within various geographical regions.

Perhaps most notably, Europe has experienced a long history of regional integration, underpinned by a strong supranational institutional framework (McKay, Armengol, & Pineau, 2005). Since the founding *Treaty of Rome* in 1957, the European Economic Community—which later became the European Union (EU)—has placed particular emphasis on agriculture (van der Meulen & van der Velde, 2008). At first, mainly directed at the creation of an internal common market for food products, European food policy underwent a first period of harmonization through vertical legislation (i.e. standards of composition), followed in the mid-1980s by a second period of harmonization through horizontal legislation. In the mid-1990s, the BSE crisis and other food scares led to the development of a third and new phase of EU food law aimed at assuring high levels of food safety. The entry into force of the cornerstone Regulation (EC) No 178/2002, which set out the general principles of food law and established an independent European Food Safety Authority (EFSA), forms the basis for food and feed legislation in the now 27-member bloc.

The North American Free Trade Agreement (NAFTA), encompassing Canada, Mexico and the USA, offers another example of regional alliance, albeit with a lower degree of formal institutional cooperation than the EU (McKay *et al.*, 2005). Overlapping with the Uruguay Round negotiations, the NAFTA negotiations raised similar concerns over the potential for arbitrary health and safety rules to serve protectionist ends (Bruinsma, 2003). As a result, the three trading partners included into NAFTA an early version of what eventually became the SPS Agreement.

Among the more ambitious regional initiatives in the area of plurilateral coordination of food regulations is the Asia-Pacific Economic Cooperation (APEC) process (Bruinsma, 2003; Josling *et al.*, 2004b). APEC considered establishing an APEC Food System, which would have included both food safety and trade liberalization instruments. The food safety part of the program has yielded a framework, the APEC Food Mutual Recognition Agreement, which builds on the SPS Agreement and allows countries to negotiate agreements to facilitate food trade in the Asia-Pacific region.

In the Southwest Pacific, the bilateral Australia-New Zealand Closer Economic Relations Trade Agreement (ANZCERTA), commonly known as CER, led to the formation of a bi-national food agency (Bruinsma, 2003). Since 1996, these two countries regulate food safety jointly through the Australia New Zealand Food Authority (ANZFA), later renamed Food Standards Australia New Zealand (FSANZ).

At the other end of the spectrum of bilateral approaches to food regulations is the attempt to use the transatlantic partnership between the United States and the EU (Bruinsma, 2003). While a number of potentially significant agreements have been negotiated, these tend to be agreements for the mutual recognition of testing and certification, rather than the recognition of the standards of the transatlantic partner. Particularly of note are the growing and unresolved trade tensions, which have ensued between the world's two largest economies over GM food regulations (Patterson & Josling, 2001). Nevertheless, both partners have long recognized the need for scientific cooperation to better protect public health. In 2007, the US Food and Drug Administration (FDA) and the European Food Safety Authority (EFSA) signed a landmark agreement to facilitate the sharing of confidential scientific information in the area of assessing food safety risk (FDA/EFSA, 2007). In this first formal step lies the promise of a closer collaboration that could help forestall future regulatory discrepancies.

3.4 THE GLOBAL HARMONIZATION[5] INITIATIVE

No matter which part of the world, consumers should benefit from adequate protection against foodborne hazards (WHO, 1998; Motarjemi et al., 2001). Despite substantial progress towards harmonization of food safety regulations, rapid globalization of the food supply, changing demographics and consumer preferences, emerging threats, and new scientific developments persistently expose weaknesses and exacerbate shortcomings in a less-than-cohesive international framework.

3.4.1 The Launch of the Global Harmonization Initiative

During a meeting between a number of food scientists at the occasion of the 2004 Annual Meeting of the Institute of Food Technologists (IFT), representatives of the International Division of IFT and of the European Federation of Food Science and Technology (EFFoST) discussed some of the adverse consequences stemming from disparities between national food safety laws and regulations (Lelieveld, Keener, & Boisrobert, 2006).

Perhaps most worrisome in a context of growing food insecurity are discrepancies in national regulatory thresholds for chemical residues and contaminants. These may lead to the undue destruction of large quantities of food or cause serious barriers to trade between countries (Keener & Lelieveld, 2004). In particular, food safety regulations may expressly prohibit the presence of certain harmful chemical substances in foods—the so-called 'zero tolerance' requirement (Lelieveld et al., 2006). As the precision and sensitivity of methods of analysis and assay continue to improve, substances detectable many years ago in parts per thousand or in parts per million are now determined in parts per billion or even in parts per trillion (Hulse, 1995; Lelieveld & Keener, 2007). Zero-tolerance of a contaminant therefore is not an absolute value but rather depends on analytical sensitivity. Although initially devised to protect public health, such regulatory provisions prove increasingly unmanageable, making a case for proper scientific risk assessment methodologies and the use of controls commensurate with the level of risk to consumers (Hanekamp, Frapporti, & Olieman, 2003).

Equally important in the current climate of concern about food safety is the challenge posed by the introduction of new technologies (WHO, 2002). While some new technologies might increase agricultural production and make food safer, their usefulness and safety must be demonstrated in a transparent manner to warrant consumer acceptance. In response to growing consumer demand for safe, fresh, and minimally processed foods, the food industry, often in conjunction with academia and governmental institutions, has invested tremendous research efforts in the development of innovative non-thermal preservation technologies (Lelieveld et al., 2006; Lelieveld & Keener, 2007). As these technologies become realistic commercial options, differences in approval procedures and safety evaluation protocols between countries often act as roadblocks to their introduction in the market (Fister Gale, 2005). Regrettably, costs and efforts associated with trying to comply

[5]Please note the US spelling of 'harmonization' as a result of GHI's inception during a meeting in the USA.

with sometimes duplicative, conflicting, and inconsistent national standards, may deter the food industry from applying these newly developed capabilities on an international scale. Food companies are indeed generally reluctant to incur increased overhead, unnecessary expenditures or bear the brunt of investing in new food safety technology that is recognized by regulatory authorities in only limited markets. Similarly, worldwide development of novel or functional foods catering to rising numbers of health-conscious consumers faces a complex and disparate international regulatory environment (Lupien, 2002). Having to prove safety only once, without undue repetition and according to globally agreed methods, would significantly reduce such hurdles and result in greater availability and faster time-to-market of new beneficial and desirable food products and technologies (Lelieveld & Keener, 2007).

In an attempt to eliminate hurdles and impediments to scientific advancement in food technology, EFFoST and the International Division of IFT, in cooperation with Food Safety Magazine and Elsevier, came to a decision to launch the Global Harmonization Initiative[6] (GHI) at this very meeting. Soon thereafter, many scientific organizations joined and supported the initiative, including the International Union of Food Science and Technology (IUFoST), the National Center for Food Safety and Technology (NCFST), the International Association for Cereal Science and Technology (ICC), the Food Chemistry Division of the European Association for Chemical and Molecular Sciences (EuCheMS–FCD), the European Hygienic Engineering and Design Group (EHEDG), as well as many universities around the world.

Initiated to help promote the worldwide harmonization of food safety regulations and legislation, GHI strongly believes that developing scientific consensus on key food safety matters is imperative to sustaining the integrity of the global food supply. Consequently, this organization proposes to facilitate discussion, globally, of the scientific issues that buttress the decisions made by individual governments and international regulatory bodies. By achieving consensus on the science of food regulations and legislation, GHI aims to ensure the global availability of safe and wholesome food products for all consumers. This concept was embodied in the first draft of the GHI charter, during its first workshop in April 2005 (Lelieveld *et al.*, 2006). The draft charter was developed and published on the GHI website for comments. The finalized version of the charter is provided in Figure 3.1. It is important to note that GHI will not attempt to effect direct change in any food safety legislation or regulation. Instead, GHI intends to provide a platform and a mechanism for individual food scientists and technologists worldwide to reach a consensus on the science that underpins such policies. It should be further noted that GHI does not seek consensus between organizations and governments, but between scientists and technologists, globally, regardless of their affiliations. GHI's philosophy is that once global consensus is obtained and published, stakeholders will use such information to achieve the desired changes.

Furthermore, GHI clearly does not purport to compete with the activities of the Codex Alimentarius Commission or its FAO/WHO expert bodies, nor does it purport to duplicate their essential work. Rather, the organization strives to develop into an international scientific expert resource and anticipates that its independent scientists and expert members will contribute tremendously via white papers and similar instruments to the discourse required to provide a transparent and unbiased scientific basis for harmonization.

---

[6]For additional information, please visit the Global Harmonization Initiative website (www.globalharmonization.net).

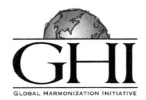

"Achieving consensus on the science of food regulations and legislation to ensure the global availability of safe and wholesome food products for all consumers."

CHARTER

The goal of the initiative is to ensure the global availability of safe and wholesome food products for all consumers.

To achieve this, undue barriers to free trade that masquerade as food safety protections must be vanquished. Such barriers include differences in regulations and legislation between countries globally. The international scientific community must, therefore, work towards achieving global consensus on the science underpinning food regulations and legislation. This will be achieved through attainment of the following objectives:

1. Identifying relevant scientific organizations.
2. Inviting and encouraging the participation of these scientific societies in the global harmonization initiative and inviting their members to join in this activity in their field of expertise.
3. Identifying relevant non-scientific stakeholders.
4. Establishing effective communication between non-scientific and scientific organizations.
5. Inviting all stakeholders (organizations and individuals) to identify and submit key issues requiring attention.
6. Prioritizing key issues with the subsequent formation of working groups to draft white papers or consensus statements regarding the scientific validity of these issues.
7. Steering working groups to assess the best available evidence and discuss their findings with the scientific community, working towards building consensus.
8. Publishing results on a per issue basis in journals, magazines and newspapers.
9. Publishing collections of resulting consensus statements in book form.
10. Presenting results and participating in appropriate conferences.
11. Making results available to all stakeholders, particularly those responsible for developing or amending regulations and legislation, global communicators, risk managers and assessors.

All of these will be done in an open, transparent manner, to avoid bias or the appearance of bias, political or otherwise.

FIGURE 3.1   Charter of the Global Harmonization Initiative (GHI).

3.4.2 GHI Association

In October 2007, the initiative gained formal legal status as a non-governmental, non-profit association, and was registered in Vienna, Austria as *'GHI Association—Globale Harmonisierungs Initiative für Gesetze und Verordnungen im Bereich Lebensmittel'*. The GHI goal of *'Achieving consensus on the science of food regulations and legislation to ensure the global availability of safe and wholesome food products for all consumers'* was carefully incorporated in the Constitution[7] (Lelieveld, 2009). Similarly, the GHI Executive Committee painstakingly ensured that the German translation and other changes necessary to comply with Austrian law did by no means alter the objectives as described in the Charter.

Figure 3.2 outlines the organizational structure[8] of the Association. Until elections take place following the procedure specified in the Constitution, the Executive Committee is currently represented by Huub Lelieveld (President,[9] The Netherlands), Larry Keener (Vice-President, USA), Gerhard Schleining (Austria), Sangsuk Oh (Korea), Vishweshwaraiah Prakash (India) and Christine Boisrobert (USA).

From its inception, GHI has recognized that impartiality of the scientific consensus process would be an essential requirement to enable cooperation with scientists from all over the world. This has led to the establishment of the Supervisory Board, which is also firmly embedded in the Constitution. Consisting of representatives of independent scientific member organizations across the globe, its main mission is to safeguard the impartiality, integrity and overall transparency of the consensus process (Lelieveld *et al.*, 2006). Dr. Roland Poms, representing ICC (the International Association for Cereal Science and Technology, a scientifically independent organization with its office in Vienna), has accepted to chair this Board, with the first task to expand the Board to meet its objective.

Furthermore, GHI intends to expand individual membership[10] principally through sister scientific organizations, also using the services of IUFoST, of which IFT is an Adhering Body and EFFoST is the European Grouping (Keener & Lelieveld, 2004). Since 2004, GHI has made great strides in garnering interest and support within the international scientific community. Both EFFoST and IFT have formed Special Interest Groups (SIGs) to support the activities of GHI. To better manage the increasing amount of correspondence about global harmonization, the responsibilities for communication have been divided geographically between members of the Executive Committee and members of the Special Interest Groups to cover Asia, North America, Latin America, Europe and Africa. Meanwhile it is clear that more scientists are willing to assist with effective communication in the regional activities, such as in the Middle East, South Africa, Russia, former Yugoslavia, Lebanon and Iran.

3.4.3 Meetings and Workshops

With the support and participation of its individual members and member organizations, GHI has convened or participated in various symposia, seminars, workshops and meetings[11] in Chicago (USA), New Orleans (USA), Sofia (Bulgaria), Paris (France), Orlando (USA), Nantes (France), Cork (Ireland), The Hague (The Netherlands), Lisbon (Portugal), Goa (India), Bologna (Italy), Seoul (Korea), Cavtat (Croatia), Shanghai (China) and Ljubljana (Slovenia).

---

[7]The GHI Constitution ('Vereinsstatuten') and corresponding English translation are posted on the GHI website (www.globalharmonization.net).

[8]While the Austrian legal terminology used in the Constitution might differ, GHI's actual structure remains identical to the one posted on the GHI website and shown in Figure 3.2 (see http://www.globalharmonization.net/structure.htm).

[9]Austrian law requires a 'President' and a 'Vice-President' in lieu of 'Co-Chairs'.

[10]Food science and technology professionals can presently apply online for an 'individual scientist membership' at http://www.globalharmonization.net/applicationform.htm.

[11]Reports on these events and presentations can be found on the GHI website (www.globalharmonization.net).

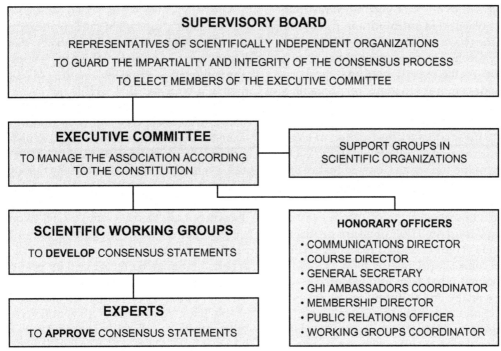

FIGURE 3.2   GHI Structure.

During these meetings, members were invited to formulate approaches to critically evaluate scientific evidence used to underpin existing regulations in the areas of product composition, processing operations, and technologies or measures designed to prevent foodborne illness. At the time of writing, GHI is planning to hold additional meetings in Amsterdam (The Netherlands), Prague (Czechoslovakia), Anaheim (USA), Copenhagen (Denmark), and Mumbai (India).

3.4.4 Working Groups

Building on the outcome of previous workshops and meetings, participants of the workshop in Lisbon, held in conjunction with the 2007 joint EFFoST-EHEDG Conference, selected four global issues to serve as examples for the proposed GHI consensus process. These issues, which respectively address microbiological food safety, toxicological safety, food preservation and harmonization of test protocols, led to the establishment of the following working groups (WGs) (Lelieveld, 2009):

Working Group on '*Listeria monocytogenes* in ready-to-eat (RTE) meals': There are significant differences in food safety requirements for *Listeria monocytogenes* in ready-to-eat (RTE) meals. While, for instance, the EU has set a maximum level of 100 colony-forming units per gram (cfu/g), the US requires its absence in 25 grams of food. Similarly, the microbiological methods used differ between countries. Clearly, a scientific consensus on what constitutes a safe maximum level and what test protocol should be used to determine that level, is essential for international trade of RTE foods. For a more detailed discussion, refer to Chapter 10 (Global Harmonization of the Control of Microbiological Risks).

Working Group on 'Safe maximum residue levels of selected antibiotics in food': Many countries have adopted a zero-tolerance policy for the presence of certain antibiotics in food. As the sensitivity of analytical methods continues to improve, probability of detecting minute trace amounts of antibiotics in the food supply increases. This can lead to the mandatory destruction of large volumes of food, as illustrated in the 2006 ruling of the European Court of Justice. The working group will consider the application of scientific risk assessment methodology to address this issue.

Working Group on 'High pressure processing of foods': High Pressure Processing (HPP) has become a fairly mature food processing technology. It has been implemented commercially and sufficient research has been conducted in the US, EU and Japan. However, regulatory requirements for HPP are still lacking or differ between countries. Particularly, the question of what process conditions will be adequate to ensure the safety of HPP-sterilized foods needs to be answered.

Working Group on 'Toxicological test protocols': Currently, toxicity is tested using whole animal models and incompetent liver cells. However, evidence has been accumulated showing that these tests are often not relevant to humans. Substances showing toxicity using these tests may be nontoxic to humans, while substances that are shown to be safe may actually be toxic. In contrast, new methods, using metabolically competent liver cells, can produce reliable results and would eliminate the need for animal testing. The objective of this WG is to achieve a consensus on such a method. This subject is not only pertinent to food producers, but also manufacturers of food processing equipment and packaging materials to establish the safety of food contact materials.

Presently, there is also much interest in setting up additional working groups on 'Nanotechnology and food,' 'Generally Recognized As Safe (GRAS) status,' the 'Precautionary principle' and 'Mycotoxins.' It should be noted that GHI is not to decide on WGs. In principle, any stakeholder group may start a WG. Each WG will collect and evaluate available scientific evidence, and circulate findings among food scientists worldwide for debate and comments. Once a scientifically founded consensus proposal has been developed and drafted, it may be submitted to GHI. That consensus document may then be sent by GHI to qualified subject-matter experts, in as many countries as possible, for review and final approval. These experts first must be recognized by peer consensus as experts in their field and be sanctioned by the GHI Supervisory Board. The intended result of this iterative process is a scientific consensus statement to be available for regulators around the world.

3.5 CONCLUSION

GHI anticipates that while developing global consensus on the science of food regulations and legislation will help narrow regulatory differences, it may also help focus food safety research on areas where supportive scientific evidence is currently lacking. Elimination of regulatory discrepancies will reduce and hopefully in time prevent the undue destruction of food. Furthermore, it will make it more attractive for the private sector to invest in food safety research and development, consequently strengthening the competitiveness of each nation's food industry and of the industries supplying the food sector (Larson Bricher, 2005). Harmonizing global regulations will aid in the uptake and application of new technologies as well as encourage the food industry to invest in new tools to enhance the safety, availability and quality of the food supply for consumers worldwide.

While global harmonization of food safety regulations is a definite challenge to the twenty-first century, it has now become an overriding necessity in an era of rapid globalization (Motarjemi *et al.*, 2001). Particularly in light of the current food crisis (FAO, 2008a), GHI recognizes that respecting, protecting and fulfilling the right of each individual to safe food requires a global and sustained collective effort by all stakeholders, including the international scientific community.

References

Bruinsma J. (Ed.). (2003). *World agriculture: Towards 2015/2030—an FAO perspective*. London: Earthscan Publications Ltd.

Chopra, M., Galbraith, S., & Darnton-Hill, I. (2002). A global response to a global problem: The epidemic of overnutrition. *B World Health Organ, 80*(12), 952–958.

Coyle, W., Hall, W., & Ballenger, N. (2001). Transportation technology and the rising share of US perishable food trade. In A. Regmi (Ed.), *Changing structure of global food consumption and trade*. WRS01-1, (pp. 31–40). Washington, DC: Economic Research Service, US Department of Agriculture.

Diakosavvas, D. (2001). *The Uruguay Round Agreement on Agriculture: An evaluation of its implementation in OECD countries*. Paris: Organisation for Economic Co-operation and Development.

Diaz Rios, L.B., & Jaffee, S. (2008). *Barrier, catalyst, or distraction? Standards, competitiveness, and Africa's groundnut exports to Europe*. Agriculture and Rural Development Discussion Paper 39. Washington, DC: World Bank.

FAO. (1997). *Report of the World Food Summit, 13–17 November 1996*. WFS 96/REP. Rome: Food and Agriculture Organization of the United Nations. Online. Available at: http://www.fao.org/wfs/index_en.htm (accessed 31 March 2009).

FAO. (2003). *Trade reforms and food security—conceptualizing the linkages*. Rome: Food and Agriculture Organization of the United Nations.

FAO. (2004). *Globalization of food systems in developing countries: Impact on food security and nutrition*. FAO Food and Nutrition Paper 83. Rome: Food and Agriculture Organization of the United Nations.

FAO. (2007). *The state of food and agriculture 2007—paying farmers for environmental services*. Rome: Food and Agriculture Organization of the United Nations.

FAO. (2008a). *The state of food insecurity in the world 2008—high food prices and food security—threats and opportunities*. Rome: Food and Agriculture Organization of the United Nations.

FAO. (2008b). *High-level conference on world food security: The challenges of climate change and bioenergy*. Report of the Conference. Rome, 3–5 June 2008. HLC/08/REP.

FAO. (2008c). *Climate change: Implications for food safety*. Rome: Food and Agriculture Organization of the United Nations.

FAO/WHO. (1992). *International conference on nutrition—world declaration and plan of action for nutrition*. Rome: Food and Agriculture Organization of the United Nations and World Health Organization of the United Nations.

FAO/WHO. (2005). *Regional conference on food safety for Africa*. Final Report. Harare, 3–6 October 2005. Rome: Food and Agriculture Organization of the United Nations.

FAO/WHO. (2006). *Understanding the codex alimentarius* (3rd ed.). Rome: World Health Organization and Food and Agriculture Organization of the United Nations.

FDA/EFSA. (2007). EFSA and FDA Strengthen Cooperation in Food Safety Science. *FDA News*. 2 July 2007. Online. Available at: http://www.fda.gov/ (accessed 31 March 2009).

Fister Gale, S. (2005). Industry waits for green light on harmonized food safety standards. *Food Safety Magazine* (October/November), 42–49.

Frazão, E., Meade, B., & Regmi, A. (2008). Converging patterns in global food consumption and food delivery systems. *Amber Waves, 6*(1), 22–29.

Hanekamp, J. C., Frapporti, G., & Olieman, K. (2003). Chloramphenicol, food safety and precautionary thinking in Europe. *Environmental Liability, 6*, 209–221.

Hawkes, C., Chopra, M., Friel, S., Lang, T., & Thow, A.M. (2007) *Globalization, food and nutrition transitions*. WHO Commission on Social Determinants of Health. Ottawa: Globalization Knowledge Network. Online. Available at: http://www.who.int/social_determinants/resources/gkn_hawkes.pdf (accessed 31 March 2009).

Hulse, J. H. (1995). *Science, agriculture, and food security*. Ottawa: National Research Council Canada, NRC Research Press.

IPCC. (2007). *IPCC fourth assessment report: Climate change 2007—synthesis report*. Geneva: Intergovernmental Panel on Climate Change.

Josling, T., Roberts, D., & Orden, D. (2004a). *Food regulation and trade: Toward a safe and open global system—an overview and synopsis*. American Agricultural Economics Association (New Name 2008: Agricultural and Applied Economics Association), 2004 Annual Meeting, Denver, 1–4 August.

Josling, T., Roberts, D., & Orden, D. (2004b). *Food regulation and trade: Toward a safe and open global system*.

Washington, DC: Peterson Institute for International Economics.

Jukes, D. (2000). The role of science in international food standards. *Food Control*, *11*(3), 181–194.

Käferstein, F., & Abdussalam, M. (1999). Food safety in the 21st century. *B World Health Organ*, *77*(4), 347–351.

Käferstein, F. K., Motarjemi, Y., & Bettcher, D. W. (1997). Foodborne disease control: A transnational challenge. *Emerging Infectious Diseases*, *3*(4), 503–510.

Keener, L., & Lelieveld, H. (2004). Global harmonisation of food legislation. *Trends in Food Science Technology*, *15*, 583–584.

Larson Bricher, J. (2005). Harmonisation: A green light for food safety? *International Food Ingredients*, *5*, 107–109.

Lelieveld, H. (2009). Progress with the global harmonization initiative. *Trends in Food Science Technology*, *20*, S82–S84.

Lelieveld, H., & Keener, L. (2007). Global harmonization of food regulations and legislation—the global harmonization initiative. *Trends in Food Science Technology*, *18*, S15–S19.

Lelieveld, H., Keener, L., & Boisrobert, C. (2006). Global harmonisation of food regulations and legislation—the global harmonization initiative. *New Food*, *4*, 58–59.

Lupien, J. R. (2002). Implications for food regulations of novel food: Safety and labeling. *Asia Pacific Journal of Clinical Nutrition*, *11*(S6), S224–S229.

McKay, J., Armengol, M. A., & Pineau, G. (Eds). (2005). *Regional economic integration in a global framework*. Frankfurt: European Central Bank.

Motarjemi, Y., van Schothorst, M., & Käferstein, F. (2001). Future challenges in global harmonization of food safety legislation. *Food Control*, *12*, 339–346.

Otsuki, T., Wilson, J. S., & Sewadeh, M. (2001). Saving two in a billion: Quantifying the trade effect of European food safety standards on African exports. *Food Policy*, *26*, 495–514.

Patterson, L.A., & Josling, T. (2001). *Biotechnology regulatory policy in the United States and the European Union: Source of transatlantic trade conflict or opportunity for cooperation?* European Forum Working Paper. Stanford University, Institute for International Studies.

Saker, L., Lee, K., Cannito, B., Gilmore, A., & Campbell-Lendrum, D. (2004). *Globalization and infectious diseases: A review of the linkages*. Social, Economic and Behavioural Research, Special Topics No.3. TDR/STR/SEB/ST/04.2, Geneva: TDR, World Health Organization of the United Nations.

UN. (2000). *United Nations Millennium Declaration*. A/RES/55/2. Online. Available at: http://www.un.org/millennium/declaration/ares552e.pdf (accessed 31 March 2009).

UN. (2006). *Report of the Special Rapporteur on the right to food*. E/CN.4/2006/44. United Nations Commission on Human Rights. Online. Available at: http://www.unhcr.org/refworld/docid/45377b1b0.html (accessed 31 March 2009).

UN. (2007). *World population prospects—the 2006 revision—highlights*. New York: United Nations Department of Economic and Social Affairs.

UN. (2008a). *The millennium development goals report 2008*. New York: United Nations Department of Economic and Social Affairs.

UN. (2008b). *World urbanization prospects—the 2007 revision—executive summary*. New York: United Nations Department of Economic and Social Affairs.

UN. (2008c). *Agriculture: Report of the Secretary-General*. E/CN.17/2008/3. United Nations Commission on Sustainable Development. Online. Available at: http://www.un.org/esa/sustdev/csd/csd16/documents/sgreport_3.pdf (accessed 31 March 2009).

UN. (2008d). *Goal 1: Eradicate extreme poverty and hunger—fact sheet*. Online. Available at: http://www.un.org/millenniumgoals/2008highlevel/pdf/newsroom/Goal%201%20FINAL.pdf (accessed 31 March 2009).

UNFPA. (2003). *State of world population 2003*. New York: United Nations Population Fund.

UNFPA. (2008). *State of world population 2008*. New York: United Nations Population Fund.

UNWTO. (2008). *Tourism highlights (2008 ed.)*. Online. Available at: http://www.unwto.org/facts/eng/pdf/highlights/UNWTO_Highlights08_en_HR.pdf (accessed 31 March 2009).

van der Meulen, B., & van der Velde, M. (2008). *European food law handbook*. Wageningen: Wageningen Academic Publishers.

Verbeke, W., Frewer, L. J., Scholderer, J., & De Brabander, H. F. (2007). Why consumers behave as they do with respect to food safety and risk information. *Analytica Chimica Acta*, *586*, 2–7.

WEF. (2008). *Global risks 2008—a global risk network report*. Geneva: World Economic Forum.

WHO. (1998). *Food safety and globalization of trade in food—a challenge to the public health sector*. WHO/FSF/FOS/97.8 Rev 1. Geneva: World Health Organization of the United Nations.

WHO. (2002). *Global strategy for food safety: Safer food for better health*. Geneva: World Health Organization of the United Nations.

4

A Simplified Guide to Understanding and Using Food Safety Objectives and Performance Objectives

International Commission on Microbiological Specifications for Foods[1]

4.1 INTRODUCTION

Diseases caused by foodborne pathogens constitute a worldwide public health problem and preventing them is a major goal of societies.

Microbiological foodborne diseases are typically caused by bacteria or their metabolites, parasites, virus or toxins. The importance of different foodborne diseases varies between countries depending on foods consumed, food processing, preparation, handling, storage techniques

[1]www.icmsf.org

© 2010 by The International Commission on Microbiological Specifications for Foods (ICMSF). All rights of reproduction in any form reserved.

employed, and sensitivity of the population. While the total elimination of foodborne disease remains an unattainable goal, both government public health managers and industry are committed to reducing the incidence of illness due to contaminated food. However, reducing the number of illnesses will always have a cost to society. 'Cost' includes money as well as considerations of culture, eating habits, etc. For example, banning a particular food commodity, such as unpasteurized milk, may be acceptable to some countries, but not to others. All countries aim at reducing foodborne illness; however, most countries have not stated explicitly to what degree they would like to reduce the number of foodborne illnesses in their country. Also, they will have different opinions about how they wish to balance costs with the reduction in foodborne illnesses.

Countries have traditionally attempted to improve food safety by setting microbiological criteria for raw or for finished processed products. However, the frequency and extent of sampling used in traditional food testing programs may not provide a high degree of consumer protection. In most cases, a microbiological criterion has been set without estimating its effect on reducing the risk of foodborne disease. Sometimes microbiological criteria established by national governments for different foods have been viewed by other countries as barriers to international trade, if a stricter level is imposed than the international level for foods in trade. More than 100 countries have signed the World Trade Organization's 'Sanitary and Phytosanitary (SPS) Agreement' (WTO, 1994). This agreement states that 'whilst a country has the sovereign right to decide on the degree of protection it wishes for its citizens, it must provide, if required, the scientific evidence on which this level of protection rests.' It follows that if a country sets a microbiological criterion—or any other limit—for a particular health hazard in a particular food product, it must be able to explain, based on scientific data,

consideration of risk and societal considerations, the rationale and justification for the criterion. Another WTO agreement, the 'Technical Barriers to Trade (TBT) Agreement' (WTO, 1995), also requires that a country must not ask for a higher degree of safety for imported goods than it does for goods produced in its own country.

4.2 GOOD PRACTICES AND HAZARD ANALYSIS CRITICAL CONTROL POINT

Realizing the many shortcomings and lack of food safety assurance provided by traditional inspection and sampling/testing of lots, the concept of Hazard Analysis Critical Control Point (HACCP) was developed in the early 1970s. The HACCP concept has provided great improvements in the production of safe foods. The goal of HACCP is to focus on the hazards in a particular food commodity that are reasonably likely to affect public health if left uncontrolled, and to design food products, processing, commercialization, preparation and use conditions that control those hazards. To be successful, HACCP needs to build on good practices such as good agricultural practices (GAPs) and good hygienic practices (GHPs), which minimize the occurrence of hazards in the product and the production environment. HACCP involves an assessment of hazards in a particular production sequence and defines steps where control measures that are critical for the safety of a product should be taken. Also, it will state limits, monitoring procedures and corrective actions. However, it is plant/factory specific and does not directly link the effectiveness of such measures to an expected level of health protection (e.g. a reduction in the number of foodborne illnesses occurring in a country).

4.3 SETTING PUBLIC HEALTH GOALS—THE CONCEPT OF APPROPRIATE LEVELS OF PROTECTION

During the past decade, there has been increased interest and effort in developing tools to more effectively link the requirements of food safety programs with their expected public health impact. This chapter introduces two such tools: the 'Food Safety Objective' (FSO) and the 'Performance Objective' (PO) (ICMSF, 2005; CAC, 2007a). These can be used to communicate food safety requirements to industry, trade partners, consumers and other countries. Good practices and the HACCP system remain essential food safety management tools for achieving FSO or PO standards.

Setting goals for public health is the right and responsibility of governments. These goals should specify the maximum number of harmful bacteria that may be present in a food. Where possible, the determination of this number should be based on scientific and societal factors. Costs may include industry costs for reformulation and changes in processing, consumer costs due to increased prices, or reduced availability of certain products, and regulatory costs in terms of surveillance.

In many countries, governments rely on disease and food surveillance data in combination with expert advice on epidemiology, food microbiology and food technology to evaluate which types and numbers of harmful microorganisms in foods will cause disease. The level of risk can be expressed in a qualitative way (e.g. high, medium or low risk), or where possible, as the number of cases of foodborne disease per number of people per year. Particularly in developing countries, disease surveillance data are limited or not available at all. In such instances, estimates of the risk level have to be based on clinical information available (e.g. how many stool samples have been found to contain salmonellae) in combination with results from microbiological surveys of foods, evaluations of the types of foods that are produced, how they are produced, and how they are stored, prepared and used. A few countries may use scientific techniques such as Quantitative Microbiological Risk Assessment (QMRA) to estimate the risk of illnesses using detailed knowledge of the relationship between the number of microorganisms in foods and the occurrence of foodborne diseases.

Whatever method is used to estimate the risk of foodborne illness, the next step is to decide whether this risk can be tolerated or needs to be reduced. The level of risk that a society is willing to accept is referred to as the 'Appropriate Level of Protection' (ALOP). Importing countries with stricter requirements for a particular hazard (e.g. harmful bacteria) may be asked to determine a value for the ALOP according to the SPS agreement. When a country is willing to accept the current risk of illnesses, that level is the ALOP. However, most countries will wish to lower the incidence of foodborne disease and may set targets for future ALOPs. For instance, the current level of listeriosis could be 6 per million people per year and a country may wish to reduce this to 3 per million people per year.

4.4 A FOOD SAFETY OBJECTIVE

When a government expresses public health goals relative to the incidence of disease, this does not provide food processors, producers, handlers, retailers or trade partners with information about what they need to do to reach this lower level of illness. To be meaningful, the targets for food safety set by governments need to be translated into parameters that can be assessed by government agencies and used by food producers to process foods. The concepts of FSOs and POs have been proposed to

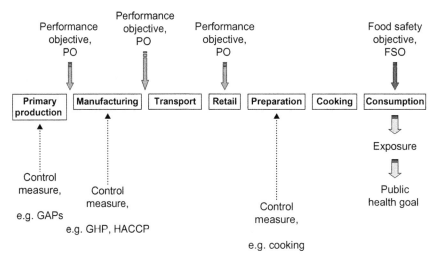

FIGURE 4.1 Model food chain indicating the position of a food safety objective and derived performance objectives.

serve this purpose. The position of these concepts appearing in the food chain can be seen in Figure 4.1.

An FSO (CAC, 2007b) is 'the maximum frequency and/or concentration of a hazard in a food at the time of consumption that provides or contributes to the appropriate level of (health) protection (ALOP).' It transforms a public health goal to a concentration and/or frequency (level) of a hazard in a particular food. The FSO sets a target for the food chain to reach, but does not specify how the target is to be achieved. Hence, the FSO gives flexibility to the food chain to use different operations and processing techniques that best suit their situation, as long as the maximum hazard level specified at consumption is not exceeded. For instance, milk is typically rendered safe by heat processing; however, in the future this may also be achieved by other technologies. This is important in international trade since different techniques may be used in different countries. The 'equivalence' of these techniques in reaching a particular level of safety must be evaluated to ensure consumer protection without imposing an unjustified barrier to trade.

4.5 A PERFORMANCE OBJECTIVE

For some food hazards, the FSO is likely to be very low, sometimes referred to as 'absent in a serving of food at the time of consumption.' For a processor that makes ingredients or foods that require cooking prior to consumption, this level may be very difficult to use as a guideline in the factory. Therefore, a level that must be met at earlier steps in the food chain should be required. This level is called a 'Performance Objective'. A PO may be obtained from an FSO, as will be explained below, but this is not necessarily always the case. A PO is defined (CAC, 2007b) as 'the maximum frequency and/or concentration of a hazard in a food at a specified step in the food chain before consumption that provides or contributes to an FSO or ALOP, as applicable.'

Foods that need to be cooked before consumption may contain harmful bacteria that can contaminate other foods in a kitchen. Reducing the likelihood of cross-contamination from these products could be important in achieving a public health goal. The level of contamination that should not be exceeded in such a situation is a PO.

For example, raw chicken may be contaminated with *Salmonella*. Although thorough cooking will make the chicken safe (the absence of *Salmonella* in a serving), raw chicken may contaminate other foods during the preparation of a meal. A PO of 'no more than a specified percentage of raw chicken carcasses may contain *Salmonella*' may reduce the likelihood that *Salmonella* will contaminate other foods. In products, such as ready-to-eat foods, the POs can be calculated from the FSO by subtracting expected bacterial contamination and/or growth between the two points.

4.6 THE DIFFERENCE BETWEEN A FOOD SAFETY OBJECTIVE, PERFORMANCE OBJECTIVE AND MICROBIOLOGICAL CRITERIA

Microbiological criteria need to be accompanied by information such as: the food product, the sampling plan, methods of examination, and the microbiological limits to be met. Traditional MCs are designed to be used for testing a shipment or lot of food for acceptance or rejection, especially in situations where no prior knowledge of the processing conditions is available. In contrast, the FSO or the PO are maximum levels and do not specify the details needed for testing. However, the MC can be based on POs in certain instances where testing of foods for a specific microorganism can be an effective means for their verification. There are several approaches to sampling (e.g. lot testing, process control testing) but they all compare the results obtained against a predetermined limit (i.e. a number of microorganisms). Approaches and tools have now been developed to relate the performance of attribute, or presence/absence testing and sampling plans to the concentration of the hazard that could be detected with a certain probability (Legan, Vandeven, Dahms, & Cole, 2001). It is hoped that these approaches will help quantify the performance of sampling plans to other risk management

metrics such as POs and FSOs which will help the use of microbial testing as a means to validate and verify that chosen control measures do, in fact, achieve the desired level of risk.

4.7 RESPONSIBILITY FOR SETTING A FOOD SAFETY OBJECTIVE

Deciding if and when to use an FSO is the responsibility of governments; the decision on what is or is not considered acceptable in terms of food safety is the traditional role of government, but the actual expression of a number and/or frequency of a hazard (e.g. bacteria or toxins) in a food at the time of consumption (the FSO) is new. Governments will typically consult with experts in foodborne disease, food microbiology and food processing, as well as other stakeholders to decide what the FSO should be. Occasionally a very quick reaction is needed—expert panels are consulted on short notice and a decision made. The SPS agreement requires that, in such instances, these values are considered as interim measures.

FSOs should only be developed in situations where they will have an impact on public health. It is, therefore, not necessary to establish FSOs for all foods. Understanding which hazards are important in which foods, predicting future food safety concerns and, importantly, designing food processing and preparation procedures that will prevent foodborne diseases from occurring, are major goals of food microbiological research conducted both in academia and in industry. Experts in these areas can assist governments in the development of realistic FSOs.

4.8 SETTING A PERFORMANCE OBJECTIVE

When an FSO has been set, POs may be set further back in the food chain by taking into account the changes that will occur in the level

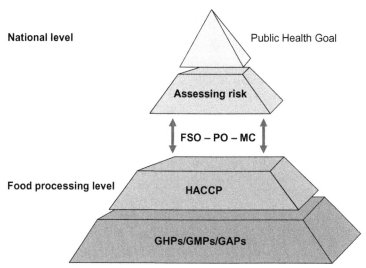

FIGURE 4.2 FSOs and POs are means of communicating public health goals to be met by food processors by good practices and HACCP. Also, industry can set POs to ensure that FSOs are met.

and/or frequency of the hazard (e.g. the harmful bacteria) between the points where POs are set and consumption. These may be stricter than the FSO to account for contamination or growth of harmful bacteria during distribution, preparation, storage and use of a particular food. On the other hand, the POs may be more lenient than the FSO; for instance, if the product is cooked just before consumption. POs may be set by both government and industry. Considering the diversity of industry, governments may decide to set POs as a means to achieve FSOs at the point of consumption. Governments may also set POs in the absence of FSOs or, for instance, in cases where raw foods are seen as a source of cross-contamination as was explained previously. POs can be set at one or more steps along the food chain where control measures can and should be applied to prevent foodborne diseases, for example, at points where it is important that all products remain below a particular level. POs, like any other microbiological limit for finished products, should take into consideration the initial level of the hazard before any treatment, as well as the decreases and possible increases of

that hazard level, if any, prior to consumption. This approach has been fundamental to safe food processing for decades and will not change with the introduction and implementation of an FSO or PO. In fact, the FSO and PO are additional tools that the food industry can use to build food safety into their products (Figure 4.2).

4.9 RESPONSIBILITY FOR COMPLIANCE WITH THE FOOD SAFETY OBJECTIVE

Marketing of food that is not harmful to consumers when used in the intended way is the responsibility of the various food businesses along the food production chain. This responsibility will not change with the introduction of FSO and PO concepts. In fact, the use of FSOs and POs will make food professionals involved in the various parts of the food chain more aware of the fact that they share this responsibility. Governments or third parties can assess programs, such as good practices and HACCP, to confirm the likelihood that the products will meet the FSOs. This can and will be extended across national boundaries, as some countries will ask that imported products are produced under food safety management programs based on GHP and HACCP.

4.10 MEETING THE FOOD SAFETY OBJECTIVE

Since the FSO is the maximum level of a hazard at the point of consumption, this level will frequently be very low. Because of this, measuring this level is impossible in most cases. Compliance with POs set at earlier steps in the food chain can sometimes be checked by microbiological testing. However, in most cases, validation of control measures, verification of the results of monitoring critical control points, as well as auditing good practices and HACCP systems, will provide the reliable evidence that POs and thus the FSO will be met. Microbiological criteria can be derived from FSOs and POs, if such levels are available. If such levels are not stated, microbiological criteria can be developed, if appropriate. The ICMSF (2002) has provided guidance on the establishment of microbiological criteria.

4.11 NOT ALL FOOD SAFETY OBJECTIVES ARE FEASIBLE

When establishing FSOs, governments should determine through discussions with relevant experts and stakeholders what feasible FSO values should be. In some cases, it may turn out that it is not possible to comply with a set FSO level in practice, and a government may decide to set a less stringent FSO. Such an FSO may be set temporarily until improvements in processing technology make it possible to set a lower (more stringent) FSO. An alternative would be

to keep the more stringent FSO and to provide a period during which processing procedures can be changed to meet the FSO. In the first case, it may be appropriate to communicate to consumers the particular risk associated with consuming the product. An alternative approach is the banning of product; e.g. banning of high-risk tissues (spinal cord, root ganglia, tonsils) of beef to be sold for human consumption due to the inability to detect and/or eliminate bovine spongiform encephalopathy (BSE).

4.12 CONCLUDING REMARKS

Food Safety Objectives and POs are new concepts that have been introduced to further assist government and industry in communicating and complying with public health goals. These tools are additional to the existing programs of GAPs, GHPs and HACCP which are the means by which the levels of POs and FSOs will be met. Hence FSOs and POs build on, rather than replace, existing food safety practices and concepts.

The new risk management approaches that are outcome based offer flexibility of operation, which can be very important when considering the most effective control measures in a particular region or operation. However, perhaps the most critical aspect of these new developments in terms of global foodborne diseases is whether such new approaches allow for food safety control measures and regulations to be developed and implemented more rapidly. Many of the food safety issues that we are facing today are more complex in nature, frequently requiring a through-chain approach and often requiring more than one control measure to effectively manage risk. It is hoped that the new risk management guidelines will offer a framework that will facilitate communication between stakeholders on the most effective food safety management options thereby speeding the development of effective risk management. A good example of a recent Codex code that benefited from these developments is the 'Code of Hygienic Practice for Powdered Formulae for Infants and Young Children' (CAC, 2008).

The emerging public health threat of *Enterobacter sakazakii* (Cronobacter species) was brought to the attention of Codex who asked FAO and WHO to convene an expert consultation on the topic in February 2004 (WHO/FAO, 2004). The consultation used risk management principles to look at a range of control strategies during both manufacture and subsequent use of powdered infant formula that could be implemented to reduce risk. Importantly, the approach facilitated the formulation of urgent advice to different stakeholders, including caregivers of infants, consumers and industry and ultimately led to a timely update of the code in 2008 (CAC, 2008).

Most importantly, these new risk-based approaches may also be used to assess whether novel processes that utilize combinations of control measures provide a level of protection equivalent to traditional processing methods. For industry, this risk-based process development approach provides a roadmap for safe innovation and will encourage the development of innovative technologies. For academia, many opportunities exist to make great contributions to the success of risk-based process development through the development of innovative process technologies, mathematical modeling, and for fundamental research in preservative-based multiple-hurdle preservation (Stewart, Tompkin, & Cole, 2002; Anderson, 2009).

ACKNOWLEDGEMENTS

This chapter is based on an original paper from the International Commission on Microbiological Specifications for Food (http://www.icmsf.iit.edu/main/articles_papers.html). ICMSF members and consultants that worked on the original paper and its translation are acknowledged.

References

Anderson, N. (2009). Risk-based process development: The Food Safety Objective approach. *Resource: Engineering and Technology for a Sustainable World* (January/February), 12–13.

CAC. (2007a). Principles and guidelines for the Conduct of Microbiological Risk Management (MRM). Codex Alimentarius Commission, CAC/GL-63. Rome: Food and Agriculture Organization.

CAC. (2007b). *Joint FAO/WHO Food Standards Programme.* Procedural Manual (17th ed), Codex Alimentarius Commission, ISSN 1020-8070.

CAC. (2008). Code of hygienic practice for powdered formulae for infants and young children, Codex Alimentarius Commission, CAC/RCP 66-2008.

ICMSF. (2002). *Microorganisms in foods 7. Microbiological testing in food safety management.* New York: Kluwer Academic/Plenum Publishers.

ICMSF. (2005). Impact of Food Safety Objectives on microbiological food safety management. Proceedings of a workshop held on 9–11 April 2003 Marseille, France. *Food Control, 16*(9), 775–832.

Legan, J. D., Vandeven, M. H., Dahms, S., & Cole, M. B. (2001). Determining the concentration of microorganisms controlled by attributes sampling plans. *Food Control, 12*(3), 137–147.

Stewart, C. M., Tompkin, R. B., & Cole, M. B. (2002). Food safety: New concepts for the new millennium. *Innovative Food Sci Emerg Technol, 3*, 105–112.

WHO/FAO. (2004) *Enterobacter sakazakii* and other microorganisms in powdered infant formula. Meeting report. http://www.who.int/bookorders/anglais/detart1.jsp?sesslan=1&codlan=1&codcol=15&codcch=606.

WTO. (1994). *Agreement on the Application of Sanitary and Phytosanitary Measures.* World Trade Organization, 16 pp. (Available at: http://www.wto.org/english/docs_e/legal_e/legal_e.htm).

WTO. (1995). *Uruguay Round Agreement, Agreement on Technical Barriers to Trade.* World Trade Organization. http://www.wto.org/english/docs_e/legal_e/17-tbt.pdf.

Further Reading

Cole, M. B., & Tompkin, R. B. (2005). Microbiological performance objectives and criteria. In J. Sofos (Ed.), *Improving the safety of fresh meat.* Cambridge: Woodhead Publishing Ltd.

FAO. (2003) Assuring food safety and quality—Guidelines for strengthening national food control systems. FAO Food and Nutrition paper number 76. ISSN 0254 4725.

ILSI-Europe. (1998). *Food Safety Management tools.* ISBN: 1-57881-034-5.

JEMRA (2005). Training and technology transfer. http://www.fao.org/es/esn/jemra/transfer_en.stm.

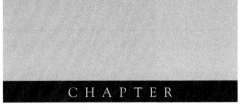

CHAPTER

5

Global Harmonization of Analytical Methods

Pamela L. Coleman and Anthony J. Fontana
Silliker Inc., Homewood, IL, USA

5.1 INTRODUCTION

'In God we trust, all others bring data.' This statement, attributed to W. Edward Deming, summarizes the importance of data and can be applied, equally well, to a myriad of different industries. The global food industry is certainly no exception. Consumer trust and satisfaction, the main concern of the food industry, is influenced and measured by application of analytical methods. Analytical data is needed for numerous and varied purposes. Data is used to quantify components, to determine value in the marketplace, to monitor key production parameters in a factory, to establish the nutrient content for labeling purposes, and to ensure the absence of harmful contaminants. The food industry relies heavily on data generated through the application of analytical chemistry methods in simple as well as complex food matrices.

Food analytical chemistry is complex and the lack of global harmonization of analytical methods and legislation makes it more complicated. The dizzying array of foods processed and manufactured around the world has led to the development of a wide variety of analytical methods for even the most basic of measurements. While the goal of each method is to generate accurate or 'correct' data, the lack of consensus on the most appropriate method often leads to trade barriers, inefficient use of resources, and economic loss. So while the utility of applying analytical chemistry techniques such as gravimetric analysis, coulometry, acid-base titrimetry, chromatography, atomic absorption or emission, and mass spectroscopy to the task of generating data concerning food is clear, the wide range of potential techniques makes the food analytical laboratory a very complex environment.

There are many areas of concern where correct analytical measurements are important, such as establishing, making, and supporting labeling claims or testing for the presence of harmful substances in food. When different analytical methods are used, they may not align with each other, in particular for new rapid methods or test kits where limited validation and the lack of reference materials for some analytes exist. Layered over the large range of methods in use are the regulatory requirements of major producing and consuming countries, sometimes harmonized, but many times divergent. Consumers ultimately suffer from this inefficiency of different countries using different methods to test foods. Whether the goal is to distribute food commodities or to develop new processed foods with nutrition benefits, the current situation of varying analytical methods and government norms is untenable.

To address this situation and reduce method variation, major commodity groups have international associations and method committees, thereby simplifying trade between states, provinces, and countries. Methods for basic quality and product parameters are generally the original focus, but eventually, key contaminants and other analytes will be addressed. For example, the International Dairy Federation (IDF) has Standing Committees on *Main Components in Milk*, on *Minor Components and Characterization of Physical Properties in Milk*, on *Quality Assurance, Statistics of Analytical Data and Sampling*, and on *Analytical Methods for Additives and Contaminants*

in Milk (IDF, 2007). These committees work with the International Organization for Standardization (ISO) to develop and harmonize standard methods.

While this chapter will not address the harmonization of regulations in any detail, it is important to note that there are numerous groups focused on this important effort. Regulatory bodies should refrain from inserting specific analytical methods into the regulations; rather they should focus on the scientific basis for the regulation. These bodies should adhere to defining the performance parameters of an acceptable analytical method instead of discussing how to show compliance. Even if international regulations were harmonized through scientific consensus, duplicate testing may be required for trade purposes if countries included specific analytical methods in the regulations themselves.

At least two prominent groups work to harmonize and validate analytical methods for foods. The International Organization for Standardization (ISO) and the Association of Analytical Communitites (AOAC International) provide guidelines with minimum recommendations on procedures that should be employed to ensure adequate validation of analytical methods. The goal of these organizations is to establish a system which allows confidence in analytical results through collaborative studies and consensus of methods. These protocols/standards require a minimum number of laboratories and test materials to be included in the collaborative trial to validate fully the analytical method.

AOAC serves the communities of analytical sciences by providing the tools and processes necessary for community stakeholders to collaborate and, through consensus building, develop fit-for-purpose methods and services for assuring quality measurements. An example of this process is the pesticide contamination of soft drinks reported by a prominent laboratory in India which resulted in these drinks being banned

TABLE 5.1   Criteria for Choice of Food Analysis Methods

Characteristic	Critical Questions
Inherent properties	
Specificity	Is the property being measured the same as that claimed to be measured? What steps are being taken to ensure a high degree of specificity?
Precision	What is the precision of the method? Is there within-batch, batch-to-batch, or day-to-day variation? What steps in the procedure contribute the greatest variability?
Accuracy	How does the new method compare in accuracy to the old or a standard method? What is the percent recovery?
Applicability of method to laboratory	
Sample size	How much sample is needed? Is it too large or too small to fit your needs? Does it fit your equipment and/or glassware?
Reagents	Can you properly prepare them? Are they stable? For how long and under what conditions? Is the method sensitive to slight or moderate changes in the reagents?
Equipment	Do you have the appropriate equipment? Are personnel competent to operate equipment?
Cost	What is the cost in terms of equipment, reagents, and personnel?
Usefulness	
Time required	How fast is it? How fast does it need to be?
Reliability	How reliable is it from the standpoints of precision and stability?
Need	Does it meet a need or better meet a need? Is any change in method worth the trouble of the change?
Personnel	
Safety	Are special precautions necessary?
Procedures	Who will prepare the written description of the procedures and reagents? Who will do any required calculations?

From Nielsen (1998).

across several Indian states.[1] Two major soft drink producers worked with AOAC, a coalition of several industry experts, and the Indian government to develop and validate methodology for detecting pesticides in soft drinks that could be utilized by both producers and regulators. Through this collaboration, no regulations were changed, but the compliance to the regulations was harmonized in that the producers and the regulators agreed on the analytical method.

Within the food industry, the concept of 'fitness of purpose' is of key importance. Many have attempted to define this concept. Table 5.1 outlines the considerations to be addressed when trying to choose a method that applies to a specific situation (Nielsen, 1998). The purpose

[1]Toxic Pesticides found in India's Soft Drinks: http://newfarm.rodaleinstitute.org/international/news/080103/081103/in_pest_drinks.shtml.

for which the data is needed should help determine the method applied.

In this chapter, three main areas of food analysis will be discussed: 1) methods meant to define the basic composition, quality, or economic value of foods; 2) methods designed to determine the nutrient value of foods; and 3) methods meant to detect or confirm the absence of contaminants in foods. For each of these three areas, at least two examples will be reviewed which highlight the importance of method selection as well as current global disagreements or compromises.

5.2 METHODS FOR ESTABLISHING THE BASIC COMPOSITION, QUALITY, OR ECONOMIC VALUE OF FOODS

Analytical methods meant to establish and monitor the basic composition and quality of foods are often used as economic value indicators. In this area of analytical concern, international agreement on what and how each component is to be measured is critical in determining the correct economic value of food products as well as in preventing harmful adulterations. The melamine incidents that occurred in 2007 and 2008 are examples of economic adulteration with dire consequences, first to animals and then to humans. While there is international standardization and regulatory agreement on the method for protein analysis, the agreed upon method is a non-specific analysis. Rather than analyzing the protein content of foods by direct methods, which can be time consuming and costly, faster and less expensive in-direct methods are generally applied. The classical Kjeldahl or Dumas methods determine the total organic nitrogen followed by conversion of total nitrogen into crude protein content using a suitable conversion factor (Mermelstein, 2009). Conversion of nitrogen into protein can only occur accurately if the nitrogen content of the protein fraction is known and if the food product includes no other nitrogen-containing matter besides protein.

Fortunately, the development of specific, rapid, and less costly methods is underway (Mermelstein, 2009). Several different approaches for protein analysis are now available, with more to follow. Improving the speed and sensitivity of the analysis for amino acids is one promising option. Since the current method requires 24 hours for the sample preparatory hydrolysis step and additional time for the detection and quantification, instrument companies are working to reduce the time required by incorporating microwave digestion. Other approaches move away from amino acid analysis by utilizing an azo-dye called Crocein Orange G, which tags by binding to the protein. The dye is added to a sample in excess. Then colorimetry is used to detect the amount of dye not bound to protein in order to calculate the amount of protein present. By analyzing specifically for protein, the economic value of nitrogenous adulterants would no longer be present and thus prevent harmful adulterations.

When payment is based on the protein content, as it is in several commodities, the incentive for fraud is high and relatively easy to achieve with nitrogenous compounds that, in fact, contain no protein at all. Thus, melamine and similar compounds can be illegally added into products for economic gain. Since we have not seen the last of these types of economic adulterations, the food industry must invest in methods to make a more accurate, fast, inexpensive, and specific protein assessment a reality. In these authors' opinion, if the focus is only on the analysis of a single adulterant, the industry will be fooled again when the culprits adulterate with another nitrogenous compound in the future.

Another example of analytical challenge is the determination of fruit juice authenticity. A single test to determine juice authenticity does not yet exist. Several different analytical procedures; organic acids, mono- and disaccharides, and minerals are compared with known levels of authentic juice to determine authenticity. While the analytical methods employed are well established, the interpretation is not. Even experienced laboratories often do not agree on the meaning of the analytical results. Juices processed from fruit grown in different geographical regions can further confuse the issue.

For this reason, numerous attempts have been made in finding suitable methods for authenticity control and determination of the fruit content in fruit-based products. The major analytical problem is due to the complexity of the products and to the substantial variance of the fruit specific components (Fügel, Carle, & Schieber, 2005). Ongoing research into DNA and mass spectrometry-based detection systems shows promise. Knight (2000) developed an analytical approach for the detection of the adulteration of orange juice by PCR technique, providing a quantification of 2.5% mandarin juice in orange juice. Fraudulent addition of sugars to authentic fruit juices and concentrates was detected using isotope ratio mass spectrometry to characterize the specific natural isotope profile of sugars and organic acids (González, Remaus, Jamin, Naulet & Martin, 1999).

Moisture content is another important food composition and quality measurement that lacks agreement on an appropriate method. Moisture is very important to food microbiological, physical and chemical stability. Moisture content is measured by direct methods, where moisture is removed by drying, distillation, extraction, or other physicochemical techniques and is measured gravimetrically or by any other direct means. Direct methods are widely used for laboratory analysis, having high accuracy and even absolute values, but are generally time-consuming and require manual operations. Some of these methods are faster and lend themselves to continuous and automated measurement in industrial processes. Loss-on-drying methods are the most common and easiest procedures for routine analysis of moisture content.

Practical application of a particular method sometimes outweighs what is correct from a scientific point of view. For the most part, the dairy industry everywhere employs the loss-on-drying method for measuring moisture content. Case studies show results can differ from the actual water content of the dairy matrices; Chapter 6 (Water Determination in Food) provides a more in-depth account of this analytical topic. However, the industry consistently applies this method, thus within the industry there is equity on a per product basis. If one part of the industry adopted the more specific and accurate Karl Fischer titration method and the rest of the industry stayed with the loss-on-drying method, there would be inequity. Perhaps this is an example of 'fitness of purpose' as the dairy industry wants to stay with a simple, chemical-free method rather than move to one that is more scientifically correct. The fact that economic decisions are made on the basis of the results adds a complication, however, within the industry all players abide by the same rules so at least there is equity, if not scientific accuracy.

It should also be noted that dairy products are not the only food matrix with this issue. To obtain the true moisture content, it is important to be aware of factors involved in the loss-on-drying technique. Factors pertaining to sample weighing, oven conditions, and post-drying operations will affect the accuracy and reproducibility of the results. The loss-on-drying methods really determine the moisture content at the specified temperature and time conditions, and not the true moisture content of many foods. However, for purposes of calculating caloric content, these methods are accepted. AOAC goes into great detail on the many permutations of the loss-on-drying method and how they apply to food matrices.

The outcome of method harmonization for the analysis of basic composition and quality tests should result in less adulteration and fewer food quality issues. Suppliers who monitor products using standard methods will help ensure buyers the value of those products. However, as shown by some examples, adulteration can have more far reaching and negative effects than economic damage, so harmonization to more specific methods would improve the situation. The industry would only have to intersperse the use of a more sophisticated measurement alongside the standard indirect methods. If only 1 per every 10 samples were tested using the direct methods and the results tracked per supplier, the threat of these specific methods would act as a deterrent. The international food community should work to collaborate and harmonize direct methods to remove the economic incentive for future adulteration issues. It is hoped that through the availability of novel analytical approaches the expense necessary for adulterating food will increase to a level which makes fraud extremely risky and increasingly uneconomical (Fügel et al., 2005).

5.3 METHODS FOR ESTABLISHING THE NUTRIENT CONTENT OF FOODS

Most foods contain a mix of some or all of the nutrient classes. For a healthy diet, some nutrients are required regularly, while others are needed only occasionally. Poor health can be caused by an imbalance of nutrients, whether excessive or deficient. These nutrient classes can be categorized as either macronutrients (carbohydrates, fats, fiber, proteins, and water) or micronutrients (minerals and vitamins). Many of the macronutrient analyses have been discussed in the previous section in this chapter as they are often used for economic or production monitoring purposes. When used for nutrition value purposes, there are often differences in the analytical methods applied. The easiest method to estimate the carbohydrate content is to utilize the 'by difference' method and then to calculate caloric content using Atwater factors.

Like proteins and lipids, carbohydrates are one of the major classes of food components. Although a well-defined group of compounds, some confusion often occurs as to what constitutes a carbohydrate and what does not. The measurement of carbohydrates in food ranges from the very simple 'by difference' method to the intensive analysis of individual mono- and disaccharides, oligosaccharides, and other complex carbohydrates. When used for nutrition labeling purposes, the 'by difference' method is allowed in several countries. However, it results in an overstatement of the actual content, especially when a significant level of fiber or sugar alcohols is present.

The Food and Agriculture Organization (FAO) and the World Health Organization (WHO) of the United Nations held a joint expert panel on carbohydrates (FAO/WHO, 1997), during which some important recommendations were issued regarding the analysis of food carbohydrates:

1. The terminology used to describe carbohydrates should be standardized by primarily classifying them by molecular size (degree of polymerization or DP) into sugar (DP 1-2), oligosaccharides (DP 3-9), and polysaccharides (DP10+). Further subdivision can be made on the basis of monosaccharide composition.
2. Food analysis laboratories should measure total carbohydrates in the diet as the sum of the individual carbohydrates and not 'by difference.'
3. The analysis and labeling of dietary carbohydrate, for whatever purpose, should be based on the chemical divisions recommended. Additional groupings such as polyols, resistant starch, non-digestible oligosaccharides, and dietary fiber can be used, provided that the included components are clearly defined.

The carbohydrate industry is rapidly changing with the advent of non-nutritive sweeteners and multiple fiber components. The reasons for determining the carbohydrate content are also evolving to now include quality control of drinks and foodstuffs, monitoring of food-labeling claims, analysis of sweeteners, and authentication. The analysis of carbohydrates sometimes involves not only the determination of the total amount of sugar present in the sample, but also the identity, configuration, and conformation of the carbohydrate components.

The American Dietetic Association (ADA) and the British Nutrition Foundation (BNF) respectively recommend a minimum fiber intake of 20–35 g/day and 12–24 g/day for healthy adults. The term 'dietary fiber' was originally synonymous with non-digestible plant matter. Even when defined in its most chemically precise form, as non-starch polysaccharides, dietary fiber is very heterogeneous and includes pectin substances, hemicellulose, cellulose, lignin, etc. With the expansion of processed and functional foods there has been an enormous increase in intakes of non-cell wall sources of dietary fiber added to foods as ingredients, and an increasing need for regulation of nutrient claims for fiber. Therefore, the concept of dietary fiber has been extended to include oligosaccharides such as oligofructans and non-digestible polysaccharides, such as pectins, gums, mucilages, and resistant starch.

The definition of dietary fiber has been revised several times and continues to evolve. A number of approaches have been taken to dietary fiber analysis, reflecting the lack of agreement on the definition. The methods developed involved chemical measurement referred to as enzymatic-gravimetric, enzymatic-chemical, enzymatic-chemical-gravimetric, and non-enzymatic-gravimetric among other methods. As the definition of dietary fiber continues to be refined, it will require further changes in methods to ensure that they provide a true measure of polysaccharides that are not digested under physiological conditions.

The final class of macronutrients is lipids, which consist of a broad group of compounds that are generally soluble in organic solvents but only sparingly soluble in water. Fatty acids are key components of lipids. Similar to moisture content, much of the food industry applies a shorthand method involving solvent extraction to quickly determine the crude fat content of foods. What is extractable includes many components like pigments, phospholipids, glycolipids, fat-soluble vitamins, and phenols that may not meet the definition of fat. Thus, a food analyzed by solvent extraction would be biased higher than one by only fatty acid analysis. The European Union uses the definition of all lipids from foods (mono-, di- and triglycerides, phospholipids, etc.), while the US FDA has adopted the definition of lipids to only include the total lipid fatty acids expressed as triglycerides. These two definitions are different and thus many times result in different amounts of lipids.

While this is close enough for many purposes, the differences between the crude fat methods and the more time and capital intensive fatty acid procedure may not warrant a move away from the crude fat methods. However, for some food matrices, the differences will be sufficient to warrant this change. In fact, the food industry continues to utilize crude fat methods to satisfy specification requirements for economic purposes and even basic quality purposes, while then turning to the sum of the fatty acids for nutrition labeling and caloric content purposes.

Nutrition labels describe the nutrient content of a food and are intended to guide the consumer in making healthy food choices. As nutrition labeling efforts continue to evolve towards harmonization of nutritional information listing, the analytical methods employed to substantiate the claims will also harmonize. The Codex Guidelines on Nutrition Labeling play an important role in providing guidance to member countries when developing or updating their national regulations and encourage harmonization of national standards with international standards.

Products marketed in different countries are currently subject to multiple regulations and formats for nutrition labeling which require specific packaging materials for each country. Chapter 17 (Nutrition and Bioavailability: Sense and Nonsense of Nutrition Labeling) provides a more in-depth account of this topic. In some cases, the same analytical methods can be employed but the results are utilized differently as with the calculation of calories and carbohydrates. Although through the harmonization efforts in the European Union, some of these differences will disappear. These disparities complicate and prolong the product development process, which ultimately increases the price of the products.

5.4 METHODS FOR DETECTING OR CONFIRMING THE ABSENCE OF CONTAMINANTS IN FOODS

Preventing acute as well as chronic harmful effects from contaminants in foods requires that foods have little to no residue of chemical contaminants that are known to be toxic. From this very simple concept, a mammoth industry has evolved. Regulators determine what exactly can be allowed and at what levels. Instrument manufacturers design ever better separation and detection devices, which command higher and higher prices. Analytical testing laboratories compete to offer the lowest sensitivity and the broadest range of analytes to their clients. Is it enough to look for 200 compounds at the ppm level or 400 analytes at the ppb level or even more compounds at even lower limits of detection? Is all of this effort resulting in food that is safer? Or does this situation drive up the cost without true benefit to the world's population?

While these questions cannot be answered here, a risk-benefit analysis approach should be employed. In no other area is regulatory harmonization needed more. The 'chasing zero' issue should be addressed and subjected to scientific

consensus on risk; simply because a compound can be detected does not mean that this compound is harmful at that low detection level. Regulations should not specify methods but rather outline the method performance parameters that should be satisfied, leaving the choice of technology open.

When employing methods for the purpose of detecting contaminants, it is vitally important to consider the entire analytical process from a holistic viewpoint. The sampling (size and protocol), sample preparation, and analytical methods need to be considered as a whole to determine the total variability associated with determining the level of contaminants. An example is mycotoxin testing where sampling represents the largest source of variation in the entire analytical process. Mycotoxins may be present in small regions randomly distributed throughout the material in question and appropriate sampling is critical. Thus, sole focus on lowering the detection limit that does not incorporate appropriate sample size and preparation parameters will not result in more accurate data (EUROCHEM, 2007).

Whitaker *et al.* (2006) and Ozay *et al.* (2006) investigated the uncertainty associated with sampling, sample preparation, and analysis for aflatoxin in almonds and hazelnuts, respectively. For hazelnuts, the sampling, sample preparation, and analytical steps of the aflatoxin test procedure accounted for 99.4, 0.4, and 0.2% of the total variability, respectively (Ozay *et al.*, 2006). For almonds, the percentages of the total variance associated with sampling, sample preparation, and analytical steps were 96.2, 3.6, and 0.2%, respectively (Whitaker *et al.*, 2006). As with the testing of other commodities for mycotoxins, the sampling step contributes the most variability, followed by the sample preparation step, and then the analytical step. The best use of resources to reduce the total variability of the aflatoxin test procedure would be to increase the size of the test sample (Whitaker *et al.*, 2006).

Due to the fact that sampling plays a critical role in the precision of the determination of the levels of contaminants in foods, the EU clearly defines the sampling methods (Commission Directive 98/53/EC). In Annex I of the Directive, the methods of sampling for official checking control of the levels of aflatoxins in certain foods are clearly defined. The following formula can be used as a guide for the sampling of lots:

$$\text{Sampling frequency (SF)} = \frac{\text{Weight (kg) of the lot} \times \text{weight of the incremental sample}}{\text{Weight of the aggregate sample} \times \text{weight of individual packing}}$$

where the weight of the incremental sample should be about 300 grams, and the number of incremental samples to be taken depends on the weight of the lot, with a minimum of 10 and a maximum of 100. Annex II of the Directive discusses the sample preparation and criteria for methods of analysis used in official checking of the levels of aflatoxins in certain foods. This is an excellent example where a regulatory body has not defined a specific analytical method; rather it has defined the sampling of lots and the criteria which the method of analysis has to comply with to ensure that laboratories obtain comparable results.

In 2004, the California Attorney General's Office filed a Proposition 65 lawsuit against 34 manufacturers whose candies tested positive for dangerous levels of lead. California's Proposition 65 law requires warnings on products that can expose the public to carcinogens or reproductive toxins. Chili powder and tamarind are popular ingredients in Mexican-style candies that are sold in California. Data have shown that some of these Mexican-style candies are contaminated with the toxic metal lead. Research has determined that some of the lead in the candies comes from the chili powder and tamarind ingredients. The US FDA is recommending that lead levels in candy products likely to be consumed frequently by small children should not exceed 0.1 ppm because such levels are achievable under good manufacturing practices and would not pose a significant risk to small children for adverse effects.

The lawsuit was settled by seven large manufacturers in June 2006. As part of the settlement, a certification process and an educational outreach fund were established. Among the companies that signed the settlement are some of the world's largest candy makers and the three leading sellers of popular spicy candies from Mexico. The certification process includes an audit of the manufacturing process to pinpoint possible sources of lead contamination, auditor's recommendations to eliminate possible sources of lead contamination, and regular testing to make certain the candy is safe. The California law does not mandate a specific technology that may change in the next 3 to 5 years; rather various analytical procedures may be used to ensure that the candy meets the required specification.

Analytical methods to detect residues and contaminants in food have significantly improved and will continue to improve with new technologies. Improving the sensitivity of the detection of the analytical method does little to ensure the safety of the food if an inappropriate sample is used or if the levels detected do not pose a safety or toxicity risk. If testing is done with the 'wrong' sample, increasing the sensitivity will not lead to improving the efficiency of the surveillance system in place. However, a risk-based strategy will improve current surveillance systems that target at reducing residues and contaminants in foods.

5.5 CONCLUSION

Global harmonization of regulations as well as standard methods of analysis would benefit the food industry, but more important, would benefit the worlds consumers significantly. Analytical methods used to analyze the basic composition and quality of food products need to be more specific in order to reduce food safety concerns as well as the threat of economic adulterants. The analytical methods for establishing the nutrient content of foods should also be harmonized to avoid lengthening the product development process and increasing the cost to introduce new products, such as fortified foods into the global market. Finally, harmonizing the analytical as well as the regulatory approach to food contaminants would focus testing efforts on ensuring food safety and would reduce the destruction of foods that may be safe to consume.

References

EUROCHEM. (2007). *Measurement uncertainty arising from sampling: A guide to method and approaches*, p. iii (www.eurachem.org/guides/ufs.2007.pdf).

FAO/WHO. (1997). *Expert consultation on carbohydrates in human nutrition*, 14–18 April, Rome.

Fügel, R., Carle, R., & Schieber, A. (2005). Quality and authenticity control of fruit purees, fruit preparations and jams – a review. *Trends in Food Science Technology*, 16, 433–441.

González, J., Remaus, G., Jamin, E., Naulet, & Martin, (1999). Specific natural isotope profile studied by isotope ratio mass spectrometry (SNIP-IRMS): 13C/12C ratios of fructose, glucose, and sucrose for improved detection of sugar addition to pineapple juices and concentrates. *Journal of Agricultural and Food Chemistry*, 47, 2316–2321.

IDF. (2007). ISO 14501/ IDF 171. Milk and milk powder—Determination of aflatoxin M1 content—Clean-up by immunoaffinity chromatography and determination by high-performance liquid chromatography.

Knight, A. (2000). Development and validation of a PCR-based heteroduplex assay for the quantitative detection of mandarin juice in processed orange juices. *Agro FoodInd Hi Tech*, 11, 7–8.

Mermelstein, N. H. (2009). Analyzing for melamine. *Food Technology*, 63(2), 70–75.

Nielsen, S. S. (1998). *Food analysis* (2nd ed.). Aspen Publishers.

Ozay, G., Seyhan, F., Yilmaz, A., et al. (2006). Sampling hazelnuts for aflatoxin: Uncertainty associated with sampling, sample preparation, and analysis. *JAOAC*, 89(4), 1004–1011.

Whitaker, T. B., Slate, A. B., Jacobs, M., et al. (2006). Sampling almonds for aflatoxin, Part I: Estimation of uncertainty associated with sampling, sample preparation, and analysis. *JAOAC*, 89(4), 1027–1034.

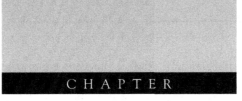

CHAPTER

6

Water Determination in Food

Heinz-Dieter Isengard

University of Hohenheim, Institute of Food Science and Biotechnology, Stuttgart, Germany

6.1 INTRODUCTION

When goods are sold beyond national borders, they must meet the requirements of the receiving country, whose requirements may differ from the regulations existing in the delivering country. Therefore, when the laws or traditional consumer expectations are not the same in the countries involved, a compromise or an agreement between the trade partners is necessary. The best solution would, of course, be to have the same regulations in both countries and, by general extrapolation, in all countries.

These considerations are particularly relevant for trade of agricultural products and food. Certain components may be characteristic for a given product and may also be decisive for the price. The content or concentration of such compounds must then be analyzed, as the method of determination may not be the same in the countries concerned. Depending on the situation, one of the partners would have an advantage if the regulation existing in one of the countries was taken as standard. Again, an agreement is necessary. Chapter 5 (Global Harmonization of Analytical Methods) gives a more general discussion on analytical methods used to establish the basic composition and quality of foods.

A further problem may be where a commonly accepted or internationally established method may exist, which may not be based on scientific research. Thus, although the results might be legally correct, they would not reflect the true value. If the existing method is replaced by another—scientifically correct—method, however, this procedure may meet the resistance of a partner should they want the existing method to be conserved. This chapter describes such a situation.

Indirect or secondary methods must be calibrated against a direct or primary method. When the primary method is not adequate, it may nevertheless be possible to establish a calibration, but the results derived from it may be erroneous or false, even though this might not be immediately obvious. Such an example is also given.

6.2 WATER CONTENT

6.2.1 Importance of Water Content

Water is one of the most important substances in food (Isengard, 2001). It is present in every foodstuff, in a range that may vary from extremely low amounts in dried products to extremely high amounts in beverages. Its content is of great significance in many respects,

affecting properties like conductivity for heat and electrical currents, density and rheological properties or corrosiveness. All of these factors must be taken into account for the design of technological processes. The amount of water in food is a determinant for its nutritive value and taste. In some cases it can also be considered as an impurity. In reference materials, the water content is important as far as specifications are given on the basis of either dry matter or initial mass. Stability and shelf life of foodstuffs are highly dependent on water content (via water activity), since water is critical for microbiological life and most enzymatic activities. Storage volume and mass also depend on water content, which can be reflected in transport costs. As water is relatively cheap, its presence in foodstuffs in general and in high-value products in particular, is of commercial interest. For this and other reasons, rules and regulations concerning water content are imposed. As a consequence of all the above, the determination of water content is certainly the most frequent analysis performed on foodstuffs.

6.2.2 Methods to Determine Water Content

The aim of water content analyses should be to detect all water and nothing but water in the sample. Direct or primary methods determine water as such. This can be done physically by separating the water contained in the sample and measuring its mass or its volume. Another possibility is to analyze water content by a selective chemical reaction. Indirect or secondary methods determine either a sample property that depends on water content, such as density, sound velocity, dielectric properties or electrical conductivity; or the response of the water molecules in the sample to a physical influence, which comprises spectrometric techniques like near-infrared (NIR) spectrometry, microwave resonance spectrometry or time-domain nuclear magnetic resonance (TD-NMR). Indirect methods need a calibration against a direct method (Isengard, 1995).

6.2.2.1 *Drying Techniques*

Water content (or what is believed to be water content)—and thus dry matter—is often determined by drying techniques, particularly by drying the product at a certain temperature for a certain time in a drying oven.

Drying techniques, be they the 'classical' oven drying, vacuum drying, freeze drying, infrared or microwave drying, do not distinguish between water and other volatile substances. The result of all of these methods is not water content, but the mass loss the product undergoes under the conditions applied. These conditions (sample size, temperature, pressure, time, energy input, criteria to stop the analysis) can principally be freely chosen. The result depends very much on these conditions but may be very reproducible. This alone shows that this technique, leading to different results when the parameters are changed, cannot be the correct one, because water content is a sample property which has a precise, though unknown value. From the scientific point of view, therefore, the results of drying methods should not be called 'water content' but rather 'mass loss on drying' with indication of the drying conditions. In past years the term 'moisture content' has more often been used as a compromise. It means the relative mass loss by evaporation of water (though possibly not all of the water) and of other volatile compounds under the drying conditions.

The problem with all drying techniques is that they do not specifically measure water. All of the volatile compounds under the analytical conditions contribute to the mass loss; even compounds that are not originally contained in the sample but formed by chemical reactions during the analysis, particularly by decomposition reactions at higher temperatures. On the other hand, strongly bound water may escape detection.

These two opposite errors, inclusion of other volatiles on the one hand and water not detected on the other hand, may compensate each other when the drying parameters are chosen appropriately (Isengard, 1995; Isengard & Walter, 1998; Isengard & Färber, 1999; Heinze & Isengard, 2001; Isengard & Präger, 2003). The appropriate choice of the parameters necessitates, of course, that the true water content has been analyzed before with a method selective for water as a primary method. The parameters of the secondary method must then be chosen in a way that the result corresponds to the water content determined with the primary method. Once the secondary method is calibrated in this way, it can be applied for this particular type of product. The calibration is product-specific and the same parameters cannot be applied for other types of samples. This procedure is particularly interesting for rapid drying techniques like microwave or infrared drying.

6.2.2.2 *Karl Fischer Titration*

The most important primary method to determine water content is the Karl Fischer titration. It is based on a chemical reaction selective for water:

$$ROH + SO_2 + Z \rightarrow ZH^+ + ROSO_2^- \qquad (1)$$

$$ZH^+ + ROSO_2^- + I_2 + H_2O + 2Z \rightarrow 3ZH^+ + ROSO_3^- + 2I^- \quad (2)$$

Overall reaction:

$$3Z + ROH + SO_2 + I_2 + H_2O \rightarrow 3ZH^+ + ROSO_3^- + 2I^- \quad (3)$$

where Z is a base (very often imidazole), and ROH is an alcohol (usually methanol).

In the first step, the alcohol is esterified with sulfur dioxide to form alkyl sulfite. The base provides for a practically complete reaction, Eq. (1). In the second step, this alkyl sulfite is oxidized by iodine to form alkyl sulfate; this reaction requires water, Eq. (2). The overall reaction, Eq. (3), shows that the consumption of iodine is stoichiometrically equivalent to water present in the sample.

6.3 WATER DETERMINATION IN DAIRY POWDERS

Dairy powders are sold on the basis of dry matter. Water determination is therefore an important analysis in this field. Practically all dairy powders contain lactose. This component causes problems when drying techniques are used.

6.3.1 The Lactose Problem—Scientific Background

Lactose exists in different forms. The α-anomer is stable at temperatures below 93°C. It crystallizes with one mole water per mole lactose. At higher temperatures the anhydrous β-anomer is more stable. Lactose also occurs in an amorphous form which may include small amounts of water. Depending on the production conditions, dried dairy powders contain mixtures of these forms. In addition to the included water and water of crystallization, the product usually contains small quantities of surface water.

The usual drying temperature for moisture determination of dairy products in drying ovens is 102°C. At this temperature the water of crystallization of α-lactose is not evaporated completely during the usual drying times. The separation of this water fraction from the matrix needs a high energy input (Rüegg & Moor, 1987; Rückold, Isengard, Hanss, & Grobecker, 2003). After the standard drying time of 2 hours, only a part of this water is detected. The consequence is that drying techniques yield results that differ more or less from the true water content.

As lactose occurs in practically all dairy products and is also used in the pharmaceutical industry,

this problem affects a wide range of products, particularly those with high lactose contents like whey powders or lactose itself.

Usually the drying results obtained are lower than the true water content. In special cases, however, they can be higher. This is possible if the lack in water detection is over-compensated by other volatile substances which are contained in the products or formed by chemical reactions of components and by decomposition processes during the drying process.

6.3.2 The Lactose Problem—Economic Aspects

Dairy powders are sold on the basis of dry matter (DM). This is (or should be) the mass of the product, m_0, minus the mass of the water, m_W, contained in it, Eq. (4). The mass of water can be calculated from water content (WC), Eq. (5). Equation (6) gives the dependence of dry matter from water content.

$$DM = m_0 - m_W \tag{4}$$

$$WC = m_W/m_0 \Rightarrow m_W = WC \cdot m_0 \tag{5}$$

$$DM = m_0 - m_W = m_0 - WC \cdot m_0$$
$$= m_0 \cdot (1 - WC) \tag{6}$$

Dry matter decreases with increasing water content. If the analytical method yields a result lower than the true water content, dry matter is then overestimated. This would give the product supplier an unjustified advantage and the buyer would pay too much for the product. This is the type of situation likely to happen in the trade of dairy powders.

6.3.3 Reference Method for Determining Moisture in Milk Powders

The International Dairy Federation (IDF) has established a method for determining the moisture content in dried milk. A new drying device was specifically designed for this purpose (de Knegt & van den Brink, 1998). The method was also adopted by the International Organization for Standardization (ISO) (ISO 5537 | IDF 26, 2004).

The introduction of this method was strongly supported by the dairy industry. Scientific arguments brought forward and results of an international inter-laboratory test (Rückold, Grobecker, & Isengard, 2000) were pushed aside. In particular—apart from possible economic interests (see above)—two arguments were put forward to introduce and establish this method. The first argument was that the results obtained by this new technique (see description below) were practically the same (but with a smaller standard deviation for replicate samples) as those received by drying the samples according to the former method using a conventional drying oven, independently from the geographic situation (altitude, air pressure, relative humidity of the environment). The second argument (against the objection that the result of this method is not the complete water content) was that the complete water content would not be the property of interest in milk powders. Rather, this would be the free water in the product (Isengard, 2006, 2008).

6.3.4 Mass Loss, Moisture Content, Water Content—Comparison of Results Obtained by Different Methods for Various Dairy Powders

Several dairy powders were analyzed for mass loss on drying and for water content: lactose, skim milk powder, full cream milk powder, whey powder, and calcium caseinate.

Two drying techniques were used: The 'classical' oven drying (OD) and the new 'reference drying' method (RD).

Water content was determined by Karl Fischer titration (KFT).

6.3.4.1 Oven Drying (OD)

The experiments were carried out according to the former IDF standard method 'Dried milk and dried cream, Determination of water content' (IDF 26A, 1993). It is remarkable to note that at that time the mass loss measured was defined as 'water content', whereas the new method, which has officially replaced this one, determines 'moisture content'.

An amount of 1–3 g of the sample—for this investigation, approximately 2 g were used—is dried at 102 ± 2°C in a ventilated drying oven. The mass loss is measured by weighing the sample before and after 2 hours of drying and cooling in a desiccator. According to this method, the sample is then to be dried for another hour and so forth until the difference between consecutive measurements is less than 0.5 mg. In this investigation, the samples were analyzed after various drying times to follow the drying process more closely (see below). The results after 2 hours were then used to compare the results with each other and with those obtained through other methods. The analyses were carried out with a drying oven FD 115 from Binder, Tuttlingen, Germany.

6.3.4.2 Reference Drying (RD)

The samples (5.0 ± 0.3 g) are placed in containers with a diameter of 20 mm and a height of 90 mm (plastics syringes without needle) between polyethylene filters and dried (up to eight in parallel per one analysis) in a heating block at 87 ± 1°C for 5 hours. Dry compressed air is passed at a rate of 33 ml/min through the containers with the samples. The mass loss determined by weighing the sample and the container before and after the drying process (after cooling in a desiccator) is defined as moisture content. It does not control if a constant mass has been reached. For this reference drying, according to the new standard method, a Referenztrockner RD 8 from Funke-Dr. N. Gerber Labortechnik, Berlin, Germany, was used.

TABLE 6.1   Results for water content by Karl Fischer titration (KFT) and for mass loss by oven drying (OD) after 2 hours and by 'reference drying' (RD); n = number of replicates

Sample	Water content by KFT (*n* = 5) [g/100 g]	Mass loss by OD (*n* = 2) [g/100 g]	Mass loss by RD (*n* = 2) [g/100 g]
Lactose	4.45 ± 0.19	2.45 ± 0.13	1.04 ± 0.03
Skimmed milk powder	3.92 ± 0.07	3.85 ± 0.00	3.94 ± 0.13
Full cream milk powder	2.65 ± 0.05	2.46 ± 0.02	2.72 ± 0.14
Whey powder	4.46 ± 0.05	2.12 ± 0.01	2.24 ± 0.07
Calcium caseinate	6.19 ± 0.11	5.62 ± 0.03	5.73 ± 0.02

6.3.4.3 *Karl Fischer Titration (KFT)*

A KF Titrino 701 from Metrohm, Herisau, Switzerland, with a titration cell with thermostatic jacket was used. The two-component technique was applied with Hydranal®-Titrant 2 as titrating solution and Hydranal®-Solvent as working medium. All chemicals were from Sigma-Aldrich, Seelze, Germany. In order to obtain a more rapid dissolution or dispersion of the samples in the working medium and, consequently, shorter titration times, the analyses were carried out at 50°C.

6.3.4.4 *General Procedure (Isengard et al., 2006a)*

The different samples were analyzed on the same day by the three methods. Five Karl Fischer titrations were carried out for every sample. The 'reference drying' was started with eight portions of each sample, two each were analyzed as duplicates after 3, 4, 5 and 6 hours (the 'official' drying time being 5 hours). Twelve portions of each sample were placed in the drying oven. Two each were analyzed in parallel after 60, 80, 100, 120, 150, and 180 minutes (the 'official' drying time being 120 minutes).

The dependence of the 'reference drying' results on the drying parameters was also examined (Isengard, Kling, and Reh, 2006b).

6.3.4.5 *Results and Discussion*

Table 6.1 (from Isengard *et al.*, 2006a) gives a juxtaposition of the results obtained by Karl Fischer titration (KFT), by conventional oven drying (OD) according to the former standard method and by the new standard method ('reference drying', RD). The OD results are—for better comparison—those obtained after 2 hours, the RD results are the values after the 'official' time of 5 hours. Values for other drying times both for oven drying and for 'reference drying' are given below. The shape of the Karl Fischer titration curves indicated a complete and correct determination of water for all the samples.

The results for the two milk powders were very similar. The KFT and the RD results were not significantly different. The OD results (obtained after 2 hours drying time) came closer to the KFT results when the drying times were longer: (3.90 ± 0.01) g/100 g after 2.5 hours for skimmed milk powder and (2.58 ± 0.01) g/100 g after 3 hours for full cream milk powder (see Figure 6.3). In the other cases, the results for water content and mass loss clearly differed. For lactose and whey powder the differences were very high.

Various drying times were tested for the two drying methods to determine the evolution of the results in the course of time. The results of these

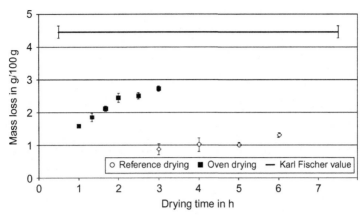

FIGURE 6.1   Mass loss by 'reference drying' and oven drying after various drying times of crystallized lactose and—for comparison and reference—the water content by Karl Fischer titration (in g/100 g).

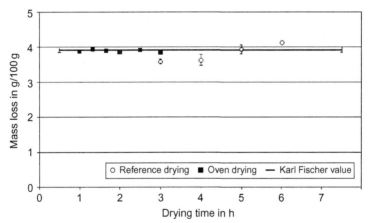

FIGURE 6.2   Mass loss by 'reference drying' and oven drying after various drying times of skim milk powder and—for comparison and reference—the water content by Karl Fischer titration (in g/100 g).

experiments are depicted in Figures 6.1 to 6.5 (from Isengard *et al.*, 2006a).

The lactose sample (Figure 6.1) is a technical product and obviously contains not only α-lactose but also anhydrous forms. The water content found by Karl Fischer titration is slightly below 5 g/100 g. This value is not easily reached using the drying techniques because the water of crystallization is strongly bound.

A very important finding is that the drying techniques do not only detect the 'free' water

(which is usually in the range of 0.1 g/100 g) but also a part of the 'bound' water. It cannot, therefore, be claimed that the new reference method will detect free water only. The measured entity is in fact not defined; it is neither free nor total water. This is a serious disadvantage for a reference method.

For the two milk powder samples (Figures 6.2 and 6.3), the mass loss on drying corresponds approximately to the water content determined by Karl Fischer titration. The 'lack'

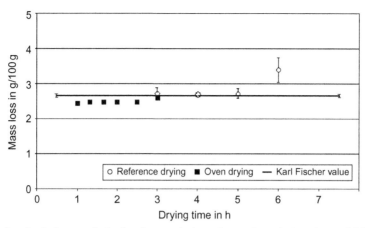

FIGURE 6.3   Mass loss by 'reference drying' and oven drying after various drying times of full cream milk powder and—for comparison and reference—the water content by Karl Fischer titration (in g/100 g).

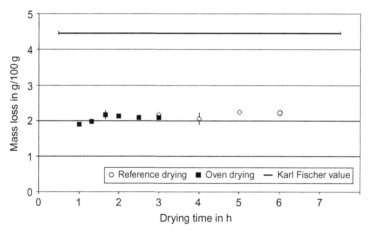

FIGURE 6.4   Mass loss by 'reference drying' and oven drying after various drying times of whey powder and—for comparison and reference—the water content by Karl Fischer titration (in g/100 g).

of water detection can be compensated by the determination of volatile substances formed by decomposition at higher temperatures (see above). This is obvious from the results by 'reference drying' which rise to numbers above the Karl Fischer results when the drying process is longer than the 'official' 5 hours. The value for both milk powders after 5 hours is, however, very consistent with the water content.

The whey powder (Figure 6.4) contains approximately 85% lactose by weight. A part of it is crystallized. Consequently, the mass loss on drying does not reach the water content. Other components with high water binding capacity may contribute to this effect.

The calcium caseinate sample (Figure 6.5) does not contain lactose. The reason for the too-low drying results, therefore, may be a slow diffusion of the water from the core of the particles to the surface. The air flow in the 'reference dryer' is obviously advantageous for the drying process as it keeps the partial pressure of

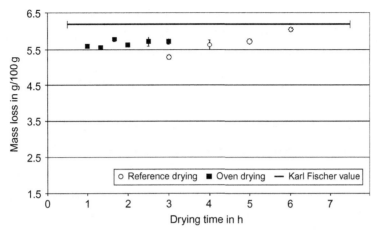

FIGURE 6.5 Mass loss by 'reference drying' and oven drying after various drying times of calcium caseinate and—for comparison and reference—the water content by Karl Fischer titration (in g/100 g).

TABLE 6.2 Mass loss of dairy powder samples determined by 'reference drying' at 87°C after 5 hours at different air flow rates and water content by Karl Fischer titration (KFT), n = number of replicates

Sample	Mass loss in g/100 g at air flow rate		Water content by KFT in g/100 g
	33 ml/min	>33 ml/min	
A	2.44 ± 0.54 ($n = 3$)	2.83 ($n = 2$)	2.58 ± 0.02 ($n = 3$)
B	3.38 ± 0.17 ($n = 3$)	4.35 ($n = 2$)	3.39 ± 0.02 ($n = 3$)
C	3.26 ± 0.34 ($n = 5$)	3.93 ($n = 2$)	2.97 ± 0.05 ($n = 3$)
D	5.91 ± 0.40 ($n = 3$)	6.06 ($n = 2$)	5.98 ± 0.13 ($n = 3$)

water above the sample extremely low. The Karl Fischer value would probably be reached if the drying time was longer.

Figures 6.1–6.5 reveal that the results obtained by 'reference drying' depend very much on drying times. Other parameters like air flow, sample size and temperature have an influence on the results as well. This is shown in Tables 6.2–6.4 (from Isengard et al., 2006b).

The mass loss detected increases with increasing flow rates. Mass loss decreases with sample size. The mass loss found at 102°C is higher than at 87°C and time-dependent. The total water content (i.e. the Karl Fischer value) is not even reached at 102°C after 7 hours.

6.3.4.6 Concluding Considerations

Results obtained for mass loss on drying and for water content by Karl Fischer titration can clearly differ. With increasing α-lactose content the difference increases and is extreme for pure lactose. The drying techniques neither determine the total water nor the free water fraction alone. Defenders of the new reference method argue that the water of crystallization is of no practical importance, because it has no influence on the flowability of the powders and almost no importance for the microbiological stability and thus the shelf life of the product. This argument does not consider the fact that this 'bound' water is set free when the product

TABLE 6.3 Mass loss by 'reference dying' at 87°C after 5 hours (air flow rate 33 ml/min) for the same sample using different sample sizes; two replicates for sample sizes 2, 3, 4 and 6 g; five replicates for sample size 5 g; water content by KFT 3.42 ± 0.02 g/100 g ($n = 3$)

Sample size in g	2	3	4	5	6
Mass loss in g/100 g	5.31	4.21	4.43	4.10 ± 0.49	3.73

TABLE 6.4 Mass loss of a lactose sample by 'reference drying' at 102°C as a function of drying time; mass loss at standard conditions (87°C, 5 hours): 1.08 ± 0.14 g/100 g ($n = 3$); $n =$ number of replicates; water content by KFT: 4.46 ± 0.10 g/100 g ($n = 4$)

Drying time in h	2	3	4	5	6	7
Mass loss in g/100 g (n)	1.79 ($n = 2$)	2.37 ± 0.56 ($n = 4$)	2.65 ± 0.51 ($n = 6$)	3.00 ± 0.32 ($n = 6$)	3.17 ± 0.30 ($n = 4$)	3.35 ($n = 2$)

is dissolved. This has to be accounted for when recipes are designed. Therefore, the total water content (including water of crystallization) is important.

The results of the 'reference method' depend strongly on drying times as well as other parameters (de Knegt & van den Brink, 1998; Isengard et al., 2006a,b). Only for ordinary milk powders are they close to the Karl Fischer results. For products with other compositions, other product-specific parameters would have to be chosen. This means that the method is limited.

The Karl Fischer method detects the total water content selectively and is independent from the lactose content. The precision of the Karl Fischer results is very good, even though the sample sizes are much smaller than those for the drying techniques. The precision of the new reference method is no better than that of oven drying.

The drying techniques are more time-consuming than the Karl Fischer method. Conventional oven drying takes several hours and real mass constancy is only rarely reached. Experience shows that terminating the measurement

after a fixed time of 2 hours is recommended. This makes the results more comparable, as in many cases additional mass loss may be due to decomposition processes. The 'reference drying' is very time-consuming (practically one day for a set of eight samples). The Karl Fischer method is by far the most rapid method for one sample (a couple of minutes). However, a disadvantage of the Karl Fischer technique is the use of chemicals.

These and other investigations (Rückold et al., 2000; Isengard et al., 2006a,b) have shown that the 'reference drying' method is correct only for ordinary milk powders but not necessarily for other dried dairy products. On the contrary, the Karl Fischer titration can generally be applied to these products and would be a more reasonable reference method.

From a scientific point of view, these considerations are clear and straightforward and cannot be doubted. Nevertheless, attempts to introduce the Karl Fischer titration as a reference method for water determination in dairy powders meets the resolute resistance of the dairy industry. A reason might be the economic interest in not 'finding' all of the water in the product being sold. The detection of the true water content would lower the price of the product if it is calculated on the basis of dry matter.

Scientific facts are, so far, not strong enough against economic arguments. Harmonizing scientific truth and accuracy with economic power and interests is necessary. Such a harmonization should, for ethical reasons, be the aim in the interest of honest and correct trade.

6.4 WATER CONTENT DETERMINATION BY NEAR-INFRARED SPECTROSCOPY

6.4.1 Rapid Water Determination by Near-Infrared Spectroscopy

Near-infrared (NIR) spectroscopy is a rapid techniques which even allows in-line measurements. Many properties of a sample can be analyzed, once an appropriate calibration against a direct method has been established. As NIR spectroscopy is based on light absorption of chemical components in the sample, a connection between one of these components or a group of components and the property to be measured must exist. This property may be a physical characteristic of the sample, or the concentration or mass concentration of a compound or group of compounds in the sample. Water is one of these compounds which can be analyzed by NIR spectroscopy.

6.4.2 Water Determination in a Whey Powder by NIR Spectroscopy (from Isengard et al., 2009)

Lactoserum Euvoserum (from Nestlé, Lausanne, Switzerland), which essentially contains whey powder, was analyzed for water content by NIR spectroscopy after calibration against mass loss on drying and against water content determination by Karl Fischer titration. Previous experiments had shown that the temperature of about 102°C usually applied for drying dairy powders in drying ovens was not sufficient to liberate the water from this product (Merkh, 2006). Higher temperatures were therefore applied. This example showed the effect at a drying temperature of 145°C. Karl Fischer titrations were carried out with a KF Titrando 841 from Metrohm, Herisau, Switzerland using the two-component technique with Hydranal®-Titrant 2 as titrating solution and a mixture of Hydranal®-Solvent and formamide in a volume ratio of 2:1 as the working medium, all chemicals being from Sigma-Aldrich, Seelze, Germany. To shorten titration times, the analyses were carried out in a double-walled titration vessel at 40°C. NIR spectra were registered using a Fourier transform NIR spectrometer NIRVIS from Bühler, Uzwil, Switzerland (now represented by Büchi, Essen, Germany).

6.4.3 Results and Discussion of NIR Measurements

Figure 6.6 shows the calibration line based on mass loss. The calibration is acceptable if the mass loss on drying is really the property to be analyzed. It is, however, useless if water content is to be analyzed. The reason is that the water content analyzed by Karl Fischer titration lies only within the range highlighted by a rectangle (Figure 6.7).

If the calibration is based on the Karl Fischer results for real water content, the line in Figure 6.8 is obtained.

The reason for this phenomenon is that the product continues to lose mass at the temperature applied. This is depicted in Figure 6.9. The dried product was analyzed for water content by Karl Fischer titration after various drying times. After some time the residual water

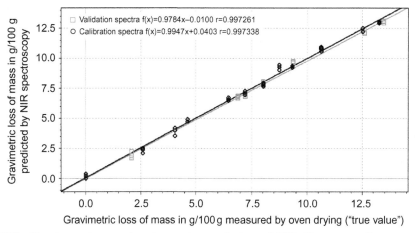

FIGURE 6.6   NIR calibration against gravimetric mass loss on drying at 145°C of Lactoserum Euvoserum from Nestlé.

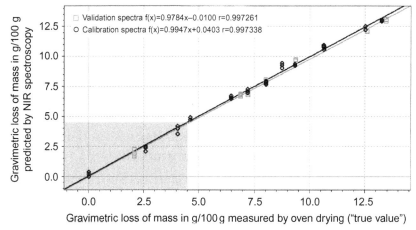

FIGURE 6.7   NIR calibration against gravimetric mass loss on drying at 145°C of Lactoserum Euvoserum from Nestlé. The water content occurring in the powders analyzed lies within the highlighted rectangle.

remained constant, although the mass loss still increased. The product obviously undergoes degradation, with formation of volatile substances. This can also be derived from its more and more darkening color. When the drying curve reached the Karl Fischer value, there was still about half of the water in the sample. Further analyses showed that the relatively constant water content found in the dried fractions was, to a great extent, due to water which was taken up by the hygroscopic dried material during handling (cooling in a desiccator, weighing and transfer into the titration vessel).

It is not possible to determine the water content of this product by NIR spectroscopy if the calibration is based on oven drying at 145°C. Such a calibration leads to mass loss results with good correlation. However, if water content is to be measured, the calibration has to be based on Karl Fischer titration. The temperatures for the

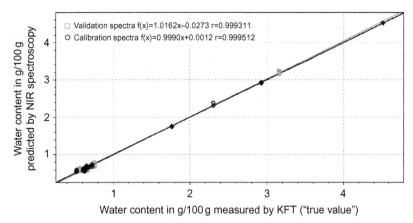

FIGURE 6.8   NIR calibration against water content determined by Karl Fischer titration of Lactoserum Euvoserum from Nestlé.

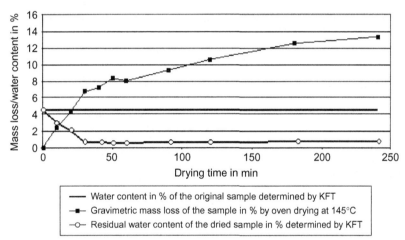

FIGURE 6.9   Drying curve of Lactoserum Euvoserum from Nestlé at 145°C and residual water content of the dried fractions.

liberation of water from α-lactose and the degradation of the product overlap. It is, therefore, not possible to choose a temperature at which water is evaporated completely without degradation of the product.

6.4.4 Concluding Considerations

Establishing a connection between a sample property to be analyzed with one method and a property measured by another method runs the risk of yielding good calibration lines without giving correct results of the sample property. This is particularly true for techniques with chemometric evaluation of the measurements like NIR spectrometry.

The whole approach depends on the 'correctness' of the reference method, because it is always possible to draw a regression line through data points. For every analytical measurement, a corresponding concentration of the analyte will be found and even a high precision is no proof of correctness. A possible error will not be detected because the results are based on the same wrong conditions and assumptions. It is therefore essential that the reference method is 'correct'. The importance of this prerequisite was shown with the example of water determination in a whey powder product.

6.5 CONCLUSION

To avoid disputes and problems in trade, analytical methods should be harmonized. The methods agreed upon must, however, be scientifically correct and correspond to the state of art. In order to be in a position to compare scientific findings, methods with which analyses have been carried out must be described in all essential details, because results depend on the methods and parameters used.

Political or economic interests may influence the choice of reference or standard methods and lead to a situation where a reference method is scientifically incorrect. At first sight this may seem harmless, since it applies to all concerned in the same way. This, however, is not the case. If the agreed analytical method does not yield correct results, this is ethically not acceptable. In addition, one of the trade partners is at an economic disadvantage. Also, the incorrect result may have negative consequences. Thus, in the example of dairy powders, incomplete detection of the water contained in the product by using the official reference method for 'determination of the moisture content' may lead the buyer of the product to think that the indicated moisture content corresponds to the true water content. But when the product is dissolved in water, the undetected water will be set free and the solution will contain less dry mass of dairy powder than was foreseen in this recipe.

When incorrect reference methods are used for calibration of secondary methods, this may lead to good calibration lines with satisfactory correlation factors, when in fact the desired property was not calibrated. This does not become apparent and false results seem to be confirmed, even if they are completely senseless.

References

de Knegt, R. J., & van den Brink, H. (1998). Improvement of the drying oven method for the determination of the moisture content of milk powder. *International Dairy Journal, 8*, 733–738.

Heinze, P., & Isengard, H.-D. (2001). Determination of the water content in different sugar syrups by halogen drying. *Food Control, 12*, 483–486.

IDF 26A (1993). Dried milk and dried cream, Determination of water content.

Isengard, H.-D. (1995). Rapid water determination in foodstuffs. *Trends Food Science and Technology, 6*, 155–162.

Isengard, H.-D. (2001). Water content, one of the most important properties of food. *Food Control, 12*, 395–400.

Isengard, H.-D. (2006). Harmonisation of analytical methods—Best solution is same regulations everywhere. *Food Engineering & Ingredients, 31*(2), 22–26.

Isengard, H.-D. (2008). Water determination—Scientific and economic dimensions. *Food Chemistry, 106*, 1393–1398.

Isengard, H.-D., & Färber, J.-M. (1999). 'Hidden parameters' of infrared drying for determining low water contents in instant powders. *Talanta, 50*, 239–246.

Isengard, H.-D., Felgner, A., Kling, R., & Reh, C. T. (2006a). Water determination in dried milk: Is the international standard reasonable? ISBN 0-8493-2993-0, 631-637. In M. del Pilar Buero, J. Welti-Chanes, P. J. Lillford, and H. R. Corti (Eds.), *Water Properties of Food, Pharmaceutical, and Biological Materials* (pp. 631–637). Boca Raton, Florida, USA: CRC Press, Taylor & Francis Group.

Isengard, H.-D., Kling, R., & Reh, C. T. (2006b). Proposal of a new reference method to determine the water content of dried dairy products. *Food Chemistry, 96*, 418–422.

Isengard, H.-D., Merkh, G., Schreib, K. et al. (2009). The influence of the reference method on the results of the secondary method via calibration. Submitted to *Food Chemistry.*

Isengard, H.-D., & Präger, H. (2003). Water determination in products with high sugar content by infrared drying. *Food Chemistry, 82*, 161–167.

Isengard, H.-D., & Walter, M. (1998). Can the true water content in dairy products be determined accurately by microwave drying? *Zeitschrift für Lebensmittel-Untersuchung und -Forschung, A 207*, 377–380.

ISO 5537 | IDF 26 (2004). Dried milk—Determination of moisture content (Reference method).

Merkh, G. (2006). Vergleichende Untersuchungen von Methoden zur Wassergehaltsbestimmung in einigen pulverförmigen Milchprodukten. *Master thesis (Diplomarbeit,)* University of Hohenheim, Institute of Food Science and Biotechnology, Stuttgart, Germany.

Rückold, S., Grobecker, K. H., & Isengard, H.-D. (2000). Determination of the contents of water and moisture in milk powder. *Fresenius' Journal of Analytical Chemistry, 368,* 522–527.

Rückold, S., Isengard, H.-D., Hanss, J., & Grobecker, K. H. (2003). The energy of interaction between water and surfaces of biological reference materials. *Food Chemistry, 82,* 51–59.

Rüegg, M., & Moor, U. (1987). Die Bestimmung des Wassergehaltes in Milch und Milchprodukten mit der Karl-Fischer-Methode, V. Die Wasserbestimmung von getrockneten Milchprodukten. *Mitteilungen Gebiete Lebensmitteluntersuchung und Hygiene., 78,* 309–319.

Testing for Food Safety Using Competent Human Liver Cells

Firouz Darroudi[1], Veronika Ehrlich[2], Axelle Wuillot[1], Thibaut Dubois[1], Siegfried Knasmüller[2] and Volker Mersch-Sundermann[3]

[1]Department of Toxicogenetics, Leiden University Medical Centre, Leiden, The Netherlands
[2]Institute of Cancer Research, Department of Medicine I, Medical University of Vienna, Vienna, Austria
[3]Department of Environmental Health Sciences, Freiburg University Medical Centre, Freiburg, Germany

OUTLINE

7.1 ASSESSMENT OF HUMAN FOOD SAFETY AND THE EXISTING PROBLEMS

It is well-documented that diet plays a crucial role in the etiology of cancer in humans (Sugimura, 1982, 2000; Knasmüller & Verhagen, 2002; Steck *et al.*, 2007). A number of epidemiological studies indicated that 40–70% of the cancer incidence in humans is due to nutritional factors (Steck *et al.*, 2007).

The nature of the food we consume and our total diet greatly influence our health and well being. Food should be tasty, nutritious and safe. The safety of our food supply is a shared responsibility, from farm to fork, of the food producing industry, regulatory authorities and consumers. As part of this safety assurance it is essential to assess the potential risks posed by food and food ingredients.

The risk assessment process, defined as the determination of the probability of harm resulting from exposure to a food component, has to be based on sound scientific data and carried out to internationally agreed standards in a transparent manner (Verhagen *et al.*, 2003). This is essential to ensure consumer confidence in the safety of the food supply, particularly when foods are traded on an international basis.

The traditional risk assessment process applied to food additives relies on toxicology testing *in vitro* and *in vivo* assays. These models, however, have important imperfections:

a. *'in vitro'* assays with metabolically incompetent cells require the addition of exogenous enzyme homogenates to catalyze the activation of genotoxic food derived carcinogens. This process is generally dependent on Cytochrome P450 enzymatic activities present in rat liver. Therefore, they may reflect only a few of the mechanisms that modulate the genotoxic effects of food carcinogens. It became evident that certain modes of action (i.e. to detect protective and synergistic effects) are not represented adequately in the *in vitro* models (Kassie *et al.*, 2003a, 2003b; Knasmüller *et al.*, 1998, 2003, 2004a; Mersch-Sundermann *et al.*, 2004).

b. *'in vivo'* assays in animals use intake levels many times higher than is likely in humans. Employing safety factors then carries out extrapolation of the data to determine the safe level for humans. Such an approach does not quantitatively assess the relationship between exposure and adverse health effects and cannot effectively deal with novel foods and macro-ingredients with high levels of intake in human diet (Knasmüller *et al.*, 1998, 2003, 2004a).

At present there is also abundant evidence that various plant constituents decrease the genotoxic and carcinogenic effects of food specific toxins (Knasmüller *et al.*, 1998; Kassie *et al.*, 2003a,b; Mersch-Sundermann *et al.*, 2004). Synergistic and antagonistic effects may have a strong impact on the cancer risk in humans but they cannot be monitored adequately in conventional *in vitro* test systems. So far, the only reliable approaches that enable the prediction of co- and anti-mutagenic effects of compounds that interfere with metabolic activation/detoxification pathways of carcinogens are *in vivo* models with laboratory animals. However, they are, in general, time-consuming and costly, and the requirement of large numbers of animals argues against their use in screening trials. Therefore, new approaches are needed to take into account the latest scientific advances.

7.2 ASSESSING GENOTOXIC POTENTIAL OF HUMAN DIETARY COMPONENTS USING HUMAN HEPATOMA HEPG2 CELLS

Unique features of active human hepatoma HepG2 cells include:

1. Human liver origin (directly relevant to humans) (Natarajan & Darroudi, 1991).
2. Mutagenic effects can be studied directly in the cells that can activate the test compound. This simplifies the test. It also allows the study of the mutagenic activity of very short-lived metabolite.
3. Subcellular fraction of human hepatoma cells (HepG2) can be obtained and used as an exogenous source for metabolic activation in Chinese hamster ovary cells, human lymphocytes and Ames *Salmonella* assay (Darroudi & Natarajan, 1993, 1994; Darroudi, Knasmüller, & Natarajan, 1998).
4. The cells used in this study are HepG2 cells that retain the activities of many relevant enzymes both Phase I (cytochromes P450) as well as Phase II (responsible for detoxification), which are lost during cultivation of any cell types used so far. The levels of activity of these enzymes in human HepG2 cells are generally similar to those present in human liver cells. Some of these enzymes play key roles in the activation/detoxification of DNA reactive

carcinogens (Wilkening, Stahl, & Bader, 2003; Westerink & Schoonen, 2007a, 2007b).
5. Various biological assays for detecting DNA damage induction following exposure to different classes of human dietary components and environmental mixture (air, water) were developed and successfully validated using HepG2 cells (Natarajan & Darroudi, 1991; Darroudi, Meijers, Hadjidekova, & Natarajan, 1996; Darroudi *et al.*, 1998; Uhl, Helma, & Knasmüller, 1999, 2000; Uhl *et al.*, 2001, 2003a, 2003b; Bezrookove *et al.*, 2003; Lu *et al.*, 2004; Filipic & Hei, 2004; Yuan *et al.*, 2005; Jondeau, Dahbi, Bani-Estivals, & Chagnon, 2006; Buchmann *et al.*, 2007).
6. In addition, state-of-the-art techniques such as microarray and proteomic were adapted to these cells and used to define the modes of action of various classes of human dietary carcinogens, non-carcinogens, and anti-carcinogens (Harries, Fletcher, Duggen, & Baker, 2001; Gerner *et al.*, 2002; Breuza *et al.*, 2004; van Delft *et al.*, 2004; Hockley *et al.*, 2006, 2009).
7. This *in vitro* model has the potential to be applied in mutagenicity testing in order to Refine, Reduce and Replace animal use (3Rs) (Russell, 1995), while ensuring protection of human and animal health and the environment (Rueff *et al.*, 1996; Kirkland *et al.*, 2007).

7.3 VALIDATION OF HUMAN HEPG2 CELLS IN DETECTING KNOWN CARCINOGENS AND NON-CARCINOGENS

HepG2 cells were used as metabolic activation systems as well as targets for evaluating DNA damage (Natarajan & Darroudi, 1991; Knasmüller *et al.*, 1998, 1999, 2004a). In addition, S9-fractions from HepG2 cells were isolated to investigate their ability to activate promutagenic carcinogens using Chinese hamster ovary cells *in vitro* and Ames *Salmonella* assay (Darroudi & Natarajan, 1993). Various biological end-points, such as sister-chromatid exchanges, micronuclei (MN) in binucleated cells, aneuploidy using MN assay in combination with a pan-centromeric probe, cytotoxicity, gene mutation (at HPRT locus), Comet assay as well as gamma-H2AX and Rad 51 foci formation were developed and validated (Darroudi & Natarajan, 1993; Darroudi *et al.*, 1996, 1998; Darroudi, Ehrlich, Tjon, & Knasmueller, 2009; Natarajan & Darroudi, 1991; Knasmüller *et al.*, 1998, 2003, 2004a; Lamy *et al.*, 2004; Mersch-Sundermann *et al.*, 2004).

The results (Table 7.1) indicate that the human hepatoma cell systems reflect the activation/detoxification of genotoxic carcinogens better than other indicator cells that are currently being used and, therefore, have an increased predictive value for the identification of mutagenic anti- and co-mutagenic constituents of human foods

(Schmeiser, Gminski, & Mersch-Sundermann, 2001; Mersch-Sundermann *et al.*, 2001, 2004; Kassie *et al.*, 2003a,b; Knasmüller *et al.*, 2004a; Wu, Lu, Roos & Mersch-Sundermann, 2005).

The HepG2 cell system was shown to be capable of detecting and discriminating between structurally related chemicals, carcinogens and non-carcinogens. Potent *in vivo* carcinogens such as 2-acetylaminofluorene, benzo(a)pyrene, and ochratoxin A have shown genotoxic potential in HepG2 cells (*in vitro*). In contrast, a structurally related chemical such as 4-acetylaminofluorene, pyrene and ochratoxin B, respectively, reported to be non-carcinogen *in vivo* has shown no genotoxic effect in HepG2 cells using micronuclei and Comet assays (Natarajan & Darroudi, 1991; Knasmüller *et al.*, 2004a, 2004b). For all chemicals tested so far a positive correlation was found between outcomes of analysis in human HepG2 cells (*in vitro*), and those obtained using vertebrate animals (*in vivo*).

TABLE 7.1 A comparative study between genotoxicity data *in vitro* using human HepG2 cell system, S9-microsomal fraction from HepG2 and rat liver, and carcinogenicity/non-carcinogenicity data *in vivo*

Chemical	Carcinogen (*in vivo*)	HepG2 (*in vitro*)	CHO cells (*in vitro*) with S9-fractions derived from		Ames *Salmonella* test	
			HepG2	Rat liver	HepG2	Rat liver
2-AAF	+	+	+	−		
4-AAF	−	−	−	−		
B(a)P	+	+	+	+		
Pyrene	−	−	−	−		
CP	+	+	+	+		
Ochratoxin A	+	+	+	−		
Ochratoxin B	−	−	−			
DMN	+	+	+	+		
HMPA	+	+	+	−	+	−
Safrole	+	+	+	−	+	−

Abbreviations: CHO, Chinese hamster ovary; 2-AAF, 2-acetylaminofluorene (carcinogen in *in vivo* test); a structurally related chemical 4-AAF, 4-acetylaminofluorene (non-carcinogen in *in vivo* test); B(a)P, benzo(a)pyrene (carcinogen in *in vivo* test); a structurally related chemical pyrene is found to be non-carcinogen in *in vivo* test; ochratoxin A is found to be a carcinogen and a structurally related chemical ochratoxin B is reported to be non-carcinogen in *in vivo* tests; CP, cyclophosphamide; DMN, dimethylnitrosamine; HMPA, hexamethylphosphoramide.

7.4 ASSESSMENT OF THE GENOTOXIC POTENTIAL OF MYCOTOXINS IN HEPG2 CELLS

Several studies were designed for validating the application of human HepG2 cells in assessment of the genotoxic potential of different classes of human dietary components (Ehrlich *et al.*, 2002a, 2002b; Knasmüller *et al.*, 2004b). The focus was primarily on chemicals (such as mycotoxins) that are known to cause cancer in animals, but so far no positive effects (except for aflatoxin B1) had been reported, neither in any mammalian tests *in vitro* nor in Ames *Salmonella* assay.

Mycotoxins of interest in naturally contaminated human foods and feeds are:

- nivalenol, 2-deoxynivalenol, T2-toxin, ochratoxin A (in wheat/barley/oats);
- fusarenone X, fumonisin B1, ochratoxin A (in maize);
- aflatoxin B1 (in maize/peanuts).

All mycotoxins are very stable during storage/milling processing and difficult to destroy at high temperatures (IARC, 1993).

Generally most of the data were generated in animal studies. Ochratoxin A was found to be a potent nephrotoxin. Deoxynivalenol caused general toxicity. Fumonisins ingestion via feed prepared from corn contaminated with *Fusarium* could cause leukoencephalomalacia (horse), pulmonary oedema (pig) and liver cancer (rat) (Ehrlich *et al.* 2002a, 2002b; Knasmüller *et al.*, 2004b). Among the tested mycotoxins, aflatoxin B1 was found to be the most potent carcinogen *in vivo* and was the only one for which its genotoxic potential has been reported in other *in vitro* assays.

In humans, there are no genotoxicity data and epidemiological studies showed that presence of mycotoxins in food can enhance the risk of esophageal cancer.

Chemicals such as nivalenol, deoxynivalenol, fumonisin B1, citrinin and ochratoxin A were tested in human HepG2 cells and were found to be potent genotoxicants (Table 7.2) (Ehrlich *et al.*, 2002a, 2002b; Knasmüller *et al.*, 2004b; Darroudi *et al.*, 2009). In a comparative study, on the basis of a dose that could enhance the biological assay (micronuclei) by a factor of 2 in comparison to the untreated samples, a ranking order was made (Table 7.2). The known carcinogen aflatoxin B1 was by far the most potent chemical; the effective concentration was found to be 0.2 μg/ml compared to 25 μg/ml for fumonisin B1.

These sets of data are the first to elucidate the genotoxic potential of the selected mycotoxins in an *in vitro* assay and, therefore, can open up the possibility of further assessments of the origin and mechanisms of genotoxicity of these chemicals in order to enhance human health. Interestingly, the non-carcinogen ochratoxin B that is a structurally related chemical to the carcinogen ochratoxin A under identical conditions, was found to be non-genotoxic in HepG2 cells (Knasmüller *et al.*, 2004b).

These data also indicate that the HepG2 cell system has the potential to discriminate between carcinogens and non-carcinogens.

TABLE 7.2   Genotoxic potential of mycotoxins in HepG2 cells

Substance	Nivalenol	Deoxynivalenol	Fumonisin B1	Aflatoxin B1
M.E.D. (μg/ml)	50	50	25	0.2
Ranking order	3	3	2	1

M.E.D. = Minimum effective dose. When frequency of micronuclei increased by 2-fold in comparison to the control (untreated) samples.

TABLE 7.3 Genotoxic potential of heterocyclic aromatic amines (cooked food mutagens in) HepG2 cells

Substance	IQ	MeIQ	MeIQx	PhIP	Trp-P-1	Trp-P-2
M.E.D. (μM)	80	50	30	30	15	5
Ranking order	5	4	3	3	2	1

M.E.D. = Minimum effective dose. When frequency of micronuclei increased by 2-fold in comparison to the control (untreated) samples.

7.5 ASSESSMENT OF THE GENOTOXIC POTENTIAL OF HETEROCYCLIC AROMATIC AMINES IN HEPG2 CELLS

Heterocyclic aromatic amines (HAAs) can be found in protein-rich food (IARC, 1993) and are known to be mutagens in prokaryotes (Sugimura, 1982, 2000). The most common ones, IQ, MeIQ, MeIQx, PhIP, Trp-P-1 and Trp-P-2 were studied in human HepG2 cells. Existing data revealed that HAAs are mutagenic in pro- and eukaryotic organisms. Experiments with laboratory rodents also showed that these food-derived compounds can cause cancer. Furthermore, epidemiological studies indicated that they might be involved in the etiology of colon cancer in humans.

HAAs have been tested extensively in microbial *in vitro* assays with rat liver microsomal fractions in Ames *Salmonella* assay and were found to be potent mutagens (Sugimura, 1982, 2000). However, the results obtained in genotoxicity tests with mammalian cell lines are highly divergent (Knasmüller, Sanyal, Kassie, & Darroudi, 1995; Knasmüller et al., 1999, 2004a; Knasmüller, Murkovic, Pfau, & Sontag, 2004c; Majer et al., 2004a, 2004b).

A number of heterocyclic aromatic amines such as IQ, MeIQ, MeIQx. Trp-P-1, Trp-P-2 and PhIP were tested in human HepG2 cells in MN as well as Comet or single cell gel electrophoresis (SCGE) assays (Knasmüller et al., 1999, 2004a, 2004c). With all of them, positive results were obtained (Table 7.3). It is notable that, in contrast to experiments with CHO cells and *Salmonella*/microsome assay, the ranking order of the genotoxic potencies of these HAAs correlated with that of their carcinogenic activities in rodents. Moreover, the sensitivity of SCGE assay towards most HAAs was found to be similar to that of MN tests.

7.6 A COMPARATIVE ANALYSIS FOR PHASE I AND PHASE II ENZYMES BETWEEN HEPG2 CELLS AND HUMAN HEPATOCYTES

Gaining knowledge on the metabolism of a drug, the enzymes involved and its inhibition or induction potential is a necessary step in pharmaceutical development of new compounds, screening of human dietary components, and environmental mutagens. Primary human hepatocytes are considered to be a cellular model of reference, as they express the majority of drug-metabolizing enzymes, respond to enzyme inducers, and are capable of generating *in vitro* a metabolic profile similar to that found *in vivo*. However, hepatocytes show phenotypic instability and have a restricted accessibility. In the past, various alternatives have been explored—such as cell lines isolated from human hepatomas. In contrast to primary cultures, hepatic cell lines are easily available and culture conditions are standardized (Westerink & Schoonen, 2007a, 2007b).

Attempts were also made to define the metabolic capabilities of the HepG2 cell line. Various housekeeping genes, such as porphobilinogen

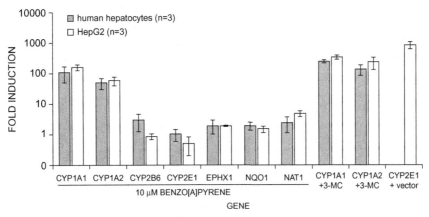

FIGURE 7.1 Quantification of gene expression profiles in HepG2 cells and/or human hepatocytes treated with benzo(a)pyrene. Induction of CYP1A1 and CYP1A2 is shown after treatment with 2 μM 3-methylcholantene (3-MC). Data show mean and standard deviation from three independent hepatocyte cultures and three different HepG2 passages.

deaminase, hypoxanthine phosphoribosyl transferase (HPRT), ATP-synthetase, glyceraldehyde-3-phosphate dehydrogenase, and elongation factor-1-alpha) are expressed equally in HepG2 cells and primary human hepatocytes (Figure 7.1). Various cytochrome P450s (CYP1A1, CYP1A2, CYP2B6), and some Phase II enzymes (e.g. glucuronosyltransferase (UGT) and N-acetyltransferase 1 (NAT1)) are also constitutively expressed (Wilkening *et al.*, 2003). Moreover, as presented in Figure 7.1, they can be induced by similar factors in HepG2 cells as in human hepatocytes following treatment with benzo(a)pyrene. This means that some carcinogens that are difficult or impossible to detect using induced rat liver S9 microsomal fraction (e.g. safrole, hexamethylphosphoramide) can be detected as inducing genotoxicity in HepG2 cells, or can induce genotoxicity in Chinese hamster ovary (CHO) cells and Ames *Salmonella* assay, when S9 microsome is prepared from HepG2 cells (Table 7.1). In both human hepatocytes and HepG2 cells, culture time is found to influence on the expression of drug-metabolizing enzymes (e.g. CYP1A1 and 2B6) (Wilkening & Bader, 2003). Therefore, it is essential to perform the analysis using early passages and to maintain uniform cell culture conditions for different sets of experiments.

S9 microsome prepared from HepG2 cells (Darroudi & Natarajan, 1993) can be particularly useful for detecting carcinogenic potential of heterocyclic aromatic amines like IQ and MeIQx. This is because they require acetylation, and this is poor in Chinese hamster cell lines such as CHO cells; it is approximately 20 times lower than in HepG2, which is equal to the level in human hepatocytes. However, even when activated by S9 from HepG2, the lack of penetration of the acetic acid ester metabolites into cells can be a problem.

Furthermore, HepG2 cells were shown to be a useful model for investigating the capacity of potential chemoprotectants to enhance g-glutamylcysteine synthetase (GCS) and Glutathione (GSH). GSH is an important antioxidant and cofactor of detoxifying metabolism. The elevation of GSH is achieved by inducing GCS (Scharf *et al.*, 2003).

Westerink and Schoonen (2007a,b) have characterized Phase II metabolism in HepG2 cells. Transcript levels and enzyme activities in HepG2 cell line were compared with those in cryopreserved primary human hepatocytes. Quantitative PCR was used to measure transcript levels of UGT1A1, 1A6, sulfotransferase (SULT) 1A1, 1A2, 1E1, 2A1, microsomal glutathione-S-transferase 1 (mGST-1), NAT1 and epoxide hydrolase (EPHX1).

In addition, the induction of Phase II enzymes in HepG2 cells was determined after treatment with aryl hydrocarbon receptor, constitutive androstane receptor and pregnane X receptor agonists.

On the basis of mRNA expression analysis, it was found that HepG2 cells have, with the exception of UGTs, a complete set of Phase II enzymes. Regulation of Phase II enzymes in HepG2 cells shows that there is good correlation with earlier results in primary human hepatocytes. Therefore, in contrast to primary hepatocytes, HepG2 cells are a relatively easy-to-handle tool for studying regulation of Phase II enzymes in human liver cells (Westerink & Schoonen, 2007a, 2007b). Consequently, because of the role of these Phase II enzymes in catalyzing the detoxification of several compounds, HepG2 cells might become a valuable tool system to predict toxicity. However, it should be noted that, for compounds in which cytochrome P450 (CYP) metabolism plays an important role in toxification, and Phase II metabolism plays a crucial role in detoxification, toxicity might be underestimated if CYPs are low in HepG2, due to a shift towards Phase II metabolism. This imbalance might explain why some compounds with known toxicity in primary hepatocytes remain non-toxic in HepG2 cells.

7.7 TOXICITY STUDIES OF COMPOUNDS AND MECHANISTIC ASSAYS ON NAD(P)H, ATP, DNA CONTENTS (CELL PROLIFERATION), GLUTATHIONE DEPLETION, CALCEIN UPTAKE AND RADICAL OXYGEN ASSAY USING HUMAN HEPG2 CELLS

An approach to reduce the cost aspects of analyzing large numbers of synthetic compounds within the pharmaceutical industry is the introduction of medium and high throughput *in vitro* screening for toxicity measurements using Alamar Blue (AB) and Hoechst 33342 coloration, and luminometric assays, using Cyto-Lite and ATP-Lite, dichlorofluorescein diacetate, monochlorobimane and calcein-AM (Schoonen, De Roos, Westerink, & Debiton, 2005a; Schoonen, De Roos, Westerink, & Debiton, 2005b).

With AB, ATP-Lite and Cyto-Lite the energy status of the cell is measured and with Hoechst 33342 the amount of DNA. Dichlorofluorescein diacetate, monochlorobimane and calcein-AM are fluorophores for the measurement of the formation of reactive oxygen species (ROS), the quantification of glutathione and the membrane stability, respectively (Schoonen *et al.*, 2005a, 2005b; Miret, De 'Groene, & Klaffke, 2006).

Further developments in this area may lead to an earlier prediction of toxic effects of compounds in cellular assay, *in vitro*, and animal studies can be largely reduced in this assay. Due to the high attrition rate of toxicity of drug candidates in development (e.g. 50% of the compounds), there is increased interest within the pharmaceutical industry to examine compounds at earlier stages and with relatively small quantities of compound. For a first glance on toxicity simple assays are needed to identify general aspects of cellular toxicity. Interference with normal cell physiology, such as energy metabolism and cellular proliferation, can be simple cell toxicity markers.

The human HepG2 cell system has been examined using the above-mentioned assays for 100–110 reference compounds with different modes of action. Also, 60 up to 100 were tested on HeLa cells, CHO cells and human endometrium (ECC-1). The highest dose tested varied between 3.16×10^{-3} and 3.16×10^{-5}, and the minimal toxicity dose obtained for different assays was found to be between 3.16×10^{-3} and 3.16×10^{-8} (Schoonen *et al.*, 2007a).

The outcome of these studies revealed that all four cell lines were responsive to the same set of drugs (classified as directly acting); however, for some drugs HepG2 cells appeared to be more sensitive, as compared to the other three cell lines. In general, in HepG2 cells it was possible to predict toxicity up to 75%. This implies that a high throughput toxicological screening can be set up with this assay, and can also be applied when tested drugs are indirectly-acting, and need an exogenous activation system. Moreover, these cells originated from human liver cells, which can increase the predictability for humans compared to the predictability based on rat, mice, hamster, or monkey cell lines.

Furthermore, it was reported that glutathione depletion and calcein uptake assays are almost equally potent and both assays are much more sensitive than the ROS measurement. Consequently it was concluded that *in vitro* screening appears to be a realistic and reliable alternative to the use of *in vivo* studies with vertebrate animals.

Miret and co-workers used other sets of *in vitro* models of cytotoxicity in human HepG2 cells. Those included Alamar Blue for the measurement of cellular adenosine triphosphate (ATP); ToxiLight as an indicator of cellular necrosis by measurement of released AK; and Caspase-3 Fluorometric Assay, Apo-ONE Caspase-3/7 Homogenous Assay, and Caspase-Glo for the determination of caspase-3/7 activity. In order to evaluate the assays, several known cytotoxic compounds such as dimethyl sulfoxide (DMSO), butyric acid, carbonyl cyanide 4-(trifluoromethoxy)phenylhydrazone (FCCP) and camptothecin were examined (Miret *et al.*, 2006). Data revealed that the best way to evaluate the potential cytotoxicity of a compound is to employ a battery of assays. The use of ATP levels, cell necrosis, and caspase-3/7 resulted in the most useful combination in HepG2 cells (Miret *et al.*, 2006).

7.8 APPLICATION OF A HUMAN HEPG2 CELL SYSTEM TO DETECT DIETARY ANTI-GENOTOXICANTS

There is increasing evidence that chemicals cannot only have adverse effects. There are many substances (e.g. human dietary components, vitamins) that can have a beneficial effect on health, and may even inhibit the effect of carcinogens in humans (Knasmüller *et al.*, 2002). However, the conventional *in vitro* assay outcomes are clearly not conclusive because many studies do not fully reflect the complex activation and detoxification processes that take place in mammals (*in vivo*). Consequently, it is not possible to extrapolate the results of such experiments to humans. Several dietary constituents that are DNA protective under *in vitro* conditions in experiments with indicator cells that require addition of exogenous activation system (liver S9-mixture) were inactive in rodent bioassays, or even led to an enhancement of the DNA damaging properties of the tested heterocyclic aromatic amines (HAAs) (Schwab *et al.*, 1999, 2000). Furthermore, certain conventional *in vivo* experiments with laboratory rodents are not adequate tools for identifying protective constituents in human food since only marginal or negative effects are obtained in these models with HAAs (IARC, 1993).

We have tested a number of HAAs (Table 7.3) in MN assay with HepG2 cells, and a ranking order was made. It is notable that, in contrast to experiments with CHO cells and Ames *Salmonella*/microsome assay, the ranking order made with HepG2 cells for the genotoxic potencies of the HAAs, positively correlated with that of their carcinogenic activities in rodents. In the follow-up studies, attempts were made to study the anti-genotoxic potential of series of human dietary components (including vitamins) against HAAs (e.g. IQ, MeIQ, MeIQx, Trp-P-1, Trp-P-2 and PhIP) in human HepG2 cells by using micronuclei and Comet assays (Sanyal *et al.*, 1997; Dauer *et al.*, 2003; Steinkellner *et al.*, 2001; Laky *et al.*, 2002; Kassie *et al.*, 2003a,b; Uhl *et al.*, 2003a, 2003b; Knasmüller *et al.*, 2004a, 2004c; Mersch-Sundermann *et al.*, 2004; Lhoste *et al.*, 2004; Majer *et al.*, 2005).

Table 7.4 summarizes the data of anti-mutagenicity studies with HAAs and B(a)P

TABLE 7.4　Anti-genotoxicity studies dealing with dietary constituents which protect against heterocyclic aromatic amines (HAAs) and benzo(a)pyrene (B(a)P) with human HepG2 cells

Putative anti-mutagen	Dose range	End-point	HAA	Results	Remarks
Ascorbic acid (Vit. C)	20 μg–20 mg/ml	SCGE	IQ, PhIP	+/+	Genotoxic at >20 mg/ml
Brussel sprout	1.0 μl/ml	SCGE	IQ	+	
Caffeine	1–500 μg/ml	MN	IQ	+	MeIQ, MeIQx, PhIP
Beta-Carotene	10 μg–10 mg/ml	SCGE	IQ, PhIP	+/+	Genotoxic at >10 mg/ml
Chrysin	1.3–33 μg/ml	MN	PhIP	+	
Coumarin	1–500 μg/ml	MN	IQ	+	
Glycine betaine	1 mM	MN	Trp-P-2	+	Anti-mutagenic in Ames *Salmonella* test + HepG2 S9-fraction
Alpha-Naphthoflavone	20 μg–20 mg/ml	MN	IQ	+	
Beta-Naphthoflavone	20 μg–20 mg/ml	MN	PhIP	+	
Phenethylisocyanate	0.25–1.0 μg/ml	MN	PhIP	+	Anti-mutagenic in *Salmonella* Ames test + HepG2 S9-fraction
Tannic acid	5–500 μg/ml	MN	IQ	+	
Vanillin	1–500 μg/ml	MN	IQ	+	MeIQ, MeIQx, Trp-P-1, PhIP
Anti-genotoxic potential of Flavonols against B(a)P [50 μM]:					
Fisetin	10–100 μM	SCGE		+	Effective at [50 μM]
Kaempferol	10–100 μM	SCGE		+	Effective at [50 μM]
Myricetin	10–100 μM	SCGE		+	Effective at [50 μM]
Quercetin	10–100 μM	SCGE		+	Effective at [50 μM]

Two biological end-points were used; SCGE and MN. SCGE: Single Cell Gel Electrophoresis (Comet assay); MN: Micronuclei in binucleated cells. +, indicates that dietary component revealed anti-mutagenic potential against selected HAA. Caffeine and vanillin also showed anti-genotoxic potential against other types of HAAs.

using HepG2 cells. The HepG2 cell system also proved to be a useful *in vitro* model for detecting human dietary anti-genotoxicants (Kassie *et al.*, 2003a,b; Knasmüller *et al.*, 2004a, 2004c; Mersch-Sundermann *et al.*, 2004; Majer *et al.*, 2005; Darroudi *et al.*, 2009). Interestingly, the results revealed that the antioxidants, ascorbic acid and beta-carotene, do give genotoxic responses in HepG2 cells at high concentration, 20 and 10 mg/ml, respectively.

7.9　THE USE OF GENOMIC AND PROTEOMIC TECHNOLOGIES IN HUMAN HEPG2 CELLS

The ability to monitor variations at the transcriptional and translational levels using DNA microarrays and proteomics is essential to improve our understanding of physiologically relevant processes at the molecular level (Gerner *et al.*, 2002; Yokoo *et al.*, 2004; Breuza *et al.*, 2004; Staal, van Herwijnen, van Schooten, & van Delft, 2006).

The DNA damage caused by chemical carcinogens is important in the initiation of carcinogenesis. However, for promotion and progression of an initiated cell to occur, other events within the cell need to take place and such events are likely to involve gene expression changes induced by the carcinogen. A broader understanding of the impact of carcinogen treatment in specific cells can be mechanistically informative and may enlarge the number of candidate genes contributing to variations in individual susceptibility to carcinogens. Microarray technology offers an attractive method to analyze globally profiles of genes (suppressed and/or expressed by carcinogen exposure). Consequently, this may give key insights into the carcinogenic, and anti-carcinogenic potential of various classes of chemicals that humans are being exposed to via food or environment (Tien, Gray, Peters, & van den Heuvel, 2003).

Gene expression profiling is also used in human HepG2 cell systems and could discriminate genotoxic from non-genotoxic carcinogens (van Delft *et al.*, 2004).

Furthermore, gene expression changes in human HepG2 and MCF-7 cell lines were studied following treatment with carcinogen benzo(a)pyrene (B(a)P) or its non-carcinogenic isomer benzo(e)pyrene (B(e)P) (Hockley *et al.*, 2006, 2009). The overall response to B(a)P consisted of up-regulation of tumor suppressor genes and down-regulation of oncogenes promoting cell cycle arrest and apoptosis. Anti-apoptotic signaling that may increase cell survival and promote tumorgenesis was also evident (Hockley *et al.*, 2006). In contrast, B(e)P did not induce consistent gene expression changes at the same concentrations. Interestingly, in another study, a number of the genes identified have been induced in normal human mammary epithelial cells by B(a)P (e.g. CYP1B1 and NQO1) (Keshava, Whipkey, &

Weston, 2005). This promises that the expression changes observed in these two cell systems are not likely to be artefacts of their cancer phenotype.

7.10 CONCLUSION

The HepG2 cell system has been demonstrated to be a useful *in vitro* model for detecting environmental and human dietary genotoxicants, and anti-genotoxicants. Furthermore, this *in vitro* cell system has the potential to discriminate between structurally related carcinogens and non-carcinogens, as well as between genotoxic and non-genotoxic carcinogens, and could discriminate between clastogens and aneugens.

Using gene expression profiling and proteomics will open the way to elucidate the kinetics and mode of action of various classes of human dietary carcinogens, such as mycotoxins, heterocyclic aromatic amines, and water contaminants, in which earlier studies using conventional tests mostly failed to reveal any DNA damaging effect.

Furthermore, certain characteristics of the commonly used rodent cell lines (e.g. CHO, CHL, V79, L5178Y, etc.), such as lack of p53, karyotype instability, DNA repair deficiencies, are recognized as possibly contributing to the high rate of false positives. The need for exogenous metabolism with these cell systems is also expected to contribute to the false positive/negative rate. In contrast, it appears that the possibility of getting false positive results is low in tests using HepG2 cells, and a wide variety of biological assays that are developed could enhance the potential of this cell system in genotoxicity studies as a model for human risk assessment, with additionally the potential to be used as an alternative to vertebrate animals in mutagenicity/carcinogenicity studies.

The human HepG2 cell system has been well-standardized and validated, and can be incorporated in research programs that are dealing with global harmonization of food safety regulations.

ACKNOWLEDGEMENTS

The studies described in this article were partly financially supported by an EU funded project HEPADNA (QLK1-CT-1999-0810) to F.D., S.K. and V.M.-S.

The authors are grateful to Dr. Huub Lelieveld for his valuable comments and support on this research program.

References

Bezrookove, V., Smits, R., Moeslein, G., et al. (2003). Premature chromosome condensation revisited: A novel chemical approach permits efficient cytogenetic analysis of cancers. *Gene Chromosome Cancer*, 38, 177–186.

Breuza, L., Halneisen, R., Jano, P., et al. (2004). Proteomics and endoplasmic reticulum-golgi intermediate compartment (ERGIC) membrane from Brefeldin A-treated HepG2 cells identifies ERGIC–32, a new cycling protein that interacts with human Erv46. *The Journal of Biological Chemistry*, 279, 47242–47253.

Buchmann, C. A., Nersesyan, A., Kopp, B., et al. (2007). DIMBOA and DIBOA, two naturally occurring benzoxazinones contained in sprouts are potent aneugens in HepG2 cells. *Cancer Letters*, 246, 290–299.

Darroudi, F., & Natarajan, A. T. (1993). Metabolic activation of chemicals to mutagenic carcinogens by human hepatoma microsomal extracts in Chinese hamster ovary cells (*in vitro*). *Mutagenesis*, 8, 11–15.

Darroudi, F., & Natarajan, A. T. (1994). Induction of sister chromatid exchanges, micronuclei and gene mutations by indirectly acting promutagens using human hepatoma cells as an activation system. *ATLA*, 22, 445–453.

Darroudi, F., Meijers, C. M., Hadjidekova, V., & Natarajan, A. T. (1996). Detection of aneugenic and clastogenic potential of X-rays, directly and indirectly acting chemicals in human hepatoma (Hep G2) and peripheral blood lymphocytes, using the micronucleus assay and fluorescent in situ hybridization with a DNA centromeric probe. *Mutagenesis*, 11, 425–433.

Darroudi, F., Knasmüller, S., & Natarajan, A. T. (1998). Use of metabolically competent human hepatoma cells for the detection and characterization of mutagens and antimutagens: An alternative system to the use of vertebrate animals in mutagenicity testing, Netherlands Centre Alternative to Animal Use. *News Letter*, 6, 6–7.

Darroudi, F., Ehrlich, V., Tjon, J., & Knasmüeller, S. (2009). The mutagenic potential of nivalenol and deoxynivalenol in human HepG2 cells and in Ames *Salmonella* test (*Mutation Research*).

Dauer, A., Hensel, A., Lhoste, E., et al. (2003). Genotoxic and antigenotoxic effects of tannins from the bark of *Hamamelis virginiana* L. in metabolically competent, human hepatoma cells (HepG2) using single cell gel electrophoresis. *Phytochemistry*, 63, 199–207.

Ehrlich, V., Darroudi, F., Uhl, M., et al. (2002a). Fumonisin B1 is genotoxic in human derived hepatoma (HepG2) cells. *Mutagenesis*, 17, 257–260.

Ehrlich, V., Darroudi, F., Uhl, M., et al. (2002b). Genotoxic effects of ochratoxin A in human-derived hepatoma (HepG2) cells. *Food and Chemical Toxicology*, 40, 1085–1090.

Filipic, M., & Hei, T. K. (2004). Mutagenicity of cadmium in mammalian cells: Implication of oxidative DNA damage. *Mutation Research*, 546(1–2), 81–91.

Gerner, Ch., Vejda, S., Gelbmann, D., et al. (2002). Concomitant determination of absolute values of cellular protein amounts, synthesis rates and turnover rates by quantitative proteome profiling. *Molecular & Cellular Proteomics*, 1(7), 528–537.

Harries, H. M., Fletcher, S. T., Duggen, C. M., & Baker, V. A. (2001). The use of genomics technology to investigate gene expression changes in cultured human liver cells. *Toxicology in vitro*, 15, 399–405.

Hockley, S. L., Arlt, V. M., Brewer, D., et al. (2006). Time and concentration-dependent changes in gene expression induced by benzo(a)pyrene in two human cell lines, MCF-7 and HepG2. *BMC Genomics*, 7, 260–283.

Hockley, S. L., Mathijs, K., Staal, Y. C. M., et al. (2009). Interlaboratory and interplatform comparison of microarray gene expression analysis of HepG2 cells exposed to benzo(a)pyrene. *OMICS*, 2, 115–118.

IARC. (1993). Some naturally occurring substances: Food items and constituents, heterocyclic aromatic amines and mycotoxins, vol. 56. Lyon: IARC Press.

Jondeau, A., Dahbi, L., Bani-Estivals, M. H., & Chagnon, M. C. (2006). Evaluation of the sensitivity of three sublethal cytotoxicity assays in human HepG2 cell line using water contaminants. *Toxicology*, 226, 218–228.

Kassie, F., Laky, B., Gminski, R., et al. (2003a). Effects of garden and water cress juices and their constituents, benzyl and phenethyl isothiocyanates, towards benzo(a)pyrene-induced DNA damage: a model study with the single cell gel electrophoresis/Hep G2 assay. *Chemico-Biological Interactions*, 142, 285–296.

Kassie, F., Mersch-Sundermann, V., Edenharder, R., et al. (2003b). Development and application of test methods for the detection of dietary constituents which protect against heterocyclic aromatic amines Review. *Mutation Research*, 523–524, 183–192.

Keshava, C., Whipkey, D., & Weston, A. (2005). Transcriptional signatures of environmentally relevant exposures in normal human mammary epithelial cells: Benzo(a)pyrene. *Cancer Letters*, 221, 201–211.

Kirkland, D., Pfuhler, S., Tweats, D., et al. (2007). How to reduce false positive results when undertaking *in vitro* genotoxicity testing and thus avoid unnecessary follow-up animal tests: Report of an ECVAM Workshop. *Mutation Research, 628*, 31–55.

Knasmüller, S., Cavin, C., Chakraborty, A., et al. (2004b). Structurally related mycotoxins, ochratoxin A, ochratoxin B, citrinin differ in their genotoxic activities, and in their mode of action in human derived liver (HepG2) cells: Implication for risk assessment. *Nutrition and Cancer, 50*, 190–197.

Knasmüller, S., Mersch-Sundermann, V., Kevekordes, S., et al. (2004a). Use of human-derived liver cell lines for the detection of environmental and dietary genotoxins; current state of knowledge. *Toxicology, 198*, 315–328.

Knasmüller, S., Murkovic, M., Pfau, W., & Sontag, G. (2004c). Heterocyclic aromatic amines – still a challenge for scientist. *Journal of Chromatography B, 802*, 1–2.

Knasmüller, S., Parzefall, W., Sanyal, R., et al. (1998). Use of metabolically competent human hepatoma cells for the detection of mutagens and antimutagens Review. *Mutation Research, 402*, 185–202.

Knasmüller, S., Sanyal, R., Kassie, F., & Darroudi, F. (1995). Induction of cytogenetic effects by cooked food mutagens and their inhibition by dietary constituents in human hepatoma cells. *Mutation Research, 335*, 62–63.

Knasmüller, S., Schwab, C. E., Land, S. J., et al. (1999). Genotoxic effects of heterocyclic aromatic amines in human derived hepatoma (HepG2) cells. *Mutagenesis, 14*, 533–539.

Knasmüller, S., Steinkellner, S., Majer, B. J., et al. (2002). Search for dietary antimutagens and anticarcinogens: Methodological aspects and extrapolation problems. *Food and Chemical Toxicology, 40*, 1051–1062.

Knasmüller, S., Uhl, M., Pfau, W., et al. (2003). Use of human cell lines in toxicology. *Toxicology, 191*, 15–16.

Knasmüller, S., & Verhagen, H. (2002). Impact of dietary factors on cancer causes and DNA integrity: New trends and aspects. *Food and Chemical Toxicology, 40*, 1047–1050.

Laky, B., Knasmüller, S., Gminski, R., et al. (2002). Protective effects of Brussels sprout towards BaP induced DNA damage: A model study with the single cell gel electrophoresis (SCGE)/Hep G2 assay. *Food and Chemical Toxicology, 40*, 1077–1083.

Lamy, E., Kassie, F., Gminski, R., et al. (2004). 3-Nitrobenzanthrone (3-NBA) induced micronucleus formation and DNA damage in human hepatoma (HepG2) cells. *Toxicology Letters, 146*, 103–109.

Lhoste, E. F., Gloux, K., De Waziers, I., et al. (2004). The activities of several detoxication enzymes are differentially induced by juices of garden cress, water cress and mustard in human HepG2 cells. *Chemico-Biological Interactions, 150*, 211–219.

Lu, W.-Q., Chen, D., Wu, X. J., et al. (2004). DNA damage caused by extracts of chlorinated drinking water in human derived liver cells (Hep G2). *Toxicology, 198*, 351–357.

Majer, B. J., Hofer, E., Cavin, C., et al. (2005). Coffee diterpenes prevent the genotoxic effects of 2-amino–1-methyl–6-phenylimidazo[4,5-b]pyridine (PhIP) and N-nitrosomethylamine in a human derived liver cell line (HepG2). *Food and Chemical Toxicology, 43*, 433–441.

Majer, B. J., Kassie, F., Sasaki, Y., et al. (2004a). Investigation of the genotoxic effects of 2-amino–9H-pyrido[2,3-b]indole (AalphaC) in different organs of rodents and in human derived cells. *Journal of Chromatography B, 802*, 167–173.

Majer, B. J., Mersch-Sundermann, V., Darroudi, F., et al. (2004b). Genotoxic effects of dietary and lifestyle related carcinogens in human derived hepatoma (Hep G2, Hep 3B) cells. *Mutation Research, 551*, 153–166.

Mersch-Sundermann, V., Knasmüller, S., Wu, X., et al. (2004). Use of a human derived liver cell line for the detection of cytoprotective, antigenotoxic and cogenotoxic agents Review. *Toxicology, 198*, 329–340.

Mersch-Sundermann, V., Schneider, H., Freywald, Ch., et al. (2001). Musk ketone enhances benzo[a]pyrene induced mutagenicity in human derived Hep G2 cells. *Mutation Research, 495*, 89–96.

Miret, S., De Groene, E. M., & Klaffke, W. (2006). Comparison of *in vitro* assays of cellular toxicity in the human hepatic cell line HepG2. *Journal of Biomolecular Screening, 11*, 184–193.

Natarajan, A. T., & Darroudi, F. (1991). Use of human hepatoma cells for *in vitro* metabolic activation of chemical mutagens/carcinogens. *Mutagenesis, 6*, 399–403.

Rueff, J., Chiapella, C., Chipman, J. K., et al. (1996). Development and validation of alternative metabolic systems for mutagenicity testing in short-term assays Review. *Mutation Research, 353*, 151–176.

Russell, W. M. (1995). The development of the three Rs concept. *Alternatives to Laboratory Animals, 23*, 298–304.

Sanyal, R., Darroudi, F., Parzefall, W., et al. (1997). Inhibition of the genotoxic effects of heterocyclic amines in human derived hepatoma cells by dietary bioantimutagens. *Mutagenesis, 12*, 297–303.

Scharf, G., Prustomersky, S., Knasmüller, S., et al. (2003). Enhancement of glutathione and g-glutamylcysteine synthetase, the rate limiting enzyme of glutathione synthesis, by chemoprotective plant-derived food and beverage components in the human hepatoma cell line Hep G2. *Nutrition and Cancer, 45*(1), 74–83.

Schmeiser, H., Gminski, R., & Mersch-Sundermann, V. (2001). Evaluation of health risks caused by musk ketone. *International Journal of Hygiene and Environmental Health, 203*, 293–299.

Schoonen, W. G. E. J., De Roos, J. A. D. M., Westerink, W. M. A., & Debiton, E. (2005b). Cytotoxic effects of 110 reference compounds on HepG2 and HeLa cells and for 60 compounds on ECC–1 and CHO cells. II. Mechanistic assays on NAD(P)H, ATP and DNA contents. *Toxicology in vitro, 19*, 491–503.

Schoonen, W. G. E. J., Westerink, W. M. A., De Roos, J. A. D. M., & Debiton, E. (2005a). Cytotoxic effects of 100 reference compounds on HepG2 and HeLa cells and for 60 compounds on ECC–1 and CHO cells. I. Mechanistic assays on ROS, glutathione depletion and calcein uptake. *Toxicology in vitro, 19*, 505–516.

Schwab, C. E., Huber, W. W., Parzefall, W., et al. (2000). Search for compounds which inhibit the genotoxic and carcinogenic effects of heterocyclic aromatic amines. *Critical Reviews in Toxicology, 30*, 1–69.

Schwab, C., Kassie, F., Qin, H. M., et al. (1999). Development of test systems for the detection of compounds that prevent the genotoxic effects of heterocyclic aromatic amines: Preliminary results with constituents of cruciferous vegetables and other dietary constituents. *Journal of Environmental Pathology, Toxicology and Oncology, 18*, 109–118.

Staal, Y. C. M., van Herwijnen, M. H. M., van Schooten, F. J., & Delft van, J. H. M. (2006). Modulation of gene expression and DNA adduct formation in HepG2 cells by polycyclic aromatic hydrocarbons with different carcinogenic potencies. *Carcinogenesis, 3*, 646–655.

Steck, S. E., Gaudet, M. M., Eng, S. M., et al. (2007). Cooked meat and risk of breast cancer – Lifetime versus recent dietary intake. *Epidemiology, 18*, 373–382.

Steinkellner, H., Rabot, S., Frewald, Ch., et al. (2001). Effect of cruciferous vegetables and their constituents on drug metabolizing enzymes involved in the bioactivation of DNA-reactive dietary carcinogens. *Mutation Research, 480–481*, 285–297.

Sugimura, T. (1982). Mutagens, carcinogens, and tumor promoters in our daily food. *Cancer, 49*, 1970–1984.

Sugimura, T. (2000). Nutrition and dietary carcinogens Review. *Carcinogenesis, 21*, 387–395.

Tien, E. S., Gray, J. P., Peters, J. M., & van den Heuvel, J. P. (2003). Comprehensive gene expression analysis of peroxisome proliferator-treated immortalized hepatocytes: Identification of peroxisome proliferator-activated receptor alpha-dependent growth regulatory genes. *Cancer Research, 63*, 5767–5780.

Uhl, M., Darroudi, F., Seybel, A., et al. (2001). Development of new experimental models for the identification of DNA protective and anticarcinogenic plant constituents. In I. Kreft & V. Skrabanja (Eds.), *Molecular and genetic interactions involving phytochemicals* (pp. 21–33).

Uhl, M., Ecker, S., Kassie, F., et al. (2003a). Effect of chrysin, a flavonoid compound, on the mutagenic activity of 2-amino–1-methyl–6-phenylimidazo[4,5-b]pyridine

(PhIP) and benzo(a)pyrene (P(a)P in bacterial and human hepatoma (HepG2) cells. *Archives of Toxicology, 77*, 477–484.

Uhl, M., Helma, C., & Knasmüller, S. (1999). Single-cell gel electrophoresis assays with human-derived hepatoma (Hep G2) cells. *Mutation Research, 441*, 215–224.

Uhl, M., Helma, C., & Knasmüller, S. (2000). Evaluation of the single-cell gel electrophoresis assays with human hepatoma (HepG2) cells. *Mutation Research, 468*, 213–225.

Uhl, M., Laky, B., Lhoste, E., et al. (2003b). Effects of mustard sprouts and allylisothiocyanate on benzo(a)pyrene-induced DNA damage in human-derived cells: A model study with the single cell gel electrophoresis/Hep G2 assay. *Teratogenesis, Carcinogenesis, and Mutagenesis* (Supplement 1), 273–282.

van Delft, J. H. M., Agen van, E., Breda van, S. G. J., et al. (2004). Discrimination of genotoxic from non-genotoxic carcinogens by gene expression profiling. *Carcinogenisis, 25*(7), 1265–1276.

Verhagen, H., Aruoma, O. I., van Delft, J. H. M., et al. (2003). The 10 basic requirements for a scientific paper reporting antioxidant, antimutagenic or anticarcinogenic potential of test substances in *in vitro* experiments and animal studies *in vivo*. *Food and Chemical Toxicology, 41*, 603–610.

Westerink, W. M. A., & Schoonen, W. G. E. J. (2007a). Cytochrome P450 enzyme levels in HepG2 cells and cryopreserved primary human hepatocytes and their induction in HepG2 cells. *Toxicology in vitro, 21*, 1581–1591.

Westerink, W. M. A., & Schoonen, W. G. E. J. (2007b). Phase II enzyme levels in HepG2 cells and cryopreserved primary human hepatocytes and their induction in HepG2 cells. *Toxicology in vitro, 21*, 1592–1602.

Wilkening, S., & Bader, A. (2003). Influence of culture time on the expression of drug-metabolizing enzymes in primary human hepatocytes and hepatoma cell line HepG2. *Journal of Biochemical and Molecular Toxicology, 17*, 207–213.

Wilkening, S., Stahl, F., & Bader, A. (2003). Comparison of primary human hepatocytes and hepatoma cell line HepG2 with regard to their biotransformation properties. *Drug Metabolism and Disposition, 31*, 1035–1042.

Wu, X., Lu, W. Q., Roos, P. H., & Mersch-Sundermann, V. (2005). Vinclozolin, a widely used fungicide, enhanced BaP-induced micronucleus formation in human derived hepatoma cells by increasing CYP1A1 expression. *Toxicology Letters, 159*, 83–88.

Yokoo, H., Kondo, T., Fujii., et al. (2004). Proteomic signature corresponding to alpha fetoprotein expression in liver cancer cells. *Hepatology, 3*, 609–617.

Yuan, J., Lu, W. Q., Dai, W. T., et al. (2005). Chlorinated drinking water caused oxidative damage, DNA migration and cytotoxicity in human cells. *International Journal of Hygiene and Environmental Health, 208*, 481–488.

8

Capacity Building: Harmonization and Achieving Food Safety

Larry Keener

International Product Safety Consultants, Seattle, WA, USA

8.1 INTRODUCTION

Global trade involving food and foodstuffs expanded rapidly during the latter decades of the twentieth century. Developing nations and newly enrolled supply chain partners, significantly benefited from the opening of new market opportunities as well as from the chance to participate in the international economy. For example, between 1980 and 1994, the contribution to the food sector from developing countries to the overall world value of international trade increased by 3.5%, while that of the European Union increased by 4.3% and that of North America by only 2.4% (UNIDO, 1997). Much of the observed growth resulted from the aggressive sourcing practices of the industrialized nations. The CEOs of multinational corporations based in Europe, the United States, and Japan and other 'Group of Eight (G8) nations' extended their supply chains into new geographic areas with a view to cultivating improved margins and new markets. Miranda-da-Cruz *et al.* (2009) of the United Nations Industrial Development Organization (UNIDO) estimate the present value of the global food industry in excess of US$5 trillion.

The much heralded stories of India, China, and Brazil's successful emergence as low cost producers and source countries are reported widely by contemporary news outlets. The economies of these nations benefited enormously from this explosion in food trade and poverty rates in each declined precipitously, according to the World Bank (Thompson, 2005). Moreover, there was also a serendipitous improvement in the public health status of the foods and foodstuffs offered by each nation for both domestic consumption and international trade. These collective gains appear to have been hard learned and expensive.

Concurrent with the reported successes were a number of sensational transnational food safety scares. The majority of the incidents have been assigned classical modes of failure (e.g. bacterial, viral or protozoan agents, and industrial, agricultural or environmental chemical contaminants). Consider, for example, the 2007 and 2008 episodes of melamine contamination in dairy products, infant formula and assorted other foodstuffs sourced from China. Likewise, in 1994, enterotoxin tainted mushrooms exported to the United States from China were implicated in a major foodborne illness outbreak (Ballentine, 1989). Similarly, in 2004 one of the largest transnational food scares in history, attributed to the industrial dye (prohibited in foods intended for human use) Sudan Red 1, is reported to have had its origins in food ingredients sourced from India (Mishra *et al.*, 2007). By no means do China, India and Brazil comprise a complete listing of the countries that have placed unsafe food into the global food supply chain. In fact, the list of culpable nations, underdeveloped or otherwise, is a long one and growing. Curtailing the occurrence of such failures is paramount for preserving the public health and for sustaining the global trade in food. Updating and upgrading the scientific capabilities and regulatory framework of all nations participating in the global food supply chain is fundamental. Collectively, these processes are referred to as capacity building.

8.2 CAPACITY BUILDING

In the process of assigning cause to food safety failures the epidemiologists and regulatory officials are beginning to acknowledge that insufficiency in both scientific and regulatory capabilities is the major contributing factor. Lacking capacity frequently translates into an inability to provide the surveillance mechanisms necessary for ensuring the safety of foodstuffs bound for international commerce. Lacking capacity is increasingly critical and problematic as global food supply chains are projected deeper into economically underdeveloped regions of the planet. Countries in Africa, Asia, and the Americas, in which the per capita income is less than US$1,000 annually, are increasingly targeted by industrialized states as potential sources for food and food ingredients (see Table 8.1).

There is an abundance of data in contemporary literature that suggests a correlation between per capita income and the likelihood

TABLE 8.1 Potential supply chain partners with per capita daily income and population data

Country	Population (Millions)[**]	Percentage <$1/day[*]	Percentage <$2/day
China	1299	16.6	46.7
India	1065	34.7	79.9
Indonesia	239	7.5	52.4
Brazil	184	8.2	22.4
Pakistan	159	13.4	65.6
Russia	144	6.1	23.8
Bangladesh	141	36.0	82.8
Nigeria	126	70.2	90.8
Mexico	105	9.9	26.3

[*]Source: World Bank. *World Development Indicators* database (Thompson, 2005).
[**]Source: US CIA Factbook, *Population and Demographic Data*, World 6,536,473,538, August 2006.

of a nation state having both of the scientific capability and regulatory infrastructures required to sustain safe exportation of food products. This finding is supported, for example, by a 2003 Pan American Health Organization/World Health Organization's food safety assessment of its regional members. The data presented in Table 8.2 show a large disparity in the food safety systems between wealthy and poor nations in the region. Brazil, Canada, Chile and USA (clusters 1 and 7 in Table 8.2), for example, received excellent scores in the PAHO/WHO assessments. By contrast, the food safety systems of the remaining 29 countries that participated in the study, less wealthy nations, did not achieve the minimum international standard (PAHO/WHO, 2003). These facts are daunting when one considers the contributions of the poor nations in this region to the global trade in food.

The PAHO/WHO study concluded the following with regard to the main weakness in food safety systems development as highlighted by the study:

1. Absence or scarcity of provisions establishing *punishing mechanisms* and control mechanisms.
2. Absence or scarcity of *transparency* in the drafting of food regulations (no integration of entities related to the food area, provisions drafted by the government without consulting all sectors involved).
3. *Insufficient harmonization with international standards* and *lack of provisions* referred to follow-up and confiscation of food in case of problems.
4. Insufficient definition and delimitation of functions of governmental authorities (*overlapping of functions or loopholes* in the appointment of competent authorities for the control of certain activities).

Similar findings have been reported by the United Nations Industrial Development Organization (UNIDO) in its assessment of food safety systems development in 25 African nations (Ouaouich, 2005). As can be seen in Table 8.3, even the best performing nations in the UNIDO assessments of their food safety programs suffered deficiencies that would cause concern for the public health status of food products emanating from those sources. The main deficiencies (Table 8.4) in food safety system development as reported by the UNIDO workers were also remarkably similar to those reported by the PAHO/WHO studies. The African nations, like those in the Americas, suffered from insufficient harmonization with international standards, poor cooperation among regulatory bodies, and a lack of national food safety policy.

Food safety experts have historically assigned food safety failures to one of three principle modes: microbiological, chemical, and foreign body contamination. Increasingly, however, lacking food safety capacity is cited as a primary or contributing factor in outbreak investigations.

TABLE 8.2 Pan-American Health Organization/World Health Organization's Food Safety Assessment of American Regional Members (2003)

Cluster (representative member)	Number of Countries/ Cluster	Performance Rating (%)
1 (Brazil, Canada, USA)	3	96–100
2	14	25–60
3 (Mexico)	5	58–81
4	4	25–60
5	3	58–81
6	3	58–81
7 (Chile)	1	58–81

Thirty-three of the 35 Nations in the Americas participated in the study (Cuba and Haiti were excluded due to insufficiency of Food Safety system data). Food safety systems in four nations (clusters 1 and 7) were defined as excellent. By contrast, the remaining 29 countries received ratings reflective of low levels of food safety system development.

TABLE 8.3   United Nations Industrial Development Organization (UNIDO) capacity building assessment in twenty-five African nations (2005)

Country	Food Safety Policy	Food Safety Information	Regulations	Food Safety Management	Auditing	Scientific Support (monitoring)	Labs
Senegal	3	3	3	3	3	3	3
Mauritania	2	3	3	2	3	2	3
Guinea	2	3	2	2	3	1	1
Uganda	3	3	3	3	3	3	3
Tanzania	3	3	3	3	3	3	3
Kenya	3	3	3	3	3	3	
Angola	2	3	2	2	3	2	2

The data in the table for the seven best performing nations of 25 involved in UNIDO food safety survey (Key 3= Satisfactory). Source: Ouaouich, 2005.

TABLE 8.4   UNIDO summary of major findings from African Survey (2005)

Frequency of food safety element's inclusion in UNIDO Programs (%)		Key finding on Implementation/Efficacy from participating nations
Food Safety Policy	68	Few countries with established national food safety policy
Food Safety Information/Awareness	100	High level of awareness and many training opportunities
Legislation, Regulations and Standards	76	50% of nations have harmonized with international standards
		25% of nations in process of developing standards
		25% of nations with no development activity
National Food Safety Management Framework	75	Poor cooperation between agencies
		7/25 nations in study have national framework
Inspection and Auditing Programs	96	18/25 nations have high competent inspectors
		750 inspectors trained in last 10 years
Scientific Support for Surveillance and Monitoring	88	Low level of development 5/25 with risk assessment capability
Laboratory Programs and Standards	84	13/25 nations with international accredited labs
		7/25 nations making progress with GLPs
		5/25 nations lack infrastructure and staff

Source: Ouaouich, 2005.

Building capacity across the transnational expanses of complex food supply chains is regarded by regulatory authorities and health officials as a major contributor in protecting public health and preserving the integrity of the global food supply.

The term 'globalization of public health' has emerged in policy discourses. It expresses the transnational or globalized nature of public health threats, including those represented by food and waterborne diseases, in an increasingly interdependent world. Because foodborne diseases and chemical contaminants have no regard for geopolitical boundaries of nation states, and because notions of state sovereignty are unknown concepts in the microbial realm, all of humanity is now (owing in part to the global trade in food) vulnerable to the emerging and re-emerging threats associated with foodstuffs improperly handled or processed.

8.3 THE ROLE OF MULTILATERAL AGREEMENTS IN ACHIEVING FOOD SAFETY

Food safety has increasingly become an important topic in international law. Its implications are far-reaching and impact a number of multilateral regimes such as the World Health Organization's (WHO) International Health Regulations (IHR), the World Trade Organization's (WTO) Trade-Related Aspects of Intellectual Property Rights (TRIPS) and Sanitary and Phytosanitary (SPS) Agreements, and the Joint FAO/WHO Codex Alimentarius Commission[1] standards on food safety. Achieving public health objectives related to preserving the integrity of the food supply present enormous global challenges that frequently transcend the capabilities of individual governments. Achieving food safety requires harmonized and global governance strategies. Historically, international law has played an important role in this dynamic, because states have used treaties and conventions to solve public health problems that are transnational in nature.

8.3.1 Historical Developments in Food Safety Management and Multilateral Agreements

The 1924 Pan-American Sanitary Code[2] is an excellent example of a multilateral agreement that was constructed with the intent of curtailing the spread of communicable diseases and other 'dangerous contagion liable to spread through international commerce' (Pan American Health Organization). It is noteworthy that surveillance and sharing epidemiological data were important elements of the Code's mandate. The 1924 sanitary code supplanted a narrowly written 1905 version that had been agreed for the expressed purpose of monitoring a specific but limited set of communicable diseases plaguing the region at that time. The success of these regional multilateral agreements set the stage for the adoption, in 1951, of the International Sanitary Regulations (ISR) of WHO. The ISRs were re-named the IHRs in 1969 and modified in 1973 and 1981. According to WHO, the IHRs are among the earliest multilateral regulatory mechanisms focusing on global surveillance for communicable diseases. As of 1997, the IHRs were legally binding on all WHO's Member States except Australia. The effectiveness and impact of the IHRs are contentious and the subject of much debate among WHO members. It is ironic that one of the main points cited in making the case against the IHRs has to do with reporting of surveillance data. For example, in 1994, after reporting a plague outbreak, India suffered nearly US$2 billion losses in trade resulting from excessive embargoes that were imposed by other nations. Similarly, in 1997, the economies of several East African nations were harmed by a ban against the importation of fresh fish into the European Community following a reported

---

[1]*Codex Alimentarius*, http://www.codexalimentarius.net/web/index_en.jsp.

[2]Pan-American Health Organization, Sanitary Food Code 1924, Chapter 1, http://www.paho.org/English/PAHO/code-1999.pdf.

outbreak of cholera (Aginam, 2002). Another frequently cited reason for the ineffectiveness of the IHRs is the regulations' inflexibility and inability to adapt to changing circumstances in international trade and public health. Indubitably, much has changed in international trade related to food and foodstuffs since the 1981 modification of the IHRs that would call into questions the regulations usefulness in terms of controlling the spread of foodborne diseases. Promoting food safety, it appears, was never the explicit intent of the IHR regulations. The regulations were promulgated and subsequently modified with the intent of providing a mechanism for the control and sharing of epidemiological information on the trans-boundary spread of cholera, plague and yellow fever; diseases that, with the exception of cholera, are not transmitted by either food or water.

8.3.2 Sanitary and Phytosanitary Agreement of the World Trade Organization

The 1995 SPS agreement of the WTO covers risk measures such as quarantine restrictions on imported agricultural products. These are intended to prevent the introduction of pests or diseases which could harm domestic industries or the natural environment within the territory of a WTO Member. Measures also include bans on imported food products given that they contain contaminants or additives which pose a risk to public health. The SPS measures potentially impact a broad range of national regulations designed to protect against health risks to humans, animals or plants. The SPS agreement was driven by a desire to minimize the impacts of national SPS measures on trade by harmonizing the WTO Members' SPS measures. Article 3.1 of the SPS Agreement requires that Members base their SPS measures on the international standards, guidelines and recommendations developed by the Codex Alimentarius

Commission (food safety), the International Office of Epizootics (animal health) and the International Plant Protection Convention (plant health). While harmonization was the objective, it was recognized that this goal could not be achieved in all cases. Consider, for example, where Members' SPS measure could not be harmonized because of lack of an agreed international standard, or because certain WTO Members opted for more stringent regulations. Article 3.3 of the SPS agreement specifically allows Members to adopt more stringent national regulations provided that they have a scientific basis. There are two provisions of the Agreement that are important in defining the criteria for measures to have a basis in science. The first is Article 2.2 which stipulates that WTO Members must base any SPS measure they wish to introduce on 'scientific principles' and to ensure that their SPS measures are 'not maintained without sufficient scientific evidence.' Article 2.2, however, is subject to an exception set out in Article 5.7. The exemption allows Members to adopt SPS measures 'on the basis of available pertinent information' in circumstance where 'relevant scientific evidence is insufficient.'

The second provision is Article 5.0 which establishes obligations for Members to ensure that their SPS measures are based on 'risk assessment'. Moreover, in conducting an assessment of risks, Members must take into account 'available scientific evidence' and risk assessment techniques developed by the international organizations whose standards are referenced in the Agreement (SPS Article 5.1).

Considering that the SPS measures are risk-based, it is worthwhile noting that nowhere in the WTO documents is there mention of risk management. It is generally accepted that the components of the risk analysis process involve the following operations: risk assessment, risk communication and risk management.

The SPS Agreement has given rise to conflicts among WTO Members. Developing nations have complained that they are held to the more onerous SPS measures, as allowed by WTO, of the developed nations and that this disparity has the effect of inhibiting participation of the poor in remunerative economic activities. The proliferation and increased level of standards pose challenges for developing countries. For example, how to cost-effectively meet external regulatory or supply chain requirements? Many in the developing world are seeking external assistance as called for under the Agreement. The provision of technical assistance and other capacity-building measures in this area are under World Bank-supported projects and there appears to be an increasing demand in this area from the Bank's clients. At the time of writing, there is no comprehensive assessment to compare or contrast the assistance that has been provided in terms of its efficacy, efficiency, or sustainability in addressing the needs of the developing nations.

As mentioned previously, 'capacity' in terms of providing adequate surveillance of the public health issues attendant to the global food supply, consists of two separate but interrelated elements. Ideally, foods safety laws and regulations are developed and underpinned by sound objective science. Capacity in terms of food safety is the construct that results from the amalgamation of science and laws. Both are fundamental for building a nation's capability to protect and preserve public health. WTO's SPS Agreement sits squarely at that intersection where scientific method meets jurisprudence.

8.3.3 FAO/WHO and *Codex Alimentarius*

In 1961, the Eleventh Session of the Conference of the Food and Agriculture Organization (FAO) of the United Nations passed a resolution to set up the Codex Alimentarius Commission. In May 1963, the Sixteenth World Health Assembly approved the establishment of the Joint FAO/WHO Food Standards Program and adopted the statutes of the Codex Alimentarius Commission. According to Codex documents, a driving force for the establishment of the Commission was

the need to harmonize standards that could be adopted in advancing public health and providing for the safe trade in food products. As previously noted, the SPS Agreement of the WTO specifically references the *Codex Alimentarius* and stipulates further that WTO Members adhere to the guidelines and standards of the Codex in developing national SPS measures. Moreover, WTO has increasingly used Codex as an international reference standard for the resolution of disputes concerning food safety and consumer protection.

Codex Alimentarius is framed and directed by the following five guiding principles:

1. Protecting the health of consumers and ensuring fair practices in the food trade.
2. Promoting coordination of all food standards work undertaken by international governmental and non-governmental organizations.
3. Determining priorities and initiating and guiding the preparation of draft standards through and with the aid of appropriate organizations.
4. Finalizing standards elaborated under (3) above and, after acceptance by governments, publishing them in a *Codex Alimentarius* either as regional or worldwide standards, together with international standards already finalized by other bodies under (2) above, wherever this is practicable.
5. Amending published standards, after appropriate survey in the light of developments.

To adopt Codex standards, countries require an adequate food law as well as a technical and administrative infrastructure with the capacity to implement it and ensure compliance. It is clear then that Codex recognizes in a fundamental way the need for those adopting its voluntary guidelines and standards to have the 'capacity' for both validations and enforcement. For many years, FAO and WHO have provided assistance to developing countries to enable them to take full advantage of the Commission's work.

According to the Commission, Codex's assistance to developing countries has included:

- *convening expert meetings*, including the Joint FAO/WHO Expert Committee on Food Additives (JECFA) and the Joint FAO/WHO Meetings on Pesticide Residues (JMPR), to advise the Codex Alimentarius Commission;
- *establishing and strengthening national food control systems*, including the formulation and revision of food legislation (acts and regulations) and food standards in accordance with Codex standards;
- *conducting workshops and training courses*, not only for transferring information, knowledge and skills associated with food control, but also to increase awareness of the *Codex Alimentarius* and activities carried out by the Commission;
- *strengthening laboratory analysis and food inspection capabilities*;
- *providing training in all aspects of food control* associated with protecting the health of consumers and ensuring honest practices in the sale of food;
- *presenting papers at conferences, meetings and symposia* on the relevance of Codex activities to the provision of safe food of acceptable quality;
- *extending guidance on matters directly related to Codex activities*, such as safety assessment of food produced using biotechnology;
- *developing and publishing manuals and texts* that are associated with food quality control and provide recommendations for the development and operation of food quality and safety systems;
- *helping with the establishment and strengthening of food control agencies* as well as with training in the necessary technical and administrative skills to ensure their effective operation;

- *developing and publishing training manuals* on food inspection and quality and safety assurance, particularly with respect to the application of the Hazard Analysis Critical Control Point (HACCP) system in the food-processing industry.

Since its inception in 1963 the Commission's demographics have changed rather dramatically. As can be seen in Figure 8.1 there has been a radical shift in the numbers of participating countries from developing nations versus those from developed nations. By 1997 membership of the developing nations outnumbered developed nations by approximately 3 to 1 (Codex Commission). While this trend has continued paradoxically it is reported that the key problem facing smaller and less-developed countries in their efforts to improve food safety capacity is due to a lack of representation in international standard setting bodies including *Codex Alimentarius*. The fact is that, for many poor nations, the cost of sending a delegation to Commission meetings is simply prohibitive.

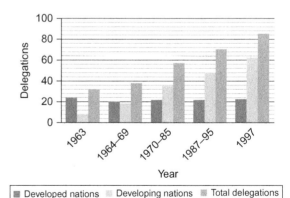

FIGURE 8.1 Codex's changing delegation demographics 1963–1997. Shift in the composition and number of delegations from developing nations versus developed nations attending Codex between 1963 and 1997 (Codex Commission).

8.4 CONCLUSION

Achieving and sustaining capacity is difficult, even for wealthy, technology rich nations. Consider that the USA, one of the wealthiest nations on the planet and certainly among the world's leaders in its technological prowess, has embarked upon a campaign to modernize and improve its food safety systems. In announcing the campaign, the US President indicated that the overall number of foodborne illness outbreaks in the US had increased from 100/year during the decade of the 1990s to upwards of 350 by 2008. The cause for the increase was attributed to inadequate surveillance of the food manufacturing and distribution supply chains (Obama, 2009). President Barack Obama indicated that a failure to adequately fund the agencies responsible for food safety oversight had created a 'hazard to the public health.' Accordingly, the US, it is reported, will invest US$1 billion in modernizing its food safety surveillance systems. China experienced similar failures in the last decades of the twentieth century during its rapid ascent to prominence as a low cost, global supplier of food and foodstuffs. Cognizant of the threat to its international reputation and its future economic development, China deployed an aggressive national program to raise the level of food safety awareness and to bolster both its scientific capability and regulatory framework to limit future foodborne illness outbreaks. There are no financial data available relating to the cost of these programs but it is reasonable to conclude that China's investment was also in billions of dollars.

Imagine the hardship that such expenditure would cause for developing nations desirous of participating in the global trade in food. The proposition is simply untenable and cost prohibitive. For example, according to the CIA's World Factbook,[3] the Republic of Chad reported a gross domestic product (GDP) of just over US$15 billion in 2004. It is difficult to conceive that this central African country of approximately 11 million people, and a contributor to the global food supply, could make a proportional investment in attaining the capacity to properly monitor its food production and distribution systems.

FAO and WHO reports concluded that the food systems of developing countries are extremely diverse and tend to be less organized, comprehensive and effective than those in developed countries. The reports go on to say that the food safety systems in these countries are challenged by problems of rapid growing population, urbanization and natural environments that expose consumers to a wide range of potential food safety risks. It is interesting to note that FAO also concluded that food safety standards in developing countries may actually attain those of international standards, but the lack of technical and institutional capacity to control and ensure compliance essentially makes the standards less effective. According to FAO this apparent paradox results from a lack of technical and scientific infrastructure, e.g. testing laboratories, human and financial resources, national legislative and regulatory frameworks, enforcement capacity, management and coordination of the food safety system. These findings are confirmed or supported by PAHO/WHO workers in their assessment of food safety systems in the Americas; and again by the outcomes of UNIDO's report from its study of food safety system development in 25 African nations.

Widespread changes in the global food economy and the rapidly evolving environment in which food safety must be considered have demonstrated the profound interdependence of all elements of the supply chain and highlighted their contribution to achieving food safety. The

[3]CIA Factbook, *GDP and Demographic Data* (2004).

historical record is replete with bilateral and multilateral conventions that have been agreed between and among nations for the purpose of preventing the transnational spread of contagion and disease causing agents. The 1924 Sanitary Agreement among the nations in the Americas, for example, offers a good case study in both the successes and failings of such agreements. The 1924 agreement was too narrowly crafted and overly ridged to keep pace with the rapid advances in science and technology. Likewise, WHO's International Health Regulations have been reported to suffer similar shortcomings. These observations withstanding it remains a fact that achieving food safety involves all elements of the food supply chain including: food production, food processing, and food distribution networks. Science and science-based regulatory constructs are also required to support and sustain the supply chain. Moreover, risk-based ex-ante (risk avoidance) measures are preferred over the more conventional ex-post strategies for achieving food safety.

Food safety has been defined as 'the biological, chemical or physical status of a food that will permit its consumption without incurring *excessive risk* of injury, morbidity or mortality' (Keener, 2004). The inequality in food safety capacity, scientific and regulatory, among various supply chain contributors places the global trade in food at risk. Building the scientific capability and regulatory framework corresponding with food safety capacity is an expensive proposition. For many developing and underdeveloped nations the costs of acquiring food safety capacity are simply too prohibitive. Yet international trading data suggest that these nations will increasingly participate as future supply chain partners.

To be successful in building scientific and regulatory capability and therefore capacity to provide for the adequate surveillance of their food and agricultural resources, developing nations will require the continued financial support of their trading partners in the 'West.' Building analytical capacity is critical for supporting and elaborating a comprehensive food safety surveillance system. Analytical capability demands people with expert skills as well as facilities and equipment. Acquiring these components represents an enormous challenge for many developing nations. Recall that both the UNIDO and PAHO/WHO studies, discussed earlier in this chapter, concluded that there was a lack of analytical skill in many of the countries involved with their surveys. Babu and Rhoe (2001) provide an excellent summary of the typical challenges facing developing countries in the organization and modernization of food safety systems. According to these workers, the problems are often related to a lack of human capacity and personnel; the lack of financial capacity to establish basic infrastructure, to conduct training and make the system sustainable over time. Acquiring laboratory capability generally and microbiological testing capability specifically, is both expensive and demanding of skilled personnel, but essential for ensuring public health and likewise for sustaining the global trade in food. In Chapter 9, Dr. M.C. Varadaraj from India's Central Food Technological Research Institute (CFTRI), provides an excellent and comprehensive treatment of the mechanics and challenges associated with building analytical and microbiological testing capacity.

References

Aginam, O. (2002). International law and communicable diseases. *Bulletin of the World Health Organization, 80,* 946–951.

Babu, S., & Rhoe, V. (2001). *Food security, regional trade, and food safety in Central Asia—Case studies from Kyrgyz Republic and Kazakhstan.* Washington, DC: International Food Policy Research Institute.

Ballentine, C. (1989). Cloud over mushrooms. *FDA Consumer Magazine, 23.*

Keener, L. (2004). Nonthermal Processing Technologies and the Global Harmonization Initiative, IFT/EFFoST NPD Conference, Cork, Ireland.

Miranda-da-Cruz, S., & Schebesta, K. (2009). Global development of the food industry—Perspective of UNIDO; http://www.futurefood6.com/files/1.Global%20development%20of%20the%20food%20industry.pdf.

Mishra, K. K., Dixit, S., Purshottam, S. K., et al. (2007). Exposure assessment to Sudan dyes through consumption of artificially coloured chilli powders in India. *Int J Food Sci Tech*, 42(11), 1363–1366.

Obama, B. (2009). *US President's Statement on Food Safety Modernization* March 14. Associated Press International.

Ouaouich, A. (2005). *A review of the capacity building efforts in developing countries: Case study Africa*; Presented at the 6th World Congress on Seafood Safety, Sydney, Australia.

PAHO/WHO. (2003). National Food Safety Systems in the Americas and the Caribbean—A Situation Analysis, http://www.fao.org/docrep/meeting/010/a0394e/A0394E20.htm.

Thompson, R.L. (2005). World Ag Trade Negotiations: Doha Development Agenda, IFT annual convention, New Orleans, LA, USA; http://ift.confex.com/ift/2005/techprogram/paper_27890.htm.

UNIDO. (1997). Trade Developments in Food and Contributions of Developing Countries, Tapia, M. IFT Presentation 2004, Las Vegas, NV, USA.

Further Reading

Berrios, M. (2003). *Participation and civic engagement in poverty reduction strategy*; 13th Inter-American Meeting PAHO/WHO Washington DC.

Food and Agriculture Organization of the United Nations. (2005). Improving the effectiveness of national food control systems in the English-speaking Caribbean (PAHO). FAO/WHO Regional Conference on Food Safety for the Americas and the Caribbean.

Food and Agriculture Organization of the United Nations. (2002). *Capacity building on Food Safety in Mongolia*. FAO/WHO Global Forum of Food Safety Regulators.

Tapia, M., De Andrade. (2004). Global regulatory situation; Case study: Regulatory development in the Americas, IFT Annual Convention, Las Vegas.

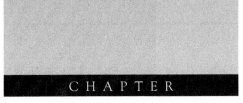

9

Capacity Building: Building Analytical Capacity for Microbial Food Safety

Mandyam C. Varadaraj

Department of Human Resource Development, Central Food Technological Research Institute, Mysore, India

9.1 INTRODUCTION

There is no capsule definition for food safety although, in general, it would mean 'the biological, chemical or physical status of a food that will permit its consumption without incurring excessive risk of injury, morbidity or mortality.'

Food safety problems are closely associated with changes evolving in society, economy, lifestyle, and eating habits (Doores, 1999). With globalization of jobs, career, and trade opportunities, there is increased travel and immigration by people. This change in lifestyle has led to outside eating habits, giving unlimited opportunities for convenience and processed foods needing less time for food preparation (Meng & Doyle, 2002). This changing situation has increased international trade in food and often raw materials are obtained globally from different places/countries and the food is processed through the use of varied unit operations. The increased globalization of the food supply chain combined with knowledgeable consumers has led to the demand for a safer food supply (Stringer, 2005).

The World Health Organization (WHO) declared that access to nutritionally adequate and safe food is a right of each individual. The WHO has urged the government health agencies, the entire food industry and the consumers to assume greater responsibility in the area of food safety. The World Health Assembly adopted a resolution on food safety in May 2000. This resolution calls upon countries to integrate food safety as one of their essential public health functions through capacity building programs. This resolution is considered as a milestone in the history of public health since, for the first time in the WHO's 50-plus years of existence, it has identified food safety as an important objective and as an essential function of the public health community (Miliotis & Bier, 2003). Globally, many regulatory agencies and organizations have been involved in the implementation of such programs in collaboration with Research and Development organizations.

9.2 SIGNIFICANCE OF MICROBIAL FOOD SAFETY

In the food safety scenario, the most important objective and function is microbial food safety. Microorganisms have replaced chemical adulterants as the major recognized agent of food poisoning in the latter part of the twentieth century and into the twenty-first century. The situation is more alarming due to a number of changes internationally. These changes include population explosion, urbanization and changes in lifestyle, consumption of minimally processed ready-to-eat foods, international trade in food and animal feed, international tourism and immigration, and a short supply of potable drinking water. Foods are prone to microbial contaminants that are known for the undesirable changes they bring about in foods, causing either spoilage and/or health hazards. A more serious aspect of microbial contamination is the possibility of serious health hazards due to the presence of potential food poisoning microorganisms and their toxic metabolites leading to food poisoning outbreaks. The recognized foodborne pathogens include multicellular animal parasites, protozoa, fungi, bacteria, and viruses. Deciding on capacity building programs requires knowledge of the major bacterial species that play a significant role in food safety.

Bacterial food poisonings are of two types: infection and intoxication. Infections are diseases caused by the presence of viable, usually multiplying microorganisms at the site of inflammation. In this case, the viable bacterial cells have been ingested with food. The dose required to produce an infection varies with the type of microorganism, even though the microorganism will usually multiply in the gastrointestinal tract or some other organ of the body to produce the infectious disease. Common bacteria involved in foodborne infections are *Salmonella* sp., *Shigella dysenteriae*, *Campylobacter jejuni*, *Clostridium perfringens*, *Escherichia coli*, *Yersinia enterocolitica*, *Listeria monocytogenes* and *Vibrio parahaemolyticus*. Intoxications are strictly poisonings implying the ingestion of a toxin produced in the ingested food. Common bacteria involved are *Staphylococcus aureus*, *Bacillus cereus* and *Clostridium botulinum*.

In most of these poisonings, the food serves only as a vehicle of transmission. The role of food here is significant, since the product may not only permit the survival of the pathogen, but may also serve as a suitable medium for the rapid proliferation of microorganisms and production of toxin, as in the case of exotoxin producing microorganisms. It is at this important juncture that the challenge for global programs lies on capacity building approaches, which need to primarily aim at creating an intellectual workforce to uncover the benefits of accurate and reliable methods for detecting potent pathogenic/virulent bacterial species.

As a primary step, food microbiologists have been using the conventional approach of isolating organism(s) of interest in pure culture and performing pre-determined biochemical tests as a means to identify the cultures, including pathogenicity/virulence (Mossel, 1986). All of the current methods have limitations in either sensitivity or specificity. Considering the changing global scenario of food safety, it is desirable to have analytical techniques that are simple to use, cost-effective, reliable and reproducible, and which could provide results in 'Real-Time.' The detection of microorganisms, particularly those known to cause health hazards, occur in very low numbers and the focus of all approaches has been to achieve a complete scenario of safety aspects of food samples through detection methods. From the growing food chain establishments and the public awareness of microbiological food safety, there exists a continued interest in development of improved commercial and feasible methods for microbiological analysis in foods. Rapid methods and automation in microbiology are dynamic fields of study that address the utilization of microbiological, chemical, biochemical, biophysical, immunological and serological methods for the study to improve isolation, early detection, characterization and enumeration of microorganisms and their products in clinical, food, industrial and environmental samples.

The following sections present methods of detection with respect to four significant bacterial pathogenic species that are commonly implicated in food related health hazards. The bacterial species focused on are *Staphylococcus aureus*, *Yersinia enterocolitica*, *Listeria monocytogenes* and *Bacillus cereus*.

9.3 *STAPHYLOCOCCUS* AND ITS SPECIES

9.3.1 Characteristics

Staphylococcus is a very significant organism because of its ability to cause a number of diseases and infections in human and animals. It causes localized supportive lesions and abscesses on skin, or deep-seated infections like osteomyelitis, endocarditis, or more serious skin infections like furunculosis. Because of their ability to develop resistance to many antibiotics, *Staphylococcus aureus* and *Staphylococcus epidermidis* form a major group of nosocomial pathogens infecting surgical wounds and causing infections associated with indwelling medical devices. *Staphylococcus aureus* is a major cause of intoxication, resulting in food poisoning due to the release of enterotoxins in foods. *Staphylococcus saprophyticus* is known to cause urinary tract infections and other *staphylococci* are infrequent pathogens.

Staphylococci are non-motile, non-sporeforming, catalase-positive, facultatively anaerobic cocci, except for *Staphylococcus saccharolyticus*, which is a true anaerobe. Growth is more rapid and abundant under aerobic conditions and acetoin is formed as an end product of glucose metabolism. Fermentation of mannitol is found to be characteristic of *S. aureus*. Colonies appear as smooth, circular and convex on agar plates (Baird-Parker, 1965). *Staphylococci* produce a number of extracellular proteins, among which the characteristic enzymes and toxins produced by *S. aureus*, hemolysins, nuclease, lipase, coagulases, staphylokinases (fibrinolysin), a large variety of cytotoxins and cytolysins and enterotoxins. Production of thermostable (heat-resistant nuclease) (TNase) is characteristic of *S. aureus, S. intermedius, S. hyicus,* while *S. carnosus* shows a delayed reaction and *S. epidermidis, S. simulans* and *S. hyicus* sub sp. *chromogenes* are negative to weakly positive (Genigeorgis, 1989).

Detection of *Staphylococcus* and its enterotoxins in foods is, of course, of prime concern. Insensitive detection methods often become bottlenecks in providing accurate results of safety aspects related to foods. The insensitivity is linked to the complexity of the food materials, wherein there is interference of a number of food components which affect the performance of detection methods. However, there has been considerable improvement in detection methods over the years in order to increase the sensitivity, specificity and rapidity of the tests.

9.3.2 Methods of Detection

Earlier workers used biological systems like feeding tests with monkeys and kittens to identify staphylococcal enterotoxins, providing a means of detecting the existence of undiscovered enterotoxins. However, these methods were unreliable, could not differentiate the types of toxins, and handling of animals was cumbersome. The earliest method based on serological/ immunological principles was the microslide method (Micro-Ouchtulony slide test), an AOAC approved method, used by FDA for the detection of enterotoxin. This has been widely used, due to its efficiency in detecting low amounts (<0.1–$0.2\mu g$) of enterotoxins in the food extract (Casman & Bennett, 1965). Reiser, Conaway, and Bergdoll (1974) modified the assay procedure so that within 1–3 days as little as 0.05 µg/ml of enterotoxin could be detected in food extracts. The disadvantages involved with microslide assay, like time consumption and lack of sensitivity, was overcome by other methods like Laurell electroimmunodiffusion (Gasper, Heimsch, &

Anderson, 1973), but the sensitivity was not adequate.

Improved serological methods such as Reverse passive hemagglutination assay (RPHA) and solid phase radioimmunoassay (RIA) evolved in due course. These were able to detect 1.5 ng of enterotoxin per ml (Bergdoll, Reiser, & Spintz, 1976). The development of enzyme immunoassays (EIA) for enterotoxin detection and typing, in particular the enzyme-linked immunosorbent assay (ELISA) methods and Reverse passive latex agglutination test (RPLA), evolved as most sensitive detection methods (Baird-Parker, 2000). An enzyme-linked immunofiltration assay (ELIFA) for the detection of staphylococcal enterotoxin was shown to detect 1 ng/ml of enterotoxin B in spiked milk samples in ≤ 1 hour (Valdivieso-Garcia *et al.*, 1996). The RPLA method uses latex particles sensitized with purified anti-staphylococcal enterotoxin immunoglobulins that agglutinate in the presence of homologous enterotoxins. Although occasional non-specific reactions have been reported, the method is simple and easy to perform (Marin, Rosa, & Cornejo, 1992).

Freed, Evenson, Reiser, and Bergdoll (1982) developed a detection method for *staphylococcal enterotoxins* based on the principle of ELISA. ELISA has proven to be an excellent immunological detection system. A very high sensitivity and specificity has been achieved by ELISA methods. An indirect double sandwich ELISA was applied in the detection of enterotoxins A, B, C1 and D in food samples using monoclonal antibodies (Lapeyre, Janin, & Kaveri, 1988). However, one limitation of ELISA was its inability to identify and characterize the antigen that reacts with the antibody to give a positive signal. Given the variety and the complexity of foods, it is difficult to rule out a cross reactivity of the antibodies with the food matrix even with proper controls.

This led to the development of nucleic acid-based detection system, which could offer a very good alternative, overcoming the problems commonly encountered with other methods of detection. These techniques are critical because they facilitate rapid, sensitive and specific analysis and therefore an appropriate choice to record foodborne disease outbreaks (Hill & Keasler, 1991). Nucleic acid probe-based methods have been developed for the detection and enumeration of foodborne pathogens. Several kits applying DNA probes are commercially available (Jones, 1991). Methods involving a polymerase chain reaction have proved to be the most promising of the rapid microbiological methods. The following section will detail the application of these methods in the detection of *Staphylococcus* and its enterotoxins in a food system.

9.3.2.1 Nucleic acid probes

An ideal probe is a single-stranded molecule with a short sequence of nucleotide bases that can hybridize only if a target is present. A probe can be either DNA or RNA. Most of the applications so far have used DNA probes (Wolcott, 1991). In order to detect the hybridization, DNA fragments have to be labeled. The label can be a radioisotope or a chemical moiety. Because of problems encountered during handling of radioisotopes, probes proved to be less popular. The availability of non-isotopic labels and efficient chemicals like Digoxigenin, psoralen and others has improved the utility of a DNA probe as a diagnostic tool. Probes can be produced either by screening of restriction genomic DNA fragments or targeting the unique sequences on genes coding for the known products or virulence genes.

Two-phase DNA hybridization formats are used in DNA probe assays. The dot-blot hybridization format requires the immobilization of crude or purified DNA containing the target on nitro-cellulose or nylon membrane. The colony hybridization method involves the impression transfer of bacterial cells from colonies on a primary isolation plate to nitrocellulose or nylon membrane (Swaminathan & Feng, 1994). A non-isotopic DNA hybridization assay was developed by Wilson *et al.*

(1994). A DIG-labeled total genomic DNA probe was used to identify *S. aureus* in their study. The GENE-TRAK™ and AccuProbe (GEN-PROBE) DNA probe assays have been developed for *S. aureus*. GENE-TRAK assay is a semi-quantitative assay, which detects *S. aureus* colorimetrically and includes a dipstick solid phase system.

9.3.2.2 Polymerase chain reaction

In the commercial set up, DNA probes could not gain the projected dominance. However, the basic principle has been utilized when developing many technologies (Feng, 2001). Polymerase chain reaction (PCR) technology has proven to be one of the most promising of the rapid microbiological methods for the detection and identification of bacteria in many food samples. This method is based on an enzymatic amplification of target nucleic acid sequences using a specific primer pair and a heat stable DNA polymerase (Lantz, Hahn-Hägerdal, & Radstrom, 1994).

Various approaches have been developed using PCR for the detection of single or multiple target genes in a single reaction. The availability of nucleotide sequences for the enterotoxin genes (A-K) has enabled the detection of enterotoxigenic *staphylococci* using PCR. Jones and Khan (1986) gave the first complete nucleotide sequence of enterotoxin B. Later, a number of researchers worked towards the same end and as a result, the nucleotide sequences of *staphylococcal enterotoxins* A, C, D, E, G, H, I, J and K were published and made available in public databases.

As a means of enhancing the sensitivity of detection, Wilson, Cooper, and Gilmour (1991) employed nested PCR, which uses internal primers for the specific gene amplicon. The nested primers for *nuc*, *ent*B and *ent*C genes of *S. aureus* could detect 1 fg of purified DNA, while 100 pg was required for the detection of these genes, when single primer pair was used. A decrease in the sensitivity was observed when applied in skimmed milk, which could be due to the presence of PCR inhibitors in milk. The problem of sensitivity was resolved by Tsen and Chen (1992), who detected enterotoxigenic *staphylococci* at the level of 10^0 to 10^1 cells per gram of various naturally contaminated food samples like beef, pork, chicken and fish, using the primers targeted to enterotoxin A, D or E genes. In another study, the same group (Tsen, Chen, & Yu, 1994) developed a PCR-based method for the direct detection of enterotoxigenic *S. aureus* in various foods, without prior enrichment and could achieve a sensitivity of <100 cfu per gram of food sample.

Khan *et al.* (1998) developed a PCR-based method targeting the *nuc* gene encoding thermonuclease of *S. aureus*. A modified rapid boil method for the isolation of DNA directly from artificially contaminated milk samples provided a sensitivity of 100%. The *nuc* gene has been widely used among microbiologists as a taxonomic tool to identify *S. aureus* in food and clinical samples (Kim *et al.*, 2001). The wide application of PCR in clinical microbiology has led to a large number of reports particularly targeting the *mec* gene, coding for the methicillinase gene of methicillin-resistant *S. aureus* (MRSA) in clinical isolates (Mehrotra, Wang, & Johnson, 2000).

The major disadvantage of uniplex PCR is that a series of separate reactions is needed to identify a single gene or subset of genes. However, multiplex PCR has the advantage of simultaneous detection and differentiation of multiple genes in a single reaction. In multiplex PCR, multiple pairs of primers specific for different DNA segments are included in the same reaction to enable amplification of multiple target sequences in one reaction. The primers used in multiplex PCR should have similar annealing temperatures or T_m. The major advantage of multiplex PCR over conventional PCR is cost effectiveness and it requires less preparation and analysis time than systems in which several tubes of simplex PCR are used (Phuektes, Mansell, & Browning, 2001). The sensitivity of PCR is dependent on the quality of the template

DNA. The extraction of DNA from *S. aureus* generally requires an enzymatic treatment and often becomes a lengthy and arduous task. Many workers have simplified the isolation of DNA from food samples in order to overcome the inhibitors and enhance the sensitivity of detection of *staphylococci* (Tamarapu, McKillip, & Drake, 2001; Ramesh, Padmapriya, Chandrashekar, & Varadaraj, 2002).

Polymerase chain reaction-ELISA is an efficient quantification tool, which combines PCR with ELISA for post-PCR analysis. The assays utilize the internal biotinylated probes to capture the amplified PCR products of toxin encoding sequences and produce quantifiable signals through enzymatic amplification of a colorimetric detection system. PCR-ELISA, sometimes called enzyme-linked oligosorbant assay (ELOSA), has been used by very few researchers for the detection of *S. aureus* and its enterotoxins (Gilligan *et al.*, 2000). Many reports are available wherein PCR-ELISA was used for the quantitative detection of bacterial pathogens like *Escherichia coli*, *Campylobacter* spp., *Listeria monocytogenes*, *Streptococcus* spp., in food and water systems (Daly, Collier, & Doyle, 2002; Ge, Zhao, Hall, & Meng, 2002; Sails *et al.*, 2002). The sensitivity of PCR was found to be enhanced when applying PCR-ELISA assay.

Real-Time PCR and biprobe assays have been used to identify and distinguish bacterial species by many researchers (Logan, Edwards, Saunders, & Stanley, 2001; Vishnubhatla *et al.*, 2001). The rapid processes for quantification of *S. aureus* cells or its enterotoxins include methods like MPN-PCR and PCR-ELISA. However, these methods are laborious and sometimes time-consuming. Another alternative rapid detection method is Real-Time quantitative PCR (RTQ-PCR), which quantifies DNA and thus has the potential for accurate enumeration of microorganisms. This system combines air thermocycler and fluorometer enabling rapid cycle PCR. Hein *et al.* (2001) used two different approaches to the RTQ-PCR based quantification of the *nuc* gene of *S. aureus* in cheese. The first approach was by using the dsDNA-binding fluorescent probe called the TaqMan probe. Quantification studies proved SYBR Green I to be less sensitive (60 *nuc* gene copies/µl) than using TaqMan probe (6 *nuc* gene copies/µl).

9.3.2.3 Molecular typing

Intraspecies differentiation of *S. aureus* and other *staphylococci* is essential during investigations into epidemiological outbreaks. Various methods of typing staphylococcal isolates are available. These include phage typing, ribotyping, comparison of plasmid profiles, restriction fragment length polymorphism (RFLP), randomly amplified polymorphic DNA (RAPD) and pulsed field gel electrophoresis (PFGE). These methods are based on the premise that clonally related organisms share traits that can differentiate them from other unrelated organisms (Fueyo, Martin, Gonźalez-Hevia, & Mendoza, 2001).

PFGE as shown by the number of workers is one of the most convenient discriminative tools not only for strain identification, but also for the resolution of the clonal relationships of *S. aureus* strains in clinical environment and in foods (Shimizu *et al.*, 2000). *Staphylococci* responsible for food poisoning outbreaks in China and Japan were studied individually for coagulase type VII and enterotoxin A profiles using PFGE. In both cases, chromosomal DNA was digested with SmaI to characterize the strains of *S. aureus* and considerable genetic diversity was observed, which could be linked to the geographic relatedness and source of the strain (Shimizu *et al.*, 2000). RFLP, in combination with PCR, has been applied for the identification of staphylococcal species (Yugueros *et al.*, 2001).

9.3.2.4 Microarrays or biochips

DNA microarrays provide a powerful tool for the parallel analysis of many genes and their expression levels (Cho & Tiedje, 2002). In one study, microarrays were designed for the identification of *Staphylococcus*, its species and methicillin resistance. The microarray contained five selective DNA capture probes for simultaneous and differential identification of five clinically important staphylococcal species (*S. aureus, S. epidermidis, S. haemolyticus, S. hominis* and *S. saprophyticus*), with a consensus capture probe to detect all *fem*A sequences, allowing the identification of genus *Staphylococcus*. The hybridization and identification processes were completed in less than 2 hours. These results help us to understand that the application of low-density microarrays, a powerful multigenotypic post-PCR analyzer could compete with conventional bacterial identification (Hamels *et al.*, 2001).

9.4 *YERSINIA ENTEROCOLITICA*

9.4.1 Characteristics

The genus *Yersinia* is composed of 11 species of which three (*Yersinia enterocolitica, Yersinia pestis* and *Yersinia pseudotuberculosis*) have clearly been shown to cause human disease. The remaining eight species (*Y. frederiksenii, Y. intermedia, Y. kristensenii, Y. bercovieri, Y. mollaretii, Y. rohdei, Y. ruckeri,* and *Y. aldovae*) are sometimes referred to as *Yersinia enterocolitica*-like organisms although they are distinct species. They have not been studied as extensively as *Y. enterocolitica, Y. pestis* and *Y. pseudotuberculosis,* and have not yet been clearly demonstrated to cause human disease (Sulakvelidze, 2000). *Yersinia enterocolitica* is a Gram-negative non-sporeforming, non-capsulated bacteria which is an oxidase-negative, catalase-positive, nitrate-reducing, facultatively anaerobic rod (occasionally coccoid) shaped bacteria. Strains belonging to *Y. enterocolitica* are urease-positive and can be differentiated from other *Yersinia* strains with a positive result for the fermentation of sucrose, and negative reactions for rhamnose and melibiose fermentation (Bercovier & Mollaret, 1984).

Pathogenic strains of *Y. enterocolitica* can be identified by specific biochemical tests such as pyrazinamidase activity (Kandolo & Wauters, 1985), autoagglutination (Gemski, Lazere, & Casey, 1980), crystal violet binding (Bhaduri, Conway, & Chica, 1987), calcium dependency (Salamah, 1990), Congo red binding (Prpic, Robins-Browne, & Davey, 1983), salicin fermentation-esculin hydrolysis and D-xylose fermentation (Farmer, Carter, & Miller, 1992). Human clinical infections with *Y. enterocolitica* ensue after ingestion of the microorganisms in contaminated food or water or by direct inoculation through blood transfusions (Bottone, 1997). In the gastrointestinal tract, *Y. enterocolitica* can cause acute enteritis (especially in children), enterocolitis, mesenteric lymphadenitis and terminal ileitis. For virulent *Y. enterocolitica* to manifest its presence through a clinical syndrome, however, it must assemble an array of attributes that enable it to successfully transcend its environmental nidus to infect a human host.

Yersinia enterocolitica is an invasive enteric pathogen but, interestingly, not all strains of this organism are virulent. Virulence in this organism is determined by virulence factors encoded in the chromosome and in a 70 kb virulence plasmid (pYV), which is required for adhesion, invasion and colonization of intestinal epithelial cells and lymph nodes; growth and survival inside macrophages, killing of neutrophils and macrophages and to confer serum resistance (Bottone, 1997).

The pathogenicity of *Y. enterocolitica* can be studied by animal tests such as the guinea pig keratoconjunctivitis model (Sereny test), suckling mouse assay, mouse intraperitoneal challenge, and mouse diarrhea and splenic infection following oral challenge (Aulisio *et al.*, 1983; Feng & Weagant, 1994). Mice infected with European serotypes of *Y. enterocolitica* via oral or intraperitoneal challenges will produce diarrhea but the more virulent American serotypes usually cause lethality (Feng & Weagant, 1994). However, since animal testing tends to be costly and is subject to increasing public opposition, it has largely been replaced by other tests.

Immunological methods, mainly agglutination tests and immune assays are also used for detection of *Y. enterocolitica*. Sory *et al.* (1990) developed a method of the detection of virulent *Y. enterocolitica* (O:3, O:5,27, O:8 and O:9) in which rabbit polyclonal antisera against pYV encoded outer membrane protein P1 was used. Latex slide agglutination and tube agglutination form the basis of commercially available kits for the detection of *Y. enterocolitica* O:3 and O:9 antibodies in serum. Immunoassays like surface adhesion immunofluorescence (SAIF), enzyme immunoassay (EIA), and enzyme-linked immunosorbent assay (ELISA) techniques are also developed for *Y. enterocolitica* detection. SAIF has been used to detect *Y. enterocolitica* in broth and also enriched meat cultures. EIA was developed for the detection of *Yersinia* immunoglobulin complexes (Ig). However, immunoblots and ELISA techniques which target the *Yersinia* outer proteins (yops) are found to be more sensitive and specific than other serological tests (Ramesh, Padmapriya, Bharathi, & Varadaraj, 2003).

9.4.2 Nucleic Acid-based Methods

9.4.2.1 DNA hybridization methods

Several DNA probes targeting virulence-associated genes of *Y. enterocolitica* have also been developed. Such gene probes can be used in colony or dot-blot hybridization for the direct detection of *Y. enterocolitica*. Colony hybridization does not require enrichment or isolation of pure cultures, and it enables the rapid detection and enumeration of all pathogenic bioserotypes. The GENE-TRAK colorimetric hybridization assay for *Y. enterocolitica* has been developed using probes targeted against specific signature sequences of 16S rRNA. This assay was found to be convenient and rapid but lacked the discrimination between virulent and non-virulent strains (Ramesh *et al.*, 2003). Weagant *et al.* (1999) used digoxigenin (DIG)-labeled PCR amplicons of *virF* and *yadA* to detect pathogenic *Y. enterocolitica* in seeded tofu and chocolate milk samples. Probes were also developed targeting the chromosomally encoded virulence factors like attachment invasion locus (*ail*), invasion (*inv*) and heat stable enterotoxin (*yst*). The *inv* gene is present in all *Yersinia* spp. whereas the *ail* gene is present only in pathogenic *Y. enterocolitica* strains. Based on this, Goverde *et al.* (1993) developed a non-radioactive colony hybridization method using DIG-labeled *inv* and *ail* probes for the detection and differentiation of pathogenic and non-pathogenic *Y. enterocolitica* strains.

9.4.2.2 PCR methods

PCR is a rapid and selective tool for the detection of pathogens in clinical, food, and environmental samples and it fulfills the criteria for specificity and sensitivity. It is faster than other methods for detecting virulence. Different PCR assays have been designed for the detection of pathogenic *Y. enterocolitica* in pure cultures and also natural samples. PCR methods targeting chromosomal virulence genes have been developed, since *Y. enterocolitica* is found to lose plasmids during sub-culturing protocols of culture maintenance (Blais & Phillippe, 1995).

Although the PCR method enables reliable and sensitive detection when applied to pure cultures, its efficiency is markedly curtailed when applied to more complex food and clinical samples. This is mainly due to the presence of potential inhibitors or high levels of background flora present in such samples (Ramesh *et al.*, 2003). Proteinases, bile and heme have been suggested to be significant PCR inhibitors in many of these samples (Rossen, Nørskov, Holmstrøm, & Rasmussen, 1992). Therefore, adequate sample preparation methods that either eliminate these inhibitors or concentrate target cells to yield satisfactory detection levels are required. Several

methods, including enrichment, dilution, filtration, centrifugation, adsorption, and floatation have been used for concentration and separation of *Y. enterocolitica* strains in natural samples. An enrichment or selective enrichment step prior to PCR, has been applied in some procedures (Jourdan, Johnson, & Wesley, 2000; Boyapalle, Wesley, Hurd, & Reddy, 2001).

DNA extraction is performed either by lysing the cell wall to release the DNA or by using more laborious DNA purification procedures. Heat is routinely used, prior to PCR, to break down the cell wall of microbes and inactivate heat-labile PCR inhibitors. However, when natural samples are studied, heat treatment alone is insufficient for *Y. enterocolitica* (Fredriksson-Ahomaa & Korkeala, 2003). Proteinase K treatment is often used before heat treatment in PCR methods designed for direct detection of *Y. enterocolitica* in natural samples (Simonova, Vazlerova, & Steinhauserova, 2007). DNA purification has been carried out by traditional phenol-chloroform extraction and ethanol precipitation in some PCR assays developed to detect *Y. enterocolitica* directly in natural samples (Özbas, Lehner, & Wagner, 2000; Simonova *et al.*, 2007).

Methods for the detection of PCR products involve agarose gel electrophoresis and the use of ethidium bromide to stain the gels. This method gives both the size and number of products and also allows a rough estimation of the concentration. However, this method does not ensure that the PCR product contains the correct sequence between primers. In addition, ethidium bromide, is a mutagen, and may not be appropriate for routine use in food-monitoring laboratories. To overcome these problems, Rasmussen, Rasmussen, Christensen, and Olsen (1995) detected the amplified products of *Y. enterocolitica* by hybridization to an oligonucleotide immobilized in microtiter wells and fluorescence detection. The developed fluorogenic 5 nuclease PCR (TaqMan) assay is an attractive option to overcome the problems of gel electrophoresis. The assay exploits the 5 1–3 nuclease activity of Taq

DNA polymerase and releases a probe which has a fluorescent reporter dye and also a quencher, which hybridizes to an internal fragment of the target gene. When the probe hybridizes with its target, the reporter dye is cleaved and becomes capable of emitting a fluorescent signal that can be detected in Real-Time (Vishnubhatla *et al.*, 2000; Boyapalle *et al.*, 2001).

Mycrs, Gaba, and Al-Khaldi (2006) developed a DNA microarray chip based on four virulence genes and 16S ribosomal DNA gene conserved regions among all Gram negative bacteria, including *Yersinia*, as a positive control and evaluated it using 22 *Y. enterocolitica* isolates. Assays using this DNA microarray showed specificity of genotyping *Y. enterocolitica*. The chip's ability to identify *Y. enterocolitica* genes from milk samples was also confirmed and the detection limit was found to be 1000 cfu per hybridization.

9.5 *LISTERIA* MONOCYTOGENES

The genus *Listeria* is a Gram positive, microaerophilic, non-sporeforming rod. The collective knowledge generated by investigation and research done over the last 25 years in the field of *Listeria* has made this organism the most important investigated Gram positive bacterium. There are six recognized species of *Listeria*: *Listeria monocytogenes*, *Listeria innocua*, *Listeria seeligeri*, *Listeria welshimeri*, *Listeria ivanovii* and *Listeria grayi*. *Listeria monocytogenes* was not a major concern from the point of food safety until the 1980s; the rapidness with which *L. monocytogenes* emerged as the etiological agent of 'listeriosis' is beyond comparison with any other foodborne pathogen.

9.5.1 Conventional Isolation Methods

Isolation of *Listeria* species including that of *L. monocytogenes*, from foods and other environments, offers a challenging task for microbiologists. Its detection, isolation and identification from inoculated and naturally contaminated foods and the recovery of sublethally injured *Listeria* from foods is quite challenging and interesting. Direct plating, cold enrichment, selective enrichment and several rapid methods have been used singly or in different combinations to detect *L. monocytogenes* in food, as well as clinical and environmental samples. Early attempts to isolate small numbers of *Listeria* from samples containing large populations of indigenous microflora relied on direct plating, and often ended in failure.

Conventionally, culture methods used for the detection of *Listeria* spp. are based on pre-enrichment, selective enrichment and plating followed by colony morphology, sugar fermentation and haemolytic properties to identify different species of *Listeria* (Janzten *et al.*, 2006). These methods are sensitive and considered as 'gold standards' compared to other methods even today. However, the time required for confirmation of positive result is usually 5–7 days from the time of sample analysis (Paoli, Bhunia, & Bayles, 2005). Various factors such as the presence of high populations of other competitive bacteria, low numbers of the test pathogen and inhibitory components of food matrices hamper the detection of *L. monocytogenes* in foods (Janzten *et al.*, 2006).

In this background, several isolation protocols have been developed over the years for the improved detection of *L. monocytogenes* in foods. Other efficient methods based on antibodies or molecular techniques (DNA hybridization or PCR) have also been developed which are equally sensitive and rapid so as to give a positive confirmation within 48 hours. Real-Time PCR is increasingly used in food diagnostics for detection of *L. monocytogenes*. Microarrays and biosensors are other newer techniques being used to detect *Listeria* spp. in foods.

The cold enrichment developed by Gray involves homogenization of samples in tryptose broth, incubation at 4°C and weekly and biweekly plating on tryptose agar during 3 months of storage. This was adopted as a standard method to detect *L. monocytogenes*, as the organism could be recovered after prolonged incubation at 4°C, even in the presence of other contaminants. Usually, cold enrichment is followed by selective enrichment, wherein the use of selective or inhibitory agents during enrichment at elevated temperatures (30–37°C), selectively inhibits other microflora, while at the same time allowing the growth of *Listeria*. The selective agents included chemicals, antimicrobials and dyes which could inhibit the growth of indigenous microorganisms and allow *L. monocytogenes* to grow. The various selective agents being used and their functions are listed in Table 9.1.

A few of the selected enrichment broths and isolation media used in recovery of *L. monocytogenes* are presented in brief. The University of Vermont (UVM) selective broth was originally recommended by FDA and USDA-FSIS for enrichment of food samples and subsequently, certain modifications were included into the medium. The modified medium designated as *Listeria* enrichment broth (LEB) by Donnelly and Baigent (1986) was used to selectively enrich *L. monocytogenes* in raw milk from other contaminants. Fraser broth (Fraser & Sperber, 1988) was a modification of UVM broth, wherein the culture of *Listeria* turns Fraser broth black due to esculin hydrolysis within 48 hours of incubation. Hence this media has now replaced LEB in USDA protocol as a secondary enrichment medium for meat, poultry and environmental samples (USDA/FSIS, 2002). The PALCAM enrichment broth developed by Van Netten *et al.* (1989) gave better results when compared to USDA-LEB as well as tryptose broth based

TABLE 9.1   Selective agents used in isolation of *Listeria*

Selective/antimicrobial agent	Conc. mg/l	Uses	References
Potassium tellurite	5–15	Selective/differential for *Listeria* that reduce tellurite to tellurium producing black colonies	Gray, Stafseth, and Thorp (1950)
Lithium chloride/Phenyl ethanol	0.5 mg/l-15 g	Amplification of *Listeria* in presence of Gram negative bacteria	Hao, Beuchat, and Brackett (1989)
Nalidixic acid	20–40	Inhibitory to Gram negative bacteria by interfering DNA gyrase except *Pseudomonas* and *Proteus*	Farber, Sanders, and Speirs (1988); Ortel (1972)
Acriflavine/trypaflavine (acridine dyes)	5–25	Inhibitory to Gram positives including *Lactobacillus bulgaricus* and *Streptococcus thermophilus*	Ralovich *et al.* (1971); Ortel (1972)
Polymyxin B	1–10^6 U	Inhibits growth of Gram negative rods and streptococci	Doyle and Schoeni (1986); Rodriguez, Fernandez, and Garayzabal *et al.* (1984).
Moxalactam	20	Broad-spectrum antibiotic, inhibits many Gram positive and Gram negative bacteria including *Staphylococcus*, *Proteus* and *Pseudomonas*	Lee and McClain (1986).
Ceftazidime	4–50	Broad-spectrum cephalosporin antibiotic	Lovet *et al.* (1987); Lovet (1988)
Cycloheximide	50	Inhibits fungi	Curtis *et al.* (1989b)

A few of the selected enrichment broths and isolation media are presented briefly.

antibiotic medium of Beckers, Soentoro, and Asc (1987) in detecting *L. monocytogenes* from naturally contaminated cheese, meat, fermented sausage, raw chicken and sausage.

McBride *Listeria* agar (MLA) was the first plating medium widely used for selective isolation of *L. monocytogenes*. It was first introduced by McBride and Girard (1960) and was prepared from phenyl ethanol agar to which lithium chloride, glycine and sheep blood were added. Subsequently, the medium has undergone several modifications. The plates with grown colonies were observed under oblique illumination for bluish to bluish-green *Listeria* colonies (Lovett, Francis, & Hunt, 1987). The lithium chloride-phenyl ethanol-moxalactam (LPM) agar was a modification of MLA medium formulated by Lee and McClain (1986). This LPM medium plus esculin and ferric iron has been in use as one of the selective agars in the FDA procedure. The Oxford agar developed by Curtis, Mitchell, King, and Griffen (1989a) eliminated oblique illumination. Modified Oxford agar (MOXA) is the modification of Oxford agar by inclusion of moxalactam and has been a recommended plating medium in the USDA-FSIS procedure. Oxford agar has been one of the selective media in the FDA method (Carnevale & Johnston, 1989).

PALCAM (Polymyxin acriflavine lithium chloride ceftazidime aesculin mannitol) agar is a selective plating medium used after primary or secondary enrichments. PALCAM agar plates are incubated at 30°C for 48 hours under microaerophilic conditions (5% oxygen, 7.5% CO_2, 7.5% hydrogen, 80% nitrogen). The colonies of *Listeria* appear as gray-green with black sunken centers. The PALCAM medium, along with L-PALCAMY enrichment broth, forms the basis of a method used for the isolation and detection of *Listeria* by the Netherlands Government Food Inspection Service (NGFIS). Gunasinghe, Henderson, and Rutter (1994) made a comparative study of two plating media (PALCAM and Oxford) to detect *Listeria* spp. in meat products. They found that the PALCAM medium was more effective in suppressing other background microflora, wherein an isolation and identification of *Listeria* spp. was easier in this medium.

In the background of several enrichment broths and selective isolation agar media, an attempt has been made to shortlist a few of these broths and agar media based on efficacy studies. Those recommended are being routinely used in the food industry worldwide; even though sensitive and reliable, they are time-consuming, almost taking 5–6 days for the results to become available. Difficulties have also been observed in these procedures, such as the inability to isolate *Listeria* from all positive samples and recover sublethally injured cells encountered during food processing.

The ISO 11290 method developed by the International Organization for Standardization (1996, 1998) is a two-stage enrichment process using Fraser broth. The presence of *Listeria* is indicated by blackening of the medium. Samples of primary and secondary enrichment broths are then plated on Oxford and PALCAM agar plates for detection of *L. monocytogenes*. The FDA method with only one enrichment step was originally developed by Lovett (1988) and has been frequently used for the isolation and detection of *L. monocytogenes* in milk and milk products (particularly ice cream and cheese), sea foods and vegetables. Food samples in 25 g quantities are pre-enriched at 30°C for 4 hours in buffered *Listeria* enrichment broth (BLEB). After 4 hours of non-selective enrichment, selective agents (acriflavine, nalidixic acid with or without cycloheximide) are added and further incubated for 48 hours for selective enrichment. The enriched sample is then plated on one of the esculin containing selective agars such as OXA or MOXA or PALCAM or LPM. The plates are incubated at 30–35°C for 24–48 hours for the development of *Listeria* colonies.

The International Dairy Federation method was developed as a reference method to recover

L. monocytogenes from dairy products (Terplan, 1988). The present AOAC approved IDF method resembles the FDA procedure (Association of Official Analytical Chemists, 1996). The enriched samples are streaked on Oxford agar. The presumptive colonies are then confirmed by other confirmatory tests. This method requires a minimum of 4 days to obtain presumptive results and is a popular method in European countries for detecting *Listeria* in dairy products. The USDA-FSIS method developed by the United States Department of Agriculture, Food Safety and Inspection Service (USDA-FSIS) is used to isolate the organism from meat and poultry products as well as environmental samples (USDA/FSIS, 2002). It involves a two-stage enrichment process. The enriched samples are then streaked onto MOXA plates for presumptive identification of black *Listeria* colonies. The presumptive *Listeria* cultures are further confirmed by the use of specific biochemical characteristics such as hemolysis, phospholipase C production, sugar fermentation, oblique illumination and growth in the presence of chromogenic substrates. Also, sensitivity and rapidity have been focal points in the detection and isolation of *L. monocytogenes* from foods. Attempts to achieve these objectives have led to the development of immunological-based and nucleic acid-based methods.

9.5.2 Immunological Detection Methods

These methods are based on antibodies specific for *Listeria* and that play an important role in the host defense mechanism. Certain unique properties of antibodies include binding to epitopes, present in living cells. Antibodies directed against surface antigens do not require that they penetrate inside the cell in order to reach the target, making them suitable for detecting live cells. ELISA is the most common immunoassay used for pathogen detection in foods. Ky *et al.* (2004) have developed monoclonal antibodies against the protein p60 encoded by the *iap* gene for the detection of *L. monocytogenes*. Several commercial kits like Transia® plate *Listeria monocytogenes* by Diffchamb AB and VIDAS® LMO by bioMérieux have been developed based on ELISA to detect *L. monocytogenes* in foods (Hitchins, 2003). Immuno-capture on immunomagnetic separation is another technique, wherein magnetic beads coated with specific antibodies are used to separate target organisms from other competing microflora and inhibitory food components. This approach has been used to capture and concentrate *Listeria* spp. directly from foods and environmental samples (Mitchell *et al.*, 1994; Hudson, Lake, & Savill, 2001).

9.5.3 Nucleic Acid-based Methods

The availability of complete genome sequences of *L. monocytogenes* (serotypes 1/2a, 4b and 6a) and *L. innocua* have led to a greater understanding of molecular features involved in pathogenesis of *L. monocytogenes* (Buchrieser *et al.*, 2003). In addition, they have also made available new diagnostic targets to detect *L. monocytogenes*. Several nucleic acid-based methods such as DNA hybridization, polymerase chain reaction (PCR) and nucleic acid-based amplification are available to detect *L. monocytogenes* and other *Listeria* spp. from innumerable samples.

9.5.3.1 *Polymerase chain reaction*

A polymerase chain reaction provides an exponential amplification of a specific DNA sequence present in the target organism. The components of a buffered PCR reaction include oligonucleotide primers, deoxyribonucleotide triphosphates, the DNA to be amplified and a thermostable DNA polymerase. Numerous studies have focused on PCR detection of *L. monocytogenes* with a good number of reviews appearing in the literature (Levin, 2003). Different types of DNA extractions, cell lysis and DNA purification techniques are applied directly to foods or to enrichment broths with varying sensitivity. PCR methods are highly sensitive, rapid and reproducible.

Various genes have been targeted for the detection of *L. monocytogenes*. They include gene *hlyA* coding for *listeriolysin O* (Mengaud *et al.*, 1988); *iap* gene coding for invasive associated protein p60 (Kohler *et al.*, 1990); *actA* gene, a surface protein required for intracellular bacterial propulsion and cell to cell invasion (Kocks, Gouin, & Tabouret, 1992); internalin *inlA* and *inlB*, surface proteins conferring invasiveness to human erythrocytes (Gaillard *et al.*, 1991); *lmaA* gene (also known as Dth-18) responsible for delayed type hypersensitivity response in *Listeria*-immune mice (Gohmaan *et al.*, 1990); *flaA* gene for flagellin which is specific to all species of *Listeria* (Dons, Rasmussen, & Olsen, 1992); *plcB* gene encoding phospholipase C (Geoffroy *et al.*, 1991); *prfA* gene responsible for the regulation of expression of cascade of virulence factors including *listeriolysin O* (Leimeister-Wachter *et al.*, 1990); and fibronectin binding protein (Gilot & Content, 2002). In addition, genus and species specific 16S rRNA and 23S rRNA sequences have also been targeted (Wesley, Harmon, Dickson, & Schwartz, 2002; Rodriguez-Lazaro, Hernandez, & Pla, 2004). A brief overview of selected genes targeted, the specific PCR primers used, generated amplicon size, sensitivity and types of foods samples tested by several researchers have been presented in Table 9.2.

Conventional PCR is the amplification of the specific gene sequence using a single primer pair for the detection of one pathogen at a time. This method is used to detect the pathogen either directly or indirectly from foods (Herman, DeBlock, & Moermans, 1995). One of the advantages of enrichment, prior to PCR, would be the elimination of false-positive results, which may arise due to DNA of non-viable bacteria in the food sample. A variety of DNA extraction methods have been employed to prepare the template for PCR amplification, which makes the method more suitable and sensitive to detecting the target organism, even if present in low numbers (Ramesh *et al.*, 2002; Liu, 2008). Nested PCR involves two sets of primers and two rounds of thermal cycling. The major advantage of nested PCR is increased sensitivity of detection by several orders of magnitude than that achieved by primary amplification and enhanced specificity, wherein it is unlikely that any non-specific amplification at the primary round will give a positive result in the second round (Levin, 2003). In multiplex PCR, two or more gene loci are simultaneously amplified in one reaction. This technique is widely used to characterize pathogens based on their antigenic traits and virulence factors. Although designing a robust multiplex assay for food is quite challenging, once optimized for specific pathogens and food products, this method has the advantage of being cost effective and highly efficient (Ramesh *et al.*, 2002).

Real-Time PCR technology is based on the ability to detect and quantify PCR products as the reaction cycle progresses. The DNA is quantified by measuring the fluorescence with respect to the binding of an intercalating dye or the binding of a fluorescent hybridization probe. SYBR green I has been the most frequently used DNA-binding dye in Real-Time PCR (Fairchild, Lee, & Maurer, 2006). Results are obtained in an hour or less, which is faster than conventional PCR. The convenience and rapidity has made Real-Time PCR very pertinent as an alternative to a conventional culture-based or immuno-based assay for the detection of *L. monocytogenes* (Norton, 2002). Various Real-Time PCR assays for the detection of *L. monocytogenes* in food have been documented in the literature (Berrada, Soriano, Pico, & Manes, 2006). Various commercial Real-Time PCR kits like Bax®-PCR (Dupont-Qualicon, Delaware, USA), Probelia® (Bio-Rad, Hercules, California, USA) and others are available.

TABLE 9.2 Overview of selected genes targeted for PCR detection of *L. monocytogenes*

Gene targeted	Primer sequence 5′ → 3′	Size of amplicon (bp)	Sensitivity (detection limit)	Samples tested	References
hlyA	F – CAC TCA GCA TTG ATT CG R – ATT TTC CCT TCA CTG ATT CG	276	–	milk	Cooray et al. (1994)
hlyA	F – CGG AGG TTC CGC AAA AGA TG R – CCT CCA GAG TGA TCG ATG TT	234	20 cfu	sea food and soft cheese	Wang, Cao, and Cerniglia (1997)
hlyA	F – GGG AAA TCT GTC TCA GGT GAT GT R – CGA TGA TTT GAA CTT CAT CTT TTGC	183	6 cfu/g	cabbage	Hough et al. (2002)
hlyA	F – TTG CCA GGA ATG ACT AAT CAA G R – ATT CAC TGT AAG CCA TTT CGTC	172	10 cfu/ml	milk	Amagliani et al. (2004)
hlyA	F – CCT AAG ACG CCA ATC GAA R – AAG CGC TTG CAA CTG CTC	701	5–10 cfu/25 ml	raw milk	Herman, DeBlock and Moermans (1995)
hlyA	F – AACCTATCCAGGTGCTC R – CTGTAAGCCATTTCGTC	267			
hlyA	F – GCA GTT GCA AGC GCT TGG AGT GAA R – GCAACGTATCCTCCAGAGTGATCG	456	–	pork beef sausage	Paziak-Domanska et al. (1999)
hlyA	F – GTGCCGCCAAGAAAAGGTTA R – CGC CAC ACT TGA GAT AT	636	10^3 cfu/0.5 ml	milk	Choi and Hong (2003)
hlyA	F – CCT AAG ACG CCA ATC GAA AAG AAA R – TAG TTC TAC ATC ACC TGA GAC AGA	858	10^3 cfu/11g	non-fat yogurt, cheddar cheese	Stevens and Jaykus (2004)
hlyA	F–CATTAGTGGAAAGATGGAATG R–GTATCCTCCAGAGTGATCGA	731	10 cfu/g	goat meat, buffalo meat	Balamurugan, Bhilegaonkar, and Agarwal (2006)
hlyA	F–GAATGTAAACTTCGGGCAATCAG R–GCCGTCGATGATTTGAACTTCATC	388			
hlyA	F–GCAGTTGCAAGCGCTTGGAGTGAA R–GCAACGTATCCTCCAGAGTGATCG	420	$10^4 \times 10^2$ cfu/ml	milk	Zeng et al. (2006)
iap	F–CAAACTGCTAACACAGTACT R–TTATACGCGACCGAAGCCAA	700	$10^4 \times 10^2$ cfu/ml	milk	Zeng et al. (2006)
iap	F – CAA ACT GCT AAC ACA GCT ACT R – GCA CTT GAA TTG CTG TTA TTG	371	3 cfu/g	cooked ground beef	Klein and Juneja (1997)
iap	F – GGGCTTTATCCATAAAATA R – TTGGAAGAACCTTGATTA	453	10^{-1}–10^{-2} cells/ml or g	meat, sausages, cheese	Manzano et al. (1997)
iap	F – CAA ACT GCT AAC ACA GCT ACT R – GCA CTT GAA TTG CTG TTA TTG	371	10^1 cfu	–	Mukhopadhyay and Mukhopadhyay (2007)
actA	F – GTGATAAAATCGACGAAATCC R – CTT GTAAAACTAGAAICTAGCG	400 or 300	4×10^{-2} to 4 cfu/g	Italian soft cheeses	Longhi et al. (2003)
actA	F – GCTGATTTAAGAGAGATAGAGGAACA R – TTTATGTGGTTATTTGCTGTC	827	10^1 cfu/25g	pork, milk	Zhou and Jiao (2005)

(Continued)

TABLE 9.2 (Continued)

Gene targeted	Primer sequence 5'→3'	Size of amplicon (bp)	Sensitivity (detection limit)	Samples tested	References
inlAB	F – CTTCAGGCGGATAGATTAGG R – TTCGCAAGTGAGCTTACGTC	902	4×10^{-1} cfu/g	frankfurters	Jung et al. (2003)
inlA	R – AGTTGATGTTGTGTTAGA F – AGCCACTTAAGGCAAT	760	10 cfu	–	Almeida and Almeida (2000)
InlA	F – ACTATCTAGTAACACGATTAGTGA R – CAAATTTGTTAAAATCCCAAGTGG	250	50–100 cfu/g	dairy products, meat products	Ingianni et al. (2001)
prfA	F – GGTATCACAAAGCTCACGAG R – CCCAAGTAGCAGGACATGCTAA	571	–	milk	Cooray et al. (1994)
prfA	F – GATACAGAAACATCGGTTGGC R – TGACCGCAAATAGAGCCAAG	215	1 cfu/25	cooked ham	Jofre et al. (2005)
16S rRNA	F – GCTAATACCGAATGATAAGA R – GGCTAATACCGAATGATGAA	–	4×10^{-2} to $\times 10^{-1}$ cfu/g	fresh and ready to eat meat and fish, potato salads, vegetable salads, pasta, ice cream	Somer and Kashi (2003)

9.5.4 Other Methods

As technology has advanced over the years, newer methods for detecting pathogens in food have been developed. Enterobacterial repetitive intergenic consensus (ERIC) sequence-based PCR assays were used to compare Listeria spp. isolated from different sources. This method was used to generate DNA fingerprints, by which Listeria spp. were divided into three major clusters and allowed differentiation among the serotypes 1/2a, 4b, 6a and 6b within each cluster (Laciar et al., 2006). Restriction enzyme analysis and pulsed-field gel electrophoresis (PFGE) was employed to detect Listeria species in raw whole milk and farm bulk tanks. This method allowed the isolated organisms to be differentiated into 16 clonal types, with the majority of them belonging to serovar 1/2a (Waak, Tham, & Danielsson-Tham, 2002). DNA microarrays are composed of many discretely located probes which are composed of a sequence that is complementary to a pathogen-specific gene sequence. This allows the analysis of thousands of gene sequences in a relatively short time. This technology has been used for the detection of L. monocytogenes in environmental samples (Call, Borucki, & Loge, 2003). Microarrays along with PFGE and serotyping have been used to study the genetic diversity of L. monocytogenes strains in dairy farms (Borucki, et al., 2005).

DNA microarrays are composed of many discretely located probes on a solid substrate such as glass, wherein each probe is composed of a sequence that is complementary to a pathogen-specific gene sequence.

Spectroscopic methods, such as Fourier Transform Infrared (FT-IR) and Raman spectroscopies, provide unique spectral fingerprints of specific cell types, so they can discriminate between bacteria at genus, species or strain levels. These are whole cell non-destructive methods; destructive methods, such as matrix-assisted laser desorption/ionization mass spectrometry (MALDI-MS), can also be used. As early as 1995, FT-IR spectrometry was used to differentiate all of the six species of *Listeria* (Holt, Hirst, Sutherland, & MacDonald, 1995).

The major players in the food supply chain would benefit enormously from the easy availability of rapid, reliable and sensitive detection methods, which enable the implementation and monitoring of food safety on a global platform. Even though newer methods are valuable tools for routinely screening food and environmental samples, they have not entirely replaced the standard cultural techniques. Rapid methods capable of differentiating living and dead cells and recovering sublethally injured cells are still needed. Nevertheless, nucleic acid-based methods do allow for efficient and reliable results within a short timeframe and have shown great promise for the detection of *L. monocytogenes* in foods.

9.6 *BACILLUS CEREUS*

Among the important bacterial pathogens, *Bacillus cereus* is of significance as it is an opportunistic organism and can dominate in any given situation, because of its ubiquitous nature and ability to occur in a wide range of foods (Reyes, Bastias, Gutierrez, & Rodriguez, 2007; Roy, Moktan, & Sarkar, 2007). The study of *B. cereus* in relation to foods has gained significance in the light of its ability to form heat-resistant endospores and its capacity to grow and produce toxins in a wide variety of foods (Ehling-Schulz, Fricker, & Scherer, 2004; Ouoba, Thorsen, & Varnam, 2008). *Bacillus cereus* food poisoning is under-reported, as both types of illnesses are relatively mild and usually last for less than 24 hours. The unique properties of *B. cereus*—like its heat-resistant endospore-forming ability, toxin production and psychrotrophic nature—give ample scope for this organism to be considered a prime cause of public health hazard (Griffiths & Schraft, 2002). Strains of *B. cereus* cause two different types of foodborne illnesses in humans, namely diarrheal and emetic (Schoeni & Wong, 2005). At present, three types of heat labile enterotoxins involved in food poisoning have been characterized at the molecular level (Tsen *et al.*, 2000). Molecular diagnostic methods based on the polymerase chain reaction have been described for the detection of potent toxigenic cultures of *B. cereus* (Radhika *et al.*, 2002; Abriouel *et al.*, 2007; Ngamwongsatit *et al.*, 2008).

9.6.1 Detection Methods

In the earlier years, studies were aimed at developing simple and rapid procedures for the enumeration, isolation and identification of *B. cereus*. Several selective and differential enumeration media have been formulated to achieve the maximum recovery of *B. cereus* from foods (Varadaraj, 1993). One of the earliest methods developed in 1955 involved surface plating on blood agar, followed by incubation for 18 hours at 37°C and the plates were observed for colonies surrounded by a halo (lecithinase activity). Later, a peptone beef extract egg yolk agar containing lithium chloride and polymyxin B as selective agents was formulated. Typical *B. cereus* colonies were surrounded by an opaque zone after 18 hours at 30°C. A further improvement in this medium was through the addition of mannitol, which enabled non-*B. cereus* colonies to be differentiated from mannitol negative *B. cereus* colonies (Mossel *et al.*, 1967). Kim and Goepfert (1971) formulated egg yolk containing medium (KG medium), which could result in sporulation within 24 hours of incubation. This medium gave a good recovery of *B. cereus* from foods with inherent background microflora. Polymyxin was used for selectivity, egg yolk to record lecithinase activity, and low levels of peptone enabled sporulation.

As a means of achieving a better recovery of the organisms from food samples, Holbrook and

Anderson (1980) developed a medium known as polymyxin pyruvate egg yolk mannitol bromothymol blue agar (PEMBA) based on the characteristics of mannitol utilization (peacock blue colored colonies) and lecithinase activity (precipitation of egg yolk) of *B. cereus* cultures. The presence of pyruvate in the medium restricts the characteristic spreading nature of sporeformers. This medium supports the growth of even small numbers of *B. cereus* cells and spores. For this reason the medium found wider application in research investigations relating to the enumeration of *B. cereus* from foods. The use of PEMBA enabled easy differentiation of *B. cereus* from other *Bacillus* species present in Indian snack and lunch foods (Varadaraj *et al.*, 1992). A later modification of PEMBA was the replacement of bromothymol blue with bromocresol blue in the medium (Szabo, Todd, & Rayman, 1984).

Although identified *B. cereus* isolates exhibited a diversified pattern with respect to virulence/toxigenic traits being harbored by them, it is important to observe that phospholipase activity was more predominant among the isolates. Phospholipase is known to cause degradation of cell and mucous membranes, which are rich in phospholipids, leading to necrosis and considered as virulence factors. In view of the importance of this character in *B. cereus*, our earlier studies resulted in obtaining a patent for the phospholipase (Pl) oligonucleotide primer designed to detect *B. cereus* among the cluster of other related species of *B. cereus* (Padmapriya, Ramesh, & Chandrashekar, 2004). Another virulence factor associated with *B. cereus* isolates was that of sphingomyelinase activity, which was recorded in 42% isolates by PCR. An earlier study concluded that phospholipase C and sphingomyelinase encoded by two tandemly arranged genes with close genetic linkage constitute a biologically functional cytolytic determinant and act in natural concert, causing lysis of target cells and are thus regarded as an effective cytolysin (Beecher & Wong, 2000).

Although diarrheal food poisoning arising from *B. cereus* is due to three enterotoxins—hemolysin BL (HBL), non-hemolytic enterotoxin (NHE) and cytotoxin K (CytK)—the major health hazard attributed to *B. cereus* is mostly related to the HBL enterotoxin complex (Hsieh, Sheu, Chen, & Tsen, 1999). The enterotoxigenicity among isolates of *B. cereus* has been attributed to the presence of all three components: a binding component B, and two lytic components L1 and L2 in the HBL complex (Schoeni & Wong, 2005). Studies have shown that the potential virulence factors (hemolysis, sphingomyelinase and phospholipase C) are under the control of a pleiotropic regulator PlcR and are expressed simultaneously. A complex interaction among

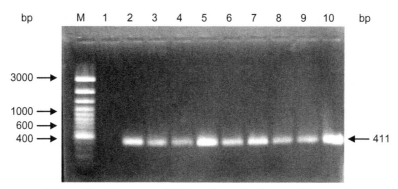

FIGURE 9.1   Agarose gel electrophoretic pattern of PCR products showing amplicons with *entB* primers in native food isolates of *S. aureus* and *S. epidermidis*. Lane M, 100 bp marker; Lanes 1–10, native food isolates of *S. aureus* and *S. epidermidis*.

these virulence factors exist, which may be cooperative, synergistic and antagonistic (Slamti *et al.*, 2004). Another study has designed eight sets of novel PCR primers to detect the wide distribution pattern of enterotoxin genes among *B. cereus* clusters (Ngamwongsatit *et al.*, 2008).

9.7 CAPACITY BUILDING INITIATIVE AT CFTRI

At the Central Food Technological Research Institute, Mysore, India, an initiative towards developing PCR-based detection methods for foodborne pathogens in the late 1990s has enabled the development of sensitive methods for detecting *S. aureus*, both in culture broth (Figure 9.1) and food systems. Further, multiplex PCR has been optimized for the simultaneous detection of *S. aureus* and *Y. enterocolitica* (Figure 9.2) in milk through the optimization of DNA extraction protocols from milk and PCR conditions (Ramesh *et al.*, 2002; Padmapriya, Ramesh, Chandrashekar, & Varadaraj, 2003). Through the use of PCR and colony hybridization protocols, targeted isolates of *B. cereus* from food samples (Figures 9.3 and 9.4) were detected (Radhika *et al.*, 2002).

Considering the expertise available at CFTRI, Mysore several collaborative programs, both at national and international levels, have been organized over the past two decades. CFTRI has

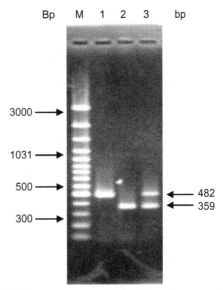

FIGURE 9.2 Agarose gel electrophoretic pattern of multiplex PCR products showing amplicons with *nuc* primers of *S. aureus* and *ail* primers of *Y. enterocolitica*. Lane M, 100 bp marker; Lanes 1, *S. aureus*; 2, *Y. enterocolitica*; 3, *S. aureus* and *Y. enterocolitica*.

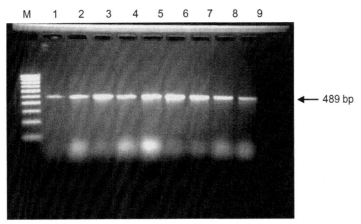

FIGURE 9.3 Agarose gel electrophoretic pattern of PCR products showing amplicons with Ha-1 primers in cultures of *B. cereus*. Lane M, 100 bp marker; Lanes 1–9, potent toxigenic native food isolates of *B. cereus*.

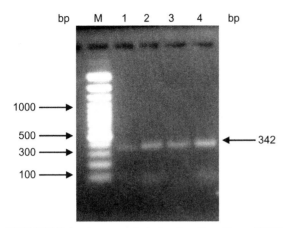

FIGURE 9.4   Agarose gel electrophoretic pattern of PCR products showing amplicons with PI primers of *B. cereus* in food samples. Lane M, 100 bp marker; Lanes 1, mustard powder; 2, turmeric powder; 3, chilli powder; 4, positive control of *B. cereus*.

been associated with international organizations of the United Nations and other related bodies in conducting training programs, workshops, symposia, one-to-one interactions, technical support and advice in setting-up of infrastructure facilities for analysis and testing, and many other focal issues related to global food safety.

Because of the large variety of methods to detect and identify microorganisms and undesirable microbial metabolites in food products, harmonization of such methods would make it easier to build the analytical capacity required for food safety surveillance. It would increase the recognition of data and reduce costs. At the same time, it would reduce the restriction of imports due to lack of availability of data produced by internationally recognized methods.

References

Abriouel, H., Ben Omar, N., Lucas López, R., et al. (2007). Differentiation and characterization by molecular techniques of *Bacillus cereus* group isolates from poto poto and dégué, two traditional cereal-based fermented foods of Burkina Faso and Republic of Congo. *Journal of Food Protection, 70*, 1165–1173.

Almeida, P. F., & Almeida, R. C. C. (2000). A PCR protocol using *inl* gene as a target for specific detection of *Listeria monocytogenes*. *Food Control, 11*, 97–101.

Amagliani, G., Brandi, G., Omiccioli, E., et al. (2004). Direct detection of *Listeria monocytogenes* from milk by magnetic based DNA isolation and PCR. *Food Microbiology, 21*, 597–603.

Association of Official Analytical Chemists. (1996). 17.10.01 AOAC official method 993.12. *Listeria monocytogenes* in milk and dairy products. In: *Official Methods of Analysis of the Association of Official Analytical Chemists*. Gaithersburg, MD: AOAC International.

Aulisio, C. C. G., Stanfield, J. T., Weagant, S. D., et al. (1983). Yersinioses associated with tofu consumption: Serological, biochemical and pathogenicity studies of *Yersinia enterocolitica* isolates. *Journal of Food Protection, 46*, 226–230.

Baird-Parker, A. C. (1965). The classification of staphylococci and micrococci from world-wide sources. *Journal of General Microbiology, 38*, 363–387.

Baird-Parker, T. C. (2000). Staphylococcus aureus. In M. B. Lund, T. C. Baird-Parker, & G. W. Gould (Eds.), *The Microbiological Safety and Quality of Food: Vol. 2* (pp. 1317–1335). Maryland: Aspen Publishers Inc.

Balamurugan, J., Bhilegaonkar, K. N., & Agarwal, R. K. (2006). A study on suitability of four enrichment broths for PCR-based detection of *Listeria monocytogenes* from raw meat. *Journal of Food Safety, 26*, 16–29.

Beckers, H. J., Soentoro, P. S. S., & Asc, E. H. M. D. -v. (1987). The occurrence of *Listeria monocytogenes* in soft cheeses and raw milk and its resistance to heat. *International Journal of Food Microbiology, 4*, 249–256.

Beecher, D. J., & Wong, A. C. L. (2000). Cooperative, synergistic and antagonistic haemolytic interactions between haemolysin BL, phosphatidylcholine phospholipase C and sphingomyelinase from *Bacillus cereus*. *Microbiology, 146*, 3033–3039.

Bercovier, H., & Mollaret, H. H. (1984). Genus Yersinia. In N. R. Krieg, & J. G. Holt (Eds.), *Bergey's Manual of Systematic Bacteriology: Vol. 1* (pp. 498–506). Baltimore: Williams and Wilkins.

Bergdoll, M. S., Reiser, R., & Spintz, J. (1976). Staphylococcal enterotoxins—Detection in Food. *Food Technology, 5*, 80–84.

Berrada, H., Soriano, J. M., Pico, Y., & Manes, J. (2006). Quantification of *Listeria monocytogenes* in salads by Real-Time quantitative PCR. *International Journal of Food Microbiology, 107*, 202–206.

Bhaduri, S., Conway, L. K., & La Chica, R. V. (1987). Assay of crystal violet binding for rapid identification of virulent plasmid bearing clones of *Yersinia enterocolitica*. *Journal of Clinical Microbiology, 25*, 1039–1041.

Blais, B. W., & Phillippe, L. M. (1993). A simple RNA probe system for analysis of Listeria monocytogenes polymerase chain reaction products. *Applied and Environmental Microbiology*, 59, 2795–2800.

Borucki, M. K., Gay, C. C., Reynolds, J., et al. (2005). Genetic diversity of *Listeria monocytogenes* strains from a high-prevalence dairy farm. *Applied and Environmental Microbiology*, 71, 5893–5899.

Bottone, E. J. (1997). *Yersinia enterocolitica*: The charisma continues. *Clinical Microbiology Reviews*, 257–276.

Boyapalle, S., Wesley, I. V., Hurd, H. S., & Reddy, P. G. (2001). Comparison of culture, multiplex and 5 nuclease polymerase chain reaction assay for the rapid detection of *Yersinia enterocolitica* in swine and pork products. *Journal of Food Protection*, 64, 1352–1361.

Buchrieser, C., Rusniok, C., Kunst, F., et al. (2003). The *Listeria* Consortium, Comparison of the genome sequences of *Listeria monocytogenes* and *Listeria innocua*: Clues for evolution and pathogenicity. *FEMS Immunology and Medical Microbiology*, 35, 207–213.

Call, D. R., Borucki, M. K., & Loge, F. J. (2003). Detection of bacterial pathogens in environmental samples using DNA microarrays. *Journal of Microbiological Method*, 53, 235–243.

Carnevale, R. A., & Johnston, R. W. (1989). Method for the isolation and identification of *Listeria monocytogenes* from meat and poultry products. US Department of Agriculture Food Safety and Inspection Service, Washington, DC, Laboratory Communication, No. 57.

Casman, E. P., & Bennett, R. W. (1965). Detection of staphylococcal enterotoxin in Food. *Applied Microbiology*, 13, 181–189.

Cho, J.-C., & Tiedje, J. M. (2002). Quantitative detection of microbial genes by using DNA microarrays. *Applied and Environmental Microbiology*, 68, 1425–1430.

Choi, W. S., & Hong, C. H. (2003). Rapid enumeration of *Listeria monocytogenes* in milk using competitive PCR. *International Journal of Food Microbiology*, 84, 79–85.

Cooray, K. J., Nishibori, T., Xiong, H., et al. (1994). Detection of multiple virulence-associated genes of *Listeria monocytogenes* by PCR in artificially contaminated milk samples. *Applied and Environmental Microbiology*, 60, 3023–3026.

Curtis, G. D. W., Mitchell, R. G., King, A. F., & Griffen, E. J. (1989a). A selective differential medium for the isolation of *Listeria monocytogenes*. *Letters in Applied Microbiology*, 8, 95–98.

Curtis, G. D. W., Mitchell, R. G., King, A. F., et al. (1989b). A selective differential medium for the isolation of *Listeria monocytogenes*. *Letters in Applied Microbiology*, 8, 95–98.

Daly, P., Collier, T., & Doyle, S. (2002). PCR-ELISA detection of *Escherichia coli* in milk. *Letters in Applied Microbiology*, 34, 222–226.

Donnelly, C. W., & Baigent, G. J. (1986). Method for flow cytometric detection of *Listeria* monocytogenes in milk. *Applied and Environmental Microbiology*, 52, 689–695.

Dons, I., Rasmussen, O. F., & Olsen, J. E. (1992). Cloning and characterization of a gene encoding flagellin of *Listeria monocytogenes*. *Molecular Microbiology*, 6, 2919–2929.

Doores, S. (1999). *Food safety: Current status and future needs*. Critical issues colloquia reports, American Academy of Microbiology, http://academy.asm.org/index.php?option=com_content&task=view&id=44&Itemid=55.

Doyle, M. P., & Schoeni, J. L. (1986). Selective-enrichment procedure for isolation of *Listeria monocytogenes* in soft, surface-ripened cheese. *Journal of Food Protection*, 50, 4–6.

Ehling-Schulz, M., Fricker, M., & Scherer, S. (2004). *Bacillus cereus*, the causative agent of an emetic type of foodborne illness. *Molecular Nutrition & Food Research*, 48, 479–487.

Fairchild, A., Lee, M. D., & Maurer, J. J. (2006). PCR basis. In J. Maurer (Ed.), *PCR Methods in Foods* (pp. 1–25). USA: Springer-Science Business Media Inc.

Farber, J. M., Sanders, G. W., & Speirs, J. I. (1988). Methodology for isolation of *Listeria* from foods—a Canadian perspective. *Journal Association of Official Analytical Chemists*, 71, 675–678.

Farmer, J. J., III, Carter, G. P., Miller, V. L., et al. (1992). Pyrazinamidase, Cr-MOX agar, Salicin fermentation-Esculin hydrolysis and D-xylose fermentation for identifying pathogenic serotypes of *Yersinia enterocolitica*. *Journal of Clinical Microbiology*, 30, 2589–2594.

Feng, P., & Weagant, S. D. (1994). Yersinia. In Y. H. Hui, Gorham., K. D. Murrell & D. O. Cliver (Eds.), *Foodborne Disease Handbook: Diseases Caused by Bacteria* (pp. 427–460). New York: Marcel Dekker.

Feng, P. (2001). Development and impact of rapid methods for detection of foodborne pathogens. In M. P. Doyle, L. R. Beuchat, & T. J. Montaville (Eds.), *Food Microbiology: Fundamentals and Frontiers* (2nd edn) (pp. 775–793). Washington DC: ASM Press.

Fraser, J. A., & Sperber, W. H. (1988). Rapid detection of *Listeria* spp. in food and environmental samples by esculin hydrolysis. *Journal of Food Protection*, 51, 762–765.

Fredriksson-Ahomaa, M., & Korkeala, H. (2003). Low occurrence of pathogenic *Yersinia enterocolitica* in clinical, food and environmental samples: A methodological problem. *Clinical Microbiology Reviews*, 16, 220–229.

Freed, R. C., Evenson, M. L., Reiser, R. F., & Bergdoll, M. S. (1982). Enzyme-linked immunosorbent assay for detection of *staphylococcal enterotoxins* in foods. *Applied and Environmental Microbiology*, 44, 1349–1355.

Fueyo, J. M., Martin, M. C., González-Hevia, M. A., & Mendoza, M. C. (2001). Enterotoxin production and DNA fingerprinting in *Staphylococcus aureus* isolated from human and food samples. Relations between genetic types and enterotoxins. *International Journal of Food Microbiology*, 67, 139–145.

Gaillard, J. L., Berche, P., Frehel, C., et al. (1991). Entry of *Listeria monocytogenes* into cells is mediated by internalin, a repeat protein reminiscent of surface antigens from Gram-positive cocci. *Cell*, *65*, 1127–1141.

Gasper, E., Heimsch, R. C., & Anderson, A. W. (1973). Quantitative detection of type A *staphylococcal enterotoxin* by Laurell electroimmunodiffusion. *Applied Microbiology*, *25*, 421–426.

Ge, B., Zhao, S., Hall, R., & Meng, J. (2002). A PCR-ELISA for detecting Shiga toxin-producing *Escherichia coli*. *Microbes and Infection*, *4*, 285–290.

Gemski, P., Lazere, J. R., & Casey, T. (1980). Plasmid associated with pathogenicity and calcium dependency of *Yersinia enterocolitica*. *Infection and Immunity*, *27*, 682–685.

Genigeorgis, C. A. (1989). Present state of knowledge of staphylococcal intoxication. *International Journal of Food Microbiology*, *9*, 327–360.

Geoffroy, C., Raveneau, J., Beretti, J. L., et al. (1991). Purification and characterization of an extracellular 29 kDa phospholipase C from *Listeria monocytogenes*. *Infection and Immunity*, *59*, 2382–2388.

Gilligan, K., Shipley, M., Stiles, B., et al. (2000). Identification of *Staphylococcus aureus* enterotoxins A and B genes by PCR-ELISA. *Molecular and Cellular Probes*, *14*, 71–78.

Gilot, P., & Content, J. (2002). Specific identification of *Listeria welshimeri* and *Listeria monocytogenes* by PCR assays targeting a gene encoding a fibronectin-binding protein. *Journal of Clinical Microbiology*, *40*, 698–703.

Gohmann, S., Leimester-Wachter, M., Schlitz, E., et al. (1990). Characterization of a *Listeria monocytogenes*-specific protein capable of inducing delayed hypersensitivity in *Listeria*-immune mice. *Molecular Microbiology*, *4*, 1091–1099.

Goverde, R. L. J., Jansen, W. H., Brunings, H. A., et al. (1993). Digoxigenin-labelled *inv-* and *ail*-probes for the detection and identification of pathogenic *Yersinia enterocolitica* in clinical specimens and naturally contaminated pig samples. *The Journal of Applied Bacteriology*, *74*, 301–313.

Gray, M. L., Stafseth, H. J., & Thorp, Jr. F. (1950). The use of potassium tellurite, sodium azide and acetic acid in a selective medium for the isolation of *Listeria monocytogenes*. *Journal of Bacteriology*, *59*, 443–444.

Griffiths, M. W., & Schraft, H. (2002). *Bacillus cereus* food poisoning. In D. O. Cliver & H. P. Riemann (Eds.), *Foodborne Diseases* (pp. 261–270). London: Academic Press.

Gunasinghe, C. P. G. L., Henderson, C., & Rutter, M. A. (1994). Comparative study of two plating media (PALCAM and Oxford) for detection of *Listeria* species in a range of meat products following a variety of enrichment procedures. *Letters in Applied Microbiology*, *18*, 156–158.

Hamels, S., Galo, J.-L., Dufour, S., et al. (2001). Consensus PCR and Microarray for diagnosis of the genus *Staphylococcus*, species and methicillin resistance. *Biotechniques*, *31*, 1364–1372.

Hao, D. Y. Y., Beuchat, L. R., & Brackett, R. E. (1989). Comparison of media and methods for detecting and enumerating *Listeria monocytogenes* in refrigerated cabbage. *Applied and Environmental Microbiology*, *53*, 955–957.

Hein, I., Lehner, A., Rieck, P., et al. (2001). Comparison of different approaches to quantify *Staphylococcus aureus* cells by Real-Time quantitative PCR and application of this technique for examination of cheese. *Applied and Environmental Microbiology*, *67*, 3122–3126.

Herman, L. M. F., DeBlock, J. H. G. E., & Moermans, R. J. B. (1995). Direct detection of *Listeria monocytogenes* in 25 milliliters of raw milk by a two-step PCR with nested primers. *Applied and Environmental Microbiology*, *61*, 817–819.

Hill, W. E., & Keasler, S. P. (1991). Identification of foodborne pathogens by nucleic acid hybridization. *International Journal of Food Microbiology*, *12*, 67–76.

Hitchins, A. D. (2003). *Listeria monocytogenes*. In: *Bacteriological Analytical Manual*, 8th edn, AOAC International, 10.01–10.13.

Holbrook, R., & Anderson, J. M. (1980). An improved selective and diagnostic medium for the isolation and enumeration of *Bacillus cereus* in foods. *Canadian Journal of Microbiology*, *26*, 753–759.

Holt, C., Hirst, D., Sutherland, A., & MacDonald, F. (1995). Discrimination of species in the genus *Listeria* by Fourier transform infrared spectroscopy and canonical variate analysis. *Applied and Environmental Microbiology*, *61*, 377–378.

Hough, A. J., Harbison, S. A., Savill, M. G., et al. (2002). Rapid enumeration of *Listeria monocytogenes* in artificially contaminated cabbage using real-time polymerase chain reaction. *Journal of Food Protection*, *65*, 1329–1332.

Hsieh, Y. M., Sheu, S. J., Chen, Y. L., & Tsen, H. Y. (1999). Enterotoxigenic profiles and polymerase chain reaction detection of *Bacillus cereus* group cells and *B. cereus* strains from foods and foodborne outbreaks. *Journal of Applied Microbiology*, *87*, 481–490.

Hudson, J. A., Lake, R. J., & Savill, M. G. (2001). Rapid detection of *Listeria monocytogenes* in ham samples using immunomagnetic separation followed by polymerase chain reaction. *Journal of Applied Microbiology*, *90*, 614–621.

Ingianni, A., Floris, M., Palomba, P., et al. (2001). Rapid detection of *Listeria monocytogenes* in foods, by a combination of PCR and DNA probe. *Molecular and Cellular Probes*, *15*, 275–280.

Janzten, M. M., Navas, J., Corujo, A., et al. (2006). Review: Specific detection of *Listeria* monocytogenes in foods using commercial methods: From chromogenic media to Real-Time PCR. *Spanish Journal of Agricultural Research*, *4*, 235–247.

Jofre, A., Martin, B., Garriga, M., et al. (2005). Simultaneous detection of *Listeria monocytogenes* and *Salmonella* by multiplex PCR in cooked ham. *Food Microbiology, 22,* 109–115.

Jones, C. L., & Khan, S. A. (1986). Nucleotide sequence of the enterotoxin B gene from *Staphylococcus aureus. Journal of Bacteriology, 166,* 29–33.

Jones, L. J. (1991). DNA probes: Applications in the food industry. *Trends Food Science & Technology, 2,* 28–32.

Jourdan, A. D., Johnson, S. C. J., & Wesley, I. V. (2000). Development of a fluorogenic 5 nuclease PCR assay for detection of the ail gene of pathogenic *Yersinia enterocolitica. Applied and Environmental Microbiology, 66,* 3750–3755.

Jung, Y. S., Frank, J. F., Brackett, R. E., et al. (2003). Polymerase chain reaction detection of *Listeria monocytogenes* in frankfurters using oligonucleotide primers targeting the genes encoding internalin AB. *Journal of Food Protection, 66,* 237–241.

Kandolo, K., & Wauters, G. (1985). Pyrazinamidase activity in *Yersinia enterocolitica* and related organisms. *Journal of Clinical Microbiology, 21,* 980–982.

Khan, M. A., Kim, C. H., Kaoma, I., et al. (1998). Detection of *Staphylococcus aureus* in milk by use of polymerase chain reaction analysis. *American Journal of Veterinary Research, 59,* 807–813.

Kim, H. U., & Goepfert, J. M. (1971). Enumeration and identification of *Bacillus cereus* in foods. I, 24-hour presumptive test medium. *Applied Microbiology, 22,* 581–587.

Kim, C.–H., Khan, M., Morin, D. E., et al. (2001). Optimization of the PCR for detection of *Staphylococcus aureus nuc* gene in Bovine milk. *Journal of Dairy Science, 84,* 74–83.

Klein, P. G., & Juneja, V. K. (1997). Sensitive detection of viable *Listeria monocytogenes* by reverse transcription-PCR. *Applied and Environmental Microbiology, 63,* 4441–4448.

Kocks, C., Gouin, E., Tabouret, M., et al. (1992). *Listeria monocytogenes* induced actin assembly requires the *actA* gene product, a surface protein. *Cell, 68,* 521–531.

Kohler, S., Leimeister-Wachter, M., Chakraborty, T., et al. (1990). The gene coding for protein p60 of *Listeria monocytogenes* and its use as a specific probe for *Listeria monocytogenes. Infection and Immunity, 58,* 1943–1950.

Ky, Y. U., Noh, Y., Park, H. J., et al. (2004). Use of monoclonal antibodies that recognize p60 for identification of *Listeria monocytogenes. Clinical and Diagnostic Laboratory Immunology, 1,* 446–451.

Laciar, A., Vaca, L., Lopresti, R., et al. (2006). DNA fingerprinting by ERIC-PCR for comparing *Listeria* spp. strains isolated from different sources in San Luis, Argentina. *Revista Argentina de Microbiología, 38,* 55–60.

Lantz, P.-G., Hahn-Hägerdal, B., & Radstrom, P. (1994). Sample preparation methods in PCR-based detection of food pathogens. *Trends Food Science & Technology, 5,* 384–389.

Lapeyre, C., Janin, F., & Kaveri, S. V. (1998). Indirect double sandwich ELISA using monoclonal antibodies for the direct detection of *staphylococcal enterotoxins* A, B, C and D in food samples. *Food Microbiology, 5,* 25–32.

Lee, W. H., & McClain, D. (1986). Improved *Listeria monocytogenes* selective agar. *Applied and Environmental Microbiology, 52,* 1215–1217.

Leimeister-Wachter, M., Haffner, C., Domann, E., et al. (1990). Identification of a gene that positively regulates expression of *listeriolysin,* the major virulence factor of *Listeria monocytogenes. Proceedings of the National Academy of Sciences of the United States of America, 87,* 8336–8340.

Levin, R. E. (2003). Application of the Polymerase Chain Reaction for Detection of *Listeria monocytogenes* in Foods: A review of methodology. *Food Biotechnology, 17,* 99–116.

Liu, D. (2008). Preparation of *Listeria monocytogenes* specimens for molecular detection and identification. *International Journal of Food Microbiology, 122,* 229–242.

Logan, J. M. J., Edwards, K. J., Saunders, N. A., & Stanley, J. (2001). Rapid identification of Campylobacter spp. by melting peak analysis of biprobes in real-time PCR. *Journal of Clinical Microbiology, 39,* 2227–2232.

Longhi, C., Maffeo, A., Penta, M., et al. (2003). Detection of *Listeria monocytogenes* in Italian-style soft cheeses. *Journal of Applied Microbiology, 94,* 879–885.

Lovett, J., Francis, D. W., & Hunt, J. M. (1987). *Listeria monocytogenes* in raw milk: Detection, incidence and pathogenicity. *Journal of Food Protection, 50,* 188–192.

Lovett, J. (1988). Isolation and identification of *Listeria monocytogenes* in dairy products. *Journal Association of Official Analytical Chemists, 71,* 658–660.

Marin, M. E., Rosa, M. C., & Cornejo, I. (1992). Entertoxigenicity of *Staphylococcus* strains isolated from Spanish dry-cured hams. *Applied and Environmental Microbiology, 58,* 1067–1069.

McBride, M. E., & Girard, K. F. (1960). A selective method for the isolation of *Listeria monocytogenes* from mixed bacterial populations. *The Journal of Laboratory and Clinical Medicine, 55,* 153–157.

Mehrotra, M., Wang, G., & Johnson, W. M. (2000). Multiplex PCR for detection of genes for *Staphylococcus aureus* enterotoxins, exfoliative toxins, toxic shock syndrome toxin 1 and methicillin resistance. *Journal of Clinical Microbiology, 38,* 1032–1035.

Meng, J., & Doyle, M. P. (2002). Introduction: Microbial food safety. *Microbes and Infection, 4,* 395–397.

Mengaud, J., Vicente, M. F., Chenevert, J., et al. (1988). Expression in *Escherichia coli* and sequence analysis of the *listeriolysin O* determinant of *Listeria monocytogenes. Infection and Immunity, 56,* 766–772.

Miliotis, M. D., & Bier, J. W. (2003). *International Handbook of Foodborne Pathogens.* Marcel Dekker, Inc.

Mitchell, B. A., Milbury, J. A., Brookins, A. M., et al. (1994). Use of immunomagnetic capture on beads to recover

Listeria from environmental samples. *Journal of Food Protection*, 57, 743–745.

Mossel, D. A. A. (1986). Developing methodology for food-borne microorganisms: Fundamentals of analytical techniques. In M. D. Pierson & N. J. Stern (Eds.), *Foodborne Microorganisms and Their Toxins: Developing Methodology* (pp. 1–22). New York: Marcel Dekker Inc.

Mukhopadhyay, A., & Mukhopadhyay, U. K. (2007). Novel multiplex approaches for the simultaneous detection of human pathogens: *Escherichia coli* 0157:H7 and *Listeria monocytogenes*. *Journal of Microbiological Methods*, 68, 193–200.

Myess, K. M., Gaba, J., & Al-Khaldi, S. F. (2006). Molecular identification of *Yersinia enterocolitica* isolated from pasturized whole milk using DNS microarray chip hybridization.. *Molecular and Cellular Probes*, 20, 71–80.

Van Netten, P., Perales, I., Van de Moosdijk, A., et al. (1989). Liquid and solid selective differential media for the detection and enumeration of *Listeria monocytogenes* and other *Listeria* spp. *International Journal of Food Microbiology*, 8, 299–316.

Ngamwongsatit, P., Buasri, W., Pianariyanon, P., et al. (2008). Broad distribution of entertoxin genes (hblCDA, nhe-ABC, cytK and entFM) among *Bacillus thuringiensis* and *Bacillus cereus* as shown by novel primers. *International Journal of Food Microbiology*, 121, 352–356.

Norton, D. M. (2002). Polymerase chain reaction-based methods for detection of *Listeria monocytogenes*: Toward real-time screening for food and environmental samples. *Journal Association of Official Analytical Chemists*, 85, 505–515.

Ortel, S. (1972). Experience with nalidixic acid-trypaflavine agar. *Acta Microbiologica Academiae Scientiarum Hungaricae*, 19, 363–365.

Ouoba, L. I., Thorsen, L., & Varnam, A. H. (2008). Enterotoxins and emetic toxins production by *Bacillus cereus* and other species of *Bacillus* isolated from Soumbala and Bikalga, African alkaline fermented food condiments. *International Journal of Food Microbiology*, 124, 224–230.

Özbas, Z. Y., Lehner, A., & Wagner, M. (2000). Development of a multiplex and semi-nested PCR assay for detection of *Yersinia enterocolitica* and *Aeromonas hydrophila* in raw milk. *Food Microbiology*, 17, 197–203.

Padmapriya, B. P., Ramesh, A., Chandrashekar, A., & Varadaraj, M. C. (2003). Staphylococcal accessory gene regulator (sar) as a signature gene to detect *enterotoxigenic staphylococci*. *Journal of Applied Microbiology*, 95, 974–981.

Padmapriya, B. P., Ramesh, A., & Chandrashekar, A. et al. (2004). Oligonucleotide primers for phosphotidyl inositol in *Bacillus cereus*. US Patent, US 6713620 dt. 30/03/2004.

Paoli, G. C., Bhunia, A. K., & Bayles, D. O. (2005). *Listeria monocytogenes*. In P. M. Fratamico, A. K. Bhunia, & J. L. Smith (Eds.), *Foodborne Pathogens: Microbiology and*

Molecular Biology. Caister (pp. 295–325). Wymondham, Norfolk, UK: Academic Press.

Paziak-Domanska, B., Boguslawska, E., Wieckowska-Szakiel, M., et al. (1999). Evaluation of the API test, phosphatidylinositol-specific phospholipase C activity and PCR method in identification of *Listeria monocytogenes* in meat foods. *FEMS Microbiology Letters*, 171, 209–214.

Phuektes, P., Mansell, P. D., & Browning, G. F. (2001). Multiplex polymerase chain reaction assay for simultaneous detection of *Staphylococcus aureus* and Streptococcal causes of bovine mastitis. *Journal of Dairy Science*, 84, 1140–1148.

Prpic, J. K., Robins-Browne, R. M., & Davey, R. B. (1983). Differentiation between virulent and avirulent *Yersinia enterocolitica* isolates using Congo red agar. *Journal of Clinical Microbiology*, 18, 486–490.

Radhika, B., Padmapriya, B. P., Chandrashekar, A., et al. (2002). Detection of *Bacillus cereus* in foods by colony hybridization using PCR-generated probe and characterization of isolates for toxins by PCR. *International Journal of Food Microbiology*, 74, 131–138.

Ramesh, A., Padmapriya, B. P., Bharathi, S., & Varadaraj, M. C. (2003). *Yersinia enterocolitica* detection and treatment. In B. L. Cabellero, C. Trugo, & P. M. Finglas (Eds.), *Encyclopaedia of Food Sciences and Nutrition: Vol. 10* (pp. 6245–6252). New York: Academic Press/Elsevier, 2nd edn.

Ramesh, A., Padmapriya, B. P., Chandrashekar, A., & Varadaraj, M. C. (2002). Application of a convenient DNA extraction method and multiplex PCR for direct detection of *Staphylococcus aureus* and *Yersinia enterocolitica* in milk samples. *Molecular and Cellular Probes*, 16, 307–314.

Rasmussen, H. N., Rasmussen, O. F., Christensen, H., & Olsen, J. E. (1995). Detection of *Yersinia enterocolitica* O:3 in faecal samples and tonsil swabs from pigs using IMS and PCR. *The Journal of Applied Bacteriology*, 78, 563–568.

Reiser, R., Conaway, D., & Bergdoll, M. S. (1974). Detection of staphylococcal enterotoxins in foods. *Applied Microbiology*, 27, 83–85.

Reyes, J. E., Bastias, J. M., Gutierrez, M. R., & Rodriguez, M. O. (2007). Prevalence of *Bacillus cereus* in dried milk products used by Chilean school feeding program. *Food Microbiology*, 24, 1–6.

Rodriguez, D. L., Fernandez, G. S., Garayzabal, J. F. F., et al. (1984). New methodology for the isolation of *Listeria* microorganisms from heavily contaminated environments. *Applied and Environmental Microbiology*, 47, 1188–1190.

Rodriguez-Lazaro, D., Hernandez, M., & Pla, M. (2004). Simultaneous quantitative detection of *Listeria* spp. and *Listeria monocytogenes* using a duplex real-time PCR-based assay. *FEMS Microbiology Letters*, 233, 257–267.

Rossen, L., Nørskov, P., Holmstrøm, K., & Rasmussen, O. F. (1992). Inhibition of PCR by components of food samples, microbial diagnostic assays and DNA-extraction solutions. *International Journal of Food Microbiology, 17*, 37–45.

Roy, A., Moktan, B., & Sarkar, P. K. (2007). Characteristics of *Bacillus cereus* isolates from legume-based Indian fermented foods. *Food Control, 18*, 1555–1564.

Sails, A. D., Bolton, F. J., Fox, A. J., et al. (2002). Detection of *Campylobacter jejuni* and *Campylobacter coli* in environmental waters by PCR enzyme-linked immunosorbent assay. *Applied and Environmental Microbiology, 68*, 1319–1324.

Salamah, A. A. (1990). Correlation of pathogenicity and calcium dependency of *Yersinia pseudotuberculosis* and *Yersinia enterocolitica* with their plasmid content. *Journal of King Saudi University, 2*, 13–19.

Schoeni, J. L., & Wong, A. C. L. (2005). *Bacillus cereus* food poisoning and its toxins. *Journal of Food Protection, 68*, 636–648.

Shimizu, A., Fujita, M., Igarashi, He, et al. (2000). Characterization of *Staphylococcus aureus* coagulase type VII isolates from staphylococcal food poisoning outbreaks (1980–1995) in Tokyo, Japan, by pulsed-field gel electrophoresis. *Journal of Clinical Microbiology, 38*, 3746–3749.

Simonova, J., Vazlerova, M., & Steinhauserova, I. (2007). Detection of pathogenic *Yersinia enterocolitica* serotype O:3 by biochemical, serological and PCR methods. *Cechoslovaca Journal of Food Science, 25*, 214–220.

Slamti, L., Perchat, S., Gominet, M., et al. (2004). Distinct mutations in Plc R explain why some strains of the *Bacillus cereus* group are non hemolytic. *Journal of Bacteriology, 186*, 3531–3538.

Somer, L., & Kashi, Y. (2003). A PCR method based on 16S rRNA sequence for simultaneous detection of the genus *Listeria* and the species *Listeria monocytogenes* in food products. *Journal of Food Protection, 66*, 1658–1665.

Sory, M., Tollenaere, J., Laszlo, C., et al. (1990). Detection of pYV+ *Yersinia enterocolitica* isolates by P1 slide agglutination. *Journal of Clinical Microbiology, 28*, 2403–2408.

Stevens, K. A., & Jaykus, L. A. (2004). Direct detection of bacterial pathogens in representative dairy products using a combined bacterial concentration-PCR approach. *Journal of Applied Microbiology, 97*, 1115–1122.

Stringer, M. (2005). Food safety objectives—Role in microbiological food safety management. *Food Control, 16*, 775–794.

Sulakvelidze, A. (2000). Yersinia other than Y. enterocolitica, Y. pseudotuberculosis and Y. pestis: The ignored species. *Microbes and Infection, 2*, 497–513.

Swaminathan, B., & Feng, P. (1994). Rapid detection of foodborne pathogenic bacteria. *Annual Review of Microbiology, 48*, 401–426.

Szabo, R. A., Todd, E. C. D., & Rayman, M. K. (1984). Twenty-four hour isolation and confirmation of *Bacillus cereus* in foods. *Journal of Food Protection, 47*, 856–860.

Tamarapu, S., McKillip, J. L., & Drake, M. (2001). Development of a multiplex Polymerase chain reaction assay for detection and differentiation of *Staphylococcus aureus* in dairy products. *Journal of Food Protection, 64*, 664–668.

Terplan, G. (1988). *Provisional IDF-recommended method: Milk and milk products—detection of Listeria monocytogenes.* Brussels: International Dairy Federation.

Tsen, H.-Y., Chen, M. L., Hsieh, Y. M., et al. (2000). *Bacillus cereus* group strains, their haemolysin BL activity and their detection in foods using a 16S RNA and haemolysin BL gene-targeted multiplex polymerase chain reaction system. *Journal of Food Protection, 63*, 1496–1502.

Tsen, H.-Y., Chen, T. R., & Yu, G.-K. (1994). Detection of B and C types enterotoxigenic *Staphylococcus aureus* using polymerase chain reaction. *Journal of the Chinese Agricultural Chemical Society, 32*, 322–331.

Tsen, H.-Y., & Chen, T. R. (1992). Use of the polymerase chain reaction for specific detection of type A, D and E enterotoxigenic *Staphylococcus aureus* in foods. *Applied Microbiology and Biotechnology, 37*, 685–690.

USDA/FSIS. (2002). Isolation and identification of *Listeria monocytogenes* from red meat, poultry, egg and environmental samples. In: *Microbiology Laboratory Guidebook*, 3rd edn, revision 3, Chapter 8.

Valdivieso-Garcia, A., Surujballi, K. D., Habib, D., et al. (1996). Development and evaluation of a rapid enzyme linked immunofiltration assay (ELIFA) and enzyme linked immunosorbent assay (ELISA) for the detection of staphylococcal enterotoxin B. *Journal of Rapid Methods and Automation in Microbiology, 4*, 285–295.

Varadaraj, M. C., Keshava, N., Nirmala Devi., et al. (1992). Occurrence of *Bacillus cereus* and other Bacillus species in Indian snack and lunch foods and their ability to grow in a rice preparation. *Journal of Food Science & Technology, 29*, 344–347.

Varadaraj, M. C. (1993). Methods for detection and enumeration of foodborne bacterial pathogens: A critical evaluation. *Journal of Food Science & Technology, 30*, 1–13.

Vishnubhatla, A., Fung, D. Y. C., Oberst, R. D., et al. (2000). Rapid 5′ nuclease (TaqMan) assay for detection of virulent strains of *Yersinia enterocolitica*. *Applied and Environmental Microbiology, 66*, 4131–4135.

Vishnubhatla, A., Oberst, R. D., Fung, D. Y. C., et al. (2001). Evaluation of a 5 -nuclease (TaqMan) assay for the detection of virulent strains of *Yersinia enterocolitica* in raw meat and tofu samples. *Journal of Food Protection, 64*, 355–360.

Waak, E., Tham, W., & Danielsson-Tham, M. L. (2002). Prevalence and fingerprinting of *Listeria monocytogenes* strains isolated from raw whole milk in farm and in dairy plant receiving tanks. *Applied and Environmental Microbiology, 68*, 3366–3370.

Wang, R. F., Cao, W. W., & Cerniglia, C. E. (1997). A universal protocol for PCR detection of 13 species of

Food-borne pathogens in foods. *Journal of Applied Microbiology, 83*, 727–736.

Weagant, S. D., Jagow, J. A., Jinneman, K. C., et al. (1999). Development of digoxigenin-labled PCR amplicon probes for use in the detection and identification of enteropathogenic *Yersinia* and shiga toxin-producing *Escherichia coli* from foods. *Journal of Food Protection, 62*, 438–443.

Wesley, I. V., Harmon, K. M., Dickson, J. S., & Schwartz, A. R. (2002). Application of a multiplex polymerase chain reaction assay for the simultaneous confirmation of *Listeria monocytogenes* and other *Listeria* species in turkey sample surveillance. *Journal of Food Protection, 65*, 780–785.

Wilson, G. I., Cooper, J. E., & Gilmour, A. (1991). Detection of enterotoxigenic *Staphylococcus aureus* in dried skimmed milk: Use of the polymerase chain reaction for amplification and detection of staphylococcal enterotoxin genes *entB* and *entC*1 and the thermonuclease gene *nuc*. *Applied and Environmental Microbiology, 57*, 1793–1798.

Wilson, I. G., Gilmour, A., Cooper, J. E., et al. (1994). A non-isotopic DNA hybridization assay for the identification of *Staphylococcus aureus* isolated from foods. *International Journal of Food Microbiology, 22*, 43–54.

Wolcott, M. (1991). DNA-based rapid methods for the detection of foodborne pathogens. *Journal of Food Protection, 54*, 387–401.

Yugueros, J., Temprano, A., Sanchez, M., et al. (2001). Identification of *Staphylococcus* spp by PCR-restriction fragment length polymorphism of *gap* gene. *Journal of Clinical Microbiology, 39*, 3693–3695.

Zeng, H., Zhang, X., Sun, Z., et al. (2006). Multiplex PCR identification of *Listeria monocytogenes* isolates from milk and milk-processing environments. *Journal of the Science of Food and Agriculture, 86*, 367–371.

Zhou, X., & Jiao, X. (2005). Polymerase chain reaction detection of *Listeria monocytogenes* using oligonucleotide primers targeting actA gene. *Food Control, 16*, 125–130.

10

Global Harmonization of the Control of Microbiological Risks

Cynthia M. Stewart[1] and Frank F. Busta[2]

[1]Silliker Food Science Center, South Holland, IL, USA
[2]University of Minnesota, St. Paul, MN, USA

OUTLINE

10.1 INTRODUCTION

Control of microbial risks, in our case related to food, involves procedures to eliminate or minimize the presence of specific groups of microorganisms, their by-products and/or their toxins. To harmonize these control measures it is essential to define the processes and procedures as well as the outcome of the control. Consequently, metrics are required to measure the procedures (e.g. times, temperatures, pressures, chemical concentrations, pH, etc.), and to measure the outcomes (e.g. absence of specific pathogenic bacteria, minimal concentrations of indicator microorganisms, inactivation of specific food enzymes, etc.). On many occasions the specific metric of measurement (e.g. the finding of a specific unacceptable concentration of a particular prohibited microorganism) serves as a motivation to implement one or more effective and appropriate interventions as control programs. Determinations of these metrics require standardization and validation of specific methods and protocols that will be used to verify the outcomes. And whenever more than one group has developed a method, procedure, process, protocol or sampling approach and these groups must reconcile their results, harmonization is an absolute requirement.

During the GHI Workshop in Lisbon, Portugal in November 2007, the Microbiology Working Group discussed topics of interest for the group to develop white papers on food microbiology. The top priority topics were the standardization of microbiological methods and protocols, the definition of the term 'pasteurization' beyond the use for heat treatment processes and dairy products, and the harmonization of global regulations for *Listeria monocytogenes* in ready-to-eat foods. The latter topic was discussed during one of the GHI symposia on global harmonization during EFFoST's First European Food Congress in Ljubljana, Slovenia in November 2008 and a working group was started. This working group was expanded, and, in collaboration with Dr. Ewen Todd (Michigan State University) who had obtained a USDA CSREES grant, held a workshop on this same topic. Following discussions in Ljubljana, a workshop with specialists in this field was organized in Amsterdam, 5–7 May 2009, hosted by Elsevier and EFFoST. The expected outcome of this workshop is a series of papers along with a consensus paper on this topic, to be published in a special edition of *Food Control*. This chapter will focus on discussing the need for harmonization of microbiological methods, criteria and standards.

10.2 MICROBIOLOGICAL FOOD SAFETY MANAGEMENT

Foodborne pathogenic microorganisms and their control has become a major worldwide public health issue. The prevention and/or reduction of foodborne disease has been, and continues to be, a major goal of societies, dating back to when food was first preserved by drying and salting (ICMSF, 2005). Food safety issues are complex and, while the appropriate policy responses are not always clear, the international harmonization of regulation is highly desirable and would facilitate trade. Changes in consumer preferences and social values play a key role in the growing importance of various policy issues. Consumers place a greater emphasis on food safety as incomes and educational levels increase in a country (OECD, 1998). Currently, there is a much greater public concern about (and less tolerance towards) health risks associated with foods than from other manufactured products (cars, tobacco), mainly because of the biological nature of foods and because such risks can impact the whole population (OECD, 1998). The consumers also insist on safety when they are not in complete control of the situation. Pressure for new and stricter enforcement of food safety regulations typically gains momentum with highly publicized incidents of food contamination, such as those that have been associated with bovine spongiform encephalopathy (BSE), *Salmonella*, *Escherichia coli* and *Listeria monocytogenes*.

The importance of different foodborne diseases varies between countries, often depending on the foods consumed, the food processing, preparation, handling and storage methods used and the sensitivity of the population to a particular pathogenic microorganism. While the total elimination of foodborne disease remains an unattainable goal, both government public health managers and the food industry are committed to reducing the number of illnesses due to contaminated food (ICMSF, 2005). The responsibility for selling food that, when used as intended, is not harmful to consumers is that of the various food businesses along the food production and distribution chain. Food safety, while a highly and vigorously discussed subject, is an elusive concept that is frequently a source of much consternation for regulatory authorities and food processors. Assessing the public health (safety) status of a food is a risk-based activity and a conundrum. That is, what is an acceptable level of risk and for whom is that level appropriate? With this as a backdrop consider the following definition of food safety: 'Food safety is the biological, chemical or physical status of a food that will permit its consumption without incurring *excessive risk* of injury, morbidity or mortality' (Keener, 2005). Logically, then, it follows that judging food safety is judging the acceptability of risks, which can be a normative, qualitative, or frequently a political activity (Stewart, Cole, Hoover, & Keener, 2009).

With regard to the food supply, a primary role of national governments is to protect their consumers, with a secondary role of facilitating trade. Over the past several decades, new outcome-based approaches, which are risk and scientific evidence-based, with a focus on food safety outcomes are being implemented by governments and the food industry alike. To communicate the (food safety) risk a country is willing to accept, as well as how it wishes to balance costs (financial costs as well as considerations of culture, eating habits, etc.) with the reduction of illness, the term 'appropriate level of protection' (ALOP) has been used. The ALOP is defined as 'the level of protection deemed appropriate by the Member (country) establishing a sanitary or phytosanitary measure to protect human, animal or plant life or health within its territory' (ICMSF, 2002). While ALOP is defined as the level of risk that a society is willing to accept, many countries have set goals to lower the incidence of foodborne disease and therefore they may propose lower limits for future ALOPs. For example, the current level of listeriosis could be 6 per million people per year and a country may want to reduce this to 3 per million people per year (ICMSF, 2005).

The Sanitary and Phytosanitary (SPS) and Technical Barriers to Trade (TBT) agreements, under the World Trade Organization (WTO), have provided an important momentum towards the use of international food safety standards, while maintaining the sovereign right of governments to provide the level of health protection they deem appropriate (OECD, 1998). The SPS agreement has been signed by more than 100 countries and states that 'whilst a country has the sovereign right to decide on the degree of protection it wishes for its citizens, it must provide, if required, the scientific evidence on which this level of protection rests'. The TBT agreement also requires that a country must not ask for a higher degree of food safety for imported foods than it does for food produced in its own country (ICMSF, 2005). The criteria used by a country to determine whether a food should be considered safe should be clearly conveyed to the exporting country and should be scientifically justifiable (ICMSF, 2001).

While a government expresses public health goals relative to the incidence of disease, this does not provide food processors, producers, handlers, retailers or trade partners with information about what specifically they need to do in order to help achieve these societal goals (ICMSF, 2005). In order for these goals to be met by the food industry, the targets of food safety set by governments need to be translated into parameters that can be used by food processors to manufacture food and parameters that can be assessed by government agencies. Food Safety Objectives (FSOs) are intended to form the link from public health-based goals to suitable control measures and allow for the equivalence of control measures to be determined. Good agricultural practices (GAPs), good manufacturing practices (GMPs), good hygienic practices (GHPs), and Hazard Analysis Critical Control Point (HACCP) remain essential for food safety management systems to achieve FSOs or performance objectives (POs) (ICMSF, 2005).

Keener (1999) has advocated and developed an integrated food safety system that focuses on the collective risk-reducing contributions of the subordinating elements to the manufacturing supply chain in delivering enhanced product safety. This integrated approach to food safety management is also reflected in the requirements of ISO standard 22000–2005 which were issued in September 2005. A more in-depth discussion of how FSOs link governmental public health goals to control measures throughout the food chain can be found in Chapter 4 (A Simplified Guide to Understanding and Using Food Safety Objectives and Performance Objectives).

The cornerstones for modern food safety management were developed in the early 1970s via the concept of Hazard Analysis Critical Control Point (HACCP). HACCP was developed to address the shortcomings and lack of food safety assurance provided by traditional inspection and sampling/microbiological testing of lots (ICMSF, 2005). The goal of HACCP is to focus on the hazards of a particular food commodity that are reasonably likely to impact public health if not controlled, and to design food products, processing, commercialization, preparation and use conditions that control those hazards. To be successful, HACCP needs to be built on practices such as GAPs, GMPs and GHPs, all of which can be viewed as basic sanitary conditions and on practices that must be maintained to produce safe foods, including support activities such as raw material selection, labeling and coding (Stewart, Tompkin, & Cole, 2002). GMPs form the basis on which HACCP programs are based. The production of safe food requires the application of GHPs and the principles of HACCP to develop and implement a total food safety management system that will control the significant hazards in the food that is being produced. An in-depth discussion of GMPs, GHPs, GAPs and HACCP can be found elsewhere.

10.3 MICROBIOLOGICAL CRITERIA

Microbiological limits that include methods and sampling plans are defined as 'microbiological criteria' (ICMSF, 2002). Microbiological criteria (MC) should specify the number of sample units to be collected, the analytical method, and the number of analytical units that should conform to the limits. Additionally, MC should be accompanied by information such as the specific food product, sampling plan, methods of examination and the microbiological limits to be met (ICMSF, 2005). Under certain circumstances, microbiological criteria may be established to determine the acceptability of specific production lots of food, particularly when the conditions of production are not known. The MC are a yardstick upon which a decision is based, and traditionally they have been designed to be used for testing a lot or shipment of food for acceptance or rejection. In contrast, FSOs and POs are maximum levels and do not specify the details needed for testing (ICMSF, 2005). However, MC can be based on POs in certain instances where testing of foods for a specific microorganism can be an effective means for their verification. While there are several approaches that can be used (e.g. lot testing, process control testing), they all compare the results against a predetermined limit. The ICMSF (2002) has provided guidance on the establishment of microbiological criteria.

MC may be established for quality as well as safety concerns (CAC, 1997) and are used in setting standards, guidelines and purchase specifications, which are defined as follows (ICMSF, 2009):

• Microbiological standards are contained in international, federal and regional laws. Relatively few standards exist in the US, with most relating to a specific pathogen, such as *Listeria monocytogenes* in ready-to-eat foods, *Escherichia coli* O157: H7 in ground beef, and

Salmonella and generic *E. coli* in meats relative to USDA's Pathogen Reduction Program. Exceeding a standard relating to a pathogen, such as *Salmonella* or *Listeria*, may lead to a product recall and/or punitive action.

- Microbiological guidelines are internal, advisory criteria established by a processor or by a trade association. Failure to meet them serves as an alert to the processor, indicating that remedial action should be taken. A wide variety of criteria fit into this category, such as results on pre-op swabs from equipment, in-process samples of product or equipment, and environmental samples tested for pathogens.
- Microbiological specifications or purchase specifications are agreements between the vendor and buyer of a product as a basis for sale. These criteria can be looked upon as mandatory since failure of the vendor to meet specifications can be used as a basis for product rejection.

While safe food is produced by adhering to GHP and HACCP programs, the level of safety these food safety systems are expected to deliver has seldom been defined in quantitative terms. The establishment of FSOs and POs (see Chapter 4) provides the industry with quantitative targets (ICMSF, 2009). Although FSOs and POs are expressed in quantitative terms, they are not MC. MC are designed to determine adherence to GHPs and HACCP (i.e. verification) when more effective and efficient means are not available. FSOs and POs are targets to be met; in this context, however, MC based on within-lot testing are meant to provide a statistically designed means for determining whether these targets are being achieved (van Schothorst, Zwietering, Ross, Buchanan, & Cole, 2009). A detailed description on setting MC is given by ICMSF (2009). The uses of MC include (ICMSF, 2009):

- verifying compliance of POs and FSOs (within the limits of sampling and testing);

- validating that a HACCP/GHP system provides the desired level of control;
- verifying control within HACCP/GHP systems;
- demonstrating the utility (suitability) of a food or ingredient for a particular purpose;
- establishing the keeping quality (shelf-life) of certain perishable foods;
- driving industry improvement when used as a regulatory tool;
- achieving market access;
- identifying unacceptable from acceptable product defined by standards, guidelines and specifications not directly related to the above applications.

MC for foods in international trade are addressed in the joint Food and Agriculture Organization/World Health Organization (FAO/WHO) food standards program, as implemented by the Codex Alimentarius Commission (CAC, 1997). This program was the direct result of conflict between national food legislation and the general requirements of the main food markets of the world. It was established in 1962, the same year as the International Commission on Microbiological Specifications for Foods was established. Serious non-tariff obstacles to trade were caused by differing national food legislation (ICMSF, 2002). At that time, the Commission's objectives were to develop international food standards, codes of practice and guidelines, anticipating that their general adoption would help remove and prevent non-tariff barriers to the food trade. The Codex Committee on Food Hygiene (CCFH) has the major responsibility for all provisions on food hygiene practice (effectively, good hygiene practice (GHP)). The CCFH requires expert advice in dealing with highly specialized microbiological matters and especially when developing microbiological criteria. Such advice has frequently been provided by the ICMSF through its publications on sampling plans and principles for the establishment and application of microbiological criteria for foods and several other discussion papers (CAC, 1997; ICMSF, 1998).

Problems with some current MC include application of sampling statistics based on random distribution to situations where contamination is not random; use of too few samples to draw valid conclusions; only meaningful if data indicate non-compliance; negative results have little value; re-sampling of product that failed initial test; many regulatory standards ignore principles of establishment of criteria, e.g. zero-tolerance; and use of indicator tests in the absence of an established relationship of the indicator to the pathogen of interest (Carter, 2008).

10.4 MICROBIOLOGICAL TESTING

Monitoring microbial contamination is a critical procedure to ensure the safety of various products, including foods, pharmaceuticals, cosmetics and healthcare items. Many methods are used in different regions of the world, depending on their local regulations. However, the lack of alignment or 'harmonization' of methods for microbiological testing creates an extra burden for manufacturers who intend to market and sell their products globally. Lack of harmonization also results in frequent conflicts and agitation between regulatory agencies of trading partners.

Microbiological testing can be a useful tool in the management of food safety. However, microbiological tests should be selected and applied with knowledge of their limitations, their benefits, and the purposes for which they are used (ICMSF, 2009). In many instances, other means of assessment of food safety assurance are faster and more effective than microbiological testing. The need for microbiological testing varies along the links of the food chain; therefore, the points in the food chain where sampling and

testing occur should be selected where information about the microbiological status of a food will prove most useful for control purposes. A number of different types of microbiological testing may be utilized by food manufacturers and governmental agencies. One of the most commonly used in relation to microbiological criteria is within-lot testing, which compares the level of a microbiological hazard detected in a food against a pre-specified limit, i.e. an MC (ICMSF, 2002).

ICMSF has written extensively on the principles of controlling microbial hazards in foods, but recognizes that those same principles are applicable to the control of microorganisms that may be associated with spoilage, or that are general indicators of good hygienic and good manufacturing practices (ICMSF, 2009). For example, the combination of pasteurization and refrigeration of milk are effective means for reducing and controlling both pathogenic and spoilage microflora, therefore producing a safe product while extending its shelf life. Good hygienic practices designed to prevent microbial contamination of the product during manufacture and packaging, prevent recontamination of the product with pathogens and spoilage organisms. Microbiological testing of pasteurized milk for pathogens is not justified because the process is effective in reducing the levels well below what can be detected with even a very extensive sampling and testing program (ICMSF, 2009). However, pasteurized milk is routinely tested to determine the Standard Plate Count (SPC)/ml and Coliform Count/ml as indicators of the efficacy of pasteurization and prevention of post-pasteurization contamination. Pasteurized milk is just one example of control measures for microbial hazards that also assure the microbial quality. Further, the microbiological testing to monitor or verify control is indicative of both quality and safety.

It is important to consider the purposes for microbiological tests because typically they are performed to reach a decision or judgment. The purpose determines the type of test (indicator or pathogen), the method (rapidity, accuracy, repeatability, reproducibility, etc.), the sample (line-residue, end-product), the interpretation of the result and action to be taken (rejection of a lot, investigational sampling, readjustment of the process, etc.) (ICMSF, 2009). If the purpose for collecting a sample cannot be defined, then the analysis should not be done. The rationale for testing falls into four general categories: to determine safety; to determine adherence to GHPs and/or GMPs; to determine the utility of a food or ingredient for a particular purpose; and to predict product stability (ICMSF, 2009). Many different aspects of microbiological testing are discussed by the ICMSF (2009).

Some of the basic steps of microbiological testing of food include collecting the samples of the food, preparing homogenates if required, and conducting either a quantitative or qualitative analysis of the subsequent sample preparation. Each of these steps has numerous procedures, depending on the purpose of the microbiological test and the type of food product being analyzed. Quantitative analysis has usually been conducted via colony counts or by the most probable number (MPN) methodology, although other methods are available if concentrations of microorganisms are sufficiently high. In qualitative analysis there is one or more enrichment steps for population amplification, followed by a detection technique and isolation of the target microorganism (confirmation, if required), with evidence of growth and identity measured by various means, such as visual, biochemical, immunological and genetic techniques (ICMSF, 2009). Modern detection technologies include enzyme immunoassay, immunocapture, immunoprecipitation, nucleic acid hybridization, use of DNA/RNA, PCR and other nucleic amplification methodologies, electrochemical techniques, enzymatic amplification, chromatographic separation, and the

list goes on. For quantitative microbial tests the approximate lower limits are (ICMSF, 2009):

- <10–100 cfu/g MPN;
- >10–100 cfu/g viable counts;
- >10^3–10^4 cfu/g DEFT;
- >10^4–10^5 cfu/g ELISA, flow cytometry, quantitative PCR;
- >10^5–10^6 cfu/g direct microscopy, spectrophotometry.

The applications of microbiological testing, both at national and international levels, are quite broad. Microbiological testing is used when: gathering epidemiological data (e.g. during outbreaks, recalls, etc.); conducting baseline studies; conducting international trade; conducting trade association studies, such as surveys of products in the marketplace; conducting retail surveys (by government); conducting comparative assays by a company across different production facilities and production lines; needed as per a customer/supplier relationship (purchase specifications); determining efficacy of a HACCP program (facility/product specific); or determining efficacy of prerequisite programs (GMPs, GHPs; facility/product specific) (ICMSF, 2009). Additionally, microbiological testing plays an essential role in food safety programs such as: conducting a hazard analysis; validating processes; monitoring critical ingredients and high-risk finished products; verifying critical control points; determining potential for post-process contamination; establishing the adequacy and frequency of cleaning and sanitation; detecting difficult areas to clean and sanitize; compliance testing; complying with mandatory regulatory programs; confirming purchase specifications; documenting situations in case of litigation; problem solving, etc. (ICMSF, 2009). Often microbiological data exists but is only being used for acceptance on a given unit of production (e.g. batch, lot, one day's production). Trend analysis of these data can frequently assist in identifying the most likely source of a problem, or pinpointing areas for further investigation. A detailed discussion about the uncertainty of microbiological data, components of sampling plans, requirements for method validation and use of lab proficiency testing as part of a quality program is given in ICMSF (2009).

Many limitations of microbiological testing revolve around sampling, i.e. it is often not practical to test a sufficient number of samples, non-random sampling may cause incorrect conclusions to be drawn and no feasible sampling plan can ensure absence of a pathogen (Carter, 2008). In addition, the results identify outcomes, not causes or controls. Irrespective of the considerations or scenario, specific methods are required for properly assessing and validating the fact that the accepted and established levels of risk, corresponding with safe food, are being achieved. Despite the limitations, microbiological testing is almost always an important component of any integrated program to assure the safety of foods at all levels of government and industry.

10.5 VALIDATION OF MICROBIOLOGICAL METHODS

Two organizations, AOAC and ISO, provide similar, yet different, procedures for the validation and certification of microbiological methods. While these organizations have helped to assist in at least allowing for the acceptance of a test method by regulatory bodies, methods have not yet been harmonized across the organizations (i.e. a method may be accredited by ISO but not by AOAC and vice-versa) thus impeding trade. While these institutions do not harmonize methodology, they do take a step in the right direction in creating procedures for determining if different microbial methods provide equivalent results, especially with regard to limits of detection, minimizing false positive and false negative results and impact of the food matrix on the test results.

10.5.1 Association of Analytical Communities

AOAC has had official observer status in *Codex Alimentarius* since its inception, allowing AOAC the ability to give input on the development of international standards for foods and agriculture; if an AOAC method is available, it will generally be accepted into a Codex standard (AOAC, 2009). As of today, the majority of analytical methods cited in Codex standards are those of AOAC, and many AOAC methods are specifically required in the enforcement of some state, provincial, municipal, and local laws and many federal food standards worldwide (AOAC, 2009). AOAC's 'Official Methods of Analysis' have been defined as 'official' by regulations promulgated for enforcement of the Food, Drug, and Cosmetic Act (21 CFR 2.19), recognized in Title 9 of the USDA-FSIS Code of Federal Regulations, and in some cases by the US Environmental Protection Agency (AOAC, 2009).

In 2002, the AOAC published guidelines on the validation process for qualitative and quantitative food microbiological official methods of analysis (Feldsine, Abeyta, & Andrews, 2002). The guidelines define the steps involved in the method validation process, including the selection of the study director, ruggedness testing, the Methods Comparison or Precollaborative Study that includes inclusivity/exclusivity testing, the Interlaboratory Collaborative Study and the approval process by AOAC (Feldsine *et al.*, 2002). These microbiological guidelines were provided by the Methods Committee on Microbiology and Extraneous Materials as part of an initiative to specify validation criteria for Methods Comparison/Precollaborative Studies and Interlaboratory Studies and to harmonize validation methodology with ISO standard 16140. These guidelines are applicable to the validation of any alternative methods, whether proprietary or non-proprietary, which are submitted to AOAC for OMA status recognition. It is the intent of the guidelines to harmonize the validation procedures with ISO standard 16140, 'Protocol for the Validation of Alternative Methods'. Data produced for an alternative method that satisfies the protocol requirements and acceptance criteria contained in ISO 16140 may be reciprocally recognized and may apply toward validation requirements specified in these guidelines; however, some additional data could be required (Feldsine *et al.*, 2002).

AOAC recommends undergoing single laboratory validation based on a study protocol that is reviewed by the Expert Review Panel (ERP) and the appropriate AOAC methods committee. Single laboratory validation shows how a method performs within one laboratory. A full collaborative study shows how a method performs in many laboratories. The value of single laboratory validation is that it can give a good indication of method performance and provide some measure of its ability to successfully complete a full collaborative study. To ensure the success of the full collaborative study involving 8–10 laboratories, the method protocol is designed using AOAC® Official Methods^SM Program guidelines and is approved by the appropriate AOAC methods committee and General Referee. The ERP also provides review comments. AOAC volunteer methods committees are composed of seven or more experts in the topic area who review recommendations of the General Referee, Study Director, and ERP, and provide overall written reviews of the study. After the study is completed, the Study Director analyzes the data and, based on the results, writes the collaborative study manuscript and submits it for methods committee review. If successfully completed, the study is then submitted to the AOAC Official Methods Board for review and first action approval of the method.

10.5.2 International Organization for Standardization

ISO 16140:2003 'Protocol for the Validation of Alternative Methods' defines the general principle and the technical protocol for the validation of alternative methods in the field of microbiological analysis of food, animal feeding stuffs and environmental and veterinary samples used for the validation of alternative methods. These can be used in particular in the framework of the official control, and the international acceptance of the results obtained by the alternative method (ISO, 2003). It also establishes the general principles of certification of these alternative methods, based on the validation protocol defined in ISO 16140:2003. Where an alternative method is used on a routine basis for internal laboratory use without the requirement to meet (higher) external criteria of quality assurance, a less stringent comparative validation of the alternative method than that set in ISO 16140:2003 may be appropriate. Alternative methods that have not been validated against a reference method in an International or European Standard are acceptable under this standard provided that:

- they have been conducted according to validation protocols approved by a recognized panel of technical reviewers and the results of such studies had been fully accepted by them;
- the technical reviewers were operating under the sponsorship of internationally recognized organizations performing method validations (for example, AFNOR, NordVal, AOAC International, AOAC Research Institute);
- the validations include studies that conform to at least the total sample number and food matrix requirements of this standard (ISO, 2003).

According to ISO 16140:2003, when the alternative method has been compared with an internationally recognized reference method (such as AOAC International) that differs in minor aspects from the reference method in the International or European Standard, and if the protocol is similar to this standard, then the results can be accepted. If the method is substantially different from the reference method in the International or European Standard, an assessment is made to determine if these differences would have a minor or major impact on method performance. An assessment is made regarding supplementary data, if any, required for the resolution of procedural and/or reference method differences (for example, primary enrichment broth). Decisions that reference methods contain major differences shall be substantiated by the organizing laboratory, with documented data. The data required to resolve the perceived differences shall be stipulated.

10.6 HARMONIZATION OF GLOBAL REGULATIONS FOR *LISTERIA MONOCYTOGENES* IN READY-TO-EAT FOODS

An outstanding example of the challenges of harmonization of global regulations is present in efforts to control public health threats from *Listeria monocytogenes*. Measurements of the presence and concentration of *Listeria monocytogenes* play a significant role in the perceived control of this specific microorganism in ready-to-eat (RTE) foods.

Listeria monocytogenes is a bacterium that can contaminate foods and cause a mild noninvasive illness (called listerial gastroenteritis) or a severe, sometimes life-threatening, illness (called invasive listeriosis). Invasive listeriosis is characterized by a high case-fatality rate, ranging from 20 to 30% (FDA, 2008). The main target populations for listeriosis are (FDA, 2009):

- pregnant women/fetus—perinatal and neonatal infections;
- persons immunocompromised by corticosteroids, anticancer drugs, graft suppression therapy, AIDS;
- cancer patients—leukemic patients particularly;

- diabetic, cirrhotic, asthmatic, and ulcerative colitis patients—less frequently reported;
- the elderly;
- normal people—some reports suggest that normal, healthy people are at risk, although antacids or cimetidine may predispose. A listerosis outbreak in Switzerland involving cheese suggested that healthy uncompromised individuals could develop the disease, particularly if the foodstuff was heavily contaminated with the organism.

The manifestations of listeriosis include septicemia, meningitis (or meningoencephalitis), encephalitis, and intrauterine or cervical infections in pregnant women, which may result in spontaneous abortion (2nd/3rd trimester) or stillbirth. The onset of the aforementioned disorders is usually preceded by influenza-like symptoms including persistent fever (FDA, 2009). It was reported that gastrointestinal symptoms such as nausea, vomiting, and diarrhea may precede more serious forms of listeriosis or may be the only symptoms expressed. The onset time to serious forms of listeriosis is unknown but may range from a few days to 3 weeks. The onset time to gastrointestinal symptoms is unknown but is probably greater than 12 hours. The infective dose of *L. monocytogenes* is unknown but is believed to vary with the strain and susceptibility of the victim. From cases contracted through raw or supposedly pasteurized milk, it can be assumed that in susceptible persons, fewer than 1000 total microorganisms may cause disease (FDA, 2009).

L. monocytogenes is widespread in the environment. It is found in soil, water, sewage, and decaying vegetation. It can be readily isolated from humans, domestic animals, raw agricultural commodities, and food processing environments (particularly cool damp areas; FDA, 2008). Control of *L. monocytogenes* in the food processing environment has been the subject of a number of scientific publications (FDA, 2008).

L. monocytogenes can grow slowly at refrigeration temperatures; therefore, refrigerated RTE foods that can support the growth of *L. monocytogenes* must be managed appropriately.

Most cases of human listeriosis occur sporadically; however, much of what is known about the epidemiology of the disease has been derived from outbreak-associated cases. With rare exceptions, foods that have been reported to be associated with outbreaks or sporadic cases of listeriosis have been foods that can support the growth of *L. monocytogenes* and that are ready-to-eat (including coleslaw, fresh soft cheese made with unpasteurized milk, frankfurters, deli meats, and butter); and are often associated with a failure during the production or processing of food (FDA, 2008). Data from a variety of sources of information show that *L. monocytogenes* has been detected to varying degrees in unpasteurized and pasteurized milk, high-fat dairy products, soft unripened cheese (cottage cheese, cream cheese, ricotta), cooked ready-to-eat crustaceans, smoked seafood, fresh soft cheese (queso fresco), semi-soft cheese (blue, brick, monterrey), soft-ripened cheese (brie, camembert, feta), deli-type salads, sandwiches, fresh-cut fruits and vegetables, and raw molluscan shellfish (FDA, 2008). However, these data also show that most RTE foods do not contain detectable numbers of *L. monocytogenes*. For many RTE foods, contamination of foods with *L. monocytogenes* can be avoided—for example, through the application of current good manufacturing practices that establish controls on ingredients, listericidal and listeristatic processes, segregation of foods that have been cooked from those that have not, and sanitation controls with effective environmental monitoring programs (FDA, 2008).

The rate of listeriosis is about the same in developed countries, independent of the policies that those countries have in place. For example, in the US there are an estimated 3.4–4.4 cases/million people, with a 20–30% mortality rate; in Australia the rate is 3 cases/million, with a 23% mortality rate; in New Zealand a rate of 5 cases/million, 17% mortality rate, and in the EU a rate of 0.3–7.5 cases/million is estimated (Todd, 2006). In 2000, the USDA Economic Research Service estimated a cost of US$2.3 billion/year for 2298 cases (ERS, 2000).

There have been three risk assessments completed for *L. monocytogenes* in RTE foods, all of which are excellent sources of information for determining a scientifically based MC for this microorganism. In 2003, the US FDA published the 'Quantitative Assessment of the Relative Risk to Public Health from Foodborne *Listeria monocytogenes* Among Selected Categories of Ready-to-Eat Foods' (HHS/USDA, 2003) and the USDA Food Safety and Inspection Service published 'Risk Assessment of *Listeria monocytogenes* in Deli Meat' (FSIS, 2003) in the same year. The following year, the FAO and WHO published a risk assessment titled 'Risk Assessment of *Listeria monocytogenes* in Ready-to-Eat Foods' (FAO/WHO, 2004).

Some of the conclusions from the USDA FSIS risk assessment for deli meats included that increased frequency of food contact surface testing and sanitation is estimated to lead to a proportionally lower risk of listeriosis; that combinations of interventions (i.e. microbiological testing and sanitation of food contact surfaces, pre- and post-packaging treatments and the use of growth inhibitors/product reformulation) appear to be more effective than any single intervention step (Todd, 2006). For example, the estimated number of deaths annually due to listeriosis could drop from 250 to <100 if industry used a combination of growth inhibitors and post-packaging pasteurization of products. Based on some of the information and scenarios from this risk assessment, the USDA FSIS, under an interim final rule released on 6 June 2003 (FSIS, 2004) afforded RTE products a different regulatory treatment. The products had to be produced using one of three alternative control programs to reduce or eliminate *L. monocytogenes*, or suppress or limit its growth.

These three programs recognize the variety of means that may be used:

- post-lethality treatment that reduces or eliminates *L. monocytogenes* and an antimicrobial agent or process that suppresses or limits its growth throughout shelf life (Alternative 1);
- post-lethality treatment that reduces or eliminates *L. monocytogenes* OR an antimicrobial agent or process that suppresses or limits its growth throughout shelf life (Alternative 2);
- sanitation procedures only to prevent *L. monocytogenes* contamination (Alternative 3; manufacturing plant using Alternative 3 will get the most frequent verification testing attention from the government regulators).

Under Alternative 1 or Alternative 2 by post-lethality treatment, FSIS would apply relatively less sampling to a product undergoing a post-lethality treatment giving $\geq$2-$\log_{10}$ reduction of *L. monocytogenes*, relatively more sampling to a product receiving a post-lethality treatment giving between 1- and 2-$\log_{10}$ reduction and would consider <1-$\log_{10}$ reduction not eligible for these two Alternatives, unless there is supporting documentation that the treatment provides an adequate safety margin (FSIS, 2004).

The HHS/USDA risk assessment (2003) estimated that those foods posing the highest risk of being associated with listeriosis support the growth of *L. monocytogenes*. In contrast, the foods that the risk assessment estimated to pose the lowest risk of being associated with listeriosis are foods that have intrinsic or extrinsic factors to prevent the growth of *L. monocytogenes*, or that are processed to alter the normal characteristics of the food (FDA, 2008). For example, it is well established that *L. monocytogenes* does not grow when: (i) the pH of the food is less than or equal to 4.4; (ii) the water activity of the food is less than or equal to 0.92; or (iii) the food is frozen.

Currently there is no international agreement on what numbers of *L. monocytogenes* in foods are acceptable to protect the consumer. In several countries, different criteria or recommendations for tolerable levels of *L. monocytogenes* in RTE foods have been established, but the rationale is not always clear (Todd, 2006). In the US, a major outbreak of listeriosis occurred in 1985, when a Mexican-style soft cheese caused over 142 cases of illness with 48 fatalities. In the same year, a survey conducted by the FDA found *L. monocytogenes* in both imported and domestic fresh cheeses. It was recognized that *L. monocytogenes* had caused foodborne diseases from food products regulated by the FDA and USDA, or had the potential to do so (Todd, 2006). Therefore, the FDA established a policy of 'zero tolerance' for *L. monocytogenes* in RTE foods, the microbiological criteria being absent in 25 g (<0.04 cfu/g).

The EU has different microbiological criteria for *L. monocytogenes* in RTE foods, based on the category of food—whether it can or does not support the growth of the microorganism and whether the food is intended for the general population or for use for special medical purposes. The EU also describes the stage where the criterion applies; either for products placed on the market and during their shelf-life or before the food has left the immediate control of the food business operator who has produced it (Table 10.1; Food Safety Authority of Ireland, 2007).

In Canada, RTE foods have been placed into three categories, based upon health risk. In the establishment of the Category 1 food list, considerations were given to RTE foods that have been causally linked to documented outbreaks of listeriosis and/or have been placed in the 'high risk' category in the HHS/USDA risk assessment (Health Canada, 2004). Products in Category 1 should receive the highest priority for inspection and compliance activities. Category 2 contains all other RTE foods which are capable of supporting growth of *L. monocytogenes* and have a shelf-life exceeding 10 days. The presence of *L. monocytogenes* in these products will

TABLE 10.1 European Union microbiological criteria for *Listeria monocytogenes* in ready-to-eat foods (Food Safety Authority of Ireland, 2007)

Food category	Sampling plan	Limit	Analytical Reference Method	Stage where the criterion applies
RTE foods intended for infants and RTE foods for special medical purposes	$n = 10$ $c = 0$	Absence in 25 g	EN/ISO 11290-1	Products placed on the market during their shelf life
RTE foods able to support the growth of *L. monocytogenes* other than those intended for infants and for special medical purposes	$n = 5$ $c = 0$ $n = 5$ $c = 0$	100 cfu/g Absence in 25 g	EN/ISO 11290-2 EN/ISO 11290-1	Products placed on the market during their shelf life Before the food has left the immediate control of the FBO* who has produced it
RTE foods unable to support the growth of *L. monocytogenes* other than those intended for infants and for special medical purposes	$n = 5$ $c = 0$	100 cfu/g	EN/ISO 11290-2	Products placed on the market during their shelf life

*Food business operator, n = number of units comprising the sample, c = number of sample units giving values over the limit.

trigger a Health 2 concern, with possible consideration of a public alert. These products receive the second highest priority in inspection and compliance activity. Category 3 contains two types of RTE food products; those supporting growth with a ≤10 day shelf-life and those not supporting growth. These products receive the lowest priority in terms of inspection and compliance action. For Category 3 RTE foods, factors such as adherence to Good Manufacturing Practices (GMPs), levels of *L. monocytogenes* in the food (action level 100 cfu/g), and/or a health risk assessment, should all be considered in determining the compliance action taken.

In the US, in 2003, fifteen trade associations submitted a petition to the FDA to amend the regulatory limit to 100 cfu/g of *L. monocytogenes* in foods that do not support the growth of this microorganism. The limit would establish a science-based standard for the presence of *L. monocytogenes* in such foods, based on new and emerging evidence that consumer protection is a function of the microorganism's level in

food, and not its mere presence; and that low levels of *L. monocytogenes* are not uncommon in the food supply and that such low levels are regularly consumed without apparent harm. In response, the FDA (2008) issued two draft documents: 'Draft Guidance for Industry: Control of *L. monocytogenes* in Refrigerated or Frozen RTE Foods' and 'Draft Compliance Policy Guideline'. The guidance document divides foods into two categories: foods that support the growth of *L. monocytogenes* are to be placed in the high-risk category, and the MC would remain at absence in 25 g (<0.04 cfu/g); and foods that do not support the growth of *L. monocytogenes* are to be placed in the low-risk category, and the MC for these foods would be <100 cfu/g. If the food contains *L. monocytogenes* at levels higher than those mentioned above, per category, the food would be considered adulterated. The MC in these draft guidelines are in alignment closer to those of the EU and Canada. The enforcement policy in the draft guidance clarifies which foods support the growth of

L. monocytogenes; this will help ensure that FDA resources are focused on these high-risk foods. FDA anticipates that it may be able to increase the number of samples that it periodically collects and tests for *L. monocytogenes* to verify compliance with the limit for this microorganism in low-risk RTE foods, while it continues to focus its inspection and outreach efforts on facilities manufacturing high-risk RTE foods. There was a 60-day comment period and, at the time of writing, no further updates were available.

Harmonization of food regulations can only be done through agreement between governments, and the Codex Alimentarius Commission is one logical international body of member countries that may allow this to be achieved. Discussions have already taken place and continue with many sub-groups and commissioned studies, including the FAO/WHO assessments. It is hoped that science-based criteria may be agreed upon. For example, that 100 cfu/g of *L. monocytogenes* at the point of consumption presents little risk to the healthy population. How governments ask the food industry to achieve this can differ. For example, some foods have industry interventions, such as added organic acid or in-package pasteurization (i.e. for sliced deli meats), but this approach will not work for all products (i.e. cheese and some fruits and vegetables) (Todd, 2006). The acceptable level of risk has a cultural component. For example, certain foods, such as raw-milk cheeses, are culturally important in European countries. A 'zero-tolerance' regulation may not be effective in reducing the number of cases of listeriosis per year. Consumer education and labeling have had some limited success (i.e. education of risk to pregnant women), but they do influence some people, and research into risk communication should continue (Todd, 2006). There are certain sub-populations of people who are at a higher risk of contracting listeriosis; for example, patients undergoing cancer therapy, AIDS patients and transplant patients. Therefore, a

different strategy/standard may be required. Some possible strategies are being considered for these populations. For example, the EU is considering more stringent policies, but most policies are likely to be internal ones developed and implemented by institutions housing these populations, rather than governments imposing national standards for *L. monocytogenes* in food served to these sub-populations (Todd, 2006).

10.7 CONCLUSION

Processes and procedures to eliminate or minimize the presence of specific groups of microorganisms or their by-products or toxins must be harmonized. Metrics required to measure the procedures and outcomes must be synchronized. Implementation of one or more effective and appropriate interventions as control programs requires standardization and validation of specific methods and protocols that will be used to verify the outcomes. Our goal must be that the plethora of methods, procedures, processes, protocols and sampling approaches reconcile their results and achieve useful harmonization.

References

AOAC. (2009). *About AOAC,* Association of Analytical Communities. http://www.aoac.org/about/aoac.htm (accessed 23 March 2009).

CAC. (1997). Codex Alimentarius Commission. Recommended international code of practice for the general principles of food hygiene. CAC/RCP 1-1969, Rev. 3.

Carter, M. (2008). The steps before PCR: Sampling and enrichment, concentration procedures, compositing, true real time PCR without enrichment. Presented during the Colorado State University Workshop on Molecular Methods in Food Microbiology, CPU Department of Animal Science, 24 June.

ERS. (2000). Economic Research Service USDA. ERS updates foodborne illness costs: Food safety v.23, i.3, USDA Sep/Dec00. http://www.mindfully.org/Food/Foodborne-Illness-Costs-USDA.htm (accessed 23 March 2009).

FAO/WHO. (2004). World Health Organization Food and Agriculture Organization and of the United Nations. Risk assessment of *Listeria monocytogenes* in ready-to-eat foods. http://www.fao.org/docrep/010/y5394e/y5394e00.htm (accessed 23 March 2009).

FDA. (2008). Food and Drug Administration, Center for Food Safety and Applied Nutrition. Guidance for industry: Control of *Listeria monocytogenes* in refrigerated or frozen ready-to-eat foods Draft Guidance. http://www.cfsan.fda.gov/~dms/lmrtegui.html (accessed 23 March 2009).

FDA. (2009). Food and Drug Administration. Foodborne pathogenic microorganisms and natural toxins handbook *Listeria monocytogenes*. http://www.foodsafety.gov/~mow/chap6.html (accessed 23 March, 2009).

Feldsine, P., Abeyta, C., & Andrews, W. H. (2002). AOAC International methods committee guidelines for validation of qualitative and quantitative food microbiological official methods of analysis. *Journal of AOAC International, 85*, 1187–1200.

Food Safety Authority of Ireland. (2007). *Listeria monocytogenes*. http://www.fsai.ie/publications/factsheet/factsheet_listeria_monocytogenes%20.pdf (accessed 23 March 2009).

FSIS. (2003). Food Safety and Inspection Service. Risk Assessment for *Listeria monocytogenes* in deli meat. http://www.fsis.usda.gov/PDF/Lm_Deli_Risk_Assess_Final_2003.pdf (accessed 23 March 2009).

FSIS. (2004). Food Safety and Inspection Service. Compliance guidelines to control *Listeria monocytogenes* in post-lethality exposed ready-to-eat meat and poultry products. http://www.fsis.usda.gov/OPPDE/rdad/FRPubs/97-013F/Lm_Rule_Compliance_Guidelines_2004.pdf (accessed 20 April 2005). – Note updated May 2006 http://www.fsis.usda.gov/oppde/rdad/FRPubs/97-013F/LM_Rule_Compliance_Guidelines_May_2006.pdf (accessed 20 March 2009).

Health Canada. (2004). Policy on *Listeria monocytogenes* in ready-to-eat foods. http://www.hc-sc.gc.ca/fn-an/legislation/pol/policy_listeria_monocytogenes_politique_toc-eng.php (accessed 23 March 2009).

HHS/USDA. (2003). HHS Food and Drug Administration and USDA Food Safety and Inspection Service. Quantitative assessment of the relative risk to public health from foodborne *Listeria monocytogenes* among selected categories of ready-to-eat foods. Available in Docket No. 1999N-1168, Vols 23–28 or http://www.foodsafety.gov/~dms/Lmr2-toc.html (accessed 23 March 2009).

ICMSF. (1998). International Commission on Microbiological Specifications for Foods. Microbial ecology of food commodities. In: *Microorganisms in foods*. London: Blackie Academic and Professional. ICMSF.

ICMSF. (2001). International Commission on Microbiological Specifications for Foods. The role of Food Safety Objective in the management of microbiological safety of food according to Codex documents. Document prepared for the Codex Committee on Food Hygiene. March 2001.

ICMSF. (2002). International Commission on Microbiological Specifications for Foods. *Microorganisms in foods, 7. Microbiological testing in food safety management*. New York: Kluwer Academic/Plenum Publishers.

ICMSF. (2005). International Commission on Microbiological Specifications for Foods. A simplified guide to understanding and using Food Safety Objectives and Performance Objectives. http://www.icmsf.iit.edu/main/articles_papers.html (accessed 23 March 2009).

ICMSF. (2009). International Commission on Microbiological Specifications for Foods. *Microorganisms in foods, 8. Use of data for assessing process control and product acceptance*. New York: Springer in press.

ISO. (2003). International Organization for Standardization. ISO 16140:2003 Microbiology of food and animal feeding stuffs—Protocol for the validation of alternative methods. http://www.iso.org/iso/iso_catalogue/catalogue_tc/catalogue_detail.htm?csnumber=30158. (accessed 23 March 2009).

Keener, L. (1999). Is HACCP Enough for ensuring food safety; *Food Testing and Analysis 5(9)*, 17–19.

Keener, L. (2005). Maximizing food safety return on investment. FI Food Safety and Innovation Seminar. Paris, France.

OECD. (1998). Organisation for economic co-operation and development. Regulatory reform in the global economy: Asian and Latin American perspectives. OECD Publishing.

Stewart, C.M., Cole, M.B., Hoover, D.G., & Keener, L. (2009). New tools for microbiological risk assessment, risk management and process validation methodology. In *Non-thermal Processing Technologies for Food*, in press.

Stewart, C. M., Tompkin, R. B., & Cole, M. B. (2002). Food safety: New concepts for the new millennium. *Innovation of Food Science Emerging Technology, 3*, 105–112.

Todd, E. (2006). Harmonizing international regulations for *Listeria monocytogenes* in ready-to-eat foods: Use of risk assessments for helping make science-based decisions. http://www.fsis.usda.gov/PDF/Slides_092806_ETodd3.pdf (accessed 20 March 2009).

van Schothorst, R., Zwietering, M. H., Ross, T., Buchanen, & Cole (2009). Relating microbiological criteria to food safety objectives and performance objectives. *Food Control, 20(11)*, 967–979.

Towards Intended Normal Use (Part I): A European Appraisal of the Chloramphenicol Case and some Thoughts on the Potential of Global Harmonization of Antibiotics Regulation

Jaap C. Hanekamp[1] and Jan H.J.M. Kwakman[2]

[1]Roosevelt Academy, Middelburg, The Netherlands; HAN-Research, Zoetermeer, The Netherlands
[2]President-Seafood Importers and Processors Alliance

11.1 INTRODUCTION

Food safety as a whole is usually defined as chemical food safety, meaning that food from whatever source is regarded as safe when man-made chemicals such as antibiotics and pesticides are absent or only present at very low concentrations. In this chapter, antibiotics as a tool in animal rearing are discussed from the perspective of the consumer end product. As antibiotics create benefits for the producers, the risks to consumers that similarly benefit from antibiotics use in terms of food abundance and concomitant lower prices, need to be balanced effectively.

We will thus focus on the topics of chemical food safety, relevant policies, and the benefits and risks when dealing with global food safety and food security. As introductory statements to this book report: 'Today's reality is that there are differences between countries that too often lead to severe measures such as the destruction of huge quantities of food to protect consumers, lacking any scientific justification, while a large part of the human population suffers from undernourishment.'

We cannot find a better illustration of this theme, including all the public, political, and moral issues, than the chloramphenicol (henceforth CAP) case, which rose to prominence in 2001 in Europe. This historic case will be our focus from which we distill three aspects. Firstly, we will review this specific CAP case and will highlight the regulatory background thereof. Secondly, we will provide context as to the reasons of the regulatory response. Lastly, we will propose a harmonized approach in terms of Intended Normal Use (INU) for regulating the use of antibiotics in the production of food.

11.2 THE 'NATURE' OF ANTIBIOTICS

With the discovery of penicillin in 1928 by Alexander Fleming, the potential to tackle bacterial infections in both humans and animals grew immeasurably. Penicillin is made by a fungus (*Penicillium notatum*), yet most antibiotics we now know today are derived from actinomycetes, nature's topmost antibiotic producers. Not only do they produce antibiotics in a huge variety, they also produce chemicals that kill fungi, parasitic worms and even insects

(Hopwood, 2007). Many other pharmaceuticals, such as anti-tumor agents and immunosuppressants, are also derived from the actinomycetes (Walsh, 2003). The antibiotics industry is valued at roughly $25 billion per year.

The streptomycetes, belonging to the actinomycetes, account for well over two-thirds of these commercially and therapeutically significant antibiotics, which are produced by means of complex 'secondary metabolic' pathways (Bibb, 2005). Streptomycetes therefore are the most important source of antibiotics for medical, veterinary and agricultural use. Streptomycetes are a group of gram-positive filamentous bacteria, ubiquitous in soil, and found worldwide. They are among the most numerous and ubiquitous soil bacteria adapted to the utilization of plant remains and are key in this environment because of their broad potential of metabolic processes and biotransformations. These include degradation of the insoluble remains of other organisms, making streptomycetes imperative organisms in carbon recycling (Bentley *et al.*, 2002). Streptomycetes are members of the same taxonomic order as the causative agents of tuberculosis and leprosy (*Mycobacterium tuberculosis* and *M. leprae*).

While secondary metabolites must in all likelihood confer an adaptive advantage, the roles of most are not fully understood. This is true even for antibiotics. Antibiotics give a competitive advantage compared to other ground-dwelling microorganisms that need to tap into the same biomass as nutrition (Shi & Zusman, 1993). An ensnarement strategy was observed as well, where competing organisms are attracted and subsequently killed by excreted antibiotics and then consumed supplying additional nutrition (Chater, 2006). Streptomycin was the first antibiotic discovered to be effective against tuberculosis (TB). Chloramphenicol (Ehrlich, Bartz, Smith, & Joslyn, 1947) was the first antibiotic to be synthetically produced and was shown to be effective against typhoid (Patel & Banker, 1949).

11.3 CHLORAMPHENICOL— HISTORY, LAW AND SCIENCE (HANEKAMP, FRAPPORTI, & OLIEMAN, 2003)

Internationally traded seafood is delimited by numerous food-safety regulations. Setting scientific and policy standards that benchmark the benefits and risks of foods is of great consequence for industry, policymakers and consumers. In Europe, the core regulatory framework in food law is Regulation 178/2002/EC (2002).[1] According to this Regulation, 'food' (or 'foodstuff') denotes 'any substance or product, whether processed, partially processed or unprocessed, intended to be, or reasonably expected to be ingested by humans.'

The scope of Regulation 178/2002/EC concerns 'all stages of the production, processing and distribution of food …' and its general objective is to provide 'a high level of protection of human life and health and the protection of consumers' interests …' This Regulation thus sets general rules for all products that are brought to market. Importantly, the Regulation also constitutes the European Food Safety Authority (EFSA) and defines the Authority's task and fields of competence and authority. With the installation of the EFSA, 'precaution' is specifically referred to as a key principle in food regulation. Especially in relation to antibiotics used in animal rearing, regulation is pervasive and precautionary. This is partly related to the need to reduce the chronic exposure through food as much as possible, but is also due in part to precautionary risk averseness. Both of these aspects are well-illustrated by the CAP case. Article 7 thereof describes the precautionary principle as follows:

1. In specific circumstances where, following an assessment of available information, the possibility of harmful effects on health is identified but scientific uncertainty persists, provisional risk management measures necessary to ensure the high level of health protection chosen in the Community may be adopted, pending further scientific information for a more comprehensive risk assessment.

2. Measures adopted on the basis of paragraph 1 shall be proportionate and no more restrictive of trade than is required to achieve the high level of health protection chosen in the Community, regard being had to technical and economic feasibility and other factors regarded as legitimate in the matter under consideration. The measures shall be reviewed within a reasonable period of time, depending on the nature of the risk to life or health identified and the type of scientific information needed to clarify the scientific uncertainty and to conduct a more comprehensive risk assessment.'

In 2001, the detection of CAP, a broad-spectrum antibiotic, in shrimp imported into Europe from Asian countries was branded as yet another food scandal. The initial European response was to close European borders to fish products, mainly shrimp, from these countries and make laboratories work overtime to analyze numerous batches of imported goods for the presence of this antibiotic. Some European countries went so far as to have food products containing the antibiotic destroyed as public health was deemed to be at stake. This regulatory response spilled over to other major seafood-importing countries such as the United States.

The legislative background to this mainly European response is found in Council Regulation

---

[1]Regulation (EC) No 178/2002 of the European Parliament and of the Council of 28 January 2002 laying down the general principles and requirements of food law, establishing the European Food Safety Authority and laying down procedures in matters of food safety. *Official Journal of the European Communities* L31, pp. 1–24.

EEC No 2377/90 (1990)[2] (now superseded by Regulation EC No 470/2009 as of the 6th of May 2009; we will comment on below), which was implemented to establish maximum residue limits of veterinary medicinal products in foodstuffs of animal origin. This so-called 'maximum residue limit (MRL) Regulation' introduced Community procedures to evaluate the safety of residues of pharmacologically active substances according to human food safety requirements. A pharmacologically active substance may be used in food-producing animals, but only if it receives a favorable evaluation. If it is considered necessary for the protection of human health, MRLs are established. They are the points of reference for setting withdrawal periods in marketing authorizations as well as for the control of residues in the Member States and at border inspection posts.

Directive 96/23/EC (the Residue Control Directive)[3] contains specific requirements, in particular for the control of pharmacologically active substances that may be used as veterinary medicinal products in food-producing animals. This includes primarily sampling and investigation procedures, requirements as to the documentation for their use, indication for sanctions in case of non-compliance, requirements for targeted investigations and for the setting up and reporting of monitoring programs. Additionally, there is the Minimum Required Performance Limit (MRPL) Regulation L221 (2002).[4] MRPL

is no more and no less than the concentration level that regulatory (reference) laboratories in the European Union should at least be able to detect and confirm. EU regulatory laboratories are obliged to try and find residues of banned substances, like CAP, at the lowest technically attainable concentration.

EEC No 2377/90 contains an Annex IV listing of pharmacologically active substances for which no maximum toxicological levels (Tolerable Daily Intake, TDI; also known as Acceptable Daily Intake, ADI) can be fixed, either from lack of toxicological or pharmacological data, e.g. the absence of a definable NOAEL (No Observed Adverse Effect Level) or LOAEL (Lowest Observed Adverse Effect Level), or because of genotoxic characteristics of the compound in question.[5] These substances are consequently not allowed in the animal food production chain. So-called 'zero-tolerance' levels are in force for Annex IV for reasons that can be subsumed as follows:

• Lack of scientific data *de facto* makes the establishment of a TDI not feasible;
• The absence of a TDI and the subsequent impossibility to establish an MRL, in regulatory terms is understood as 'dangerous at any dose' requiring zero-tolerance regulation;
• With the introduction of zero-tolerance, a veterinary ban on Annex IV compounds (such as CAP) is in place, whereby the listed

[2]Council Regulation (EEC) No 2377/90 of 26 June 1990 laying down a Community procedure to set up maximum residue limits of veterinary medicinal products in foodstuffs of animal origin. *Official Journal of the European Communities* L224, pp. 1–8. Regulation (EC) No. 470/2009 of the European Parliament and of the Council of 6 May 2009 laying down Community procedures for the establishment of residue limits of pharmacologically active substances in foodstuffs of animal origin, repealing Council Regulation (EEC) No. 2377/90 and amending Directive 2001/82/EC of the European Parliament and of the Council and Regulation (EC) No. 726/2004 of the European Parliament and of the Council. *Official Journal of the European Communities* L152, pp. 11–22.
[3]Council Directive 96/23/EC of 29 April 1996 on measures to monitor certain substances and residues thereof in live animals and animal products and repealing Directives 85/358/EEC and 86/469/EEC and Decisions 89/187/EEC and 91/664/EEC. *Official Journal of the European Communities* L125, pp. 10–32.
[4]Commission decision of 12 August 2002 implementing Council Directive 96/23/EC concerning the performance of analytical methods and the interpretation of results. *Official Journal of the European Communities* L221, pp. 8–36.
[5]Genotoxic agents (chemicals, ionizing radiation) are those capable of causing damage to DNA. Such damage can potentially lead to the formation of a malignant tumor.

compounds, when producers compliance is achieved, would disappear from the food chain;

- When zero-tolerance was implemented, analytical equipment was only capable to detect at the Limit of Detection (LOD) of ppm (parts per million; mg per kg); nowadays LODs are at least ppb (parts per billion; μg per kg), obviously depending on analyzed chemicals.

No TDI could be established for CAP due to the lack of scientific information to assess its carcinogenicity and effects on reproduction, and because the compound showed some genotoxic activity (IPCS-INCHEM).[6] Overall, CAP—and other Annex IV substances—should not be detected in food products at all, regardless of concentrations. The presence of CAP in food products,[7] which can be detected by any type of analytical apparatus, is a violation of European law and moreover deemed to be a threat to public health. In consequence, food containing the smallest amount of these residues is considered unfit for human consumption. For all intents and purposes, zero-tolerance is best understood as zero concentration, a molecular prohibition. Only when Annex IV substances are completely absent from food are the risks deemed completely absent. The presence of CAP in food products is solely related to illicit veterinary use; other sources are not taken into account, or indeed considered, as they are not included in the legislation. Chloroform, chlorpromazine, colchicine, dapsone, dimetridazole, metronidazole, nitrofurans (including furazolidone) and ronidazole are the other compounds in Annex IV.

11.4 TOXICOLOGY—POTENTIAL RISKS OF CAP EXPOSURE THROUGH FOOD

Despite a ban in animal food production, CAP is still used as human medication. It has a wide spectrum of activity against gram-positive and gram-negative bacteria. CAP therapy is usually restricted to serious infections when other drugs are not as effective. Internal infections are only rarely treated with CAP. Ophthalmic infections, however, are still treated with CAP. A number of registered pharmaceutical products containing CAP that are used to treat eye infections are on the market in the Western World. In Asian countries, it is still widely used against, for example, typhoid.

Aplastic anemia, a form of anemia when the bone marrow ceases to produce sufficient red and white blood cells, is the most dangerous effect produced by CAP. Its occurrence is extremely rare, albeit fatal and is only observed as a result of therapeutic treatment with CAP (Benestad, 1979). The minimum dose of CAP associated with the development of aplastic anemia is not known. The total aplastic anemia incidence estimated by the JECFA (Joint FAO/WHO Expert Committee on Food Additives) is about 1.5 cases per million people per year (IPCS-INCHEM).[8] Only about 15% of the total number of cases was associated with drug treatment and, among these, CAP was not a major contributor. These data roughly gave an overall incidence of therapeutic CAP-associated aplastic anemia in humans of less than one case per 10 million per year. In considering epidemiological data derived from the ophthalmic

---

[6]IPCS-INCHEM (Chemical Safety Information from Intergovernmental Organizations). See webpage http://www.inchem.org/documents/jecfa/jecmono/v23je02.htm (accessed 3 February 2009).

[7]Instituto Technológico Agroalimentario (Agri-food Technology Institute: AINIA), 2003. *Presence of chloramphenicol in foods.* (This report can be obtained through the authors.)

[8]IPCS-INCHEM (Chemical Safety Information from Intergovernmental Organizations). See webpage http://www.inchem.org/documents/jecfa/jecmono/v33je03.htm (accessed 3 February 2009).

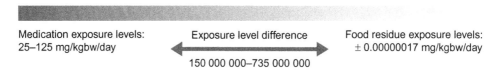

FIGURE 11.1 Exposure level—differences between medication and food.

use of CAP, systemic exposure to this form of treatment was not associated with the induction of aplastic anemia. Because of the limited data available, however, it is unfeasible to determine a genuine dose–response correlation for the occurrence of aplastic anemia (IPCS-INCHEM).

Then again, when considering the difference between therapeutic exposure, where aplastic anemia has been observed (albeit rarely), and food residues, where aplastic anemia has never been observed, it seems clear that CAP is unlikely to present a substantial hazard assuming a linear dose–response correlation (see below), if at all. The food residue exposure levels shown in Figure 11.1 are taken from the RIVM study (Rijksinstituut voor Volksgezondheid en Milieu; Dutch National Institute for Public Health and the Environment) on CAP in shrimp. These indicate that low-level exposure to CAP, either as a result of ophthalmic use or of residues in animal food, is not related to aplastic anemia (Janssen, Baars, & Pieters 2001).[9]

Limited evidence exists for the genotoxic carcinogenicity of CAP in humans exposed to therapeutic doses (Doody *et al.*, 1996). CAP is categorized by the IARC (International Agency for Research on Cancer)[10] as probably carcinogenic in humans; group 2A. However, the available data on the genotoxicity of CAP show mainly negative results in bacterial systems and

mixed results in mammalian systems. It was concluded that CAP must be considered genotoxic, but only at concentrations about 25 times higher than those occurring in patients treated with the highest therapeutic dose (Martelli *et al.*, 1991). Moreover, no adequate studies are available to evaluate the carcinogenicity of CAP in animals used for experimentation.

The RIVM, in their above-mentioned study, estimated the cancer risk as a result of the consumption of shrimp containing CAP. The concentrations in imported shrimp varied roughly between 1 and 10 ppb (parts per billion; 1 and 10 µg/kg product). The estimated 'reasonable worst-case risk' as a result of eating shrimp containing CAP is lower than the maximum tolerable risk (MTR) level (being an added risk of disease or death of 1 individual in a population of 1 million, usually put forward as 1:1,000,000 or $1:10^6$) by at least a factor of 5000. The RIVM, in their final analysis, deemed the CAP exposure cancer risk negligible.

11.5 TOXICOLOGY—MODELS OF ANALYSIS

Paradigmatically, the regulatory zero-tolerance has a basis in default toxicology modeling. The risks of exposure to CAP through the

---

[9][*Recommendations on chloramphenicol in shrimp*]. The food exposure was calculated from the 'reasonable worst-case' scenario of a weekly shrimp consumption of 8.4 g contaminated with 10 µg CAP per kg shrimp. Kgbw stands for kilogram of body weight. Toxicological data are usually related to this unit.

[10]IARC (International Agency for Reasearch on Cancer), 1997, *Volume 50 Pharmaceutical drugs. Summary of data reported and evaluated.* See webpage http://monographs.iarc.fr/ENG/Monographs/vol50/volume50.pdf (accessed 3 February 2009).

food chain are regarded as dose-independent, meaning that any dose might give rise to disease, primarily cancer. This is related to the dominant linear non-threshold dose–response model (A; LNT), which is reserved for (genotoxic) carcinogenic compounds (Figure 11.1). The potential effects of CAP at very low-level exposures are derived from this model as, of course, actually observing those effects in human populations would be out of the question (as the effects are so small). B—the linear threshold (LT) curve—is reserved for non-carcinogenic compounds, which have a threshold for toxicity.

It is argued, however, that the most fundamental shape of the dose–response is neither threshold nor linear, but U-shaped (C), and hence both current models A and B provide less reliable estimates of low-dose risk as in the case of CAP and other Annex IV antibiotics. This U-shape is usually referred to as 'hormesis' (Moustacchi, 2000; Calabrese & Baldwin, 2003; Parsons, 2003; Tubiana & Aurengo, 2005; Calabrese, Staudenmayer, Stanek, & Hoffmann, 2006). Hormesis is in many ways the physiological equivalent of the philosophical notion that 'what does not kill you makes you stronger.' Hormesis is best described as an adaptive response to low levels of stress or damage (for example, from chemicals or radiation), resulting in enhanced robustness of some physiological systems for a finite period. More specifically, hormesis is defined as a moderate overcompensation to a perturbation in the homeostasis of an organism. The fundamental conceptual facets of hormesis are, respectively: (1) the disruption of homeostasis; (2) the moderate overcompensation; (3) the re-establishment of homeostasis; (4) the adaptive nature of the overall process (Calabrese & Baldwin, 2001).

We need to define hormesis in a continuum of the dose–response curve. There are low-dose effects and high-dose effects of exposed organisms (Rozman & Doul, 2003). Low doses could be stimulatory or inhibitory, in either case prompting living organisms to be dissociated from the homeostatic equilibrium that in turn leads to (over)compensation. For example, heavy metals such as mercury prompt synthesis of enzymes called metallothioneins that remove toxic metals from circulation and probably also protect cells against potentially DNA-damaging free radicals produced through normal metabolism (Kaiser, 2003). Conversely, low doses of anti-tumor agents commonly enhance the proliferation of the human tumor cells in a manner that is fully consistent with the hormetic dose–response relationship (Calabrese, 2008).

High doses push the organism beyond the limits of kinetic (distribution, biotransformation, or excretion) or dynamic (adaptation, repair, or reversibility) recovery. This is the classical toxicological object of research usually required as a result of public and regulatory concerns whereby hormetic responses are by default regarded as irrelevant, or even contrary to policy interests, and therefore unlooked for. Public concern about synthetic chemicals exposure seems to infuse public reluctance to view hormesis as a viable description of toxicological reality. Policymakers, similarly, are eager to address this concern and see no room for exploring hormesis and the possibilities of regulatory implementation (US EPA, 2004).

Therefore, regulatory-driven hazard assessments focus their primary, if not exclusive, attention on the higher end of the dose–response curve in order to estimate the NOAEL and LOAEL levels, subsequently modeled with linear assumptions (Crump, 1984; Weller, Catalano, & Williams, 1995). Risks of chemicals exposure should therefore be excluded from the public realm (Calabrese, 2001). Acceptance of hormesis suggests that low doses of toxic/carcinogenic agents may reduce the incidence of adverse effects observed at higher dosages.

In Figure 11.2 tumors per animal are depicted on the y axis (response), with the related dose on the x axis. The animal control group (not exposed to the carcinogen) is depicted by the horizontal dotted line. The hormetic model C predicts a lower amount of tumors than the control group

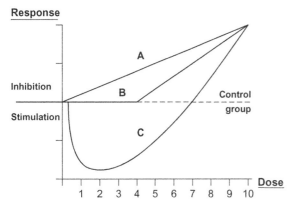

FIGURE 11.2   Three toxicological dose–response models.

when exposure levels of the carcinogen are below dose 7. The hormesis concept challenges the axiom and use of low-dose linearity in estimating cancer risks, and emphasizes that there are thresholds for carcinogens (Wiener, 2001). The particular choice of the LNT dose–response model in the assessment of the exposure risks of CAP and the role of the precautionary principle (Regulation EC No 178/2002) will be considered in the final section of this chapter.

It seems safe to conclude that CAP, at the levels found in different food products which not only included shrimp but also milk and milk powder, posed no risk to the general public,[11] either considering aplastic anemia or cancer, even when operating on the LNT assumption. Nevertheless, the flurry of activity related to the analysis of numerous batches of food products imported into the European Union between 2002 and 2005 is indicative of a combination of interpreting zero-tolerance on a molecular level (the precautionary 'when in doubt, keep it out' related to the 'high level of health protection' as expounded in Regulation 178/2002/EC) (Hanekamp *et al.*, 2003) and the evolution of analytical technology, which is now capable of

measuring in the ppb (parts per billion; μg/kg) and even ppt (parts per trillion; ng/kg) range.

The sensitive detection of analytes has improved dramatically over the past few decades, including methods used for the detection of CAP. Screening methods based on immunochemistry showed on average a tenfold improvement of sensitivity for the detection of CAP in milk powder every 7 years. The developments in instrumental methods, which are used for confirmation, have been less prominent. On average they needed 14 years to increase tenfold in sensitivity. However, it is not unlikely that the instrumental methods will show a more rapid evolution in the future. The sensitivity of LC-MS-MS has improved at least tenfold in the last couple of years and a fundamental limit has not yet been reached (Hanekamp *et al.*, 2003). This development makes zero-tolerance as a regulatory standard problematical as the notion of risk disappears out of the food safety equation.

11.6 REGULATORY DEVELOPMENTS—EUROPE AND BEYOND (HANEKAMP, 2005)

In Australia, the matter of veterinary residues without an MRL was—contrary to the European response of banning and destroying food containing ppb of banned antibiotics—contextualized within the risk instead of the precautionary framework. In October 2003, data became available indicating that very low levels of a furazolidone metabolite, 3-amino-oxazolidinone, had been found in certain imported prawns.[12] Where residues had been detected, they were only at a few parts per billion (μg/kg). However, in the absence of a specific MRL, these residues were not permitted.

[11]See court decision LJN: AU4248, Rechtbank Breda, 004817-02, webpage http://zoeken.rechtspraak.nl/resultpage.aspx?snelzoeken=true&searchtype=ljn&ljn=AU4248 (accessed 3 February 2009).
[12]*Joint FAO/WHO technical workshop on residues of veterinary drugs without ADI/MRL*, 2004, 24–26 August, Bangkok, Thailand, pp. 37–42.

The risk assessment indicated that the risk arising from these trace residues in prawns was very low and that they were safe to eat. It was not considered necessary to recall prawns that had entered into distribution within Australia. However, given that these residues were not compliant with the Food Standards Code, the enforcement authorities were advised to introduce import testing of prawns for nitrofurans. A relatively low frequency of testing has been implemented, commensurate with the level of food safety risk to the consumer.

The Australian example showed that, with the aid of risk assessment tools, food products containing low levels of veterinary residues without an MRL—which are banned—could still be marketed. The contextualization of the legal issue of forbidden veterinary products detected in food and feed products elucidates the issue of risk beyond the tautological legal inference espoused by the Annex IV list of Council Regulation 2377/90. To some extent, however, this legal flaw has been alleviated by new European regulation.

Laying down harmonized standards for the testing for certain residues in products of animal origin imported from third countries has proven to be an arduous task for which current regulation did not provide clear cut and consistent directions. The Commission's decision of 11 January 2005[13] tries to close this regulatory gap. As restated in this decision: 'Regulation (EEC) No 2377/90 does not provide MRLs for all substances and in particular not for those substances whose use is prohibited or not authorized in the Community. For those substances, the presence of any residue may present grounds to reject or destroy the relevant consignment at import.' However, in order to amend the observed problems with import from third countries as a result of regulation, isolated detection of residues of a substance below the Minimum Required Performance Limits (MRPLs) set by Decision 2002/657/EC[14] should be construed as not of immediate concern. For CAP the MRPL is set at 0.3 ppb, and for nitrofuran metabolites the MRPLs are set at 1 ppb.

As stated earlier, MRPLs were no more and no less than the concentration levels that regulatory laboratories in the European Union should at least be able to detect and confirm; the MRPLs should not be mistaken for a tolerance limit, or any similar terminology. However, with this new decision MRPLs are given some legal status in terms of levels of concern. Indeed, where the results of analytical tests on products are below the MRPLs laid down in Decision 2002/657/EC, the products will not be prohibited from entering the food chain. The European Commission will bring matters to the attention of the competent authority of the country or countries of origin and shall make appropriate proposals only when a recurrent pattern of detection of prohibited veterinary residues arises. Evidently, MRPLs only hold for regulated substances without an MRL. Substances that do not have MRLs and are not part of any regulatory structure, and therefore do not fall under the current MRPL regulation, are still regulated at zero-tolerance levels. A basic resolution is required that is not based on regulatory lists of analyzable compounds, but on the science of toxicology itself.

[13]Commission decision of 11 January 2005 laying down harmonized standards for the testing for certain residues in products of animal origin imported from third countries. *Official Journal of the European Communities* L16, pp. 61–63.
Regulation EC No 470/2009, as the new regulatory standard for the establishment of residue limits of pharmacologically active substances in foodstuffs of animal origin we referred to above, specifically refers to the issue of LODs when it states in the preamble that 'as a result of scientific and technical progress it is possible to detect the presence of residues of veterinary medicinal products in foodstuffs at ever lower levels.' This has caused considerable problems, as we have shown here, that need to be amended, of which this new regulation, superseding among others EEC No 2377/90, is regarded as a step forward. Basic resolutions, however, require more than just this regulation. This we will deal with subsequently.
[14]Commission decision of 13 March 2003 amending Decision 2002/657/EC as regards the setting of minimum required performance limits (MRPLs) for certain residues in food of animal origin. *Official Journal of the European Communities* L71, pp. 17–18.

11.7 BASIC RESOLUTIONS— INTENDED NORMAL USE[15]

Existing regulations list CAP and other antibiotics as substances prohibited in animal food production as no acceptable daily intake could scientifically be derived. Through zero-tolerance, regulatory bodies propagate the view that residues of non-allowed compounds in food constitute a hazard to consumer health; a view at odds with scientific knowledge. Efforts to enforce zero-tolerance for antibiotics have evoked concerns for reliable analytical methods able to generate transparent and reproducible results,[16] regulatory harmony, practical modes of prevention and useful risk assessments. Sensitivity of analytical methods in effect determines the operational definitions for 'zero' (LODs), and as the analytical sensitivities reach ppb and ppt levels, the costs for equipment and tests limit surveillance and furthermore increase the probability of detection. Detection as such says very little, if anything, of the toxicological relevance thereof.

Furthermore, with advancing analytical scrutiny, other sources than anticipated (or regulated) might come to the fore. For instance, semicarbazide (SEM), a marker for nitrofurazone listed in the Annex IV of Council Regulation 2377/90, proved to have other sources than the banned substances whereby its legal status for demonstrating illicit use of this group of antibiotics is ambiguous, to say the least. SEM can occur naturally in shrimps and eggs and is formed from natural substances such as arginine and creatine. A significant formation of SEM

occurs in samples treated with hypochlorite (Hoenicke et al., 2004).

Additionally, when considering increasing analytical capabilities, CAP and many other antibiotics have been detected in different aquatic environments at different locations such as hospital effluents, sewage, wastewater treatment plants, river water and drinking water (Hirsch, Ternes, Haberer, & Kratz, 1999; Lindberg et al., 2004; Loraine & Pettigrove, 2006; Papa et al., 2007; Watkinson, Murby, Kolpin, & Costanzo, 2009). Thereby another, much more diffuse source, has come to the fore that might potentially contaminate food. These contaminants are sometimes referred to as PPCPs (Pharmaceuticals and Personal Care Products). PPCPs comprise all drugs, diagnostic agents (such as X-ray contrast media), 'nutraceuticals' (bioactive food supplements), and other consumer chemicals, such as fragrances and sunscreen agents (Kummerer, 2008). From the perspective of the point of entry into the aquatic environment, namely wastewater and wastewater treatment plant discharge, PPCPs are referred to as organic wastewater contaminants (OWCs) (Kolpin et al., 2002). The human and veterinary use of pharmaceuticals results in a diffuse dispersion in the environment, comparable to, for instance, pesticides. These can be traced in food and food products.

A more contentious subject is related to the possibility of natural background concentrations of antibiotics[17]; although the fact that almost all antibiotics have a natural source is quite uncontentious, as we very briefly discussed above (Walsh, 2003). The overall natural production of antibiotics

[15]Joint FAO/WHO technical workshop on residues of veterinary drugs without ADI/MRL, 2004, 24–26 August, Bangkok, Thailand, pp. 37–42, 81–86.
[16]Final report on chloramphenicol—laboratory comparison study, Schröder, U., 2002. Bundesforschungsanstalt für Fischerei, Institut für Fischereitechnik und Fischqualität, GFR, Hamburg. (This report can be obtained through the authors.)
[17]See http://toxnet.nlm.nih.gov/cgi-bin/sis/search/f?./temp/~FE3uhM:1 (accessed 3 of February 2009).

(such as CAP) (Piraee, White, & Vining, 2004) by streptomycetes under natural conditions is not clear, and whether or not these natural background concentrations can actually be detected is equally unclear (van Pée & Unversucht, 2003; Adriaens, Gruden, & McCormick, 2007).

With the Commission decision of 11 January 2005, the European Commission tried to clear the air in Europe and the international community in relation to the trade of food and feed products between developing countries and the European trade zone. Detection *per se* of forbidden veterinary products and their metabolites in food or feed should not immediately be seen as a concern for human or animal health. Indeed, the MRPL is now functioning as a tolerance limit by which the problems that surfaced in 2001 with the detection of CAP in shrimp will be reduced. However, ambiguity remains, as the toxicological relevance of these concentrations is not addressed as such. With analytical technology advancing, MRPLs will be lowered whereby problems may develop anew. Ambiguity persists with Regulation EC No 470/2009 as toxicological relevance is not addressed. Therefore, in order to fundamentally address food safety in relation to veterinary medicinal products irrespective of source, we propose the following schemes based on 'Intended Normal Use.' By that we mean that clinical substances applied in the animal-producing field are authorized products used with an intentional normal purpose. This means that food safety regulation is not meant to tackle intended misuse. Again, its focus is on safeguarding public health. Figure 11.3 depicts a decision tree by which future regulation could best be organized.

The buttress of the decision tree is the risk approach. A number of effective risk tools are on hand, namely: the MTR level, the TDI, the related MRL and the toxicologically insignificant exposure (TIE) level. With the latter, the concept of hormesis is embraced as a means to advance a rational approach of low-level exposures of chemicals in food, which need not be zero (Hanekamp & Calabrese, 2007). With the concept of a TIE, the hormetic part of the dose–response curve is 'translated' into a toxicological threshold. Insignificance is understood *not* as an evaluatory outcome based on an MTR level of 1:1,000,000 as is done with the threshold of toxicological concern (TTC) concept (Kroes *et al.*, 2004), but as a direct toxicological dose–response matter (Calabrese & Cook, 2005). Exposure at some (low) level is therein not regarded as potentially hazardous but understood within the framework of a hormetic adaptive response. As Renn (2008) observes:

> 'With respect to hormesis it is ethically mandated that potential beneficial aspects of low exposure to potentially hazardous material are incorporated in the risk–benefit balancing procedure. The potential harm done by pollutants does not justify the invocation of a categorical principle. Minimization of risk is not required if health benefits are also at stake. Society needs to find an informed consent on the threshold of risk below which compensation of goods is legitimate and morally justified. Such a threshold can be defined context-specific but any human action associated with potential health impacts makes such an acceptability judgment – implicitly or explicitly. Incorporating hormesis into risk management forces regulators to make such thresholds explicit. Once risk is below this threshold, all positive and negative impacts are subject to a relative balancing towards reaching a final judgment on acceptability and necessary risk management options.'

As shown in the depicted decision tree (Figure 11.3), INU is not limited to authorized veterinary use but also includes human clinical use as the aquatic environment can potentially be a source of excreted clinical residues for the food-production chain.

Obviously, concentrations present in food as a result of exposure of clinical products through the aquatic environment are much lower than

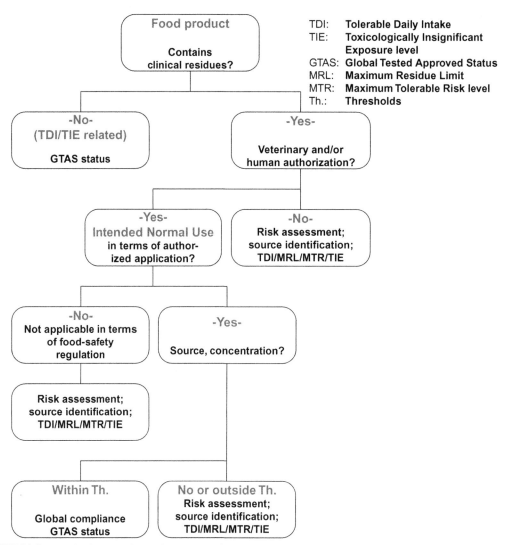

FIGURE 11.3   Food safety regulatory decision tree for clinical residues.

normal intended veterinary use. Drinking water derived from either surface or groundwater contains numerous excreted clinical compounds at very low levels not associated with any measurable risk for human health; whereby a strict risk-avoiding approach in terms of zero-tolerance within the food sector is disproportionate and unnecessary.[18]

[18]Comments on the discussion paper on risk analysis principles and methodologies in the CODEX Committee on Residues of Veterinary Drugs in Foods, 2001. Joint FAO/WHO Foods standards Programme CODEX Committee on Residues of Veterinary Drugs in Foods. Thirteenth Session, Charleston, SC, USA, 4–7 December 2001, CX/RVDF 01/9-Add.1.

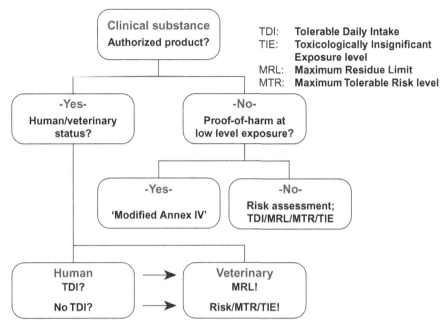

FIGURE 11.4 Relationship between human and veterinary clinical substances regarding food.

The inclusion of the INU of human medication as a result of which the food chain is exposed to these substances (through the aquatic environment) is a logical consequence of the risk-based approach proposed here and resolutely widens the window of risk-based food safety regulations. Therefore, the relationship between human and veterinary clinical substances could best be depicted in Figure 11.4, when risk assessment strategies are used as a central theorem.

It is essential that proof-of-harm of low-dose toxicity supersedes the current Annex IV regulation. When proof-of-harm as a result of food residue exposure surfaces, then the substance needs to be listed on an amended 'Annex IV'— a Universally Banned Substances List (UBSL). This is related to the fact that proof of a negative is scientifically impossible and will generate a legal *probatio diabolica* (Hanekamp *et al.*, 2003). Lack of data to establish an MRL as such is not sufficient grounds to ban certain veterinary products; even more so when those products are authorized as human medication and damaging effects surface only as a result of human therapeutic use. Indeed, with any authorized human and veterinary medications, a balance is struck between toxicity and beneficial effects at the biological active dosage. Risks materializing at the human therapeutic level cannot be indicative of a veterinary ban.

The risk approach should have a global jurisdiction in order to avoid trade barrier issues based on analysis non-compliance. Therefore, a 'Global Tested Approved Status' is introduced in the decision tree. Tools of analysis need to be horizontally unified in order to generate global compliance and a level playing field as to preclude trade barriers. Trade between nations will benefit from international cross-compliance, in which properly analyzed goods will be accepted unreservedly by importing nations. In cases where non-authorized substances are detected, a risk analysis of observed concentrations needs to be undertaken with food safety as the sole objective.

11.8 CONCLUSIONS

Globally acceptable maximum allowable concentrations of contaminants such as CAP require an internationally harmonized risk assessment approach, using globally agreed methodology. Regulations should refer to a UBSL, which in turn ought to be based on proof of toxicity at relevant food-exposure levels. Here, the proposed framework of food safety regulation—as founded on scientific principle—necessitates a move towards analytical harmonization. Exporting and importing countries and the various internal markets are in need of general compliance rules as to preclude unwarranted trade barriers or, to put it constructively, to generate a truly free and open market for all food-producing countries.

Tools of analysis need to be unified on an international level in order to generate international compliance and a level playing field. Trade between nations will benefit from international cross-compliance, in which properly analyzed goods will be accepted unreservedly by importing nations—Global Tested Approved Status. In cases where banned substances are detected, a risk analysis of observed concentrations and potential exposure routes needs to be undertaken with food safety as the leading objective. With the aid of the TIE, endless analytical exercises will thereby become nonoperational. In our view, this will further add a renewed pharmaceutical interest in applying for authorization for innovative veterinary medication (Hanekamp & Kwakman, 2004). Proof of no harm—as intrinsically espoused by precautionary zero-tolerance strategies—generates a chilly climate for innovation typical of a cautious culture (Hanekamp & Bast, 2008).

The CAP case is the first policy example in which a regulatory shift is observed from zero tolerance to a threshold approach, which could hopefully pave the way for the incorporation of a hormetic perspective into, not only food safety

regulations, but also into environmental regulations. This is clearly needed to rationalize safety and conservation regulations at large. Hormesis redefines our concept of pollution and contamination; questions the premise that pollutants are unconditionally bad; and therefore, acknowledges that the human organism does have adaptive capabilities. This is innovative because modern environmental and public health legislation is built not only in large part on the moral dichotomies of good versus evil, clean versus dirty, natural versus unnatural, but also safety versus health. Chemical substances—be it natural or synthetic—are generally neither bad nor good; they are both, depending on exposure levels and adaptive responses from the exposed organisms (Hanekamp, 2008). Policies on chemicals safety, as proposed here in relation to antibiotics in food, need to abandon the simplistic moral dichotomy of good and evil in order to be able to mature into a regulation that truly addresses the safety and health of citizens in relation to food consumption.

References

Adriaens, P., Gruden, C., & McCormick, M. L. (2007). Biogeochemistry of halogenated hydrocarbons. In B. Sherwood Lollar (Ed.), *Treatise on geochemistry, Vol 9, Environmental Geochemistry*. New York, NY: Elsevier.

Benestad, H. B. (1979). Drug mechanism in marrow aplasia. In C. G. Geary (Ed.), *Aplastic anaemia* (pp. 26–42). London: Balliere Tindall.

Bentley, S. D., Chater, K. F., Cerdeño-Tárraga, A.-M., et al. (2002). Complete genome sequence of the model actinomycete *Streptomyces coelicolor* A3(2). *Nature, 417*, 141–147.

Bibb, M. J. (2005). Regulation of secondary metabolism in streptomycetes. *Current Opinion in Microbiology, 8*, 208–215.

Calabrese, E. J. (2001). The future of hormesis: Where do we go from here? *Critical Reviews in Toxicology, 31*(4/5), 637–648.

Calabrese, E. J. (2008). Hormesis and medicine. *British Journal of Clinical Pharmacology, 66*(5), 594–617.

Calabrese, E. J., & Baldwin, L. A. (2001). Hormesis: A generalizable and unifying hypothesis. *Critical Reviews in Toxicology, 31*(4/5), 353–424.

Calabrese, E. J., & Baldwin, L. A. (2003). Toxicology rethinks its central belief. Hormesis demands a reprisal of the way risks are assessed. *Nature, 421,* 691–692.

Calabrese, E. J., & Cook, R. R. (2005). Hormesis: How it could affect the risk assessment process. *Human & Experimental Toxicology, 24,* 265–270.

Calabrese, E. J., Staudenmayer, J. W., Stanek, E. J., & Hoffmann, G. R. (2006). Hormesis outperforms threshold model in national cancer institute antitumor drug screening database. *Toxicological Sciences, 94*(2), 368–378.

Chater, K. F. (2006). *Streptomyces* inside-out: A new perspective on the bacteria that provide us with antibiotics. *Philosophical Transactions of the Royal Society B, 361,* 761–768.

Crump, K. S. (1984). A new method for determining allowable daily intakes. *Fundamental and Applied Toxicology, 4,* 854–871.

Doody, M. M., Linet, M. S., Glass, A. G., et al. (1996). Risks of non-Hodgkin's lymphoma, multiple myeloma, and leukemia associated with common medications. *Epidemiology, 7,* 131–139.

Ehrlich, J., Bartz, Q. R., Smith, R. M., & Joslyn, D. A. (1947). Chloromycetin, a new antibiotic from a soil actinomycete. *Science, 106,* 417.

Hanekamp, J. C. (2005). Veterinary residues and new European legislation: A new hope? *Environmental Liability, 2,* 52–55.

Hanekamp, J. C. (2008). Micronutrients, hormesis and the aptitude for the maturation of regulation. *American Journal of pharmaceutical Toxicology, 3*(1), 141–148.

Hanekamp, J. C., & Bast, A. (2008). Why RDAs and ULs are incompatible standards in the U-shape micronutrient model. A philosophically orientated analysis of micronutrients standardisations. *Risk Analysis, 28*(6), 1639–1652.

Hanekamp, J. C., & Calabrese, E. J. (2007). Chloramphenicol, European legislation and hormesis. *Dose Response, 5,* 91–93.

Hanekamp, J. C., Frapporti, G., & Olieman, K. (2003). Chloramphenicol, food safety and precautionary thinking in Europe. *Environmental Liability, 6,* 209–221.

Hanekamp, J. C., & Kwakman, J. (2004). Beyond zero-tolerance: A new approach to food safety and residues of pharmacological active substances in foodstuffs of animal origin. *Environmental Liability, 1,* 33–39.

Hirsch, R., Ternes, T., Haberer, K., & Kratz, K.-L. (1999). Occurrence of antibiotics in the aquatic environment. *The Science of the Total Environment, 225,* 109–118.

Hoenicke, K., Gatermann, R., Hartig, L., et al. (2004). Formation of semicarbazide (SEM) in food by hypochlorite treatment: Is SEM a specific marker for nitrofurazone abuse? *Food Additives and Contaminants, 21,* 526–537.

Hopwood, D. A. (2007). *Streptomyces in nature and medicine. The antibiotic makers.* Oxford: Oxford University Press.

Janssen, P. A. H., Baars, A. J., & Pieters, M. N. (2001). *Advies met betrekking tot chlooramfenicol in garnalen.* Bilthoven, The Netherlands: RIVM/CSR.

Kaiser, J. (2003). Sipping from a poisoned chalice. *Science, 320,* 376–378.

Kolpin, D. W., Furlong, E. T., Meyer, M. T., et al. (2002). Pharmaceutical, hormones, and other organic waste water contaminants in U.S. streams, 1999–2000: A national reconnaissance. *Environmental Science & Technology, 36,* 1202–1211.

Kroes, R., Renwick, A. G., Cheeseman, M., et al. (2004). Structure-based thresholds of toxicological concern (TTC): Guidance for application to substances present at low levels in the diet. *Food and Chemical Toxicology, 42,* 65–83.

Kummerer, K. (Ed.). (2008). *Pharmaceuticals in the environment. Sources, fate, effect and risks.* Berlin: Springer Verlag.

Lindberg, R., Jarnheimer, P.-A., Olsen, B., et al. (2004). Determination of antibiotic substances in hospital sewage water using solid phase extraction and liquid chromatography/mass spectrometry and group analogue internal standards. *Chemosphere, 57,* 1479–1488.

Loraine, G. A., & Pettigrove, M. E. (2006). Seasonal variations in concentrations of pharmaceuticals and personal care products in drinking water and reclaimed wastewater in Southern California. *Environmental Science & Technology, 40,* 687–695.

Martelli, A., Mattioli, F., Pastorino, G., et al. (1991). Genotoxicity testing of chloramphenicol in rodent and human cells. *Mutation Research, 260,* 65–72.

Moustacchi, E. (2000). DNA damage and repair: Consequences on dose–responses. *Mutation Research, 464,* 35–40.

Papa, E., Fick, J., Lindberg, R., et al. (2007). Multivariate chemical mapping of antibiotics and identification of structurally representative substances. *Environmental Science & Technology, 41,* 1653–1661.

Parsons, P. A. (2003). Metabolic efficiency in response to environmental agents predicts hormesis and invalidates the linear no-threshold premise: Ionizing radiation as a case study. *Critical Reviews in Toxicology, 33*(3/4), 443–449.

Patel, J. C., & Banker, D. D. (1949). Chloramphenicol in typhoid fever. A preliminary report of clinical trial in 6 cases. *British Medical Journal, 22*(2), 908–909.

Piraee, M., White, R. L., & Vining, L. C. (2004). Biosynthesis of the dichloroacetyl component of chloramphenicol in *Streptomyces venezuelae* ISP5230: Genes required for halogenation. *Microbiology, 150,* 85–94.

Renn, O. (2008). An ethical appraisal of hormesis: Towards a rational discourse on the acceptability of risks and benefits. *American Journal of Pharmaceutical Toxicology*, 3(1), 165–181.

Rozman, K. K., & Doul, J. (2003). Scientific foundations of hormesis. Part 2. Maturation, strengths, limitations, and possible applications in toxicology, pharmacology, and epidemiology. *Critical Reviews in Toxicology*, 33(3/4), 451–462.

Shi, W., & Zusman, D. (1993). Fatal attraction. *Nature, 366*, 414–415.

Tubiana, M., & Aurengo, A. (2005). Dose–effect relationship and estimation of the carcinogenic effects of low doses of ionising radiation: The Joint Report of the Académie des Sciences (Paris) and of the Académie Nationale de Médecine. *I Journal of Low Radiation*, 2(3/4), 1–19.

US EPA. (2004). Environmental Protection Agency. *An examination of epa risk assessment principles and practices*, EPA/100/B-04/001.

van Pée, K.-H., & Unversucht, S. (2003). Biological dehalogenation and halogenation reactions. *Chemosphere, 52*, 299–312.

Walsh, C. (2003). *Antibiotics. Actions, origins, resistance.* Washington, DC: ASM Press.

Watkinson, A. J., Murby, E. J., Kolpin, D. W., & Costanzo, S. D. (2009). The occurrence of antibiotics in an urban watershed: From wastewater to drinking water. *The Science of the Total Environment, 407*, 2711–2723.

Weller, E. A., Catalano, P. J., & Williams, P. L. (1995). Implications of developmental toxicity study design for quantitative risk assessment. *Risk Analysis, 15*(5), 567–574.

Wiener, J. B. (2001). Hormesis and the radical moderation of law. *Human & Experimental Toxicology, 20*, 162–164.

12

Mycotoxin Management: An International Challenge

Rebeca López-García

Logre International Food Science Consulting, México, DF, México

12.1 INTRODUCTION

Mycotoxins are a group of diverse toxic secondary fungal metabolites that contaminate cereal grains as well as other agricultural products and are of concern to human and animal health. The total number of mycotoxins is not known but according to reports by the Council for Agricultural Science and Technology (CAST) on mycotoxins (CAST, 2003), toxic fungi metabolites could potentially number in the thousands. However, the number of mycotoxins actually known to be involved in disease is considerably less. The major classes of mycotoxins of concern are: aflatoxins, tricothecenes, fumonisins, zearalenone, ochratoxin A and ergot alkaloids. Consuming foods contaminated with high levels of certain mycotoxins can cause the rapid onset of mycotoxicosis, a severe illness characterized by vomiting, abdominal pain, pulmonary edema, convulsions, coma, and in some rare cases death (Dohlman, 2003). However, lethal cases are not common and in many cases are associated with lack of food security since the affected food would be considered inedible under conditions where food supply is adequate. Among mycotoxins, the most widely recognized risk comes from aflatoxins; particularly aflatoxin B_1 (AFB$_1$) since it is listed as a known human carcinogen by the International Agency for Research on Cancer (IARC) (IARC, 1997). In addition, aflatoxins are of particular toxicological concern for populations with a high incidence of hepatitis B because the rate of liver cancer is up to 60 times greater in people with hepatitis B than in healthy people who are exposed to aflatoxins (Miller, 1996). Other mycotoxins have also been considered as suspected carcinogens (IARC, 1997) and human exposure may be directly through the consumption of contaminated agricultural commodities or indirectly through the consumption of animal products from animals that have been fed with contaminated feed. Mycotoxins can be detected in meat, milk and eggs and can also result in economic losses from animal health and productivity problems (CAST, 2003). Thus, mycotoxin contamination of food and feedstuffs causes food safety and economic concerns and control has a huge impact on grain and agricultural product trade.

12.2 MYCOTOXIN REGULATIONS

Countries have the legitimate right to protect their consumers from the toxic effects of these naturally-occurring compounds. However, setting limits for unavoidable contaminants is not an easy task—it is not always straightforward since minimizing the risk may not be economically feasible. Therefore, regulatory bodies must continually assess the levels of allowable exposure to humans by using a sound risk assessment process (CAST, 2003). Risk assessment is defined as the scientific evaluation of the probability of occurrence of known or potentially adverse health effects resulting from human exposure to foodborne hazards. It is the primary scientific basis for the establishment of regulations (FAO, 2004). Its main components include hazard identification, a qualitative indication that a contaminant can cause adverse effects on health that depends on the availability

of toxicological data; and hazard characterization, a qualitative and quantitative evaluation of the nature of the adverse effects that depends on the availability of exposure data.

In addition to data used for the risk assessment process, risk management of mycotoxins is affected by other scientific and socio-economic factors such as the distribution of mycotoxin concentrations within a lot, the availability of analytical methods, legislation in other countries that are trading partners, and availability of a sufficient food supply (FAO, 2004). Although the World Trade Organization's Sanitary and Phytosanitary (SPS) agreement states that standards must be based on sound risk assessments; economic and sociological implications of regulations are also very important since there are diverging perceptions of tolerable health risks largely associated with the level of economic development and the susceptibility of a nation's crops to contamination. The availability of sampling and analytical methods also plays an important role in establishing limits since tolerance levels that do not have a reasonable expectation of being measured may waste resources and condemn products that are perfectly fit for consumption (Smith, Lewis, Anderson, & Solomons, 1994). The regulatory philosophy may also change in different areas of the world since it should not jeopardize the availability of basic commodities at reasonable prices. So, in developing countries, the adequate level of protection must take into consideration the amount of food available. If food supplies are already limited, drastic legal measures may cause food shortages and excessive consequences. Thus, there is a wide range of varying standards among different national or multilateral agencies (Dohlman, 2003). According to a survey of worldwide mycotoxin regulations by the Food and Agriculture Organization of the United Nations (FAO), the number of countries that have mycotoxin regulations has been steadily increasing (FAO, 2004). In 2003, approximately 100 countries were known to have established specific limits for various combinations of mycotoxins and commodities, often accompanied by prescribed or recommended procedures for sampling and analysis.

12.3 HARMONIZED REGULATIONS

Until around the late 1990s, the setting of regulatory limits was mainly a national affair. However, gradually, several economic communities have harmonized their regulations. According to the 2004 FAO report, the following trading blocks: Australia/New Zealand, the European Union (EU), MERCOSUR (*Mercado Común del Sur* – Common Market of the South) and the Association of Southeast Asian Nations (ASEAN) have harmonized regulations.

12.3.1 Australia/New Zealand

In 2002, Australia and New Zealand initiated a joint regulatory approach to be codified in the Australia New Zealand Food Standards Code. This transition occurred parallel to an evolution from hazard to risk-based standards. Common limits are now applied for total aflatoxins in peanuts and tree nuts, and ergot (the sclerotium of *Claviceps purpurea*, not actually a mycotoxin but a dormant winter form of the fungus containing the ergot alkaloids mycotoxins). The harmonized standards also include limits for phomopsins in lupin seeds and products thereof and for agaric acid in food containing mushrooms and alcoholic beverages. These limits are unique to Australia and New Zealand and have not been reported anywhere else in the world. Although some analytical methods are recommended in import regulations, mycotoxin testing in Australia and New Zealand is based on a performance approach. For this, laboratories must be accredited and use appropriate, suitably validated methods. Ochratoxin A and the *Fusarium* toxins (T-2, nivalenol, acetodeoxynivalenol,

zearalenone and fumonisins) were also included in the original risk assessment but it was concluded that it was premature to establish maximum permitted concentrations in food for these mycotoxins. There have been no subsequent amendments to date to include these toxins in the harmonized regulations (Cressey, 2008).

12.3.2 European Union

The European Union has harmonized regulations for aflatoxin B_1 in various feeds since 1976 including official protocols for sampling and analysis. In 1998, harmonized regulations for mycotoxins in foods that included sampling protocols and methods of analysis came into force and have been gradually expanding. In 2004, a significant expansion was initiated for several mycotoxin/food combinations. For foods, harmonized regulations include patulin, aflatoxin B_1, aflatoxin M_1, ochratoxin A and deoxynivalenol (DON) in infant and follow-up formulae; ochratoxin A in coffee, wine, beer, spices, grape juice, cocoa and cocoa products; several *Fusarium* mycotoxins, i.e. tricothecenes (T-2 and HT-2 toxins in addition to DON), fumonisins and zearalenone and ochratoxin A.

12.3.3 MERCOSUR

MERCOSUR includes Argentina, Brazil, Paraguay and Uruguay. Bolivia, Chile, Colombia, Ecuador and Peru have associate member status. Venezuela signed a membership agreement on 17 June 2006 but, before becoming a full member, its entry has to be ratified by the Paraguayan and Brazilian parliaments. A formal process of harmonization of national regulations took place in 1994. Through this process, common maximum limits were established for aflatoxins B_1, B_2, G_1 and G_2 for peanuts and corn and for aflatoxin M_1 in dairy products. These limits included sampling plans and analytical methods for each mycotoxin/commodity combination.

The general criteria and guidelines followed for the harmonization of regional mycotoxin regulations include: the definition of priority products in relevance to health and trade; the comparison of national regulations with international standards or regulations; the use of risk assessment data as reference; and the application of equivalency principles and risk analysis. After all the specific steps were taken to develop the final approval of the common regulations for mycotoxin maximum limits, the approved regulations were incorporated into the four members' legal bodies and became mandatory. However, implementation of the regulations may be challenging due to a lack of data that represent all member countries. To date, full member countries apply common limits for total aflatoxins in peanuts, maize and products thereof, and for aflatoxin M_1 in fluid and powdered milk. In addition, each member country can publish its own legislation for other non-harmonized products; such is the case of Uruguay where maximum levels for other mycotoxins have been established to address specific mycotoxins of concern for the country. Brazil has a proposal on maximum limits for other relevant mycotoxins as well. In special cases, international references can be used (Lindner Schreiner, 2008).

12.3.4 ASEAN

Current member countries include Brunei Darussalam, Cambodia, Indonesia, the Lao People's Democratic Republic, Malaysia, Myanmar, the Philippines, Singapore, Thailand and Viet Nam. Most of these countries have specific regulations for mycotoxins. Harmonized regulations are not yet established. However, an ASEAN Task Force on *Codex Alimentarius* has taken a common position to support the 0.5 µg/kg level for aflatoxin M_1 in milk. ASEAN Reference Laboratories (ARLs) have been established for mycotoxins as well as pesticide residues, veterinary drugs, microbiology, heavy

metals and genetically modified organisms. In addition, other documents such as the ASEAN Common Food Control Requirements (ACFCR), the ASEAN Common Principles for Food Control Systems, the ASEAN Common Principles and Requirements for the Labeling of Prepackaged Food, and the ASEAN Common Principles and Requirements for Food Hygiene have been finalized and will serve as guiding principles for the ASEAN relevant food bodies (Le Chau, 2006).

12.3.5 *Codex Alimentarius*

The Codex Alimentarius Commission (CAC), supported by FAO and the World Health Organization (WHO), aims to facilitate world trade and protect the health of consumers through the development of international standards for foods and feeds. Within the CAC, the Codex Committee on Food Additives and Contaminants (CCFAC) derives maximum limits (standards) for additives and contaminants in food, which are decisive in trade conflicts. The Joint FAO/WHO Expert Committee on Food Additives (JECFA) is the scientific body that develops advisory documents on food additives and contaminants for the CAC. JECFA uses the formal risk assessment approach to evaluate contaminants. Information presented to JECFA includes the hazard identification and characterization data. JECFA then evaluates all the toxicological information and gives a Provisional Tolerable Weekly Intake (PTWI) or a Provisional Tolerable Daily Intake (PTDI). The term 'provisional' is used to express the tentative nature of the evaluation in view of the paucity of reliable data on the consequences of human exposure at levels approaching those with which JECFA is concerned. The evaluation is based on the determination of a No Observed Adverse Effect Level (NOAEL) in toxicological studies and the application of an uncertainty factor that is calculated using the lowest NOAEL in animal studies divided by a factor of

100 (10 for the extrapolation from animal studies or interspecies differences and 10 for the variation among different individuals or intraspecies differences). If the availability of toxicological data is inadequate, then a higher safety factor is used. This calculation derives a tolerable intake level. This approach is not considered appropriate for toxins where carcinogenicity is the basis for concern (i.e. aflatoxins). A no-effect concentration limit cannot be established for genotoxic compounds since any small dose will have a proportionally small effect. The imposition of a complete elimination of the carcinogen would be appropriate. However, natural contaminants cannot be completely eliminated from a food or feed without outlawing the commodity they contaminate. For these particular cases, JECFA has established the As Low as Reasonably Achievable (ALARA) level. This may be considered as the level where the contaminant has been minimized to an irreducible level. ALARA is formally defined as the concentration of a substance that cannot be eliminated from a food without involving the discard of the food altogether or seriously compromising the food supply (CAST, 2003; FAO, 2004).

12.4 TRADE IMPACT OF REGULATIONS

It is difficult to establish the overall cost of mycotoxin contamination in a consistent and uniform manner since the lack of information on the health costs and other economic losses from mycotoxin-related human illness is not easy to establish due to the complication in exactly determining cause-and-effect relationships between mycotoxins and the chronic diseases they are suspected of causing (Dohlman, 2003). Mycotoxin contamination is associated with economic losses due to their impact on productivity and world trade. Globalization of trade has complicated the regulatory control of mycotoxins since

regulatory standards may become bargaining chips in trade negotiations. While developed countries have well-developed infrastructures for monitoring food safety and quality; people in developing countries may not be as protected due to the lack of food safety, quality monitoring, and available resources for an effective enforcement infrastructure (Cardwell, Desjardins, Henry, Munkvold, & Robens, 2001). In some cases, it has been clear that developing countries have experienced market losses due to persistent mycotoxin problems or the imposition of new, stricter regulations by importing countries (Dohlman, 2003). One study has estimated that crop losses (corn, wheat and peanuts) from mycotoxin contamination in the United States amount to $932 million annually, in addition to losses averaging $466 million annually from regulatory enforcement, testing and other quality control measures (CAST, 2003). However, large economic losses due to stricter regulations may have greater impact on the major exporters of commodities susceptible to contamination. Trade disputes from mycotoxin contamination arise because it is recognized as an unavoidable risk and there are several factors that influence the level of contamination in cereals and grains that are purely environmental (weather and insect infestation), and thus are difficult or impossible to control. In addition, perception of tolerable risks is based largely on the level of economic development and the susceptibility of the nation's crops to contamination (Dohlman, 2003). A study by Wilson and Otsuki (2001) estimated that, for a group of 46 countries, including the United States, the adoption of a harmonized standard based on the Codex guidelines would increase trade of cereals and nuts by more than $6 billion or more than 50% compared with the divergent standards in effect during 1998. However, the European Union (EU) regulation is among the strictest in the world (4 ng/g total aflatoxins in foods other than peanuts and 15 ng/g in peanuts) with these concentrations well under the harmonized Codex standards (Wu, 2008).

When these European harmonized limits were communicated, the international trade community was afraid of the impact of this regulation from an importing commercial block on the economies of the exporting countries. In fact, several studies indicated that the standards could cause severe economic losses in the United States (US), Argentina and Africa, without any considerable gain in health benefits for European consumers (Otsuki, Wilson, & Sewadeh, 2001; Wu, 2004). A World Bank (2005) study indicated that Otsuki and co-workers had overestimated the impact of the EU aflatoxin standard on Africa due to the lack of productivity and other commercial factors that influenced African exports. This trade study showed, however, that the major losses were incurred by the more successful exporters of these commodities, Turkey, Brazil and Iran. Wu (2008) estimated that these studies do not take into account the multiple stakeholders and price fluctuations that are inherent in adjusting to the EU standard and do not account for the fact that in certain circumstances, a stricter food standard can actually result in economic benefits to high-quality export markets.

On the other hand, there is a well-recognized fear that the imposition of stricter standards in higher value markets could have a more negative impact on the health of the population in the exporting countries that have, in fact, more vulnerable populations. This is because the best commodities are selected for the demanding export market while the lower quality, more contaminated products, may stay in the domestic market; and consumed by those with low incomes and who may be more susceptible due to higher incidences of hepatitis B. Wu estimated (2004) that, in the EU, a change in aflatoxin standards from 20 to 10 ng/g, much less from 10 to 2 ng/g, would likely reduce the risk of mortality by an amount so small that it would not be detected. However, areas with high incidences of hepatitis B and C (China and Sub-Saharan Africa) could be at greater health risk.

Most countries recognize that placing standards on the level of mycotoxin entering the food chain is prudent, but there are still diverging perceptions on how to balance economic costs and health benefits. This issue is especially relevant for countries that lack the means to implement stronger quality control measures. One generalized conclusion of all of these studies is that, regardless of the level of economic impact calculated using different models, it is important for policymakers to consider the implications of both health and economic outcomes when developing harmonized standards for mycotoxins. It is clear that the creation of these standards will continue since regulating mycotoxin contamination is a clear goal for the twenty-first century.

12.5 TECHNICAL ASSISTANCE

The setting of stricter regulatory limits should always be paired with the technical assistance required to minimize the initial risk of mycotoxin contamination and thus, lessen the likelihood of exceeding the regulatory limits. A World Bank trade analysis (Diaz Rios & Jaffee, 2008) reported that after 6 years of harmonized standards for mycotoxins in Europe, the 'lost' trade for the Sub-Saharan countries attributed to the EU standards is very low in contrast to the original estimates. For most of these countries, the EU standards were significant neither as a barrier to trade nor as a catalyst for proactive action since Sub-Saharan Africa's edible groundnut export sector had been gradually losing competitiveness for decades. The stricter EU standards were counteracted by competitive countries with the implementation of control systems. Since there is now better knowledge of the factors associated with the prevention and control of aflatoxin contamination; upgrades to production of susceptible commodities can gradually incorporate Good Agricultural Practices (GAPs) and the Hazard Analysis and Critical Control Point (HACCP) system. These improvements are combined with end-product inspections at different stages of the supply chain, implemented by officials before exporting. The World Bank study (Diaz Rios & Jaffee, 2008) shows that even if the EU had adopted the less stringent Codex standards, Africa's groundnut exports to the EU would not have been higher. Analysis of the notifications reported in the European Rapid Alert System for Food and Feed (RASFF) shows that nearly 80% of African consignments intercepted by EU authorities over 2004–2006 would have failed even the Codex standards. If the EU had adopted the Codex standards, however, the major beneficiaries would have been the more competitive ground nut exporters, Argentina, the US, Brazil, China and Egypt. All of these countries have made investments in upgrading their production system to not only boost quality and productivity, but also achieve better control with subsequent beneficial impact on food safety. However, some exporting countries may not have the technical resources to upgrade their systems accordingly. Such has been the case of coffee exporting countries that had to face the more stringent European requirement for Ochratoxin A (OTA). In this case, FAO acknowledged the need to support these countries with technical assistance so that they could develop systems that were appropriate for improving the quality of coffee sent to the export market and controlling the contamination with OTA. The implementation of an Integrated Mycotoxin Management System in Ecuador (López-García, Mallmann, & Pineiro, 2008) showed that technical assistance is important, but the effectiveness of such systems relies on the ability to reach producers and demonstrate the benefits of applying proper controls. This may be difficult because other economic factors may prevent the producer from getting a higher price for a seemingly higher value product. However, it is important to show producers that the use of proper controls does in fact have a beneficial economic impact in the long-term and for them, the benefit may only be future market access.

12.6 CONCLUSION

The impact of mycotoxin contamination around the world is well-recognized and it is only natural that countries will continue to set regulatory limits to protect public health as well as their access to different markets. However, the setting of these regulations must always be based on sound risk assessment processes combined with the development of adequate sampling and analysis methods. In addition, policymakers should always take into account the economic impact of setting different standards. In harmonization processes, it is important to find a delicate equilibrium between the economic impact and an adequate level of protection at all levels. Risk perception and the desired level of protection are most definitely different in countries with different resources and food availability. However, it is the duty of international organizations to protect public health overall, including that of the most vulnerable populations that may not even be aware of the risks associated with mycotoxin contamination. The development and implementation of proper control systems is also important not only to decrease mycotoxin contamination and maintain access to higher value markets but also to achieve higher quality products that will hopefully fetch better values in world trade with the subsequent benefit to producers.

References

Cardwell, K. F., Desjardins, A., Henry, S. H., Munkvold, & Robens, (2001). Mycotoxins: The costs of achieving food security and food quality. ASPSnet. American Phytopathological Society. August 2001. www.apsnet.org/online/feature/mycotoxin/top.html (accessed 10 March 2009).

CAST. (2003). Mycotoxin: Risks in plant, animal and human systems. In J. L. Richard & G. A. Payne (Eds.), *Council for Agricultural Science and Technology Task Force* Report No. 139, Ames, Iowa.

Cressey, P. (2008). Fungal downunder: mycotoxin risk management in New Zealand and Australia. Presented at The Fifth World Mycotoxin Forum. 17–18 November 2008. Noordwijk, the Netherlands.

Diaz Rios, L. B., & Jaffee, S. (2008). Barrier, catalyst or distraction? Standards, competitiveness and Africa's groundnut exports to Europe. Agriculture and Rural Development Discussion Paper 39, World Bank. http://siteresources.worldbank.org/INTARD/Resources/AflatoxinPaperWEB.pdf (accessed 10 March 2009).

Dohlman, E. (2003). Mycotoxin hazards and regulations: impacts on food and animal feed crop trade. In J. Buzby (ed.), *International Trade and Food Safety: Economic Theory and Case Studies*, Agricultural Economic Report No. 828, USDA, ERS.

FAO. (2004). Worldwide regulations for mycotoxins in food and feed in 2003. FAO Food and Nutrition Paper 81. Rome, Italy: Food and Agriculture Organization of the United Nations.

IARC. (1997). Some naturally occurring substances: food items and constituents, heterocyclic aromatic amines and mycotoxins. Summary of data reported and evaluation. International Agency for Research on Cancer Monographs on the Evaluation of Carcinogenic Risks to Humans. Volume 56 last updated 08/21/1997. http://monographs.iarc.fr/ENG/Monographs/vol56/volume56.pdf (accessed 16 March 2009), Lyon, France.

Le Chau, G. (2006). ASEAN Approaches to Standardization and Conformity Assessment Procedures and their Impact on Trade. Presented at: Regional Workshop on the Importance of Rules of Origin and Standards in Regional Integration, 26–27 June 2006, Hainan, China.

Lindner Schreiner, L. (2008). Mycotoxins: Regulatory measures in MERCOSUR, the common market of the Southern Cone. Presented at The Fifth World Mycotoxin Forum, 17–18 November 2008, Noordwijk, The Netherlands.

López-García, R., Mallmann, C. A., & Pineiro, M. (2008). Design and implementation of an integrated management system for ochratoxin A in the coffee production chain. *Food Additives Contaminants, 25*(2), 231–240.

Miller, J. D. (1996). Foodborne natural carcinogens: Issues and priorities. *African Newsletter*, 6 (Supplement 1). http://www.ttl.fi/Internet/English/Information/Electronic+journals/African+Newsletter/1996-01+Supplement/06.htm (accessed 16 March 2009).

Otsuki, T., Wilson, J. S., & Sewadeh, M. (2001). What price precaution? European harmonization of aflatoxin regulations and African groundnut exports. *European Review of Agricultural Economics, 28*, 263–283.

Smith, J. W., Lewis, C. W., Anderson, H. G., & Solomons, G. L. (1994). Mycotoxins in Human and Animal Health. Technical report. European Commission, Directorate XII: Science, Research and Development, Agro-Industrial Research Division, Brussels, Belgium.

Wilson, J., & Otsuki, T. (2001). Global trade and food safety: Winners and losers in a fragmented system. The World Bank. October 2001. http://www-wds.worldbank.org/external/default/WDSContentServer/IW3P/IB/2001/12/11/000094946_01110204024949/Rendered/PDF/multi0page.pdf (accessed 27 February 2009).

World Bank (2005). Food safety and agricultural health standards. Challenges and opportunities for developing country exports. Report No. 31207, Washington, DC, USA.

Wu, F. (2004). Mycotoxin risk assessment for the purpose of setting international standards. *Environmental Science & Technology, 38*, 4049–4055.

Wu, F. (2008). A tale of two commodities: How EU mycotoxin regulations have affected US tree nut industries. *World Mycotoxin Journal, 1*(1), 95–101.

Monosodium Glutamate in Foods and its Biological Effects

Kalapanda M. Appaiah

Food Safety and Analytical Quality Control Laboratory, Central Food Technological
Research Institute, Mysore, India

13.1 INTRODUCTION

Monosodium glutamate (MSG) is a flavor enhancer in foods. In 1908, Kikunae Ikeda, a Japanese scientist, was first to extract it from the seaweed *Laminaria japonica* and discover its flavor-enhancing properties (Ikeda, 1908). The chemical name is monosodium L-glutamate monohydrate ($C_5H_8NNaO_4.H_2O$) and it has a molecular weight of 187.13. It is a practically odorless, white crystalline powder. It is freely soluble in water, sparingly soluble in ethanol, and practically insoluble in ether. The arsenic and lead content in the product shall be not more than 2 and 5 mg per kg, respectively. The total heavy metal content shall be not more than 10 mg/kg (MSG Standard, 2007). Glutamate is naturally produced in human bodies and also exists in many of the foods we eat such as Parmesan cheese, tomatoes, mushrooms, walnuts, eggs, chicken, beef, pork, carrots, peas and other vegetables. MSG is created by fermenting starch, corn sugar or molasses from sugarcane or sugar beets. There are three types of commercial glutamates. The first type is when hydrolyzed protein is refined to approximately 99% glutamate, and the glutamate is identified on a label as monosodium glutamate. The second type is when the refinement of hydrolyzed protein contains less than 99% glutamate, and the product is called hydrolyzed protein product (HPP). The third type of MSG is created by adding protease enzyme to a product during processing. This kind of glutamate production does not require disclosure (US FDA). MSG is the sodium salt of the non-essential amino acid L-glutamic acid (L-GA) and is the most abundant amino acid found in nature. It exists both as free glutamate and bound with other peptides and proteins. Glutamate is also produced in the body and plays an essential role in human metabolism. It has been calculated that a man weighing 70 kg has a daily glutamic acid intake of 28 g that is derived from his diet and from the breakdown of gut proteins. The body cannot distinguish between glutamate added to foods and those naturally occurring in foods. The body produces an average of 50 g of free glutamate for the body to metabolize daily. It stimulates taste buds and brings out the flavor in food. However, MSG does not enhance the flavors of all foods and is more effective when added to foods such as poultry, seafood, meats and many vegetables.

13.2 THE UMAMI TASTE

In nature, there are three umami substances: MSG, disodium 5'-guanosine monophosphate (GMP), and disodium 5'-inosine monophosphate (IMP). These umami substances are present in abundance in various foods including vegetables (tomato, potato, cabbage, mushroom, carrot, soybean, green tea); seafood (fish, kelp, seaweed, oyster, prawn, crab, sea urchin, clam and scallop); meat and cheese; and contribute greatly to the characteristic tastes of these foods. There are four basic tastes namely sweet, sour, salty and bitter. The umami taste is the fifth taste which is unique (Kumiko, 2002). The hypothesis is that glutamate taste sensors may be glutamate receptors bearing structural and pharmacological similarities to those characterized in the brain (Brand, 2000). Glutamate taste transduction may involve one or more receptors that are similar, but probably not identical, to brain glutamate receptors (Brand, 2000). The neuronal glutamic acid is released by many stimuli and can be measured *in vitro* and *in vivo* by microdialysis. There are two major groups of glutamate receptors: ionotropic and metabotropic. The ionotropic receptors include the α-amino-3-hydroxy-5-methyl-4-isoxazole propionate (AMPA) receptors containing $iGluR_1$ and $iGluR_4$ subtypes, kainate receptors ($iGluR_5$, $iGluR_7$ and KA_1 KA_2 subtypes) and N-methyl-D-aspartate (NMDA) receptors (NR_1, NR_{2A-D}, NR_3 subtypes). AMPA and kainate receptors mediate fast excitatory synaptic transmission and are associated with voltage-independent channels that gate a depolarizing current carried by an influx of Na^+ ions (Cotman *et al.*, 1995). The NMDA receptor activation results in the development of a relatively slow rising, long-lasting current mediated primarily by the influx of Ca^{++} ions. The metabotropic receptors are coupled to intracellular second messengers via G protein and fall into three groups as follows: the first group contains $mGluR_{1a,b,c}$ and $mGluR_{5a,b}$; the second group contains $mGluR_{2,3}$; and the third group contains $mGluR_{4,6,7,8}$ (Nakanishu & Masu, 1994). The response to umami substances such as MSG is independent of other basic tastes (Kenzo & Makoto, 1998). Remarkable synergism between MSG and IMP or GMP has been reported (Kuninaka, 1967). The umami taste fulfills the basic taste concepts such as: 1) a characteristic taste that is clearly different from any other basic taste; 2) it is not reproduced by mixing the other basic taste stimuli; and 3) it is a universal taste induced by components of many foods.

MSG influences the expression of the strain difference in MSG acceptance in mice. There are two hypotheses which explain umami taste transduction (Brand, 2000). One states that umami is transduced by an N-methyl-D-aspartate (NMDA)-type glutamate ion channel receptor; the other that this taste is transduced via a metabotropic-type glutamate receptor. Chaudhari, Landin, and Roper (2000) discovered that the L-glutamate taste receptor, taste-mGluR$_4$, regulated the so-called firing of taste receptor cells. Sodium in MSG may activate the glutamate to produce the umami effect (Hegenbart, 1992). Umami acts as a flavor partner, flavor layer, flavor balance, and flavor catalyst in foods. The results of an experiment conducted on humans indicate that the high glutamate and low glutamate in saliva groups did not differ in the parameters of taste such as electro-gustometric thresholds, rated intensity of the MSG samples and pleasantness of distilled water, and the lower MSG concentrations. The low glutamate saliva group rated the higher MSG concentrations as more unpleasant (Scinska-Bienkowska, Wrobel, & Turzynska, 2006). It was also reported that a chemical stimulus such as in umami substances (MSG) is first adsorbed by receptor membrane in the taste buds. This evokes a receptor potential in receptor cells, ending in the release of a chemical transmitter which, in turn, triggers an impulse in one of the nerves mediating gustatory sensitivity. Successive brain relays convey the message to the primary and secondary cortex where it is processed and recognized (Bellisle, 1999). MSG in small amounts in a low sodium product can make it taste as good as its high salt content. This makes the food acceptable.

13.3 MSG IN HUMAN AND ANIMAL METABOLISM

Glutamate occupies a central position in human metabolism. It comprises between 10 and 40% by weight of most proteins and can be synthesized *in vivo*. Glutamate supplies the amino group for the biosynthesis of other amino acids, is a substrate for glutamine and glutathione synthesis, and is the key neurotransmitter in the brain as well as an important energy source for certain tissues. Hormones are exposed to dietary glutamate from two main sources: either from ingested dietary protein or by the ingestion of foods containing a significant amount of free glutamate which can be naturally present or added in the form of MSG/hydrolyzed protein. Dietary glutamate is absorbed from the gut by an active transport system into mucosal cells where it is metabolized as a significant energy source. Glutamic acid is transformed in the intestinal mucosal cells to alanine, and in the liver to glucose and lactate (Stegink et al., 1979). Intestinal tissues are responsible for the significant metabolism of dietary glutamate and glutamine (Munro, 1979). Very little dietary glutamate actually reaches the portal blood supply. The net effect of this is that plasma glutamate levels are only moderately affected by the ingestion of MSG and other dietary glutamates. It is only when very large doses (>5g MSG) are ingested will significant increases occur in plasma glutamate concentrations. In general, foods providing metabolizable carbohydrates significantly attenuate peak plasma glutamate levels at doses up to 150 mg/kg body weight. Breast milk concentrations of glutamate are influenced by the ingestion of MSG. Although glutamate is an important neurotransmitter in the brain, the blood–barrier effectively excludes passive influx of plasma glutamate. The ingestion of large amounts of (>3g) of MSG in the absence of food may be responsible for provoking symptoms similar to Chinese Restaurant Syndrome (CRS) in a small number of individuals. As MSG is always consumed in the presence of food, such incidences are not reported. There is no evidence that MSG is a significant factor in causing systemic reactions resulting in severe illness or mortality. Glutamic acid is metabolized in the tissues by oxidative deamination or by transamination with pyruvate to yield oxaloacetic acid which, via alpha-ketoglutarate, enters the citric acid cycle (Meister, 1965). Glutamate metabolism involves decarboxylation to gamma-aminobutyrate (GABA) and amidation to glutamine (Meister, 1979). Decarboxylation to GABA is dependent on pyridoxal phosphate, a coenzyme of glutamic acid decarboxylase, as is glutamate transaminase. Vitamin B6-defficient rats have elevated serum glutamate levels and delayed glutamate clearance. Glutamate is absorbed from the gut by an active transport system specific for amino acids. This process is saturable, can be competitively inhibited, and is dependent on sodium ion concentration (Schultz, Yu-Tu, Alvafez, & Currans, 1990). During intestinal absorption, a large proportion of glutamic acid is transaminated and consequently, alanine levels in portal blood are elevated. If large amounts of glutamate are ingested, portal glutamate levels increase. This elevation results in increased hepatic metabolism of glutamate, leading to the release of glucose, lactate, glutamine and other amino acids into systemic circulation (Steginck, Filer, Jr., & Baker, 1983). Glutamic acid in dietary protein together with endogenous protein secreted into the gut is digested to free amino acids and small peptides, both of which are absorbed into mucosal cells where peptides are hydrolyzed to free amino acids and some of the glutamate is metabolized. As a consequence of the rapid metabolism of glutamate in intestinal mucosal cells and the liver, systemic plasma levels are low, even after ingestion of large amounts of dietary protein. Oral administration of high doses of glutamate results in elevated plasma levels. The plasma glutamate levels are dose and concentration dependent. An increase in concentration of MSG from 2 to 10% in neonatal rats caused a five-fold increase in plasma. Age related differences between neonates and adults were also observed and the plasma levels were higher in infants than adults. The plasma levels of glutamate were markedly lower when MSG was fed to mice along with infant formula than with water. Similar effects of food on glutamate absorption and plasma levels have been observed in humans. As mentioned

earlier, dietary carbohydrates result in a lower rise in plasma levels. Carbohydrates provide pyruvate as a substrate for transamination with glutamate in mucosal cells so that more alanine is formed and less glutamate reaches the portal circulation (Steginck et al., 1983). Infusion of MSG into pregnant rhesus monkeys at a rate of 1 g/hr led to a 10–20-fold increase in maternal plasma glutamate, but fetal levels remained unchanged. In vitro perfusion studies using human placenta indicated that the placenta served as an effective metabolic barrier to the transfer of glutamic acid (Schneider, Moehlenkii Challier, & Danicis, 1979). Studies conducted to understand the effect on the blood–brain barrier revealed that the glutamate levels are far higher in brain than in plasma in mice, rats, guinea pigs and rabbits. Efflux of glutamate from the brain has been reported to be seven times greater than influx, reflecting biosynthesis in brain. The transport rate of glutamate from blood to the brain is much lower than basic amino acids. The blood–brain barrier which controls the type of molecules that enter the brain does not allow the passage of glutamate, so that the brain has to make its own glutamate from glucose and other amino acids. Normal plasma glutamate levels are nearly four times the Michaelis-Menten constant (Km) of the transport rate to the brain, so that glutamate transport systems are virtually saturated under physiological conditions (Pardridge, 1979). In animal experiments, brain glutamate increased significantly only when plasma levels were 20 times basal values, following an oral dose of 2g MSG/kg body weight. L-glutamate and GABA act as excitatory and inhibitory transmitters, respectively, in the central nervous system. Glutamate is also involved in the synthesis of proteins. Glutamic acid is an excitory neurotransmitter, suggesting that the precursors of neurotransmitter glutamic acid are glucose, glutamine and/or L-ketoglutarate (Shank & Aprison, 1979).

Glutamate acts as a co-substrate in the transamination and deamination of several amino acids. These reactions provide a carbon skeleton for glucogenesis or ATP generation (Brosnan,

2000). Glutamate is important in intracellular nitrogen transfer reactions whereas the opposite is true for glutamine (i.e. the amino acid appears to have as a focus the shifting of nitrogen among cells and organs) (Watford, 2000). The placenta utilizes glutamate as an important source of energy (Battagalia, 2000). The placenta accounts for >60% of the total fetal glutamate disposal rate. The fetal liver has been identified as the key provider of glutamate, although placenta is fully capable of utilizing maternal-derived glutamate. In the brain, the endogenous glutamate functions as an excitatory neurotransmitter (it causes depolarization of neurons). The dietary glutamate (MSG) might also be excitotoxic to brain neurons (Meldrum, 1993). Potent mechanisms that strictly compartmentalize the amino acid locally exist within the brain. The glutamate present in and used by the brain as a neurotransmitter has been found to be synthesized within neuronal, and actively removed from the synapse to be recycled to neurons in nonneurotransmitter (Daikhin & Yudkoff, 2000). The low rate of glutamate penetration combined with the occurrence in brain of the metabolic machinery for compartmentalizing the actions of glutamate evidently affords great protection to brain neurons from accidental or purposeful vagaries in systemic and local brain glutamate concentrations (Walker & Lupien, 2000).

13.4 NUTRITIONAL STUDIES

Nutritional studies in rats have shown glutamic acid to be a non-essential amino acid that is required in substantial amounts to ensure high growth rate in rats. The free amino acid pools in the tissues constitute about 70 g in adults, of which the major components are alanine, glutamic acid, glutamine and glycine. The daily turnover of glutamic acid in a man weighing 70 kg has been estimated as 4800 mg (Munro, 1979). Human plasma contains 4.4–4.5 mg/l of free glutamic acid and 9 mg/l of bound glutamic acid. Total glutamate in organs and tissues are 6000 mg in muscles, 2250 mg in brains, 680 mg in kidneys, 670 mg in livers and 40 mg in plasma. The free glutamic acid in human milk is 300 mg/l. However, cow's milk contains just 30 mg/l glutamic acid. The daily intake of free glutamic acid in a breast-fed infant has been estimated to be about 36 mg/kg body weight, which is equivalent to 46 mg/kg body weight as MSG. High levels of glutamic acid are found in cantaloupe (0.5 g/kg) and grapes (0.4 g/kg). Daily intake of free and bound glutamate in breast-fed 3-day-old infants was 1.1 g bound and 0.115 g free. Infants aged 5–6 months receiving 500 g cow's milk and two jars baby food per day would have a daily intake of 4 g bound and 0.075 g free glutamic acid equivalent to 0.62 g/kg body weight of glutamic acid. The mean daily intake of MSG of individuals over 2 years of age has been estimated as 100–225 mg per capita. Stable isotope studies show that dietary glutamate is a major energy source for the intestines, accounting for half of the energy consumed during digestion (Reeds, Burrin, Stoll, & Jahoor, 2000). Nutritional status in humans or animals is a strong determinant of food preferences (Booth & Davis, 1973). Aversions are created following a single exposure to a new food whose ingestion precedes the development of digestive malaise. By contrast, preferences develop for the sensory qualities of substances whose ingestion predicts satiety or the repletion of a specific nutrient. It has been established that the rats' preference for the umami taste is dependent upon nutritional status. A deficiency in one of the essential amino acids in an ingested protein restricts the utilization of this protein to the level of the limiting amino acid which can compromise growth (Leung & Rogers, 1987). It was reported that rats fed a diet deficient in lysine do not prefer MSG solutions. Severe protein malnourished rats prefer NaCl as well as glycine sources (Leung, Rogers, & Harper, 1968). After animals are re-fed a balanced amino acid diet, and recover from amino acid deficiency, the preference for umami tasting substances reappears. MSG enhances taste sensitivity to NaCl (Yamaguchi & Kimizuka, 1979). Addition of MSG did augment the intake of target foods. After admission to a renutrition center, protein malnourished children displayed greater preference for vegetable soup fortified with MSG (Vazquez, Pearson, & Beauchamp, 1982). Glutamate can be a helpful contribution to the diet of elderly people by making many foods more appetizing and appealing. Food-derived glutamate is required together with cysteine and glycine for the production of glutathione—an antioxidant molecule that plays an important role in the body's defense mechanism.

13.5 TOXICOLOGICAL STUDIES

L-glutamic acid was not mutagenic when tested against *Salmonella typhimurium* strains TA98, TA100, TA1537; and *Saccharomyces cerevisiae* in the presence or absence of S-9 mix (Litton Bionetics, 1977). An amount of 2% of intra-arterial sodium glutamate increased epileptic fits and intracisternal L-glutamic acid caused tonic-clonic convulsions in animals and humans. An intraperitoneal injection of MSG at a level of 3.2 g/kg body weight caused reversible blockage of beta waves in the electroretinogram in immature mice and rats indicating retinotoxicity (Potts, Modrell, & Kingsbury, 1960). Glutamate treatment decreases glutaminase activity and increases glutamic aspartate transaminase activity. Subcutaneous injection of L-monosodium glutamate at 4–8 g/kg into mice caused retinal damage with ganglion cell necrosis. Degradation of neonatal mouse retina has been reported following parenteral administration of MSG. It was reported that there was irreversible damage to neurons in the arcuate nucleus and rapid cell necrosis in mice. Similar results were also observed in guinea pigs and birds. Long-term studies in mice fed with 1 or 4% L-glutamic acid and monosodium L-glutamate

in their diet did not show any malignant tumors after 2 years (Little, 1953). The induction of brain lesions may highly depend upon the administration route of MSG. It was demonstrated that the transient accumulation of glutamate in the arcuate nucleus of the hypothalamus was attained following the forerunning elevation of plasma glutamate after a single subcutaneous injection of MSG to mice, indicating that this might relate to the selective destruction of arcuate neurons. This also suggests that the plasma glutamate concentration over a certain level is necessary to induce brain lesions (Yuichi, Seinosake, Masamiche, & Makoto, 1977). Studies have shown that the body uses glutamate as a nerve impulse transmitter in the brain and that there are glutamate-responsive tissues in other parts of the body as well. Abnormal function of glutamate receptors has been linked with certain neurological diseases, such as Alzheimer's disease and Huntington's chorea. Injections of glutamate in laboratory animals have resulted in damage to nerve cells in the brain. However, consumption of glutamate along with food did not cause this effect. The glutamate receptors are present in the central nervous system as the major mediators of excitatory neurotransmission and excito-toxicity (FAO/WHO, 2006). Subcutaneous injections of glutamic acid in infant mice caused degeneration of neurons in the inner layers of the retina (Lucas & Newhouse, 1957). Neuron lesions are also observed in the brain, particularly in the arcuate nucleus of the hypothalamus (Olney, 1969). Perinatal MSG treatment significantly attenuated fasting-induced reductions in heart rate and oxygen consumption in rats. This effect was specific to reduced caloric availability, since MSG-treated rats exhibited an intact capacity to both increase and decrease in heart rate, and oxygen consumption in response to cold and thermoneutrality (Michelina, Stephanie, Steven, & Michael, 2005). It has been demonstrated that high concentrations of monosodium glutamate (4 mg/kg body weight) in the central nervous system induce neuronal necrosis and damage in retina and circumventricular organs (Ortiz, Bitzer, & Quintero, 2006). This concentration was also toxic to liver and kidneys in rat experiments.

13.6 MSG SENSITIVITY

MSG sensitivity is a sensitivity to free glutamic acid that occurs in foods as a consequence of a manufacturing process. Virtually all proteins contain bound glutamic acid, but only when glutamic acid has been freed from protein prior to ingestion do MSG-sensitive people react. The MSG sensitivity is also known as Chinese Restaurant Syndrome (CRS), and the symptoms include burning tightness and numbness. MSG-sensitive people also show reactions ranging from simple skin rashes to severe depression and life-threatening physical conditions. The reactions are dose-related and vary from person to person and diet and cumulative effect. There is considerable evidence to suggest that consumption of MSG places humans at risk and that the greatest risk is faced by children. It is reported that MSG may be linked to brain tumors and neurodegenerative diseases such as ALS, Alzheimer's disease, and Parkinson's disease (Andreas & Pullanipally, 2000).

13.7 HEALTH EFFECTS ON INFANTS

MSG has been shown to cause lesions on the brain especially in children. These lesions cause cognitive, endocrinological and emotional abnormalities. In children, excess glutamate affects the growth cones on neurons. Growth cones are vital in laying down chemical pathways in the brain to enable the brain to operate effectively. Studies show that rats who had been fed MSG since birth could not escape mazes or discriminate between stimuli as well as non-MSG fed rats. The implications for children are that MSG could seriously affect their cognitive skills and cause learning difficulties (Leber, 2008).

13.8 OTHER EFFECTS

Independent research has identified adverse effects such as headaches/migraines, lethargy, sleepiness, anxiety, panic attacks, mental confusion, insomnia, nausea, diarrhea, stomach cramps, irritable bowel syndrome, bloating, asthma, shortness of breath, running nose, sneezing, and dryness of mouth (Leber, 2008).

13.9 SAFETY EVALUATION OF MSG

The US FDA has confirmed that the use of MSG is safe for the general population and it has classified MSG as GRAS. The safety aspects were reviewed by the American Medical Association (AMA), the Joint FAO/WHO (1988) Expert Committee on Food Additives (JECFA), and the Scientific Committee for Food of the European Union (SCF, 1991); and the conclusion was similar to JECFA. JECFA concluded that the total dietary intake of glutamates arising from their use at levels necessary to achieve the desired technological effect and from their acceptable background in foods do not represent a hazard to health. MSG has been allocated an ADI not specified by JECFA, which indicates that no toxicological concerns arise when used as a food additive in accordance with good manufacturing practices (GMPs). For that reason, the establishment of an acceptable daily intake (ADI) was not deemed necessary. JECFA reported that the intestinal and hepatic metabolism results in elevation of MSG levels in systemic circulation only after extremely high doses given by gavage (>30 mg/kg body weight). Human infants metabolized glutamate similar to adults. Ingestion of MSG was not associated with elevated levels in mother's milk and glutamate did not pass the placental barrier. In

2003, the Food Standards Australia New Zealand (FSANZ)[1] reaffirmed the safety of MSG. Total intake of glutamate from food in European countries ranged from 5 to 12 g/day. A maximum intake of 16 mg/kg body weight is regarded as safe (Beyreuther, Biesalski, & Fernstrom, 2007).

13.10 LABELING ISSUES

The US FDA recommends labeling of foods which contain MSG in the ingredient list (FR 57467, 1992). The Australia New Zealand Food Standards Code requires that MSG and other glutamates (monopotassium L-glutamate, calcium di-L-glutamate, monoammonium L-glutamate, magnesium di-L-glutamate) to be specifically declared by their name or code number in the ingredient list when they are added to food as flavoring. This is because the Federation of American Societies for Experimental Biology (FASEB, 1995) has reported that an unknown percentage of the population may be prone to MSG symptom complex. This is done to protect public health and safety, to enable consumers to make informed choices, and to prevent misleading or deceptive conduct. The Joint FAO/WHO Codex Alimentarius Commission has included MSG under GSFA[2] provisions for use in food in general except infant formulae, follow-up formulae, formulae for special medical purposes for infants, and complementary foods for infants and young children (FAO/WHO, 2007).

13.11 FUTURE PERSPECTIVES

Today's rapid global industrialization, urbanization, and changing life styles have spurred increased consumption of processed foods and foods prepared in restaurants. These foods may contain substantial amounts of MSG. As a result, people of all age groups who live in cities are continuously exposed to MSG and MSG sensitivity has been reported as Chinese Restaurant Syndrome (CRS). Adverse health effects such as neurodegenerative diseases, brain lesions, and retinal damage were also observed in animal experiments. Toxicity of any chemical to humans and animals is dose related. Present dietary habits may result in MGS intake levels and serum glutamate levels being several times higher than the threshold limits, with potential deleterious effects on humans. Admittedly, there is a need to investigate the long-term effects of continuous exposure to MSG on people from a global perspective. As stated above, Codex does not allow MSG in infant formulas, follow-up formulae, and formulae for special medical purposes for infants and young children (FAO/WHO, 2005). Several countries in the world have also recommended labeling of packaged foods containing MSG. Under this situation, there is an urgent need for international organizations and federal governments to re-evaluate the safety of MSG for consumers, taking present dietary patterns and intake levels into consideration. Risk analysis may be done based on the prevailing food habits of vulnerable subgroups in the population.

References

Andreas, P., & Pullanipally, S. (2000). Glutamate transport and metabolism in dopaminergic neurons of substantia nigra: implications for the pathogenesis of Parkinsons disease. *Journal of Neurology*, 247(14), 1125–1135.

Battagalia, F. C. (2000). Glutamine and glutamate exchange between the fetal liver and the placenta. *The Journal of Nutrition*, 130, 974S–977S.

Bellisle, F. (1999). Glutamate and umami taste: sensory, metabolic, nutritional and behavioural considerations.

[1] Food Standards Australia New Zealand, June, http://www.foodstandards.govt.nz/standardsdevelopment/notificationcirculars/current/notificationcircular2182.cfm.

[2] General Standard for Food Additives (CODEX STAN 192-1995, Table 3).

A review of the literature published in the last 10 years. *Neuroscience and Biobehavioral Reviews, 23,* 423–438.

Beyreuther, K., Biesalski, H. K., & Fernstrom, J. D. (2007). Consensus meeting: monosodium glutamate: An update. *European Journal of Clinical Nutrition, 61,* 304–313.

Booth, D. A., & Davis, J. D. (1973). Gastro-Intestinal factors in the acquisition of oral sensory control of satiation. *Behavioral Biology, 11,* 23–29.

Brand, J. G. (2000). Receptors and transduction processes for Umami taste. *The Journal of Nutrition, 130,* 942S–945S.

Brosnan, J. T. (2000). Glutamate at the interface between amino acid and carbohydrate metabolism. *The Journal of Nutrition, 130,* 988S–990S.

Chaudhari, N., Landin, A. M., & Roper, S. D. (2000). A metabolic glutamate receptor variant functions as a taste receptor. *Nature Neuroscience, 3*(2), 113–119.

Cotman, C. W., Kahle, J. S., Miller, S. E., *et al.* (1995). Excitory amino acid neurotransmission. In F. E. Bloom & D. J. Kupfer (Eds.), *Psychopharmacology: The Fourth Generation of Progress* (pp. 75–85). New York, NY: Raven Press.

Daikhin, Y., & Yudkoff, M. (2000). Compartmentalization of brain glutamate metabolism in neurons and glia. *The Journal of Nutrition, 130,* 1039S–1042S.

FAO/WHO. (2005). CAC/STAN 192–199, Rev. 6.

FAO/WHO. (1988). Joint Expert Committee on Food Additives (JECFA). L-glutamic acid and its ammonium, calcium monosodium and potassium salts. WHO Food Additive Series 32, Toxicological Evaluation of Certain Food Additives, Geneva.

FAO/WHO. (2006). Join Expert Committee on Food Additives. A report on the toxic effects of the food additive monosodium glutamate. Presented by John Erb of Canada.

FAO/WHO. (2007). 30th Session of the Codex Alimentarius Commission.

FASEB. (1995). *Analysis of adverse reactions to monosodium glutamate (MSG), Report.* Washington, DC: Life Sciences Research Office, Federation of American Societies for Experimental Biology.

Hegenbart, S. (1992). Flavor enhancement: Making the most of what's there. *Prepared Foods, 159*(2), 83–84.

Ikida, K. (1908). Method of producing a seasoning material whose main component is the salt of glutamic acid. Japanese patent No. 14,805.

Kenzo, K., & Makoto, K. (2000). Physiological studies on umami taste. *The Journal of Nutrition, 130,* 931S–934S.

Kumiko, N. (2002). Umami. A universal taste. *Food Revue Internationale, 18*(1), 23–38.

Kuninaka, A. (1967). A flavor potentiator. In H. W. Schultz, E. A. Day, & L. M. Libbey (Eds.), *The Chemistry and Physiology of Flavors* (pp. 517–535). Washington: AVI Publications.

Leber, M. J. (2008). Umami and MSG controversy: Cooks know the power of taste but are the ingredients safe? *Food Market Place Review,* 1–4.

Leung, P. M. B., Rogers, Q. R., & Harper, A. E. (1968). Effect of amino acid imbalance on dietary choice in the rat. *The Journal of Nutrition, 95,* 483–492.

Leung, P. M. B., & Rogers, Q. R. (1987). The effect of amino acids and protein on dietary choice. In Y. Kawarmura & M. R. Kare (Eds.), *Umami, a basic taste.* (pp. 565–610). New York: Marcel Dekker.

Little, A. D. (1953). Report submitted to International Mineral and Chemical Corporation dated 13 January 1953, submitted to WHO in 1970.

Litton Bionetics. (1977). Mutagenic evaluation of compound FDA 75-65, L-glutamic acid.HCl. US Department of Commerce, National Technical Information Sciences, P.B. 266, 889.

Lucas, D. R., & Newhouse, J. P. (1957). The toxic effect of sodium l-glutamate on the inner layer of retina. *American Medical Association Archives of Ophthalmology, 58,* 193–201.

Meister, A. (1965). *Biochemistry of the Amino Acids* (Vol. 1 and 2) (2nd edn). Academic Press.

Meister, A. (1979). Biochemistry of glutamate, glutamine and glutathione. In L. J. Filer, S. Garattini, M. R. Kare (Eds.), *Glutamic Acid: Advances in Biochemistry* (pp. 69–84). New York, USA: Raven Press.

Meldrum, B. (1993). Amino acids as dietary excitotoxins: a contribution to understanding neurodegenerative disorder. *Brain Research Reviews, 18,* 293–314.

Michelina, M. M., Stephanie, A. E., Steven, J. S., & Michael, O. J. (2005). Perinatal MSG treatment attenuates fasting—induced bradycardia and metabolic suppression. *Physiology & Behavior, 86,* 324–330.

MSG Standard (2007). GB/T8967-2007. Linghua International (Hongkong) Co. Ltd. E-1 Building Bihai Shanzhuang No. 254 East Hongkong Road, Quingdao, China.

Munro, H. N. (1979). Factors in regulation of glutamate metabolism. In F. J. Filer, Jr., S. Garattine, M. R. Kare (Eds.), *Glutamic Acid: Advances in Biochemistry and Physiology* (pp. 55–68). New York, NY: Raven Press.

Nakanishi, S., & Masu, M. (1994). Molecular diversity and functions of glutamate receptors. *Annual Review of Biophysics and Biomolecular Structure, 23,* 319–348.

Olney, J. W. (1969). Brain lesions, obesity and other disturbances in mice treated with monosodium glutamate. *Science (Washington, DC), 164,* 719–721.

Ortiz, G. G., Bitzer, O. K., & Quintero, C. (2006). Monosodium glutamate-induced damage in liver and kidney: a morphological and biochemical approach. *Biomedical Pharmatherapy, 60,* 86–91.

Pardridge, W. M. (1979). Regulation of amino acid availability to brain; Selective control mechanisms for glutamate. In L. J. Filer, S. Garattini, M. R. Kare (Eds.),

Glutamic Acid: Advances in Biochemistry (pp. 125–137). New York, USA: Raven Press.

Potts, A. M., Modrell, R. W., & Kingsbury, C. (1960). Permanent fractionation of the electroretinogram by sodium glutamate. *American Journal of Ophthalmology, 50*, 900–907.

Reeds, P. J., Burrin, D. G., Stoll, B., & Jahoor, F. (2000). International glutamate metabolism. *The Journal of Nutrition, 130*, 978S–982S.

SCF. (1991). Reports of the Scientific Committee for Food on a first series of food additives of various technological functions. Commission of the European Communities Reports of the Scientific Committees for food, 25th Series. Brussels, Belgium.

Schneider, H., Moehlenkii Challier, J. C., & Danicis, J. (1979). Transfer of glutamic acid across the human placenta perfused *in vitro*. *British Journal of Obstetrics and Gynaecology, 86*, 299–306.

Schultz, S. G., Yu-Tu, L., Alvafez, O. O., & Currans, P. F. (1970). Dicarboxylic aminoacid influx across brush border of rabbit ileum. *The Journal of General Physiology, 56*, 621–639.

Scinska-Bienkowska, B. A., Wrobel, E., & Turzynska, D., (2006). Glutamate concentration in whole saliva and taste responses to monosodium glutamate in Humans. *Nutritional Neuroscience, 9*(1/2), 25–31.

Shank, R. P., & Apison, M. H. (1979). Biochemical aspects of the neurotransmitter function of glutamate. In L. J. Filer, S. Garattini, M. R. Kare (Eds.), *Glutamic Acid: Advances in Biochemistry* (pp. 139–150). New York, NY: Raven Press.

Stegink, L. D., Filer, L. J., Jr., Baker, G. L. et al., (1979). Factors affecting plasma glutamate levels in normal levels in normal adult subjects. In L. J. Filer, S. Garaltini, M. R. Kare (Eds.), *Glutamic Acid: Advances in Biochemistry* (pp. 333–351). New York, NY: Raven Press.

Stegink, L. D., Filer, L. J., Jr., & Baker, G. L. (1983). Plasma amino acid concentrations in normal adults fed meals with added monosodium L-glutamic and aspartame. *The Journal of Nutrition, 113*, 1851–1860.

Vazquez, M., Pearson, P., & Beauchamp, G. K. (1982). Flavor. Preference in malnourished Mexican infants. *Behavior, 28*, 513–519.

Walker, R., & Lupien, J. (2000). The safety evaluation of monosodium glutamate. *The Journal of Nutrition, 130*, 1049S–1052S.

Watford, M. (2000). Glutamate at the interface between amino acid and carbohydrate metabolism across the liver sinusoid. *The Journal of Nutrition, 130*, 983S–987S.

Yamaguchi, S., & Kimizuka, A. (1979). Psychometric studies on the taste of monosodium glutamate. In L. J. Filer, S. Garaltini, M. R. Kare (Eds.), *Glutamic Acid: Advances in Biochemistry and Physiology* (pp. 35–54). New York, NY: Raven Press.

Yuichi, O., Seinosake, I., Masamiche, I., & Makoto, S. (1977). Effect of administration routes of monosodium glutamate on plasma glutamate levels in infant, weanling and adult mice. *The Journal of Toxicological Sciences, 2*(3), 281–290.

14

Food Packaging Legislation: Sanitary Aspects

Gisela Kopper[1] and Alejandro Ariosti[2]

[1]University of Costa Rica, San José, Costa Rica

[2]INTI (National Institute of Industrial Technology), Plastics Center, Buenos Aires, Argentina

14.1 INTRODUCTION

14.1.1 Scope

This chapter will cover the legislation and regulations applying to the sanitary aspects of food contact materials (FCMs), a category of objects that usually comprises packages, articles and generic materials intended to come into contact with foodstuffs. Legislation on labeling (except cases related directly to sanitary aspects of FCMs) and metrology of packaged foodstuffs is beyond the scope of this chapter. See Chapter 17 (Nutrition and Bioavailability: Sense and Nonsense of Nutrition Labeling) for a wider discussion on labeling.

Along with legislative aspects of food packaging, this chapter includes information on FCMs that may be used for the development of international regulations.

14.1.2 Food-packaging-environment Interactions

Interactions between a foodstuff, its package, and the environment to which it is exposed during storage, have been extensively studied. An effort to understand the physicochemical principles involved and thus being able to control these interactions, results in the assurance of a longer product shelf-life, improved food nutritional and sensory quality, and better consumer health protection.

The main interactions for each type of packaging materials are briefly described below.

14.1.2.1 Plastics and Elastomeric Materials

Plastic and elastomeric materials intended to come into contact with foodstuffs are composed mainly of the **basic polymer** or **resin** and **non-polymeric components**. Resins include polyethylene (PE), polypropylene (PP), polystyrene (PS), polyvinyl chloride (PVC), polyethylene terephthalate (PET), etc. in the case of plastics; and natural and synthetic rubber, nitrile rubber, thermoplastic elastomers (TPE), etc. in the case of elastomeric materials.

Non-polymeric components generally consist of:

a) **polymerization residues** such as monomers, oligomers, solvents, emulsifiers, etc.
b) **additives**, which are substances intentionally added to the basic polymer to facilitate the manufacture of commercial materials or articles (stabilizers, antioxidants, etc.), and/or to impart to them certain technical and desired final properties (impact modifiers, plasticizers, pigments, colorants, etc.). Though some polymers can be used as additives to the basic polymer in low percentages, their probability of migrating into the foodstuffs is generally considered as negligible.

Polymers are rather inert, in the sense that the macromolecular chains of high molecular weight or molecular mass form a polymer matrix in the FCMs and do not migrate to the contained foodstuff. In the case of thermoplastic materials (e.g. polyethylene, polypropylene, polystyrene, PVC, PET, etc.), the principal ways in which the polymeric chains interact with each other to form the matrix are mechanical entanglements in the amorphous regions and crystal formation in the crystalline regions; both types of interactions being non-covalent in nature. In the case of thermoset materials (e.g. epoxy resins, polyurethanes, unsaturated polyesters, etc.), those interactions are covalent bonds between the main macromolecules.

Generally, non-polymeric components are low molecular weight substances that, depending on contact time(s) and temperature(s), may migrate into foodstuffs. It is important to note that the US Food and Drug Administration (FDA) regulate both basic polymers and their additives as 'indirect food additives.'

The main food-package-environment interactions in these materials are:

- **Permeability or permeation**: transfer of gases, water vapor and aromas, from the environment to the foodstuff or *vice-versa*, through the package or container wall.
- **Migration**: transfer of non-polymeric components from the package or container wall to the contained foodstuff or to the environment. From the sanitary point of view, only migration into the foodstuff is important, and consequently, these are the substances to be determined quantitatively, by means of analytical validated methods.
- **Sorption or negative migration**: dissolution of major food components (e.g. water, oil, fat, blood, etc.) or minor food components (e.g. aromas, essential oils, etc.) into the package or container wall. The first case is known as 'swelling' which normally alters the polymeric matrix and the second case is known as 'scalping' which does not normally alter the polymeric matrix.
- **Desorption or re-migration**: transfer of sorbed substances from the package or container to a product during refilling (in the case of refillable plastic packages) or in the packaging of foods in packages or containers manufactured with recycled materials. The sorbed substances may be food components as mentioned above; but also potentially harmful substances such as pesticides, herbicides, cleaning agents, etc., associated with misuse of the package or container by the consumer.

These are submicroscopic physicochemical phenomena, involving mass transfers that do not require a macroscopic discontinuity in the plastic or elastomeric material (pore, micro-pore, fracture or crack), due to a diffusion mechanism, and can be predicted by Fick's laws (Catalá & Gavara, 2002; Hernández & Gavara, 1999; Katan, 1996).

In brief, it is very important for package designers, FCMs manufacturers, food processors, public or private laboratories, researchers and public health authorities to study and measure:

- **permeability**: in the design of packages and prediction of shelf-life of packaged foodstuffs;
- **migration**: to establish compliance with food safety regulations;
- **sorption and desorption**: to evaluate whether refillable plastic packages and recycled plastic materials intended to come into contact with foodstuffs, comply with food safety regulations.

14.1.2.2 Metallic Materials (Tinplate, Tin-Free Steel, Aluminum)

14.1.2.2.1 Corrosion A galvanic cell develops when two metals acting as electrodes (e.g. tin and iron, in the case of tinplate), and the canned foodstuff acting as an electrolyte, come into contact; due to, for example, discontinuities in the tin coating and the polymeric lacquer or varnish. A redox pair of reactions takes place, leading to the oxidation of the metal with a more negative potential (normally tin, dissolving as Sn^{2+}); and thus protecting the metal with a less negative potential (inert electrode-normally iron). The oxidation process releases electrons, and the electron flow in the metal surface corresponds to an ion flow in the foodstuff (Robertson, 1993).

Sometimes, the nature of canned foodstuff produces the inversion or depolarization of the electrodes, changing the pattern of the oxidation. In the case of tinplate, under a depolarized corrosion process, tin does not protect the iron base, which dissolves into the product (as Fe^{2+}).

In aluminum and tin-free steel (TFS) (electrolytic—also referred to as chromium coated steel, ECCS) cans, aluminum (Al^{3+}) and chromium (Cr^{3+}) ions, respectively, appear in the foodstuff due to corrosion.

The consequences of the presence of these ions are mostly sensory changes in the products: metallic taste, sulphide-black stains (by Sn^{2+} and Fe^{2+}), discoloration of anthocyanins by Sn^{2+} in canned vegetables and fruits, etc. The use of a thicker metal (tin or chromium) coating and the use of polymeric sanitary lacquers or varnishes on the internal surface of the metallic can help to diminish, but not to completely eliminate, the corrosion process.

As another consequence of the corrosion process, some impurities in the basic metals can contaminate the food. Heavy metals and metalloids (arsenic (As), cadmium (Cd), mercury (Hg), lead (Pb), etc.) are of special toxicological interest in canned foodstuffs. Food regulations establish maximum levels for these elements and for tin (Sn) in food products.

14.1.2.3 Glass and Ceramics

14.1.2.3.1 Lixiviation The most common type of glass used in food packaging is soda-lime glass. Its basic ingredients are: vitreous silicon oxide (SiO_2); alkaline oxides (mainly of sodium (Na) and potassium (K)) to lower the working temperature in the glass-melting furnace; and alkaline-earth oxides (mainly of calcium (Ca), magnesium (Mg), and elements of higher nuclear charges or 'valences') to stabilize the glass structure and prevent excessive dissolution of glass into water or aqueous solutions. Recycled glass, known as cullet, is commonly used in high percentages (up to 70–80%) in the manufacture of soda-lime glass. It is very important to control the source of cullet, in order to keep the heavy metals and metalloids content as low as possible.

In soda-lime glasses, the chemical bond to oxygen (O) in the case of Si-O is covalent in nature, and quite strong. The ionic bonds Na-O or K-O are weaker in comparison. When glass comes into contact with water or acidic or basic solutions, as in the case of foodstuffs and beverages, Na^+ and K^+ ions are involved in a mass transfer process associated with an interchange of charged species. These ions migrate from the package or container glass wall to the foodstuff in contact; and protons (H^+) or hydrated protons ($H^+.H_2O$) enter the vitreous mass, altering its

structure and resulting (to a certain degree) in its dissolution. The greater the amount of alkali in soda-lime glass the less resistant it is to chemical attack (it has lesser hydrolytic resistance).

In the case of divalent ions (e.g. Ca^{2+} and Mg^{2+}) or higher valence ions, the ionic bonds to oxygen are stronger than in the case of the monovalent alkaline ions, and their migration is lower.

This process of differential migration of charged species through the interface glass-foodstuff is usually called 'lixiviation'.

In the case of glazed glass, ceramics or metals, vitreous enamels or glazes are used to coat the food-contact surface. These glazes are also glasses, but with the difference that some substances are used to impart a special transparency or color, to modify the viscosity of the glaze during the coating process, or to lower its melting temperature. These substances are commonly lead and cadmium oxides, and therefore the main regulations establish specific migration limits for these ions in the case of glazed glass, ceramics or metals.

Non-glazed porous ceramics are generally forbidden in the manufacture of food packages and containers (Mari, 2002).

Crystal glasses (containing a minimum of 10% of lead and barium oxides) and lead crystals (containing a minimum of 24% of lead oxide) are used in the manufacture of high-quality tableware or hollowware intended for brief contact times with foodstuffs. However, they are generally forbidden for the manufacture of food packages, due to the potential migration of lead during longer contact times (MERCOSUR, 1992).

14.1.2.4 Cellulose-Derived Materials (Paper, Paperboard, Cardboard)

14.1.2.4.1 Extraction Cellulose-derived materials, mainly paper, paperboard and cardboard, are manufactured with pulp (mechanical, semi-chemical, chemical, etc.) from wood, sugar cane bagasse, and other natural resources.

The composition of cellulose-derived materials include first-use cellulose fibers (primary fibers), recycled cellulose fibers (secondary fibers), as well as synthetic fibers (plastic fibers), various types of additives (including pigments) and inorganic fillers. The fibers bind together with the aid of additives, to form a cellulose matrix or network, with pores, whose diameters can be reduced by applying mechanical operations, thus rendering the cellulose substrate less permeable to gases, water vapor, water and fat. Sizing agents and oil repellents are also used to improve resistance to the penetration of water and grease.

Cellulose-derived materials are basically intended to come into direct contact with dry solid foodstuffs. Nevertheless, if food, water, or fat come into contact with the cellulose substrate, they can penetrate through the pores by capillarity, changing the cellulose network and resulting in the migration of additives, fillers and fiber fragments into foods. This process is called 'extraction'.

Due to the higher residues of heavy metals, dioxins, pentachlorophenol and PCBs in cellulose materials manufactured with recycled fibers (Söderhjelm & Sipiläinen-Malm, 1996), their use is generally restricted to applications for dry foods without surface fat (MERCOSUR, 1999). As in glass, it is very important to control the source of recycled fibers, in order to keep these contaminants as low as possible (Council of Europe, 2005; USFDA, 2008b).

Another point to consider is the migration of volatile compounds from the cellulose substrates to foodstuffs (Söderhjelm & Sipiläinen-Malm, 1996). Preventive sensory analysis is a very useful tool to avoid taint problems of this kind.

14.1.3 Importance of Evaluating and Controlling the Interactions

In summary, every type of FCM interacts with the contained foodstuffs. The general

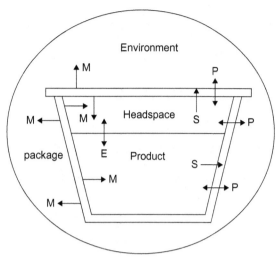

P : Permeability
M : Migration (General)
S : Sorption
E : Headspace-product Equilibrium

FIGURE 14.1   Main food-packaging-environment interactions.

phenomenon is called 'migration', though, as described, the mechanisms involved in the mass transfer vary, depending on the type of material.

A schematic summary of these interactions can be seen in Figure 14.1 and Table 14.1.

Elements and substances migrated from FCMs to foodstuffs are ingested by the consumer. Therefore, to control the migration phenomenon, a realistic risk-exposure evaluation is of vital importance (Arvidson, Cheeseman, & McDougal, 2007; Oldring, 2007), making legislation on FCMs necessary.

14.1.4 Hygienic Requirements of Food Contact Materials

The hygienic requirements of packages and materials intended to come into contact with foodstuffs should be established by specific regulations, depending on the application.

TABLE 14.1   Main migrations in FCMs

Migrants	Examples	FCMs
Gases and vapors	ethylene monomer	polyethylene
	vinyl chloride monomer	PVC
	acetaldehyde	PET
	solvents	plastic laminates, printed substrates, coated substrates
Ions	Na, K, Li, Ca, Mg	glass
	Pb, Cd	glazed ceramics, glasses and metals
	Pb	Crystals, lead crystals
	Sn, Fe	tinplate
	Al	aluminum
	Cr	TFS (ECCS), stainless steel
Liquids and solids of low molecular weight	additives	Plastics, varnishes or lacquers, coatings, elastomers, paper and board, regenerated cellulose

14.1.4.1 Basic Hygienic Requirements of FCMs

In particular plastic FCMs have been the subject of ample hygiene regulations in the past decades.

Some of the concepts described below for plastic FCMs can, with precaution, be extrapolated to other types of materials.

To have a general understanding of these hygienic requirements, two similar legislations on plastic FCMs were reviewed: the European Union and the Common Market of the south (MERCOSUR, Mercado Común del Sur) in South America. The hygienic requirements can be summarized as follows (Ariosti, 2002a):

- **Positive lists:** the basic polymer or resin (MERCOSUR), or its monomer(s) and other starting components (European Union),

and the additives used are regulated by positive lists of authorized substances. These lists are restrictive, and mandatory. Available positive lists contain substances that have been submitted to a process of risk assessment, mainly biological assays. Their use is considered safe for FCMs applications, sometimes subject to specific restrictions.

- **Overall, global or total migration limit(s):** maximum quantities of non-polymeric components transferred from a plastic FCM to the foodstuffs or corresponding food simulants. To verify the compliance of the plastic FCM with these limit(s), overall migration tests must be performed, according to standardized and validated methods using foods or preferably their simulants, under various contact time(s) and temperature(s).

A simulant is a substance or a simple mixture of substances that during the migration tests, under standardized conditions of contact time(s) and temperature(s), has an interaction with a plastic FCM, considered equivalent to that of a foodstuff or a group of foodstuffs. Aqueous non-acidic, aqueous acidic, alcoholic and fatty simulants are described in legislations and standards.

The overall migration limits (OMLs) are expressed in the following units:

- mg of non-polymeric components/kg of food or simulant;
- mg of non-polymeric components/dm^2 of surface area of FCM.

- **Specific migration limit(s):** maximum quantities of a particular non-polymeric component (monomer or additive) transferred from a plastic FCM to the foodstuffs or food simulants. To verify the compliance of the plastic FCM with these limit(s), specific migration tests must be performed, as described above. To the same end, calculations of the potential migration of the specific migrant (assuming a 100% transfer to the foodstuff or simulant), or predictions of its migration using a validated mathematical model, based on Fick's laws of diffusion, are allowed.

The specific migration limits (SMLs) are expressed in the following units:
- mg of non-polymeric component migrated/kg of food or simulant.

- **Concentration limit(s)**: maximum quantity of the substance (monomer or additive) allowed in the very plastic FCM. To verify the compliance of the plastic FCM with these limit(s), no specific migration tests are performed, because the determination of the concentration of the substance is done on the plastic FCM directly.

The concentration limits, QM (quantity in material) and QMA (quantity per surface area) are expressed in the following units:

- mg of non-polymeric component/kg of FCMs (QM);
- mg of non-polymeric component/6 dm^2 of surface area of FCMs (QMA).

- **Group limit(s)**: there are also three additional and interesting (though difficult to use) types of limits: the group migration limits (SML(T)); and the group concentration limits (QM(T) and QMA(T)).These are the maximum allowed quantities of related substances that belong to a common chemical group (e.g. isocyanates, glycols, etc.).

The group limits are expressed in the following units:

- mg of non-polymeric components migrated with the same chemical group/ kg of food or simulant (SML(T));
- mg of non-polymeric components with the same chemical group/kg of FCMs (QM(T));
- mg of non-polymeric components with the same chemical group/6 dm^2 of surface area of FCMs (QMA(T)).

The analytical difficulty mentioned above can be illustrated with the following example: if several substances with the glycol group (ethylene glycol, diethylene glycol, and stearic acid esters with ethylene glycol) are used in a given plastic FCM formulation, and the positive list establishes an SML(T) for them, the specific migration of each substance must be determined. Subsequently, the specific migration results must be added, and the obtained value must be compared with the SML(T) to verify that the FCM complies with the legislation.

- **Sensory characteristics of the foodstuffs**: the color, aroma, taste, flavor and texture of the foodstuffs must not be adversely affected by migration of neither regulated substances nor non-intentionally added substances (NIAS). Regulated substances are compounds that are included in the positive lists and therefore in the original formulation of the plastic FCM. Non-intentionally added substances are compounds that appear as artifacts of the manufacture process of the plastic FCM, or are impurities of regulated substances, etc.

Taint problems affecting packaged foods can be studied by instrumental analysis (GC or GC/MS), sensory analysis (e.g. ISO Standard 13302:2003 or IRAM Standard 20021:2004), or by combined techniques such as olfactometry. These techniques are very useful for the prevention and correction of taint problems (Fernández & Cacho, 2002).

- **Other requisites:** other requirements, however, may also be established:
  - regulated use of a substance in certain types of plastics;
  - regulated use of a substance in plastics in contact with certain types of foodstuffs;
  - purity criteria for certain substances.

14.1.4.2 *Pigments and Colorants*

Requisites on pigments and colorants for plastic FCMs have been established, for instance, by the European Union, MERCOSUR, and the USA.

14.1.4.3 Functional Barriers, Threshold of Regulation and Food Grade Recycled Materials

In the final FCM, **non-intentionally added substances** (NIAS) may also appear. These substances may largely be impurities and/or isomers of the regulated components; compounds that appear as artifacts of the manufacture process of the plastic FCM; potential contaminants present in recycled materials (Ariosti, 2002b; Bayer, 1997, 2002; Castle, 2007; Franz, Bayer, & Welle, 2003, 2004a, 2004b; van Dongen *et al.*, 2007; Welle & Franz, 2007); components of inks on promotional labels and painted toys which are used as a marketing tactic inside food packages (Ariosti, 2002b), etc.

In order to have better control over these unknown, or non-regulated or poorly regulated substances that can appear in foods as a result of their migration, the concept of functional barriers has been developed. It is now a well-established theoretical tool with technological applications, described in the US-FDA regulations since 1995 with the introduction of the Threshold of Regulation (TOR); in the European Union legislation (Directive 2002/72/EC on plastic FCMs); and in the MERCOSUR legislation (Resolution GMC (Common Market Group) 25/99 on trilayer PET soft-drinks bottles containing recycled PET, and Resolution GMC 30/07 on food grade recycled PET (covering multilayer and monolayer bottles)) (Ariosti, 2002b; Bayer, 1997, 2002; Franz *et al.*, 2003; Franz, Bayer, & Welle, 2004a; Franz, Mauer, & Welle, 2004b; Welle & Franz, 2007).

In a multilayer plastic package, a **functional barrier** is a layer (Ariosti, 2002b; Bayer, 1997, 2002; Franz *et al.*, 2003, 2004a, 2004b; Welle & Franz, 2007) that:

- is generally in contact with the foodstuff;
- separates it from an outer layer of the plastic package that may have been manufactured with non-regulated substances or that can retain potential contaminants (after a process of decontamination and recycling);

- is efficient in reducing the migration of these substances to the foodstuff, during its shelf-life, to quantities that neither pose any toxicological risk to human health nor alter the nutritional and sensory characteristics of the foodstuff.

According to Article 7a of Directive 2002/72/EC (EU, 2002a), the key quantity that defines when a substance (not classified as carcinogenic, mutagenic or toxic to reproduction) poses no toxicological risk to human health is a migration value no greater than 0.01 mg substance/kg of food or simulant (10µg/kg) measured with statistical certainty by a validated method. In a multilayer plastic FCM with a functional barrier, such substance (even if it is not included in the positive list) can be used in the manufacture of a layer that is not in contact with a foodstuff, provided that the final FCM complies with the overall and specific migration limits established for the regulated substances used in its formulation.

This last value has not been explicitly included in the European Union Regulation (EC) 282/2008 (EU, 2008a) on recycled plastic materials and articles intended to come into contact with foods. Article 4 (c) (ii) states that:

> 'it must be demonstrated in a challenge test, or by other appropriate scientific evidence that the (recycling) process is able to reduce any contamination of the plastic input to a concentration that does not pose a risk to human health.'
>
> EU, 2008a

One possible interpretation is that this concentration in the output plastic material, by analogy with the case of a multilayer FCM, must not allow a migration resulting in a concentration in the foodstuff of more than 10µg/kg of potential contaminants.

In the case of the FDA (1995, 2006) that key quantity is the Threshold of Regulation (TOR), defined as 0.5µg of the substance/kg human diet. With certain assumptions, two parameters can be derived from the TOR:

- one parameter comparable to a QM, a maximum quantity of the substance per kg of plastic;
- one parameter comparable to an SML, a maximum specific migration of the substance per kg of food or simulant.

In the case of recycled food grade PET, the values of these parameters are, respectively, 220 µg/kg of plastic and 10 µg/kg of food or simulant.

If a manufacturer can demonstrate to the FDA that a substance present in a FCM ends up in the human diet in quantities below the TOR, or complies with its derived parameters, it is considered a component of non-toxicological concern, and therefore, it is not a food additive.

It is important to note that the end points for contaminant migration in the US and European legislations are the same (10 µg/kg of food or simulant), though they differ in their conceptual basis.

During the development of the MERCOSUR legislation (Resolution 30/07 on food grade recycled PET), the FDA approach was followed, thus adopting both the derived parameters from the TOR.

14.2 FOOD CONTACT MATERIALS LEGISLATION IN THE EUROPEAN UNION

In the EU, two types of FCMs legislation coexist: the harmonized EU legislation; and the national legislations of the Member States that apply only in the fields not harmonized at the EU level (Heckman, 2005; Schäffer, 2007). In this chapter, only the EU legislation on FCMs is discussed.

In the EU, FCMs legislation was enacted to overcome possible technical barriers to trade between the Member States, and comprises mainly of two types of legal instruments: Directives and Regulations. The former come into the Member States National Legislations only after a process of transposition (internalization), and can have deadlines up to 18 months; the latter can be implemented immediately.

The authorization of FCMs substances undergoes a risk assessment process guided by the European Food Safety Authority (EFSA, 2008; EU, 2002b), followed by a risk management decision from the EU Commission or the Council of the European Union and the European Parliament. Within the EFSA, a Scientific Committee is formed by the presidents of the technical–scientific commissions or panels and six independent experts. As of July 2008, there are 11 technical–scientific commissions or panels responsible for the scientific studies; one being the CEF Panel on FCMs, enzymes, flavorings and processing aids.

The EFSA's final resolutions are given to comply with EU regulations, as a response to requests from the EU Commission, the European Parliament, a Member State, or in some cases on its own initiative.

In cases of justified urgency due to an imminent risk to human or animal health, EFSA takes the necessary measures to give a fast response to an appeal. EFSA has a high transparency in all of its activities, and makes all of its resolutions public, as well as those of the scientific-technical commissions and the results of scientific studies performed.

In summary, at the EU level, FCMs and articles are regulated by (EU, 2008c, e):

- Regulation (EC) No 1935/2004, which establishes general requirements for all FCMs, and is considered the framework Legislation for all of them;
- Regulation (EC) No 2023/2006 on good manufacturing practices for materials and articles intended to come into contact with food;
- Legislation on specific materials covering groups of materials and articles listed in the Framework Regulation;

- Directives on individual substances or groups of substances used in the manufacture of materials and articles intended for food contact.

Detailed information on FCMs research and analysis is available on the website for the Contact Materials Group at the Joint Research Centre (JRC) in Ispra (Italy): http://crl-fcm.jrc.it/index.php?option=com_content&task=view &id=31&Itemid=62.

14.2.1 Framework EU Legislation on FCMs

In November 1976, the EU Commission adopted a framework Directive which established the general principles for all FCMs and objects, as well as criteria and procedures which should be followed for the elaboration of specific Directives such as those for plastics, ceramics, etc., and for specific substances such as vinyl chloride monomer in PVC (Robertson, 1993).

Historically, the aforementioned framework Directive 76/893/EEC (EU, 1976), established the principle that all materials and objects intended to come into contact directly or indirectly with foodstuffs, must not transfer any of their constituents to the food product in quantities that could endanger human health and produce an unacceptable change in the composition of the foods or alter their sensory characteristics (Heckman, 2005; Robertson, 1993; Schäfer, 2007). It also introduced the principle of 'positive labeling', according to which all FCMs and articles (with exceptions), must indicate the words 'for food' or an appropriate symbol, such as the one defined in Directive 80/590/EEC (EU, 1980; Robertson, 1993) (see Figure 14.2).

In 1989, the framework Directive was substituted by Directive 89/109/EEC (EU, 1989) in which 10 material groups were defined for further EU Regulations and specific Directives. The specific Directives must include the positive lists which comprise of authorized materials and

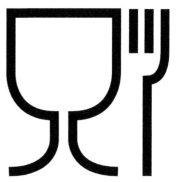

FIGURE 14.2 European Community Symbol for labeling of food contact materials and objects.

substances; purity criteria for some substances as well as conditions for its use; specific migration limits for certain components (mainly when a TDI has been established); and a total migration limit for these components to the foods. This Directive also establishes the guidelines for sampling and analytical methods of control.

Besides mandatory labeling (with exceptions) of the materials and articles intended to come into contact with foods, these must be accompanied by a written certificate called the 'Declaration of compliance' from the manufacturer, which indicates that they comply with the applicable regulations.

Directive 89/109/EEC (EU, 1989) was substituted in October 2004 by Regulation (EC) 1935/2004 (EU, 2004a) of the European Parliament and Council, therefore converted into European Law. As of July 2009, this Regulation is the last framework Legislation generated on FCMs by the European Union and considers the general requisites for active and intelligent food packaging (EU, 2008b, c).

This inclusion represents a change in approach while accepting that certain beneficial components may be transferred from the packaging to the food to enhance its preservation and control.

Regulation (EC) 1935/2004 sets mechanisms to ensure traceability of FCMs at all stages in the production chain, to facilitate the control and recall of products and to identify responsibilities. Special consideration is given to Good Manufacturing Practices when producing FCMs that comply with specifications and the important role of the food industry to cooperate with national authorities for product recall.

It also establishes a list of materials that can generate specific EU regulations. The list includes 17 different materials and packaging systems (e.g. active and intelligent materials) and, as of July 2009, only a few of them are covered by harmonized EU regulations (plastics, ceramics, regenerated cellulose and rubber teats and soothers).

It is important to remember that, whereas no EU Legislation exists, each Member State may apply its own National Legislation, following the general rules described in Regulation (EC) 1935/2004 (EU, 2004a). The FCMs thus cleared in the harmonized and non-harmonized fields can be commercialized in the whole EU under the principle of mutual recognition (Heckman, 2005; Schäfer, 2007).

14.2.2 EU Legislation on Specific FCMs

14.2.2.1 *Plastics*

Plastic materials and objects were the first materials covered by the EU harmonization. Even though this harmonization is not yet complete, several regulations exist at the national and EU level.

Directive 2002/72/EC about plastics covers monolayer and multilayer plastic structures. Multilayer structures made up with non-plastic materials, such as composite cartons for beverage packages, are not included in this Directive. In these cases, the National Laws are applied, where in general, it is required that every layer complies with the specific material regulation and the overall structure complies with Regulation (EC) 1935/2004. Nevertheless, Directive 2007/19/EC allows the use of plastic layers formulated

with non-approved substances that do not comply with specific restrictions when they are separated from the food by a plastic functional barrier in a way that the material or finished object complies with the specific and total migration limits. The above-mentioned substances must be non-carcinogenic, non-mutagenic and non-toxic to reproduction (EU, 2008d).

Directive 2002/72/EC contains a harmonized positive list of monomers and starting substances for the production of plastic materials and articles, and an incomplete list of additives for plastics materials; where applicable, the lists include specific restrictions (mainly specific migration limits (SMLs), maximum residual levels in the material (QMs), restrictions of use, etc.). It also includes lists of substances that can be provisionally used at the national level, pending EFSA's evaluation and final opinion. This Directive also establishes an OML of 60 mg of substances/kg of foodstuff or food simulants or 10 mg/dm^2 of surface area of the FCMs for all substances migrating from a material into foodstuffs. Finally, the Directive includes procedures for updating and completing the lists of authorized substances (EU, 2008d).

As of July 2009, Directive 2002/72/EC has been amended by (EU, 2008d, e):

- *Directive 2004/1/EC* which suspends the use of the blowing agent azodicarbonamide as of 2 August 2005.
- *Directive 2004/19/EC* (EU, 2004b) which updates the positive lists of authorized substances and establishes that the list of authorized additives will become a positive list, setting specified deadlines.
- *Directive 2005/79/EC* (EU, 2005a) which updates the positive lists of authorized substances.
- *Directive 2007/19/EC* which establishes requisites for phthalates in gaskets in lids, and introduces a fat consumption reduction factor to be considered in the migration tests and the functional barrier concept.

It also updates the positive lists of authorized substances and confirms the prohibition of the use of azodicarbonamide in the manufacture of expanded plastic materials and articles.

- *Directive 2008/39/EC* which updates the list of authorized substances used in the manufacture of plastic materials and articles intended to come into contact with food, and clarifies the criteria for the removal of an additive from the provisional list. It also establishes that the EU list of additives becomes a positive list on 1 January 2010. This means that after this date only those additives listed will be permitted for the manufacture of plastic FCMs in the EU. However, substances on the provisional list may continue to be used subject to National Laws after that date until a final decision is taken on their possible inclusion in the positive list of additives. This provisional list includes all additives under present evaluation by EFSA and for which a petition was submitted in December 2006.

Council Directive 82/711/EEC establishes the basic rules necessary for testing migration of the components of plastic materials and articles intended to come into contact with foodstuffs. It has been amended by *Directive 93/8/EEC* and *Directive 97/48/EC* (EU, 2008e).

Council Directive 85/572/EEC (EU, 1985) originally established the simulants to be used for testing migration of components of plastic materials and articles intended to come into contact with foodstuffs, and has been amended by *Directive 2007/19/EC*. These Directives, in combination with *Council Directive 82/711/EEC* amended by *Directive 93/8/EEC* and *Directive 97/48/EC*; and with *Directive 2002/72/EC* amended by *Directive 2007/19/EC*, have established in detail the nature of the present food simulants and the basic rules for migration tests (EU, 2008e).

Food simulants representing the different extraction properties of foods or group of foods are defined. The main simulants used to verify the migration limits of plastic FCMs are:

(a) aqueous non-acidic simulant: distilled water;
(b) aqueous acidic simulant: acetic acid 3% (w/v) in aqueous solution;
(c) alcoholic simulants: ethanol 10% (v/v) in aqueous solution, or ethanol in solutions at higher concentrations;
(d) fatty foods simulants: rectified olive oil, or alternatively a mixture of synthetic triglycerides or sunflower oil.

In the latter case (d), in order to make the migration tests easier, *substitute fatty foods simulants* can be used, such as ethanol 95% (v/v) in aqueous solution, or isooctane, or MPPO (modified polyphenylene oxide).

Council Directive 85/572/EEC amended by *Directive 2007/19/EC*, presents a table in which the established simulants correspond to different foods or groups of foods. The food list is ample and comprises of beverages, cereals, chocolate products, sugars and confectionery products, fruit and vegetables, fats and oils, animal and dairy products, amongst others. One interesting point is that in the last amendment, the simulant assigned to milk is an aqueous solution of ethanol 50% (v/v).

Commission Regulation (EC) No 372/2007 establishes transitional migration limits for plasticizers in gaskets in lids intended to come into contact with foods. It has been amended by *Commission Regulation (EC) No 597/2008* (EU, 2008e).

Regulation (EC) 282/2008, as previously mentioned in this chapter (see section 14.1.4.3, Functional barriers), establishes requisites on recycled plastic materials and articles to be used in FCMs, requisites about the manufacture processes of recycled material and final packages and articles, and an authorization procedure of recycling processes used in the manufacture of recycled plastics for food contact use (EU, 2008a, e).

14.2.2.2 Ceramics

Ceramics are regulated by *Council Directive 84/500/EEC* as amended by *Directive 2005/31/EC* (EU, 2005b). The heavy metals oxides used in the production of ceramic articles intended to come into contact with foods may pose a risk for the consumer. Lead and cadmium are of major concern, due to the possibility of their release from decoration and/or glazing enamels, so specific migration limits for these elements are given in the Directives. Analytical methods for the determination of the specific migration of these elements are provided. It is mandatory to present a declaration of compliance as specified in Regulation (EC) 1935/2004 (EU, 2008e; Schäfer, 2007).

14.2.2.3 Regenerated Cellulose

Regenerated cellulose films are regulated by *Directive 93/10/EEC* amended by *Directive 93/111/ EC*, *Directive 2004/14/EC* and *Directive 2007/42/ EC* (EU, 2007b). Synthetic regenerated cellulose casings are excluded and must comply with the corresponding national regulations. A positive list for the production of *Cellophane*® films is given, but does not include pigments, inks or adhesives (EU, 2008e; Schäfer, 2007).

14.2.3 EU Legislation on Individual Substances

Some specific Directives have been sanctioned regarding the toxicity of vinyl chloride monomer (VCM), its presence as a residue into the materials and objects manufactured from polymers or copolymers of this monomer, such as PVC, and its possible migration to foodstuffs. *Council Directive 78/142/EEC* (EU, 1978) establishes a QM of 1 mg VCM/kg in the finished product and an SML of 0.01 mg VCM/kg of food or food simulant. *Directive 80/766/EEC* and *Directive 81/432/ EEC* lay down, respectively, the methods of analysis of VCM levels in materials and articles which are intended to come into contact with foodstuffs, and of VCM specific migration into foodstuffs or simulants (EU, 2008e).

Directive 93/11/EEC establishes maximum levels for the release of N-nitrosamines and N-nitrosatable substances from rubber teats and soothers (EU, 2008e; Schäfer, 2007).

For coatings, plastics and adhesives of epoxy base, specific migration limits are given in *Regulation 1895/2005* (EU, 2005c) for substances of toxicological concern (epoxy derivatives) such as BADGE (Bisphenol A Diglycidyl Ether), BFDGE (Bisphenol F Diglycidyl Ether) and NOGE (Novolac Glycidyl Ethers). For BADGE and its hydrolysis products BADGE. H_2O and BADGE.$2H_2O$, a group migration limit of 9 mg/kg of food or food simulant is given; for BADGE.HCl, BADGE.2HCl and BADGE.H_2O.HCl, a group migration limit of 1 mg/kg of food or food simulant is given; whereas BFDGE and NOGE are prohibited from use (EU, 2008e; Schäfer, 2007).

14.2.4 Active and Intelligent FCMs

Taking into consideration the new functions of active packaging and to ensure its safe application, the principle of inert materials was modified in Regulation 1935/2004 (EU, 2004a). Active FCMs and articles are intended to extend the shelf-life or to maintain or improve the condition of packaged food. They are designed to deliberately incorporate components that would release or absorb substances into or from the packaged food or the environment surrounding the food. On the other hand, intelligent FCMs and articles are intended to monitor the conditions of packaged food or the environment surrounding the food (Wilson, 2007).

Active materials may release substances to the food under certain circumstances. The released substances must be authorized in the Food Laws (as allowed additives or flavorings) according to the approved usage and quantities. Consumers must not be misled through changes in food or information given about the quality condition of food. Active and intelligent materials must be declared in the label, and special labeling shall identify non-edible parts such as sachets with absorbers, (e.g. oxygen or ethylene scavengers).

Discussions took place with all interested parties at the European Union level for further development of the basic requisites on active and intelligent materials already established by Regulation (EC) 1935/2004.

Finally, Regulation (EC) 450/2009 on active and intelligent materials intended to come into contact with food was sanctioned on 29 May 2009 (EU, 2009).

The main Articles are related to:

– definitions (Article 3);
– requisites for placing on the market of active and intelligent FCMs (Article 4);
– Community (EU) list of substances that may be used in active and intelligent components (Articles 5 to 8);
– specific labeling (Article 11). The non-edible parts or components must be labeled

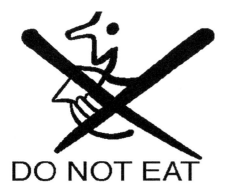

DO NOT EAT

FIGURE 14. 3　European Community Symbol for labeling of non-edible parts or components of active and intelligent food contact materials.

with the words "DO NOT EAT", and always where technically possible, must be accompanied by the symbol reproduced in Figure 14.3;
– declaration of compliance with the regulations that apply (Article 12);
– requisites on supporting documentation (Article 13).[1]

14.3 FOOD CONTACT MATERIALS LEGISLATION IN THE UNITED STATES OF AMERICA

In 1938, the Federal Food, Drug and Cosmetic Act (FFDCA) was introduced, and with it the prohibition of unsafe foods and non-sanitary packages. The Food and Drug Administration (FDA) was also established then. But it was not until 1958, with the passage of the Food Additives Amendment Act, that the formal food packaging regulation in the USA was introduced (Heckman, 2005).

The Code of Federal Regulations (CFR) publishes the legal requirements of the USA, divided into titles or areas of control. Title 21 contains all of the general regulations to assure the compliance of the FFDCA and the Fair Packaging and Labeling Act (USFDA, 2008a). FCMs are regulated mainly in two acts: The Food Additives Amendment of the FFDCA of 1958 and the National Environmental Policy Act (NEPA) of 1969 (Robertson, 1993; Twaroski, Batarseh, & Bailey, 2007).

In 1958, the US Congress (1969) gave authority to the FDA to regulate food additives, defined as any substance whose intended use could result or reasonably is expected to result, direct or indirectly, as part of the food or affect

---

[1]A copy of the consultation documents including a copy of the draft EU Regulation is available online at: http://www.reading.ac.uk/foodlaw. G/SPS/N/EEC/340 is a Draft Commission Regulation by the Committee on Sanitary and Phytosanitary Measures—Notification—European Communities—Food contact materials. It can be found at: http://docsonline.wto.org/gen_home.asp.

its characteristics (FFDCA section 201). This definition excludes colorants, substances generally recognized as safe (GRAS), and prior sanctioned substances (whose use was accepted before 1958) (Twaroski *et al.*, 2007). Under this definition, FDA considers FCMs as indirect food additives (USFDA, 2007c).

As detailed in the FFDCA, a food additive is considered unsafe unless:

- it is subjected to an exemption, for instance if its migration to food is below the TOR;
- it is included in a regulation list (positive list); or
- it has an effective Food Contact Notification (FCN).

In addition, food additives in the USA must follow a pre-market evaluation before entering into interstate commerce. The FDA established the Division of Food Contact Notification and Review within the Office of Food Additive Safety, at the Center for Food Safety and Applied Nutrition (CFSAN), to ensure that components of FCMs, including food packaging and processing equipment, are safe for their intended use.

The approval process for a food additive begins with a petition and concludes in the publication of its regulatory use. The petition process is codified under Title 21 Part 171 of the CFR (USFA, 2002). The general and specific regulations for all food ingredients and packaging materials are established in Title 21 CFR Parts 170 through 189 (see Table 14.2).

One of the possible substitutions of a petition is the Threshold of Regulation (TOR) exemption process, established by FDA in 1995 (21 CFR 170.39). It exempts certain substances used in FCMs from the requirement of an authorizing regulation before its use. To obtain a TOR exemption, the estimated daily intake (EDI) of the substance must be less than or equal to 1.5 μg/person/day (or an equivalent of 0.5 μg/kg of food consumed). The substance must be non-carcinogenic and must not contain any carcinogenic impurity. Guidance for industry to submit a request for a

TOR exemption can be found at: http://www.cfsan.fda.gov/~dms/torguid.html. (USFDA, 2005).

In 1997, the Food and Drug Administration Modernization Act (FDAMA), amended the Federal Food Drug and Cosmetic Act (FFDCA) to renew the way in which the FDA conducted the approvals. One of the new procedures established to accomplish this goal was a notification process for food contact substances (FCSs). The amended FFDCA defined a FCS as 'any substance intended for use as a component of materials used in manufacturing, packing, packaging, transporting, or holding food if such use is not intended to have

TABLE 14.2 Title 21 of the US Code of Federal Regulations dealing with food contact materials

Part	Description
170	Food additives
171	Food additive petitions
172	Food additives permitted for direct addition to food for human consumption
173	Secondary direct food additives permitted in food for human consumption
174	Indirect food additives: General
175	Indirect food additives: Adhesives and components of coatings
176	Indirect food additives: Paper and paperboard components
177	Indirect food additives: Polymers
178	Indirect food additives: Adjuvants, production aids, and sanitizers
179	Irradiation in the production, processing and handling of food
180	Food additives permitted in food or in contact with food on an interim basis pending additional study
181	Prior-sanctioned food ingredients
182	Substances generally recognized as safe
184	Direct food substances affirmed as generally recognized as safe
186	Indirect food substances affirmed as generally recognized as safe
189	Substances prohibited from use in human food

a technical effect in such food' (CFSAN Office of Food Additive Safety, December 2007. Available at: http://www.cfsan.fda.gov/~dms/fcnbkg.html).

The FCN process is intended to replace the petition process as the primary means for authorizing new uses of food additives that are FCSs (21 CFR Sections 170.100 to 170.106). However, discretion is given to the FDA for deciding when the petition process is more appropriate for evaluating data to provide an adequate safety assurance.

A petition must be submitted to FDA for a FCS when the cumulative estimated daily intake (CEDI) is greater than 3 mg per person per day (or 0.6 mg per person per day for biocidal compounds), or when FDA has not reviewed bioassays which are not clearly negative for carcinogenic effects (Twaroski et al., 2007).

It shall be highlighted that, in contrast with the TOR exemption and the petition processes, the FCN process results in an authorization for only the notifier and the manufacturer or supplier listed (USFDA, 2007a, b). Besides, all FCN processes are subjected to NEPA regulations (Twaroski et al., 2007). FDA maintains a list of effective FCNs and TOR exemptions on its website: http://www.cfsan.fda.gov/dms/opa-fcn.html and http://www.cfsa.fda.gov/dms/opa-torx.html.

The limitations of use of a FCS may include the concentration limits in the FCM itself as well as the type of foods and time-temperature conditions under which these FCMs must be used. At 21 CFR 176.170 nine types of foods are described (fresh or processed) and classified as aqueous, acid, alcoholic and fatty foodstuffs. Conditions of use are also defined regarding thermal treatment and storage.

For the migration analysis, FDA recommends the use of different food simulants such as:

- ethanol 10% (v/v) in aqueous solution (with exceptions), for aqueous and acidic foods;
- ethanol 10% (v/v) or 50% (v/v) in aqueous solution, for low- and high-alcoholic foods (actual ethanol concentration may be used);
- edible oil (e.g. corn), HB307 or Miglyol 812 for fatty foods.[2]

The most important consideration with regard to the overall regulatory status of a FCM is the concern of the regulatory status of each individual component that comprises the FCM. The CFSAN has a food additive evaluation program that covers more than 3000 substances mentioned in Title 21 of CFR that may be considered as indirect additives. Special attention must be given to Part 175 (adhesives and coatings), Part 176 (paper and paperboard), Part 177 (Polymers) and Part 178 (Adjuvants, production aids and sanitizers), since all of them are substances that may come into contact with food as part of packaging or processing equipment.

14.4 FOOD CONTACT MATERIALS LEGISLATION IN JAPAN

Japan is a very important and demanding exporter of fresh and processed food which must be adequately conditioned, so it is of prime importance to be aware of the main features of its FCMs Legislation.

JETRO is the Japan External Trade Organization, a government-related agency. One of its main objectives is to promote and facilitate mutual trade and investment between Japan and the rest of the world.

Of particular importance are three documents published by JETRO in English version:

1. JETRO (2006a). **Food Sanitation Law in Japan.** This contains the Food Sanitation Law (Law No 233 dated 24-12-1947; last

---

[2]HB307 is a mixture of synthetic triglycerides (also accepted in the EU Legislation as fatty foods simulant), with fatty acid composition mainly corresponding to C_{12}, and also C_{10} and C_{14}. Miglyol 812 is a simulant derived from coconut oil.

amendment: Law No 87 dated 26-07-2005), the Food Sanitation Law Enforcements Ordinances and the Food Law Enforcements Regulations.

2. JETRO (2006b). **Specifications, Standards and Testing Methods for foodstuffs, implements, containers and packaging, toys, detergents.** Chapter II: Standards and Testing Methods for Implements, Containers and Packaging. This contains a detailed summary of standards and testing conditions specified in the section 'Implements, Containers and Packaging' of the Ministry of Health and Welfare Notice No 370, dated 28-12-1959, final version Ministry of Health and Welfare Notice No 499, dated 29-11-2005, which comply with Article 10 of the Food Sanitation Law.

3. JETRO (2007). **Specifications and Standards for Foods, Food Additives, etc., under the Food Sanitation Law (Summary).** Chapter IV: Apparatus and Containers/Packages. This summarizes standards and methodology for FCMs testing.

The Food Sanitation Law specifies general hygienic requirements on apparatus and containers/packages (as defined by Article 4) intended to come into contact with foodstuffs. The category 'apparatus' includes tableware, kitchen utensils and machine implements.

The objective of the Law, stated in Article 1, is the protection of human health from hazards arising from food consumption. The introductory Articles are outstanding in promoting science, education, training and industrial voluntary effort:

- **Article 2** summons the State to take measures through educational activities and public relations, in order to promote research relating to food sanitation, to improve control facilities, such as registered laboratories, concerning food sanitation, to train men of ability and to improve their talent.

- **Article 3** states that food and FCMs manufacturers shall make a voluntary effort to get knowledge and techniques relating to the safety of their products and to the practice of self-imposed examination.

In the regulated field, the Ministry of Health, Labor and Welfare (MHLW) is the risk management authority, and the Pharmaceutical Affairs and Food Sanitation Council is the risk assessment authority (JETRO, 2006a; Kawamura, 2008). FCMs manufacturers also apply voluntary standards issued by Industrial Hygienic Associations, such as the Japan Hygienic Olefin and Styrene Plastics Association (JHOSPA), the Japan Hygienic PVC Association (JHPA), and the Japan Hygienic Association of Vinylidene Chloride (JHAVC). For instance, JHOSPA Standards cover 29 types of plastic resins (Kawamura, 2008).

- **Article 25** of the Food Sanitation Law establishes a case by case obligatory approval system of food and FCMs that comply with the Legislation, and the obligatory use of a label stating that they passed the technical examinations performed by State or Registered Laboratories.
- **Article 26** establishes the procedures for official inspections of food and FCMs.

In the JETRO Document (3) previously cited (JETRO, 2007), different requisites on FCMs can be found, classified as standards on materials in general and standards by specific materials. In the last case, the following FCMs are covered: glass; ceramics; synthetic resins in general; specific plastics (PVC, PE, PP, PS, PVDC, PET, PMMA, PA, PMP, PC, PVA); phenolic, melamine, urea and formaldehyde resins; rubber (including nursing utensils); and metal cans.

The general OML in the case of resins, plastics, rubbers and coated cans is 30 mg/kg. If n-heptane is used as fatty foods simulant, the following OMLs apply:

- for PE and PP: 150 mg/kg;
- for PMP: 120 mg/kg;

- for PS: 240 mg/kg;
- for PVC: 150 mg/kg.

In October 2007, new specifications for PLA (polylactic acid), a biodegradable plastic, were established (Kawamura, 2008).

In the case of glass and ceramics, specific migration limits for cadmium and lead were established. There is a proposal to change these limits according to Standard ISO 6486:1999 in the case of ceramic ware, to Standard ISO 6486:1999 and Standard ISO 7086:2000 in the case of glassware and bottles, and to Standard ISO 4531:1998 in the case of enameled ware (Kawamura, 2008).

For metal cans, specific migration limits for arsenic and cadmium are established.

The FCMs Legislation establishes also standards by applications, specifically on pressure and heat-sterilized packaged foods (except canned and bottled foods); soft drinks (except fruit juice as ingredient) packages manufactured with glass, metal, plastics, and composite materials; automatic vending machines; and FCMs in contact with flavored ice and stock solutions of soft drinks. It is important to note that for some categories, mechanical properties specifications and performance requisites are established.

Finally, the FCMs Legislation specifies requisites on manufacturing standards and dairy products packages; in the last case, for milk, fermented milk, prepared milk powder, cream, etc.

An important work is being done for the revision of specifications and methodology. The Japanese Government is also engaged in the revision of the approval system from 2008 (Kawamura, 2008).

14.5 FOOD CONTACT MATERIALS LEGISLATION IN MERCOSUR

The Protocol of Ouro Preto (Brazil) (December 17, 1994) fixed the present institutional structure of MERCOSUR. The maximum decision-making political body is the Common Market Council (CMC), and the executive body is the Common Market Group (GMC). The Administrative Secretary has its headquarters in Montevideo, Uruguay.

The activities on FCMs Legislation are organized in the following hierarchical way (Padula & Ariosti, 2002):

- **Packaging Group**: which discusses and prepares drafts on technical issues;
- **Food Commission**: which coordinates the work of the Packaging Group and other Groups within the Commission (that deal with food contaminants, food additives, claims, etc.), and prepares Resolutions on FCMs and other food issues;
- **Working Sub-Group 3 (SGT 3)**: which coordinates the technical work of the Food Commission and other Commissions within the SGT 3 (that deal with pharmaceutical products, toys, etc.);
- **Common Market Group (GMC)**: which sanctions the Resolutions.

The harmonized GMC Resolutions must be transposed (incorporated) into the National Laws of the Member States. For example, in Argentina, they must be incorporated into the Argentine Food Code ('Código Alimentario Argentino' in Spanish); and in Brazil, in Federal Decrees ('Portarias' in Portuguese).

The harmonization work began in 1991 on the basis of the two main FCMs Legislations available in the region, the Argentine and Brazilian ones. Since 1991, one of the authors (Ariosti) has been participating within the Packaging Group–Food Commission, in technical discussions with his colleagues from other Member States, at the periodical meetings held in the four countries. The technical references are the EU and US-FDA FCMs Legislations. These are mainly used to periodically update the MERCOSUR FCMs Legislation.

The MERCOSUR FCMs Legislation is, in general, similar to the EU FCMs Legislation. This is due to the fact that the Argentine and Brazilian FCMs Legislations previous to MERCOSUR were both based on the FCMs Italian Legislation. But it is rather eclectic, because it also incorporates some concepts, such as the TOR, and certain positive lists of substances and their restrictions, such as those corresponding to rubber and paper and board, from the US-FDA FCMs Legislation.

The positive lists are transcribed from the EU and US-FDA FCMs Legislations. If a FCS is present in the positive lists of both Legislations, it enters the MERCOSUR positive list with the EU FCMs positive lists restrictions. For a new substance to be incorporated in the MERCOSUR FCM positive lists, it must be previously included in the FCMs positive lists of one of these two international references, or in those of European countries or other countries recognized by the MERCOSUR national sanitary authorities, after the opinion of the Packaging Group–Food Commission. In the case of the European Union, plastics additives not yet incorporated in the EU positive list, but legally used in the Member States, can be included in the MERCOSUR plastics additives positive list. The same applies in the case of certain substances covered by FCNs recognized by the US-FDA, and not included in the 21CFR positive lists.

The MERCOSUR Framework Resolution GMC 3/92 on FCMs establishes a pre-market approval of food packages and articles before its commercialization. It means that the manufacturer must demonstrate the compliance of their products with the Legislation, to the sanitary authorities, which then issue an approval/authorization certificate, case by case. At the same time, the food manufacturer must use only the food packages and articles already approved by the sanitary authorities. Since the 1980s, the system has been in full application in Argentina, even before the obligatory enforcement of the MERCOSUR Legislation (from 1995). Presently in Brazil, however, only the food packages and articles manufactured with recycled materials must be submitted to this system of pre-market approval (Padula & Ariosti, 2002; Ministry of Agriculture, 2006).

Mutual recognition of FCMs approval certificates issued by the national sanitary authorities of the Member States is working quite well (Padula and Ariosti, 2002). FCMs imported into Argentina and Brazil from other countries must comply with the MERCOSUR legislation. The pre-market approval requisites apply as in the case of national FCMs, as commented previously for both countries.

The main similarities with the EU FCMs Legislation are the existence of positive lists, OMLs ($50\,mg/kg$ and $8\,mg/dm^2$), QMs and SMLs. The MERCOSUR OMLs are rather similar to the US-FDA OMLs ($50\,mg/kg$ and $0.5\,mg/in^2$ ($=7.75\,mg/dm^2$)), and a little bit different from the EU OMLs ($60\,mg/kg$ or $10\,mg/dm^2$). These differences pose no practical problems if the analytical tolerances established by the EU Directive 2002/72/EC are taken into account.

As the GMC Resolutions are issued in Spanish or in Portuguese, to our knowledge, no English version is available yet. Since 1991 several GMC Resolutions have been sanctioned on the following issues:

- General criteria on FCMs hygienic requirements (Framework Resolution);
- Plastics;
- Metals (tinplate, TFS, aluminum, etc.);
- Cellulose based materials (paper, paperboard, cardboard);
- Glasses and ceramics;
- Elastomers;
- Regenerated cellulose (films and casings);
- Food coatings;
- Adhesives;
- Refillable PET bottles;
- Recycled post-consumer PET for food packages (mono and multilayer).

A more detailed reference can be found in Table 14.3, where only the last versions of the GMC Resolutions for each kind of FCMs appear (MERCOSUR, 2008; Ministry of Economy, 2008; Padula & Ariosti, 2002). The repealed GMC Resolutions are not referenced in Table 14.3, but can be found in the Internet sites mentioned in the references.

TABLE 14.3   MERCOSUR GMC Resolutions

Material	Subject	GMC Resolution No
General	Framework Resolution: general requisites for FCMs	3/92
	General requisites for positive lists up dating	31/99
	Reference analytical methodology for the control of FCMs	32/99
Plastic FCMs	General requisites	56/92
	Positive list of resins and polymers	24/04
	Positive list of additives	32/07
	Food and simulants classification	30/92, 32/97
	Overall migration methods	36/92, 10/95, 33/97
	Colorants and pigments	56/92, 28/93
	Method for the determination of residual vinyl chloride monomer content in PVC	47/93, 13/97
	Method for the determination of residual styrene monomer content in polystyrene	86/93, 14/97
	Method for the determination of specific migration of mono- and diethylene glycol	11/95, 15/97
	Fluorinated polyethylene	56/98
	Polymeric and resinous coatings for foods	55/99
	Refillable PET packages for carbonated non-alcoholic beverages	16/93
	Multilayer PET packages, with central layer containing recycled material, for carbonated non-alcoholic beverages	25/99
	Recycled PET for food packages (multilayer and monolayer packages)	30/07
Metallic FCMs	General requisites	46/06
Glass and ceramic FCMs	General requisites	55/92
Cellulose based FCMs (paper, paperboard and cardboard)	General requisites	19/94, 35/97, 20/00
	Positive list of components	56/97
	Overall migration method	12/95
	Papers for filtration and hot cooking	47/98
	Recycled cellulose fibers	52/99
Regenerated cellulose FCMs	Films	55/97
	Casings	68/00
Elastomeric FCMs	General requisites	54/97
	Positive list of components	28/99
Adhesives	General requisites	27/99
Paraffins for food contact	General requisites	67/00

Nomenclature: GMC Resolutions are referred to by the designation XX/YY, where XX is the GMC Resolution number and YY are the two last digits of the year of sanction.

14.5.1 Last Reviews and Novelties (2004–2010)

The last up date of the positive list of polymers for food contact plastics was finished in 2004, and was sanctioned as GMC Resolution 24/04. The MERCOSUR positive list for plastics regulates polymers, not monomers as the equivalent EU positive list. The update of this Resolution began in May 2009, as part of the Packaging Group–Food Commission activities program for 2009–2010.

The 1993 GMC Resolution on metallic packages was revised in 2006 and an up dated technical document was sanctioned as GMC Resolution 46/06.

The last up date of the positive list of additives for plastics (that incorporates the novelty of being in Spanish and Portuguese at the same time in one document) was finished in 2007, and was sanctioned as GMC Resolution 32/07.

In December 2007, the technical document on recycled post-consumer PET for food grade packages was sanctioned as GMC Resolution 30/07. It covers multilayer packages with functional barriers and monolayer packages (MERCOSUR, 2007).

The last technical harmonized document regarding colorants and pigments for plastic materials, finished in June 2008, was based on the Council of Europe 'Resolution AP (89) 1 on the use of colorants in plastic materials coming into contact with food (dated 13.09.1989)' (see below). It was being submitted in 2009 to a public consult process and was expected to be sanctioned as a GMC Resolution by the end of 2009.

Since August 2008, the GMC Resolutions that deal with the overall and specific migrations determination methods have been under a review process. The objective is to adopt the EU Legislation and the CEN (European Committee for Standardization) standards on this subject. The final document is also being submitted in 2009 to a public consult process. It was expected that the technical document would be sanctioned as a GMC Resolution during the second semester of 2009.

The update of the positive list of cellulose-derived FCMs also began in May 2009 as part of the Packaging Group–Food Commission activities program for 2009–2010.

14.6 COUNCIL OF EUROPE TECHNICAL RECOMMENDATIONS ON FOOD PACKAGING MATERIALS

The Council of Europe (CoE) was founded by the Treaty of London in May 1949, being thus the oldest European Organization. Its headquarters are located in Strasbourg (France), and as of December 2008, it has 47 Member States.

The activities on FCMs recommendations are organized in the following hierarchical way (Council of Europe, 2008a; Rossi, 2007):

- **Ad-hoc Working Groups**: which discuss and prepare drafts on technical issues;
- **Committee of Experts on materials coming into contact with food**: which prepares the Resolutions and Technical Documents;
- **Public Health Committee**: which adopts the Technical Documents;
- **Committee of Ministers**: is the Council of Europe decision-making body, composed by the Member States Foreign Ministers or their Strasbourg-based deputies (ambassadors or permanent representatives), which adopts the Resolutions.

The results of this harmonization process on FCMs are the following types of recommendations: Policy Statements, Resolutions, Guidelines and Technical Documents.

The CoE recommendations are not binding for the Member States, unless they are transposed into the National Laws. Several European countries have instructed the use of the CoE recommendations as reference documents to enforce the clause on safety of Article 3 of the EU Framework Regulation (EC) 1935/2004 on FCMs (Rossi, 2007). MERCOSUR technical document on colorants and pigments for plastics (expected to be sanctioned as a GMC Resolution during 2009) follows CoE Resolution AP (89) 1 on this issue.

The CoE has traditionally taken initiatives in technical issues not yet harmonized by the EU, and the CoE recommendations are considered as appropriate references in the absence of European Union or National Laws (Rossi, 2007; Schäfer, 2007).

Several recommendations have been issued over the years. They are summarized in Table 14.4, where only the last versions for each kind of FCMs appear (Council of Europe, 2008b). Previous versions are not referenced in Table 14.4, but can be found in the Internet sites mentioned in the references.

14.7 FOOD CONTACT MATERIALS IN THE *CODEX ALIMENTARIUS*

The *Codex Alimentarius* is a group of food standards accepted internationally and presented in a uniform way, by means of codes of practices, guidelines and other measures which establish detailed requirements for specific foods or food groups. There are no specific standards or guidelines related directly to FCMs in general or specifically to packaging materials, though some general norms may apply. For example, the *Code of Practice for the Prevention and Reduction of Tin Contamination in Canned Foods* (Codex Alimentarius Commission, 2005) gives recommendations to the producers and users of tin cans. It is to be noted that the recommended maximum levels of heavy metals are established according to specific foodstuffs. For example, tin content is regulated for different canned foods, but there is no specific reference to the packaging material.

The *General Standard for Contaminants and Toxins in Foods* contains the principles and procedures applied and recommended by the Codex regarding foods and feed; it also sets up the maximum permitted level of contaminants and toxic substances (Codex Alimentarius Commission, 1995b). The regulated contaminants are some mycotoxins, compounds and heavy metals such as arsenic, cadmium, lead, mercury, methylmercury, tin, radionucleids, acrylonitrile, dioxins and vinyl chloride monomer in foods and packaging materials. It establishes maximum reference levels of $0.02\,mg/kg$ for acrylonitrile in foods, $0.01\,mg/kg$ for vinyl chloride monomer in foods, and $1.0\,mg/kg$ for vinyl chloride monomer in packaging materials.

The *General Standard for Food Additives* (Codex Alimentarius Commission, 1995a) establishes the conditions of use of food additives. The Standard defines food additive as a substance intentionally added to food for a 'technological purpose in the manufacture, processing, preparation, treatment, packing, packaging, transport or holding of such food, that results, or may be reasonably expected to result (directly or indirectly) in it or its by products becoming a component of, or otherwise affecting the characteristics of such foods.' According to this definition, FCMs are not considered as food additives since they are not intentionally added to food, and so, they are not included in the list.

The principal objective of the *Code of Practice Concerning Source Directed Measures to Reduce Contamination of Foods with Chemicals* (Codex Alimentarius Commission, 2001) is to increase awareness of sources of chemical contamination of food and feed, and of source-prevented measures to avoid this contamination. It deals mainly with environmental contamination, and no reference is made either to pesticides, veterinary medicines, food additives or processing aids that are regulated in other Codex standards, or to FCMs or articles.

The *General Standard for the Labelling of Prepackaged Foods* (Codex Alimentarius Commission, 1985) applies to the standard and mandatory labeling of all foods so as not to mislead the consumer. There is no reference to food

TABLE 14.4 Council of Europe Technical Recommendations

Subject	Recommendation	Last version dated	Content
Colorants for plastic materials	Resolution AP (89) 1 on the use of colorants in plastic materials coming into contact with food.	13.09.1989	Resolution AP (89) 1
Plastics polymerization aids	Resolution AP (92) 2 on control of aids to polymerization (technological coadjuvants) for plastic materials and articles intended to come into contact with foodstuffs.	19.10.1992	Resolution AP (92) 2
Metals and alloys	Policy Statement concerning metals and alloys.	version 1 dated 13.02.2002	Technical document: Guidelines on metals and alloys used as food contact materials.
Rubbers	Policy Statement concerning rubber products intended to come into contact with foodstuffs.	version 1 dated 10.06.2004	- Resolution ResAP (2004) 4 on rubber products intended to come into contact with foodstuffs. - Technical document No 1. List of substances to be used in the manufacture of rubber products intended to come into contact with foodstuffs (to be prepared). - Technical document No 2. Practical Guide for users of Resolution ResAP (2004) 4 on rubber products intended to come into contact with foodstuffs. - Appendix 1. Inventory list of substances to be used in the manufacture of rubber products intended to come into contact with foodstuffs.
Silicones	Policy Statement concerning silicones used for food contact applications.	version 1 dated 10.06.2004	- Resolution ResAP (2004) 5 on silicones to be used for food contact applications. - Technical document No 1. List of substances to be used in the manufacture of silicones used for food contact applications.
Glass	Policy Statement concerning lead leaching from glass tableware into foodstuffs.	version 1 dated 22.09.2004	- Guidelines for lead leaching from glass tableware into foodstuffs. - Appendix 1. Parameters influencing lead leaching. - Appendix 2. Excerpt for lead from Resolution AP (96) 4 on maximum and guideline levels and on source-directed measures aimed at reducing the contamination of food by lead, cadmium and mercury.

(Continued)

TABLE 14.4 (*Continued*)

Subject	Recommendation	Last version dated	Content
Cellulose based materials	Policy Statement concerning tissue paper kitchen towels and napkins.	version 1 dated 22.09.2004	– Guidelines (covering: specifications, raw materials, test conditions and methods of analysis, use of recycled fibers, good manufacturing practices). – 4 Technical Appendixes.
	Policy Statement concerning paper and board materials and articles intended to come into contact with foodstuffs.	version 3 dated 11.12.2007	– Resolution ResAP (2002) 1 on paper and board materials and articles intended to come into contact with foodstuffs. – Technical document No 1. List of substances to be used in the manufacture of paper and board materials and articles intended to come into contact with foodstuffs. – Technical document No 2. Guidelines on test conditions and methods of analysis for paper and board materials and articles intended to come into contact with foodstuffs. – Technical document No 3. Guidelines on paper and board materials and articles, made from recycled fibers, intended to come into contact with foodstuffs. – Technical document No 4. CEPI (Confederation of European Paper Industries) Guide for GMP for paper and board for food contact. – Technical document No 5. Practical Guide for users of Resolution ResAP (2002) 1 on paper and board materials and articles intended to come into contact with foodstuffs.
Cork	Policy Statement concerning cork stoppers and other cork materials and articles intended to come into contact with foodstuffs.	version 2 dated 05.09.2007	– Resolution ResAP (2004) 2 on cork stoppers and other cork materials and articles intended to come into contact with foodstuffs. – Technical document No 1. List of substances to be used in the manufacture of cork stoppers and other cork materials and articles intended to come into contact with foodstuffs. – Technical document No 2. Test conditions and methods of analysis for cork stoppers and other cork materials and articles intended to come into contact with foodstuffs.

Ion exchange resins	Policy Statement concerning ion exchange and adsorbent resins in the processing of foodstuffs.	version 2 dated 05.09.2007	– Resolution ResAP (2004) 3 on ion exchange and adsorbent resins used in the processing of foodstuffs. – Technical document No 1. List of substances to be used in the manufacture of ion exchange and adsorbent resins used in the processing of foodstuffs.
Inks	Policy Statement concerning packaging inks applied to the non-food contact surface of food packaging	version 2 dated 10.10.2007	– Resolution ResAP (2005) 2 on packaging inks applied to the non-food contact surface of food packaging materials and articles intended to come into contact with foodstuffs. – Technical document No 1. Requirements for the selection of packaging ink raw materials applied to the non-food contact surface of food packaging materials and articles intended to come into contact with foodstuffs. – Technical document No 2. Part 1. GMP for the production of packaging inks formulated for use on the non-food contact surface of food packaging materials and articles intended to come into contact with foodstuffs. – Technical document No 2. Part 2. Code of GMP for flexible and fiber-based packaging for food. – Technical document No 3. Guidelines on test conditions for packaging inks applied to the non-food contact surface of food packaging materials and articles intended to come into contact with foodstuffs.
Coatings	Policy Statement concerning coatings intended to come into contact with foodstuffs.	version 2 dated 29.01.2008	– Resolution ResAP (2004) 1 on coatings intended to come into contact with foodstuffs. – Technical document No 1. List of substances to be used in the manufacture of coatings intended to come into contact with foodstuffs.

packaging or FCMs. The *Guidelines Procedures for the Visual Inspection of Lots of Canned Foods* (Codex Alimentarius Commission, 1993a) are established for the detection of different kinds of defects in the packages (cans and cardboard boxes) but, as in the Labeling Standard, no reference is made to FCMs or articles.

Last but not least, the *Codex Alimentarius*'s various codes of hygienic practices for the processing of different foods have chapters regarding good manufacturing practices and hygiene for buildings, equipment and personnel (Codex Alimentarius Commission, 1993b, 1999). Recommendations are given to every processing step, storage and transport of specific foods. Packaging considerations include the:

- keeping of sanitary conditions and cleanliness of the packaging material during storage;
- appropriate selection of packaging materials according to the food and process to be used;
- use of packaging materials that do not transfer any objectionable substances to the food beyond the limits acceptable to the official agency having jurisdiction upon it;
- observance of appropriate programs of sampling and inspection of packages to assure compliance with specifications.

14.8 COMPARISON OF FCMS LEGISLATIONS

A detailed comparative analysis of the Legislations already described is beyond the scope of this chapter, and can be found in several technical publications and conferences. Therefore, a general scenario only will be described in this section.

The *Codex Alimentarius* does not establish requisites on FCMs, except in the case of general recommendations (in the voluntary field) for tin in canned foodstuffs and vinyl chloride monomer in packaging materials.

The Council of Europe has issued recommendations, mainly on subjects not covered yet by the EU Legislation, considered of great technical value, that follow the European Union approach to safety assessment based on toxicology, and that have been taken as references by several EU Member States (Rossi, 2007) and by the MERCOSUR.

The Japanese Legislation's outstanding point is that, in order to assure public health, FCMs that include by definition packages, containers, utensils and tableware, are covered not only by the Food Sanitation Law issued by the government (Ministry of Health, Labor and Welfare) in the regulatory field, but also by voluntary standards issued by several private industrial hygienic Associations. The Japanese Food Sanitation Law establishes horizontal FCMs requisites, valid for different kinds of foodstuffs, and some vertical FCMs requisites for special types of foodstuffs such as milk and milk products, certain types of retortable packages, soft drinks packages, automatic vending machines, manufacturing equipment for flavored ice, etc. (Kawamura, 2008).

The focus of the comparisons in the available publications is centered, no doubt due to their international standing, in the differences between the EU and the US-FDA FCMs Legislations (Eisert, 2008; Heckman, 2005; Kuznesof, 2002; Schäfer, 2007; Twaroski *et al.*, 2007). A brief summary related to both Legislations follows.

According to the US-FDA, polymers and additives as well as other food contact substrates are considered as indirect food additives, when present in the human diet, due to migration, in quantities greater than the TOR. Excluded from the indirect food additives category are color additives, GRAS substances and substances cleared prior to 1958 (6 September). In addition, tableware and utensils, as well as drinking water supply equipment are exempt from the FCMs Legislation. In contrast, the EU Legislation does not define FCMs as food additives, and it applies to all the FCMs (including tableware and utensils), except those used to transport and store drinking water. Different types of FCMs have been regulated by both Legislations.

The US-FDA has established two systems by means of which FCSs enter the positive lists. The older one mainly comprises the cleared substances following the Petition-Regulation procedure, which are thus included in a positive list (Regulation) which is public and of general use. The most recent system, in force since 1997, comprises the substances cleared following the Pre-Market Notification system, by means of FCNs, which are of public access in general aspects, but have restrictions in proprietary information. In this last system, the clearances are issued for the petitioner (e.g. a particular FCMs manufacturer), case by case. This means that the food manufacturer must buy the cleared FCMs only from their producers and not from another one.

In the EU Legislation, the substances enumerated in the positive lists are of general use: that means that the food manufacturer may buy the cleared FCMs from different producers, as long as each FCM complies with the restrictions established. However, in the EU, the recycled and active and intelligent FCMs are going to have case by case (proprietary) clearance based lists.

The conceptual basis of the FCSs clearance for their inclusion in the positive lists differs in both Legislations. The US-FDA approach is an exposure-based risk assessment of the FCSs, which takes into account:

- the **consumption factors** (CFs), which are the fractions of the daily diet (assumed as 3 kg per day per person) of a 60 kg body weight consumer, expected to contact each specific FCM; and
- the **food-type distribution factors** (f_Ts), defined as the fractions, for each FCM, of different types of foodstuff (aqueous, acidic, alcoholic and fatty) packaged in the FCM.

These factors (CFs and f_Ts) and the migration data for FCSs in different simulants are used to calculate their **dietary concentrations** (DCs) and their **estimated daily intakes** (EDIs). If different uses of the FCS are already regulated for similar or different technological purposes, a **cumulative estimated daily intake** (CEDI) must be calculated. The EDI or CEDI values, and a comparison of them with the FCS acceptable daily intake (ADI), determine the kind of toxicology data needed to be submitted to the US-FDA. The intended use for each FCM, either for single or repeated use, the type(s) of foodstuffs and the contact time(s) and temperature(s) conditions, an estimated M/S ratio (ratio of mass of foodstuff contained/contact surface area of FCM) and an estimated FCM thickness, must also be declared. The cleared FCSs are then included in the positive lists, along with the main physico-chemical parameters that allow their easy characterization by the purchaser of the FCMs (the food manufacturer). If the purchaser checks that the FCM complies with these specifications, the FCM is considered to pose no health risk if used in the conditions established in the positive list, and that correspond to the assumptions made in the exposure evaluations. No other uses are allowed for the FCS, other than that stated in the positive lists.

The EU approach, instead, is a toxicological-based risk assessment, which involves the determination of the no-observed effect-level (NOEL) and the tolerable daily intake (TDI) of the FCS under evaluation (monomer, additive, etc.). A conservative assumption is made; that is, that a 60 kg body weight person consumes daily 1 kg of foodstuff packaged in an FCM containing this FCS. The FCS TDI and the aforementioned assumption are used to calculate a specific migration limit (SML). No exposure considerations involving CFs, f_Ts and EDIs or CEDIs are made. Generally, the use of the cleared FCS is allowed in different types of FCMs and in different situations of use (S/M ratios, contact time(s) and temperature(s) conditions, etc.), providing that the specific migration of the FCS complies with its SML, or other restrictions, in the case they exist. This last point can pose a considerable analytical effort for the FCMs manufacturer. Some kind of exposure consideration has been introduced in Directive 2007/19/EC relating to the specific migration determination of certain lipophilic substances, by means of the use of three correction factors: the **fat reduction factor** (FRF), the **simulant D reduction factor** (DRF) and, when it corresponds, the product of both of them, defined as the **total reduction factor** (TRF) (EU, 2007a).

These two divergent approaches, naturally, may pose different types of problems and uncertainties to the FCMs and food manufacturers. In the USA, the procedure adopted, minimizes the analytical effort for the FCMs manufacturer, but may imply a reduction of flexibility for the food manufacturer to FCSs possible novel uses. In the EU, the procedure adopted maximizes the consumer protection, assuming a greater exposure to the FCSs, but may imply a greater analytical effort to verify SMLs for the FCMs manufacturer. Besides, through the conceptual dissociation of FCS and the FCM in which it is used (neither CFs nor f_Ts are applied), there are generally more options of final uses for the food manufacturer, including the novel ones. In the US, the FCMs manufacturer first makes an exposure evaluation (EDIs or CEDIs), and according to its result, proceeds, if necessary, to perform toxicological studies. In the EU, the FCSs or FCMs manufacturer is expected to provide toxicological data, which are the basis of SMLs calculations, without an exposure evaluation (Heckman, 2005; Schäfer, 2007).

Finally, it must be noted that the US-FDA has a double role, because it performs risk assessments by evaluating the Petitions or Notifications, and risk managements by issuing Regulations and an accepted FCN list. In the EU, the risk assessment is the duty of the EFSA, and the risk management is the task of the EU Commission, the EU Council of Ministers and the EU Parliament.

The MERCOSUR Legislation is eclectic, taking elements from the EU and US-FDA Legislations, and also from the Council of Europe recommendations, and the positive lists and other requisites are transposed from them. Certain Member States enforce a pre-market approval system for all FCM types. The Legislation is obligatory for the manufacturer of the final product which by definition includes: packages, containers, materials, utensils and tableware, but does not include articles used to transport or store drinking water. When compliance is verified, the sanitary authorities of the Member States clear them generally by issuing approval/authorization certificates, case by case (Ariosti, 2007; Padula & Ariosti, 2002). Thus, no uncertainties related to the final use (e.g. contact time(s) and temperature(s) conditions; types of foodstuff(s); FCMs medium thickness and its distribution in the object; real S/M ratios; etc.) arise for the raw FCMs or foodstuffs producer, since the approval/authorization is given for the final package or article manufacturer. This requires a considerable analytical effort, but it has been assumed by the FCMs manufacturer industries in the last three decades, as well as by the Member States governments, whose Technical Institutes (such as INTI (Argentina), CETEA-ITAL (Campinas, São Paulo, Brazil), INTN (Asunción of Paraguay) and LATU (Montevideo, Uruguay)) have trained personnel in FCMs hygienic requirements evaluation (Ariosti, 2007).

A comparative summary of the different Legislations is presented in Table 14.5.

14.9 CONCLUSIONS— HARMONIZATION, MUTUAL RECOGNITION, AND NEW LEGISLATION

As has been seen in the EU and MERCOSUR, a harmonization process precedes the sanction of FCMs Legislation, and in the non-harmonized fields, there is also a system of mutual recognition of the products cleared in the origin Member

TABLE 14.5   Comparison of FCMs Legislations

Subject	European Union	USA	MERCOSUR	Japan
Level	Supranational (27 Member States)	National	Supranational (4 full Member States; 2 applying Member States; 5 Associated States)	National
Legal status of FCMs	Regulated.	Regulated.	Regulated.	Regulated.
	Drinking water supply equipment is excluded from the Regulation.	Drinking water supply equipment is excluded from the Regulation.	Drinking water supply equipment is excluded from the Regulation.	Covered also by voluntary standards issued by Industrial Hygienic Associations.
	Houseware and utensils are not excluded.	FCMs are considered as indirect food additives.	Houseware and utensils are not excluded.	Houseware and utensils are not excluded.
		Houseware and utensils are excluded.		
Type of Legislation related to FCMs hygienic requirements	Directives (must be transposed into the National Legislations).	Federal Law	Resolutions (must be transposed into the National Legislations).	Food Sanitation Law
	Regulations (direct application without transposition).			
General FCMs Legislation/ Regulation	Regulation (EC) 1935/2004	Federal Food, Drug and Cosmetic Act (FFDCA)	Resolution GMC 3/92	Food Sanitation Law (1947)
		Code of Federal Regulations (CFR) - Title 21		Food Safety Basic Law (2003)
Main regulated FCMs	Plastics	Plastics	Plastics	Plastics
		Paper and board	Paper and board	
	Elastomers	Elastomers	Elastomers	Elastomers
	Ceramics			Metal cans
	Regenerated cellulose (films)	Recycled plastics	Metals	Glass
		Active and intelligent materials	Glass	Ceramics
	Recycled plastics		Ceramics	

(Continued)

TABLE 14.5   (*Continued*)

Subject	European Union	USA	MERCOSUR	Japan
	Active and intelligent materials		Regenerated cellulose (films and casings) Recycled PET	
Cleared FCMs logo or label	Obligatory and standardized logo or obligatory label (with exceptions).	–	–	Obligatory and standardized label.
	Obligatory label on recycled plastic FCMs.		Obligatory label on refillable and recycled PET packages, indicating these conditions.	
	Obligatory label and standardized logo (this last where possible) for active and intelligent materials.			
Legal obligation for the FCMs manufacturer	Obligatory Declaration of Compliance with the Legislation.	Compliance with the Legislation.	Compliance with the Legislation.	Compliance with the Legislation.
	Case by case obligatory approval system for recycled, and active and intelligent FCMs.		Case by case obligatory approval system for FCMs that comply with the Legislation (partially applied in Brazil).	Compliance with voluntary standards.
				Case by case obligatory approval system for FCMs that comply with the Legislation.
Positive lists	General use positive lists, non proprietary.	General use positive lists, non proprietary (under the Petition-Regulation system).	General use positive lists, non proprietary.	General use positive lists, non proprietary.
		Case by case positive list (FCNs list), proprietary (under the FCN system).		
Plastics positive list	Monomers and other starting substances (fully harmonized).	Polymers	Polymers (fully harmonized).	Polymers
	Additives (partially harmonized).	Additives	Additives (fully harmonized).	Monomers and other starting substances.

TABLE 14.5 (*Continued*)

Subject	European Union	USA	MERCOSUR	Japan
	SML (based on toxicological risk assessment data (NOEL, TDI))	Several purity criteria and specifications of use (based on exposure risk assessment, CF, f_T, EDI, CEDI, ADI).	SML (=LME)	Additives.
	QM		QM (=LC)	Polymerization aids.
	Very few purity criteria and specifications of use.		Purity criteria and specifications of use transposed from EU and US-FDA FCMs Legislations.	Colorants.
				SML
				QM
				Purity criteria and specifications of use.
Overall migration limits (plastics)	60 mg/kg	50 mg/kg	50 mg/kg	30 mg/kg (general); different values for different plastics when using n-heptane as fatty food simulant
	10 mg/dm^2	7.75 mg/dm^2 (=0.5 mg/in^2)	8 mg/dm^2	
TOR	Not established	0.5 μg/kg (dietary base)	0.5 μg/kg (dietary base), only in the case of post-consumer decontaminated recycled PET.	–
Functional barrier concept	Adopted	Adopted	Adopted	–
Non-toxicological concern migration limit (s)	10 μg/kg	Derived from the TOR, different values for different plastics.	Derived from the TOR, and accepted only in the case of decontaminated recycled PET (=10 μg/kg).	–
Risk Assessment Authority	EFSA	US-FDA	Food Commission-SGT 3	Pharmaceutical Affairs and Food Sanitation Council. Industrial Hygienic Associations
Risk Management Authority	EU Commission	US-FDA	GMC	Government (MHLW).
	EU Council of Ministers			
	EU Parliament			Industrial Hygienic Associations.

States (Ariosti, 2007; Eisert, 2008; Heckman, 2005; Montfort, 2007; Padula & Ariosti, 2002; Schäfer, 2007).

The differences between the US-FDA and EU Legislations on FCMs are so significant that they pose real hurdles to the harmonization process of these two major regulatory bodies, and to global trade. A harmonization process seems rather difficult to achieve quickly, due to the differences commented on in the previous section. An alternative step should be a mutual recognition system; but also in this subject, possibilities of non-compliance of products to diverging Legislations with a different basis, may pose severe concerns to the sanitary authorities of the EU and the US (Eisert, 2008; Heckman, 2005).

Therefore, no clear scenario can be envisaged for the near future, as has been discussed extensively at international Conferences held in 2007, 2008 and 2009 (INTERTECH-PIRA Conferences on Global FCMs Legislation). In the meantime, a mutual recognition system has an increasing interest between the actors involved all over the world. Also a better sharing of information between them has been identified as a necessity.

For the emerging FCMs Legislations of countries in Africa, Asia and Latin America and the Caribbean, it is important to recognize the global benefits of having their own FCMs Legislative systems, to analyze the two main international Legislative bodies with their strengths and drawbacks, in order to be able to decide if they can be adopted as references, with adaptations if necessary, to the local realities. In order to facilitate a future harmonization process or a mutual recognition system, the less divergent Legislations there are, the easier the implementation of these strategies will be.

The same could also be applied in the European area, in countries that do not belong to the EU— such as Iceland, Liechtenstein, Norway and Switzerland—that form an association (European Free Trade Association (EFTA)) within the occidental area; in some Eastern Europe countries; dental area; in some Eastern Europe countries; and in the former USSR eastern countries; that have developed or are on the way to developing their own FCMs Legislations.

The worldwide recognized food regulation system developed by the Codex Alimentarius Commission may be an interesting alternative for a global legislation on food packaging issues. Member countries could submit specific proposals to the Commission for initiating a debate regarding the development of a new code of practice on food packaging issues to protect consumers' health and ensure fair commercial practices in the food trade.

References

Ariosti, A. (2002a). Aptitud sanitaria de envases y materiales plásticos en contacto con alimentos. In R. Catalá & R. Gavara (Eds.), *Migración de componentes y residuos de envases en contacto con alimentos* (pp. 85–100). Valencia, Spain: Instituto de Agroquímica y Tecnología de Alimentos (IATA).

Ariosti, A. (2002b). Uso de materiales plásticos reciclados en contacto con alimentos. Barreras funcionales. In R. Catalá & R. Gavara (Eds.), *Migración de componentes y residuos de envases en contacto con alimentos* (pp. 261–279). Valencia, Spain: Instituto de Agroquímica y Tecnología de Alimentos (IATA).

Ariosti, A. (2007). Aptitud sanitaria de materiales en contacto con alimentos. Exigencias legislativas para envases en el MERCOSUR. In: *Memorias del Primer Seminario Internacional de Envases Activos para Alimentos*—CYTED (Iberoamerican Program of Science and Technology for Development)—USACH (University of Santiago de Chile). Santiago de Chile (28 March) and Puerto Varas (30 March).

Arvidson, K. B., Cheeseman, M. A., & McDougal, A. J. (2007). Toxicology and risk assessment of chemical migrants from food contact materials. In K. A. Barnes, C. Richard Sinclair, & D. H. Watson (Eds.), *Chemical migration and food contact materials* (pp. 158–179). Cambridge, UK: Woodhead Publishing Ltd.

Bayer, F. L. (1997). The threshold of regulation and its application to indirect food additive contaminants in recycled plastics. *Food Additives and Contaminants, 14*(6–7), 661–670.

Bayer, F. L. (2002). PET recycling for food-contact applications: Testing, safety and technologies: A global perspective. *Food Additives and Contaminants, 19*(Suppl), 111–134.

Castle, L. (2007). Chemical migration into food: An overview. In K. A. Barnes, C. Richard Sinclair, & D. H. Watson (Eds.), *Chemical migration and food contact materials* (pp. 1–13). Cambridge, UK: Woodhead Publishing Ltd.

Catalá, R., & Gavara, R. (Eds.), (2002). *Migración de componentes y residuos de envases en contacto con alimentos.* Valencia, Spain: Instituto de Agroquímica y Tecnología de Alimentos (IATA).

Codex Alimentarius Commission. (1985). CODEX STAN 1-1985. General Standard for the Labelling of Prepackaged Foods. Available at: http://codexalimentarius.net/search/advanced.do?lang=en

Codex Alimentarius Commission. (1993a). CAC/GL 17-1993. Guidelines procedures for the visual inspection of lots of canned foods. Available at: http://codexalimentarius.net/search/advanced.do?lang=en

Codex Alimentarius Commission. (1993b). CAC/RCP 40-1993. Code of hygienic practice for aseptically processed and packaged low-acid foods. Available at: http://codexalimentarius.net/search/advanced.do?lang=en

Codex Alimentarius Commission. (1995a). CODEX STAN 192-1995. General standard for food additives. available at: http://codexalimentarius.net/search/advanced.do?lang=en

Codex Alimentarius Commission. (1995b). CODEX STAN 193-1995, Rev 3-2007. General standard for contaminants and toxins in foods. Available at: http://codexalimentarius.net/search/advanced.do?lang=en

Codex Alimentarius Commission. (1999). CAC/RCP 46-1999. Code of hygienic practice for refrigerated packaged foods with extended shelf-life. Available at: http://codexalimentarius.net/search/advanced.do?lang=en

Codex Alimentarius Commission. (2001). CAC/RCP 49-2001. Code of practice concerning source directed measures to reduce contamination of foods with chemicals. Available at: http://codexalimentarius.net/search/advanced.do?lang=en

Codex Alimentarius Commission. (2005). CAC/RCP 60-2005. Code of practice for the prevention and reduction of tin contamination in canned foods. Available at: http://codexalimentarius.net/search/advanced.do?lang=en

Council of Europe. (2005). Committee of experts on materials coming into contact with food. Resolution ResAP (2002) 1 on paper and board materials and articles intended to come into contact with foodstuffs. In: *Policy statement concerning paper and board materials and articles intended to come into contact with foodstuffs.*

Council of Europe. (2008a). www.coe.int/T/e/com/about_coe/ (for general information).

Council of Europe. (2008b). www.coe.int/soc-sp (for specific technical documents).

Eisert, R. (2008). Comparing Food Contact Legislation. In: *Proceedings of the INTERTECH-PIRA conference on global legislation for food contact packaging.* Washington, USA, April 2–4.

European Food Safety Authority. (2008). Opinion of the Scientific Panel on food additives, flavourings, processing aids and materials in contact with food (AFC) on Guidelines on submission of a dossier for safety evaluation by the EFSA of a recycling process to produce recycled plastics intended to be used for manufacture of materials and articles in contact with food. Adopted on 21/05/2008. *The EFSA Journal, 717,* 1–12.

EU. (1976). Council Directive 76/893/EEC on the approximation of the laws of the Member States relating to materials and articles intended to come into contact with foodstuffs. Available at: http://eur-lex.europa.eu/en/index.htm.

EU. (1978). Council Directive 78/142/EEC on the approximation of the laws of the Member States relating to materials and articles which contain vinyl chloride monomer and are intended to come into contact with foodstuffs. Available at: http://eur-lex.europa.eu/en/index.htm.

EU. (1980). Commission Directive 80/590/EEC determining the symbol that may accompany materials and articles intended to come into contact with foodstuffs. Available at: http://eur-lex.europa.eu/en/index.htm.

EU. (1985). Council Directive 85/572/EEC laying down the list of simulants to be used for testing migration of constituents of plastic materials and articles intended to come into contact with foodstuffs. Available at: http://eur-lex.europa.eu/en/index.htm.

EU. (1989). Council Directive 89/109/EEC on the approximation of the laws of the Member States relating to materials and articles intended to come into contact with foodstuffs. Available at: http://eur-lex.europa.eu/en/index.htm.

EU. (2002a). Commission Directive 2002/72/EC relating to plastic materials and articles intended to come into contact with foodstuffs, amended by Commission Directive 2004/1/EC, Commission Directive 2004/19/EC, Commission Directive 2005/79/EC, Commission Directive 2007/19/EC and Directive 2008/39/EC. Available at: http://eur-lex.europa.eu/en/index.htm.

EU. (2002b). Regulation (EC) No 178/2002 of the European Parliament and of the Council laying down the general principles and requirements of food law, establishing the European Food Safety Authority and laying down procedures in matters of food safety. Available at: http://eur-lex.europa.eu/en/index.htm.

EU. (2004a). Regulation (EC) No 1935/2004 of the European Parliament and of the Council on materials and articles intended to come into contact with food and repealing Directives 80/590/EEC and 89/109/EEC. Available at: http://eur-lex.europa.eu/en/index.htm.

EU. (2004b). Commission Directive 2004/19/EC amending Directive 2002/72/EC relating to plastic materials and articles intended to come into contact with foodstuffs. Available at: http://eur-lex.europa.eu/en/index.htm.

EU. (2005a). Commission Directive 2005/79/EC amending Directive 2002/72/EC relating to plastic materials and articles intended to come into contact with food. Available at: http://eur-lex.europa.eu/en/index.htm.

EU. (2005b). Commission Directive 2005/31/EC amending Council Directive 84/500/EEC as regards a declaration of compliance and performance criteria of the analytical method for ceramic articles intended to come into contact with foodstuffs. Available at: http://eur-lex.europa.eu/en/index.htm.

EU. (2005c). Commission Regulation (EC) No 1895/2005 on the restriction of use of certain epoxy derivatives in materials and articles intended to come into contact with food. Available at: http://eur-lex.europa.eu/en/index.htm.

EU. (2007a). Commission Directive 2007/19/EC amending Directive 2002/72/EC relating to plastic materials and articles intended to come into contact with food and Council Directive 85/572/EEC laying down the list of simulants to be used for testing migration of constituents of plastic materials and articles intended to come into contact with foodstuffs. Available at: http://eur-lex.europa.eu/en/index.htm.

EU. (2007b). Commission Directive 2007/42/EC relating to materials and articles made of regenerated cellulose film intended to come into contact with foodstuffs. Available at: http://eur-lex.europa.eu/en/index.htm.

EU. (2008a). Commission Regulation (EC) 282/2008 of 27 March 2008 on recycled plastic materials and articles intended to come into contact with foods and amending Regulation (EC) No 2023/2006. Available at: http://eur-lex.europa.eu/en/index.htm.

EU. (2008b). Europa, The EU at a glance. Available at: http://europa.eu/index_en.htm.

EU. (2008c). Food Contact Materials, EU Legislation. Available at: http://ec.europa.eu/food/food/chemical-safety/foodcontact/eu_legisl_en.html.

EU. (2008d). Food Contact Materials, Legislation on specific materials. Available at: http://ec.europa.eu/food/food/chemicalsafety/foodcontact/spec_dirs_en.html.

EU. (2008e). Food Contact Materials, Legislative List. Available at: http://ec.europa.eu/food/food/chemical-safety/foodcontact/legisl_list_en.html.

EU. (2009). "Commission Regulation (EC) 450/2009 of 29 May 2009 on active and intelligent materials and articles intended to come into contact with food". Available at: http://eur-lex.europa.eu/en/index.htm.

FAO. (2008). Corporate Document Repository. Agriculture and Consumer Protection. 'The Codex Alimentarius', Available at: http://www.fao.org/docrep/U3550T/u3550t0p.htm.

FDA. (1995). Food additives: Threshold of regulation for substances used in food-contact articles (Final Rule). US food and drug administration. Fed Reg, 60(136), 36582–36596.

FDA. (2006). Points to consider for the use of recycled plastics in food packaging: Chemistry considerations, US Food and Drug Administration. http://www.cfsan.fda.gov/~dms/guidance.html.

Fernández, M. R., & Cacho, J. (2002). Efectos sensoriales de la migración. In R. Catalá & R. Gavara (Eds.), Migración de componentes y residuos de envases en contacto con alimentos (pp. 101–125). Valencia, Spain: Instituto de Agroquímica y Tecnología de Alimentos (IATA).

Franz, R., Bayer, F. L., & Welle, F. (2003). Guidance and criteria for safe recycling of post-consumer polyethylene terephthalate (PET) into new food packaging applications. In Program on the recyclability of food packaging materials with respect to food safety considerations – Polyethylene terephthalate (PET), paper and board and plastics covered by functional barriers. Freising, Germany: Fraunhofer Institute for Process Engineering and Packaging (IVV).

Franz, R., Bayer, F. L., & Welle, F. (2004a). Guidance and criteria for safe recycling of post consumer polyethylene terephthalate (PET) into new food packaging applications. Report EU-Project FAIR-CT98-4318 Recyclability, European Commission, Brussels.

Franz, R., Mauer, A., & Welle, F. (2004b). European survey on post-consumer poly(ethylene terephthalate) materials to determine contamination levels and maximum consumer exposure from food packages made from recycled PET. Food Additives and Contaminants, 21(3), 265–286.

Heckman, J. H. (2005). Food packaging regulation in the United States and the European Union. Regulatory Toxicology and Pharmacology, 42, 96–122.

Hernández, R. J., & Gavara, R. (1999). Plastics packaging. Methods for studying mass transfer interactions. Leatherhead, Surrey, UK: PIRA International.

JETRO. (2006a). Food Sanitation Law in Japan. http://www.jetro.go.jp/en/reports/regulations/pdf/food-e.pdf.

JETRO. (2006b). Specifications, standards and testing methods for foodstuffs, implements, containers and packaging, toys, detergents. http://www.jetro.go.jp/en/reports/regulations/pdf/testing2009-e.pdf.

JETRO. (2007). Specifications and standards for foods, food additives, etc., under the food sanitation act (summary).

Katan, L. L. (Ed.). (1996). Migration from food contact materials (pp. 159–180). Cambridge, UK: Blackie Academic and Professional.

Kawamura, Y. (2008). Food contact legislation in Japan. In: Proceedings of the INTERTECH-PIRA Conference on Global Legislation for Food Contact Packaging. Washington, USA, April 2–4.

Kuznesof, P. M. (2002). Legislación sobre envases para alimentos en los Estados Unidos. In R. Catalá & R. Gavara (Eds.), *Migración de componentes y residuos de envases en contacto con alimentos* (pp. 65–83). Valencia, Spain: Instituto de Agroquímica y Tecnología de Alimentos (IATA).

Mari, E. A. (2002). Migración en envases de vidrio y de cerámica esmaltada. In R. Catalá & R. Gavara (Eds.), *Migración de componentes y residuos de envases en contacto con alimentos* (pp. 329–346). Valencia, Spain: Instituto de Agroquímica y Tecnología de Alimentos (IATA).

MERCOSUR. (1992). Resolución GMC 55/92 'Envases y equipamientos de vidrio y cerámica destinados a entrar en contacto con alimentos'.

MERCOSUR. (1999a). Resolución GMC 25/99 'Reglamento Técnico MERCOSUR sobre envases de PET multicapa (único uso) destinados al envasado de bebidas analcohólicas carbonatadas'.

MERCOSUR. (1999b). Resolución GMC 52/99 'Reglamento Técnico MERCOSUR sobre material celulósico reciclado'.

MERCOSUR. (2007). Resolución GMC 30/07 'Reglamento Técnico MERCOSUR sobre envases de polietilentereftalato (PET) postconsumo reciclado grado alimentario (PET-PCR grado alimentario) destinados a estar en contacto con alimentos.'

MERCOSUR. (2008a). www.mercosur.org.uy.

MERCOSUR. (2008b). www.mercosur.int.

Ministry of Agriculture. (2006). Secretary of Agriculture, Brazil, Instrução Normativa 49.

Ministry of Economy. (2008). Argentina, www.puntofocal.gob.ar.

Montfort, J.-P. (2007). Key issues to marketing food-contact materials and articles in the EU. In *Proceedings of the INTERTECH-PIRA conference on global legislation for food contact packaging*. Barcelona, Spain, July 11–12.

Oldring, P. K. T. (2007). Exposure estimation—the missing element for assessing the safety of migrants from food. In K. A. Barnes, C. Richard Sinclair, & D. H. Watson (Eds.), *Chemical migration and food contact materials* (pp. 122–157). Cambridge, UK: Woodhead Publishing Ltd.

Padula, M., & Ariosti, A. (2002). Legislación MERCOSUR sobre la aptitud sanitaria de los envases para alimentos. In R. Catalá & R. Gavara (Eds.), *Migración de componentes y residuos de envases en contacto con alimentos* (pp. 45–64). Valencia, Spain: Instituto de Agroquímica y Tecnología de Alimentos (IATA).

Robertson, G. L. (1993). *Food packaging. Principles and practice.* New York: Marcel Dekker, Inc.

Rossi, L. (2007). Status of the Council of Europe Resolutions and Future Programmes. In *Proceedings of Food Contact Polymers 2007. First International Conference*. Paper 1, pp. 1–28. Smithers RAPRA Ltd, Shawbury, Shrewsbury, U.K.

Schäfer, A. (2007). Regulation of food contact materials in the EU. In K. A. Barnes, C. Richard Sinclair, & D. H. Watson (Eds.), *Chemical migration and food contact materials* (pp. 43–63). Cambridge, UK: Woodhead Publishing Ltd.

Twaroski, M. L., Batarseh, L. I., & Bailey, A. B. (2007). Regulation of food contact materials in the USA. In K. A. Barnes, C. Richard Sinclair, & D. H. Watson (Eds.), *Chemical migration and food contact materials* (pp. 17–42). Cambridge, UK: Woodhead Publishing Ltd.

US Congress. (1969). 'Congressional Declaration of National Environmental Policy. Nacional Environmental Protection Act of 1969'. Available at http://www.nepa.gov/nepa/regs/nepa/nepaeqia.htm.

USFDA. (2002). 'Guidance for Industry. Preparation of Food Contact Notifications and Food Additive Petitions for Food Contact'. Substances: Chemistry Recommendations. Final Guidance. Available at: www.cfsan.fda.gov/~dms/opa2pmna.html.

USFDA. (2005). 'Guidance for Industry. Submitting Request Under 21 CFR 170.39 TOR for substances used in food contact materials'. CFSAN/Office of Food Additive Safety, April 2005. Available at: http://www.cfsan.fda.gov/~dms/torguid.html.

USFDA. (2007a). CFSAN/Office of Food Additive Safety. (2007a). 'Inventory of effective food contact substance notifications'. Available at: http://www.cfsan.fda.gov/~dms/opa-fcn.html.

USFDA. (2007b). CFSAN/Office of Food Additive Safety, 'Inventory of effective food contact substance notifications. Limitations specifications and use'. Available at: http://www.cfsan.fda.gov/~dms/opa-fcn2.html.

USFDA. (2007c). CFSAN/Office of Food Additive Safety, 'Food Ingredients and Packaging Terms'. Available at: www.cfsan.fda.gov/~dms/opa-def.html.

USFDA. (2008a). 'Code of Federal Regulations. Title 21 Food and Drugs Database'. Available at: http://www.fda.gov/cdrh/aboutcfr.html.

USFDA. (2008b). 'Code of Federal Regulations. Title 21, Part 176, Indirect Food Additives: paper and paperboard components. Section 176.260 Pulp from reclaimed fiber'.

van Dongen, W., Coulier, L., Muilwijk, B. et al. (2007). Analytical strategy to assess the safety of food contact materials. In *Proceedings of Food Contact Polymers 2007. First International Conference*, Paper 7, pp. 1–10. Smithers RAPRA Ltd, Shawbury, Shrewsbury, U.K.

Welle, F., & Franz, R. (2007). Recycled plastics and chemical migration into food. In K. A. Barnes, C. Richard Sinclair, & D. H. Watson (Eds.), *Chemical migration and food contact materials* (pp. 205–227). Cambridge, UK: Woodhead Publishing Ltd.

Wilson, C. L. (2007). *Intelligent and active packaging for fruits and vegetables* (pp. 321–326). Boca Raton: CRC Press.

CHAPTER

15

Nanotechnology and Food Safety

Syed S.H. Rizvi[1], Carmen I. Moraru[1], Hans Bouwmeester[2]
and Frans W.H. Kampers[3]

[1]Department of Food Science, Cornell University, Ithaca, NY, USA
[2]RIKILT-Institute of Food Safety, Wageningen UR, Wageningen, The Netherlands
[3]Wageningen UR, Wageningen, The Netherlands

15.1 INTRODUCTION

Nanoscale objects are not new; they have been known to exist for decades. Yet, it was the ability of scientists to see and engineer nanostructures via self- or directed-assembly in the 1980s that catalyzed their rapid development. Nanotechnology has now evolved into a convergent discipline involving a variety of sciences (physical, chemical, biological, engineering and electronic) designed to understand and manipulate structures and devices at nanoscale. The use of nano-based consumer products is growing rapidly and many such products are available in the market. To date, more than 600 consumer products that are self-identified by the manufacturers as containing nanotechnology are included in the public database (PEN, 2009). Nano-based goods are projected by various sources to be an estimated $2.6 trillion global industry by 2014 (ScienceDaily, 2007) and a nano-dominated future is not too distant.

A nanomaterial is generally defined as 'a discrete entity that has one or more dimensions of the order of 100 nm or less' (SCENIHR, 2007b). Unique properties of these materials arise at the nanoscale where they do not behave like their macroscale counterparts. The physico-chemical properties of nanostructures are not governed by the same laws as larger structures, but by quantum mechanics. Color, solubility, diffusivity, material strength, toxicity and other properties will be very different at the nanoscale as compared to the macroscale. Other important properties include increased reactivity because of quantum mechanical effects in combination with the high (relative) surface area of nanostructures, which allows the creation of genuinely new properties and materials with desired functionalities. The potential benefits for application of nanotechnologies in food have been widely discussed and cover many aspects such as efficient nutrient delivery, formulations with improved bioavailability, new tools for molecular and cellular detection of contaminants and food packaging materials (Chaudhry *et al.*, 2008; Chen, Weiss, & Shahidi, 2006; Das, Saxena, & Dwivedi, 2008; Moraru *et al.*, 2003, 2009; Weiss, Takhistov, & McClements, 2006).

As new applications emerge, there is also growing concern, both from the public and the scientific community, about the potential risks and toxicity of nanotechnology products, or the environmental and personal safety aspects of their use. The fact that size matters as it influences efficacy and safety, the question arises

whether a nanoscale particle that has unique material properties should be deemed new or non-natural for purposes of safety evaluation. A lack of knowledge of how nanoscale structures may interact with biological systems and potentially create safety issues is often cited as the last hurdle to overcome in their acceptability in food and pharmaceutical applications.

The purpose of this chapter is to explore the global safety and regulatory issues associated with the application of nanotechnology to food systems. Emphasis is placed on the toxicological knowledge needed to perform a hazard assessment and the lack of measurement technologies for exposure assessment. Additionally, the current state of the regulatory food safety framework is described, and the consequences of the scientific knowledge gaps that exist in the application and enforcement of the current regulations are highlighted.

15.2 NANOTECHNOLOGY AND FOOD SYSTEMS

Food science and technology has made many micro- and often nano-size food particles by utilizing either the top-down (e.g. grinding, microparticulation, micronizing) or bottom-up (e.g. molecular aggregation) approaches. The advent of nanotechnology has ushered in new scientific and technological opportunities for the food industry, but the uncertainty remains whether small sized material should be treated as new entities when compared to their larger forms (Chau, Wu, & Yen, 2007). Efforts are underway worldwide to most responsibly realize the benefits of nanomaterials without exposing the public and environment to harm. Controlled cross-linking, inhibition of droplets coalescence, generation of multi-layered structures are just a few generic examples of the role of nanotechnology. To date, the key areas of food nanotechnology research, development and application include the following.

15.2.1 Structure and Function Characterization and Modification

Macro components of food, protein, carbohydrates and fat constitute a set of nanostructures that are ideally suited for targeted advances via nanotechnology. A vast majority of food carbohydrates and lipids are one-dimensional nanostructures of less than 1 nm in thickness, while globular proteins are nanoparticles of 10 to 100 nm in size. An understanding of the behavior and functionality of these nanostructures can be profitably used to set up processing strategies to improve food structure. Availability of new physical tools like the atomic force microscope (AFM) to study nanostructures has proven invaluable in understanding food structure-function relationships. AFM has been successfully used to quantify properties like stiffness, hardness, friction, elasticity or adhesion at the molecular level. The ability to manipulate individual biomolecules using AFM has allowed the study of structural and phase transitions, nanorheological and nanotribological properties of polymers (Boskovic, Chon, Mulvaney, & Sader, 2002; Morris *et al.*, 2001; Nakajima, Mitsui, Ikai, & Hara, 2001; Strick, Allemand, Croquette, & Bensimon, 2000; Terada, Harada, & Ikehara 2000). The gelation ability, the mechanisms of gelation, and the microstructure of the resulting gels were studied for biopolymers such as gums and proteins (Gajraj & Ofoli, 2000; Ikeda, Morris, & Nishinari, 2001; Morris *et al.*, 2001).

The development of new generation scanning probe microscopy (SPM) instrumentation, including the near-field scanning optical microscope, scanning thermal microscope, scanning capacitance microscope, magnetic force and resonance microscopes, and scanning electrochemical microscope, further enhanced the capability of investigations at the nanoscale. By combining SPM and AFM with other imaging, mechanical and spectroscopic methods, it is now possible to quantitatively characterize the structures of polymers at the micrometer and nanometer level,

as well as the intra- and intermolecular forces that stabilize such structures. Non-intrusive determination of local phase behavior and structure in complex biopolymer matrices could ultimately lead to improved control and design of the quality and stability of foods.

Fabrication at the nanoscale opened windows of opportunity for the creation of new, high performance materials with applications in food processing, packaging and storage. For example, nanotechnology approaches have been used to develop nanoparticles enhanced polymeric membranes for applications such as purification of ethanol and methanol (Jelinski, 1999; Kingsley, 2002). Another novel solution for enhancing membrane functionality is based on the use of nanotubes.

Nanotubes are long and thin tubes that can be assembled in extremely stable, strong, and flexible honeycomb structures. Nanotubes are the strongest fibers known—one nanotube is estimated to be 10 to 100 times stronger than steel per unit weight. By functionalizing nanotubes in a desired manner, membranes could be tailored to efficiently separate molecules both on the basis of their molecular size and shape, and on their chemical affinity. High selectivity nanotube membranes can be used both for analytical purposes, as part of sensors for molecular recognition of enzymes, antibodies, proteins and DNA, or for the membrane separation of biomolecules (Huang *et al.*, 2002; Lee & Martin, 2002; Rouhi, 2002).

Another application of nanotubes is the fabrication of nanotube-reinforced composites with high fracture and thermal resistance. Such materials could replace conventional materials in the manufacture of a wide range of machinery, including food-processing equipment (Gorman, 2003; Zhan, Kuntz, Wan, & Mukherjee, 2003). While such technologies are still too expensive for commercial scale food applications, it can be foreseen that they would become feasible for food-related applications in the not so distant future.

15.2.2 Nutrient Delivery Systems

Nanostructures in foods can be designed for the targeted delivery of nutrients in the body for the most beneficial effects. By facilitating a precise control of properties and functionality at the molecular level, nanotechnology enabled the development of highly effective encapsulation and delivery systems. Examples include nanometer sized association colloids such as surfactant micelles, vesicles, bilayers, reverse micelles, or liquid crystals. Such systems could be used in food applications as carrier or delivery systems for vitamins, antimicrobials, antioxidants, flavorings, colorants, or preservatives (Weiss et al., 2006).

Nanospheres have been proven to have superior encapsulation and release efficiency as compared to traditional encapsulation systems (Riley et al., 1999; Weiss et al., 2006). Nanoscale encapsulation systems can be produced using food biopolymers such as proteins or polysaccharides, which then can be used to encapsulate functional ingredients and release them in response to specific environmental triggers. Dendrimer-coated particles and cochleates can also be used as efficient encapsulation and delivery systems (Gould-Fogerite, Mannino, & Margolis, 2003; Khopade & Caruso, 2002; Santangelo et al., 2000). Cochleates can be used for the encapsulation and delivery of many bioactive materials, including compounds with poor water solubility, protein and peptide drugs, and large hydrophilic molecules (Gould-Fogerite et al., 2003). Another solution for encapsulation of functional components is via nanoemulsions. The advantage of nanoemulsions is that they can enable the slowdown of chemical degradation by engineering the properties of the interfacial layer surrounding them (McClements & Decker, 2000). Such systems could potentially be used for the encapsulation and targeted delivery and controlled release of functional food molecules.

15.2.3 Sensing and Safety

Nanotechnology has benefited the area of food safety mostly through the development of highly sensitive biosensors for pathogen detection and the development of novel antimicrobial solutions. Fellman (2001) reported the development of a method to produce nanoparticles with a triangular prismatic shape for detecting biological threats such as anthrax, smallpox and tuberculosis, and a wide range of genetic and pathogenic diseases. Latour et al. (2003) investigated the ability of two types of nanoparticles to irreversibly bind to certain bacteria, inhibiting them from binding to and infecting their host. One type was based on inorganic nanoparticles functionalized with polysaccharides and polypeptides that promote the adhesion of the targeted bacterial cells. This research has the potential to reduce the infective capability of human food borne enteropathogens such as Campylobacter, Salmonella and Escherichia coli in poultry products (Latour et al., 2003).

Kuo, Wang, Ruengruglikit, & Huang (2008) successfully developed a bioconjugation procedure that allows the attachment of water-soluble cadmium tellurium semiconductor quantum dots to anti-E.coli antibody. Such quantum dots are promising probe materials in the development of antibody-based immunosensors with high stability, sensitivity, and reproducibility, that could allow the detection of a single pathogenic cell (Kuo et al., 2008). Jin et al. (2009) showed that quantum dots made out of zinc oxide could be effective at inhibiting pathogens such as Listeria monocytogenes, Salmonella enteritidis, and Escherichia coli O157:H7, which further demonstrated the promise of nanoparticles for food safety applications.

15.2.4 Food Packaging and Tracking

The use of nanostructured materials, particularly nanocomposites, could considerably enhance the functional properties of packaging materials, and thus improve the shelf life of packaged foods. Nanocomposites are made out of nanoscale structures with unique morphology, increased modulus and strength, as well as good barrier properties. For example, a packaging material made out of potato starch and calcium carbonate that has good thermal insulation properties, lightweight, and biodegradability, was proposed as a replacement for the polystyrene 'clam-shell' used for fast food (Stucky, 1997). Nanocomposites are also regarded as a potential solution for plastic beer bottles (Moore, 1999). Natural smectite clays, particularly montmorillonite, a volcanic material that consists of nanometer-thick platelets, can be used as an additive that makes plastics lighter, stronger, more heat-resistant, with improved oxygen, carbon dioxide, moisture and volatile barrier properties (Quarmley & Rossi, 2001). Nanocomposites based on starch and reinforced with tunicin whiskers (Mathew & Dufresne, 2002) or clay nanocomposites (Park *et al.*, 2003) have also been developed in recent years. A nanocomposite material based on chitosan and reinforced with exfoliated hydroxyapatite layers was developed by Weiss *et al.* (2006).

Coatings or films for food packaging materials could also be made using nanolaminates and nanofibers. Nanolaminates consist of two or more layers of material with nanometer dimensions physically or chemically bonded to each other. Nanolaminates can be made using the layer-by-layer (LbL) deposition technique, which allows precise control of the thickness and properties of the nanolaminates (Weiss *et al.*, 2006). Nanofibers are polymeric strands of sub-micrometer diameters produced by interfacial polymerization and electrospinning. Electrospun polymer fibers have unique mechanical, electrical, and thermal properties, and have applications in filtration, manufacturing of protective clothing and biomedical applications. Production of nanofibers from food biopolymers in the future might increase their use in the food industry for a range of applications, including packaging materials (Weiss *et al.*, 2006).

15.3 CURRENT STATUS OF REGULATION OF NANOMATERIALS IN FOOD

The need for information and scientific advice on the safety implications that may arise from the use of nanotechnology in food and agriculture was recognized by the World Health Organization (WHO) and the Food and Agriculture Organization (FAO) of the United Nations. These organizations decided to work together on identifying knowledge gaps in areas related to food safety, risk assessment procedures, as well as on developing global guidance on adequate and accurate methodologies to assess potential food safety risks that may arise from nanoparticles. This collaborative effort will focus on both the application of nanotechnology in the primary production of foods, in food processing, packaging and distribution, as well as the use of nano-diagnostic tools for detection and monitoring in the food and agriculture production. According to information posted on the FAO website (http://www.fao.org), the issues that will be addressed jointly by the two agencies include: a) on-going research and development on nanotechnologies for use in the food and agriculture sectors that are expected to reach market within the next 10 years; b) investigations of nanoparticle migration from food contact materials into foods; c) purity, particle size distribution and properties of nanoparticulate substances for use in foods and food contact surfaces; d) mechanistic understanding of the behavior of nanoparticles in the body; e) nano-forms of vitamins and nutrients in relation to their bio-availability, interference with the absorption of other nutrients and consideration of safe-limits; f) interactions of nanoparticles with biomolecules, nutrients and contaminants, and their relevance to human health; g) techniques for detecting, characterizing and measuring nanoparticles in foods and food contact materials; h) risk assessments of nanomaterials for use in foods and food contact surfaces; i) information on nano-diagnostic tools in the food and agriculture sectors; j) public perceptions of the applications of nanotechnologies to the food and agriculture sectors; and k) identification of needs and priority areas for scientific advice needed in safety management and regulation by national authorities.

The last issue listed above is of particular importance, as regulation of nanotechnology is still in its infancy, and there is a great deal of variability in how this topic is addressed from country to country. A brief overview of the current status of regulating nanotechnology products that are relevant for the food and agriculture sectors is provided below.

15.3.1 North America

In the United States, the government agency responsible for regulating food, dietary supplements, and drugs is the Food and Drug Administration (FDA). However, it must be noted that dietary supplements fall under a different set of regulations than those covering 'conventional' foods and drug products. The fact that some of these products, especially dietary supplements, are currently manufactured using nanotechnology creates an additional layer of complexity, as size has not been addressed so far by existing regulations. Under current US legislation, an ingredient or substance that will be added to foods is subject to premarket approval by FDA, unless its use is generally recognized as safe (GRAS). Yet, at this point there is no information or guidance on how existing listings for food additives and GRAS substances apply to nanoscale materials. Clarification in this area has been identified by many policy experts as

an urgent need, because otherwise products that contain nanoscale ingredients could be placed on the market without FDA clearance.

In a statement posted on its official website (http://www.fda.gov), the FDA states that it regulates products, not technologies, and that 'nanotechnology products will be regulated as "Combination Products" for which the regulatory pathway has been established by statute'. At the same time, recognizing the challenges associated with the development of nanoproducts, FDA issued in July 2007 a 'Nanotechnology Task Force Report'. The report is public and also available on the FDA's website. This report acknowledges that nanoscale materials could be potentially used in most product types regulated by FDA and that such materials present challenges because properties relevant to product safety and effectiveness may change at the nanoscale. This report recommends that FDA provides guidance regarding when the use of nanoscale materials changes the regulatory status of foods, food additives, food contact substances, or dietary supplements.

Efficient and strict regulations about nanotechnology cannot be passed, however, without a proper understanding of the potential risks associated with nanoproducts. The House Science and Technology Committee is currently looking into the need to strengthen federal efforts to learn more about the potential environmental, health and safety risks posed by engineered nanomaterials. This was done following Environmental Protection Agency (EPA) recommendations for improving federal risk research and oversight of engineered nanomaterials by EPA, FDA and the Consumer Product Safety Commission. The report, 'Nanotechnology Oversight: An Agenda for the Next Administration', published by the Project on Emerging Nanotechnologies (PEN) (Davies, 2008), offers a range of proposals on how Congress, federal agencies and the White House can improve oversight of engineered nanomaterials.

The report 'Review of the Federal Strategy for Nanotechnology-Related Environmental,

Health and Safety Research' (National Research Council, 2008), identified serious weaknesses in the National Nanotechnology Initiative (NNI) plan for research on the potential health and environmental risks posed by nanomaterials. Among other observations, the report states that the NNI plan fails to identify important areas that should be investigated, such as a more comprehensive evaluation of how nanomaterials are absorbed and metabolized by the body and how toxic they are at realistic exposure levels. Significant criticism stemmed from the fact that the NNI plan does not address the current lack of studies on how to manage consumer and environmental risks, or mitigate exposure through consumer products. The report called for a revamped and comprehensive national strategic plan to minimize the potential risks of nanotechnology, which will allow the society to fully benefit from the discoveries of this technology in areas like medicine, energy, transportation and communications.

In a significant development, Canada is planning to become the first country in the world to require companies to detail their use of engineered nanomaterials. This information is meant to help evaluate the risks of engineered nanomaterials and will be used towards the development of a regulatory framework (Heintz, 2009). This action came shortly after the Office of Pollution Prevention and Toxics of the US EPA released in January 2009 an interim report on the Nanoscale Materials Stewardship Program (NMSP) (EPA, 2009). NMSP was developed to help provide a firmer scientific foundation for regulatory decisions by encouraging submission and development of information about nanoscale materials. Under the NMSP Basic Program, EPA invited participants to voluntarily report information on the engineered nanoscale materials they manufacture, import, process or use. Under the NMSP In-Depth Program, EPA invited participants to work with the Agency and others on a plan for the development of data on representative nanoscale materials over a longer time frame.

15.3.2 Europe

It is clear from a number of regulatory reports that there is currently no nano-specific regulation in the European Union (EU) (Chaudhry *et al.*, 2008), or other countries (Hodge *et al.*, 2007). However, the EU's approach to nanotechnology is that 'nanotechnology must be developed in a safe and responsible manner' (European Commission, 2008). To that end, the EU has commissioned the Scientific Committee on Emerging and Newly Identified Health Risks (SCENIHR) to make an inventory to check whether nanotechnologies are already covered by other community legislation, thus defining the legislative framework, considering both implementation and enforcement tools for this specific framework. It was concluded that the EU regulatory framework in principle also covered nanotechnologies (SCENIHR, 2007a). In line with this, EU member states will aim to modify existing laws and rules as and when developments within the fields of nanoscience and nanotechnology render such measures necessary (Franco, Hansen, Olsen, & Butti, 2007; Health Council Netherlands, 2006). The European Food Safety Authority (EFSA) was asked for a scientific opinion on the need for specific risk assessment approaches for technologies, processes and applications of nanoscience and nanotechnologies in the food and feed area. While EFSA recognized the limited knowledge on possible food applications and the limited knowledge on the nanotoxicology, it considered the currently used risk-assessment paradigm applicable for nanoparticles in food (EFSA, 2009).

15.3.2.1 Nano-size and regulations

The European General Food Law (GFL) is the umbrella of EU's food safety regulations (EC/178/2002) (EU, 2002). According to the GFL all foods placed on the Community market must be safe ('Food shall not be placed on the market if it is unsafe'; where unsafe is defined as 'injurious to health' or 'unfit for human consumption' article 14, sub 1). In making an assessment of food safety, producers, among others, are required to take into account the probable immediate, short-term and/or long-term effects on the consumer and subsequent generations. The GFL stipulates that it is the responsibility of 'food business operators' to ensure that their foods satisfy the requirements of food law. This regulation clearly stipulates that in decision making, scientific risk assessment should be central. The GFL stipulates that if after assessing the available information a possibility of harmful effects on health is identified but scientific uncertainty persist, risk management measures to ensure a high level of health protection may be adopted. Pending gathering and developing further scientific information for a more comprehensive risk assessment, the GFL allows the application of the precautionary principle.

Chemicals or substances intentionally added to food need to be authorized, meaning that in general a safety assessment of the material has been made before its market entry. In order to conduct a safety assessment, sufficient toxicological hazard information should be made available by the producers of the substance. This will also be the case for nano-substances subjected to authorization. However, in the existing European food safety legislation, no reference is made to nanotechnology or the nano-size of chemicals.

Authorization procedures, legislation, guidelines and guidance documents describe how and which toxicity tests should be performed. Adjustments of legislation in particular, guidelines and guidance documents concerning the testing of nanoparticles are considered to be necessary (SCENIHR, 2007a). In particular, information concerning the physico-chemical parameters—e.g. particle size, particle form, surface properties and other properties that may impact the toxicity of the substance—should be included. In addition, the validity of currently used toxicological assays—such as in the Organisation for Economic Co-operation and Development (OECD) safety test protocol—for the detection of 'novel' nanoparticle related effects needs to be determined. The currently used assays are validated for the toxicity testing of bulk chemicals. Furthermore, appropriate dose metrics to use in the hazard characterization and consumer exposure assessments of nanostructured materials should be developed. Thresholds or limits already set may not be appropriate for nano-sized variants of the particular substances.

If a substance in its conventional form has been evaluated, re-evaluation of the nano-sized form may be necessary. One should be aware, that each new nano-sized form of a certain chemical probably has to be considered as a separate new compound, as long as size-effect relationships are not established for that compound. This underscores the need for taking into account the effect of particle size (including distribution of the size) in toxicological studies.

15.3.2.2 Monitoring the products containing nanotechnology on the market

A requirement in the GFL is that member states should monitor to verify if the requirements of food law are fulfilled by food business operators. Also the EFSA should establish monitoring procedures to identify emerging risks. The monitoring of nanoparticles will require the development of new analytical detection and confirmation techniques.

The Novel Food Regulation (EC/258/97) can be very relevant for nanotechnology in food. This regulation addresses 'production processes not currently used', making it likely that this regulation also covers nanotechnology because of its novelty. It is not clear, however, whether the use of nano variants of chemicals in foods already on the market makes these foods 'novel' and thus requiring authorization. The Novel Food Regulation is under revision at this moment, which creates an opportunity to sort out nanotechnology related issues.

In conclusion, the current food safety legislative system should be adapted but not rewritten to cover nanotechnologies, while it continues to protect the European consumer. The discussions on definitions of nanotechnologies and nanoparticles continue within, for example, the scientific committees of the European Commission but also globally within ISO (IRGC, 2008). The outcome will have a direct effect on the regulatory framework within Europe. However, there are serious concerns on the sensitivity of current toxicity assays, these concerns are addressed in the next section.

15.4 HURDLES IN EVALUATION AND REGULATION OF THE USE OF NANOTECHNOLOGY IN FOODS

Food safety regulations require scientific safety assessments of foods and their ingredients, and this applies to nano-sized substances as well. While EFSA considered the currently used risk-assessment paradigm also applicable to nanoparticles in food (EFSA, 2009), it is also clear that this is severely hampered by the limited scientific knowledge of the biological interactions of nanoparticles and on consumer exposure (Bouwmeester et al., 2009; EFSA, 2009). The following section will focus on the main scientific knowledge gaps that currently hinder the safety assessment of nanoparticles in food and related products.

15.4.1 Lack of a Good Definition

The lack of a good definition of nanotechnology is problematic from a governance point of view. There are currently many definitions of nanotechnology available. Unfortunately, these either are too rigid to be applicable for food applications, or they are too flexible to be useful in legislation since they do not specify clear boundaries.

The rigid definitions, e.g. the ones that specifically mention that nanotechnology refers to dimensions of less than 100 nm, open the possibility that applications that use structures of slightly more than 100 nm need not conform to the regulation. If the definition is too flexible—e.g. if it refers to sizes of 'about 100 nm', although it is scientifically more accurate—it cannot be used in legal texts. Something as simple as labeling cannot be enforced at the moment because of the lack of a clear definition of nanomaterials, which allows industry to maintain a lack of transparency. For instance, the food industry is actively exploring the applicability of nanotechnology in food products, but is reluctant to admit to that.

15.4.2 Detection of Manmade Nanomaterials in Complex Matrices, Including Foods

Governance of applications of nanotechnology requires regulation of its use. Regulation in turn requires legislation and enforcement. Without means to enforce the regulation, the governance is useless and only constitutes an administrative process that does not really provide the protection against unwanted effects that the governance is seeking. Unfortunately, one key issue that hinders the enforcement of regulations related to the use of nanotechnology products is the capacity to detect nanostructures. Enforcement implies that manmade nanomaterials can be detected even if manufacturers of the products deny the use of nanotechnology.

Whereas the characterization of bulk chemical compounds in foods is usually relatively straightforward, characterization of nanoparticles is much more complex, due to several reasons. First, from an analytical point of view, there is not a single (or a handy) analytical tool-kit that allows the full characterization of nanoparticles in food. At present there is a vast array of analytical techniques available to characterize nanoparticles, both single-particle techniques and techniques for characterizing the assembly of engineered nano materials (ENM) (Hassellov, Readman, Ranville, & Tiede, 2008; Luykx, Peters, van Ruth, & Bouwmeester, 2008; Powers *et al.*, 2006; Tiede *et al.*, 2008). Generally, these methods are only able to determine one single characteristic; and currently, it is practically impossible to fully characterize nanoparticles. Therefore, research should primarily focus on method development for the detection and characterization of nanoparticles. Ideally, such methods should be relatively easily performed, and use equipment that is currently present at laboratories equipped for detection of chemicals in food. Interestingly, some of the definitions of nanoparticles introduce the specific functionalities of nanoparticles compared to the larger scale equivalents. While it might be difficult to define specific functionalities in general terms, this opens an alternative avenue for the characterization of nanoparticles: effect characterization. For this approach, *in vitro* assays searching for biomarkers for exposure might be a very elegant alternative.

Secondly, at the moment it is virtually impossible—apart from some very specific cases—to distinguish between manmade and natural nanoscale structures. And lastly, from a toxicological point of view, there is a lack of knowledge on how to describe biological dose-response relations, i.e. which metrics need to be used to express these relations. Up to now it has not been possible to establish a single dose-describing parameter that best describes the possible toxicity. It is likely that mass alone is not the good metric (SCENIHR, 2007a), but other characteristics such as size specific surface area, surface charge (Zeta potential), number of particles per particle size, as well as the number of particles per particle size might be very useful for describing the dose (Hagens *et al.*, 2007; McNeil, 2009; Oberdörster, Oberdörster, & Oberdörster, 2007a). Given the complexity of the matter, it is reasonable to say that the scientific requirements for analytical tools for nanostructures cannot be fully formulated yet.

15.4.3 Assessment of Exposure to Nanoparticles

Exposure assessment is defined as the qualitative and/or quantitative evaluation of the likely intake of biological, chemical or physical agents via food, as well as exposure from other sources if relevant (FAO/WHO, 1997). The reliability of the exposure assessment is critically depending on the availability of analytical tools to determine the presence or absence of nanoparticles in food. Basically, the principle of assessing exposure to nanoparticles via food will be comparable to the exposure assessment of conventional chemicals. Usually one of the following three approaches is applied for integration of data: 1) point estimated; 2) simple distributions; and 3) probabilistic analyses (Kroes *et al.*, 2002). Issues like food sampling and variability within composite samples, variation in concentrations between samples and consumption data on specific food products are not different from those encountered when assessing the exposure to conventional chemicals. Alternatively, food processors should provide reliable data on the use of nanoparticles in their products. The quality and reliability of the exposure assessment will be greatly improved if the concentration data is collected in an occurrence database. The last step in performing exposure assessment is the integration of occurrence and food consumption data. The procedures used here are not different from the ones used for conventional chemicals.

15.4.4 Toxicity of Nanoparticles

Knowledge on the potential toxicity of nanoparticles is limited but rapidly growing. So far, very few studies focused on elucidating what happens when nanoscale materials, some designed to be biologically active, enter the human body or are dispersed in the environment (Kuzma & VerHage, 2006). There is a body of review papers available (Donaldson *et al.*, 2001; Nel, Xia, Madler, &

Li, 2006; Oberdörster et al., 2005a; Oberdörster, Stone, & Donaldson, 2007b) that suggest that nanoparticles may have a deviating toxicity profile when compared to their bulk equivalents.

Most of the work that has been done so far addresses primarily the occupational hazards associated with the manufacture and handling of nanostructured materials. Some nanomaterials may initiate catalytic reactions and increase their fire and explosion potential and could potentially present a higher risk than similar quantities of a coarser material with the same chemical composition (Barlow et al., 2005; Duffin et al., 2002; Lison et al., 1997; Oberdörster, Ferin, & Lehnert, 1994; Pritchard, 2004). Experimental studies in rodents and cell cultures have shown that the toxicity of nanoparticles is greater than that of the same mass of larger particles of similar chemical composition. In addition to particle surface area, other particle characteristics may influence the toxicity, including solubility, shape, and surface chemistry (Donaldson et al., 2006; Duffin et al., 2002; Oberdörster et al., 2005a).

Based on several animal studies, nanoparticles have the greatest potential to enter the body if they become airborne or come into contact with the skin, from where they can translocate to other organs (CDC/NIOSH, 2006; Nemmar et al., 2002; Oberdörster et al., 2002; Ryman-Rasmussen et al., 2006; Takenaka et al., 2001). Experimental studies in rats have shown that at equivalent mass doses, particles smaller than 100 nm are more potent than larger particles of similar composition in causing pulmonary inflammation and fibrosis, tissue damage, and lung tumors, and that toxicity increases with decreasing particle size/increasing surface area (Barlow et al., 2005; Duffin et al., 2002; Lison et al., 1997; Oberdörster et al., 1992, 1994; Tran et al., 2000). In vitro studies performed on single- and multi-walled carbon nanotubes showed that they can enter cells and cause release of pro-inflammatory cytokines, oxidative stress, and decreased viability (Maynard et al., 2004; Monteiro-Riviere et al., 2005). Based on their findings in mice, Shvedova et al. (2005) estimated that workers may be at risk of developing lung lesions if exposed to single-walled carbon nanotubes for 20 days at the current Occupational Safety and Health Administration (OSHA) Permissible Exposure Limit for graphite (5 mg/m^3). According to the Centers for Disease Control/The National Institute for Occupational Safety and Health (CDC/NIOSH) report, epidemiological studies in workers exposed to aerosols of ultrafine particles have revealed depreciation of lung function, adverse respiratory symptoms, chronic obstructive pulmonary disease, and fibrosis, and even elevated levels of lung cancer (CDC/NIOSH, 2006).

The quality of many studies, however, is disputable, severely limiting the use of this information for risk assessment purposes (EFSA, 2009). For example in most studies only a single sized, poorly-characterized nanoparticle is used or nanoparticles are administered at unrealistically high doses, or a narrow range of effects are generally studied (Oberdörster et al., 2007b). In addition, when evaluating the plethora of in vitro studies with nanoparticles, caution has to be exercised when extrapolating their results or mechanisms for the hazard characterization to subsequent human risk assessment (Oberdörster et al., 2007b). The in vitro studies might be suitable for searching mechanistic explanations of toxic effects, or as screening methods in combination with profiling studies in a tiered hazard assessment approach (Balbus et al., 2007; Lewinski, Colvin, & Drezek, 2008).

One of the most important questions for the safety assessment is the sensitivity and validity of currently used test assays. While the knowledge on potential toxicity of nanoparticles is growing, at the time of writing only studies following acute (single dose) oral exposure are available. There is a great demand for studies using chronic oral exposure to nanoparticles combined with a broad screen for potential effects. Information from toxicity studies with other routes of exposure indicate that several systemic effects on different organ systems may occur after long-term exposure to nano-particles, including the immune, inflamma-tory and cardiovascular system. Effects on the immune and inflammatory systems may include oxidative stress and/or activation of pro-inflammatory cytokines in the lungs, liver, heart and brain. Effects on the cardiovascular system may include pro-thrombotic effects and adverse effects on the cardiac function (acute myocardial infarction and adverse effects on the heart rate). Furthermore, genotoxicity, and possible carcinogenesis and teratogenicity may occur but no data on the latter is available as yet (Bouwmeester et al., 2009).

15.4.5 Characteristics and Behavior of Nanoparticles in Food

According to the Woodrow Wilson Center's Project on Emerging Nanotechnologies, 84 con-sumer products from the food and beverage sector are currently available on the market (PEN, 2009). The list contains a range of items that come in direct contact with food, such as from aluminum foil or antibacterial kitch-enware, but also dietary supplements (i.e. Nanoceuticals™ Artichoke Nanoclusters) or canola oil fortified with free phytosterols. Such products allow, directly or indirectly, nanoparti-cles to enter the human body via ingestion.

Engineered nanoparticles in food may encom-pass many forms. Here the focus will be on persistent nanoparticles, i.e. non-soluble or bio-degradable particles, since potential risks are predominantly associated with these types of particles. It is likely that nanoparticles are used in foods in an agglomerated form, but it can-not be excluded that these agglomerates will break down and that the consumer will finally be exposed to free nanoparticles. Due to their specific chemico-physical properties, it is to be expected that nanoparticles could interact with proteins, lipids, carbohydrates, nucleic acids, ions, miner-als and water in food, feed and biological tissues. Experimental data available so far indicates that the characteristics of nanoparticles are likely to influence their absorption, distribution metabo-lism and excretion (ADME) (Ballou et al., 2004; des Rieux et al., 2006; Florence, 2005; Jani, Halbert, Largridge, & Florence, 1990; Roszek, de Jong, & Geertsma, 2005; Singh et al., 2006). For nanoparti-cles present in food their interactions with proteins are important (Linse et al., 2007; Lynch & Dawson, 2008). Protein adsorption to engineered nano-materials may enhance membrane crossing and cellular penetration (John et al., 2001, 2003; Pante & Kann, 2002). Furthermore, interaction with engineered nanomaterials may affect the tertiary structure of a protein, resulting in malfunctioning (Lynch, Dawson, & Linse, 2006). Therefore, it is important that the effects and interactions of nan-oparticles are characterized in the relevant food matrix (Oberdörster, Oberdörster, & Oberdörster 2005b; Powers et al., 2006; The Royal Society and the Royal Academy of Engineering, 2004).

Translocation of particles through the gastro-intestinal wall is a multi-step process, involving diffusion through the mucus lining the gut wall, contact with enterocytes or M-Cells, cellular or paracellular transport, and post-translocation events (des Rieux et al., 2006; Hoet, Bruske-Hohlfeld, & Salata, 2004). After passage of the intestinal epithelium, nanoparticles can enter the capillaries and enter the portal circulation to the liver, a major site for metabolism, or they can enter the lymphatic system which empties directly into the systemic blood circulation. The interactions with blood components might itself affect the fate of the nanoparticles. Unfortunately, there is little information regarding the distribu-tion of nanoparticles following oral exposure (Hagens et al., 2007). But following other expo-sure routes, a widespread distribution of nano-particles has been identified, where as a general pattern it appears that the smallest nanoparticles have the most widespread distribution (De Jong *et al.*, 2008; Hillery, Jani, & Florence, 1994; Hillyer & Albrecht, 2001; Hoet *et al.*, 2004; Jani *et al.*, 1990). Information on the potential of the nanoparticles to cross natural barriers like cellular, blood–brain, placenta and blood–milk barriers are important for the safety assessors.

Very little is known regarding biotransformation of nanoparticles after oral administration. The metabolism of nanoparticles should depend, among other properties, on their surface chemical composition. Polymeric nanoparticles can be designed to be biodegradable. For metal and metal oxide nanoparticles the slow dissolution will be of importance. Even less is known about the excretion of nanoparticles. As indicated, the potency of nanoparticles to interact with normal food constituents has raised speculation whether some nanoparticles may act as carriers (a 'Trojan horse' effect) of contaminants or foreign substances present in food (Shipley, Yean, Kan, & Tomson, 2008). This could result in aberrant exposure to these compounds, with severe implications on consumer health.

Generally, the focus is placed on non-soluble free nanoparticles. But another category of nanotechnology applications in food is represented by nano-encapsulates. These are specially designed to deliver their content with increased bioavailability. This type of application also needs to be considered by safety assessors.

To perform a robust safety assessment more information needs to be gathered on the mechanisms of absorption, distribution, metabolism and excretion of nanoparticles and other nanostructures. Only when this information is available will it be possible to initiate extrapolation and modeling approaches that will allow a more generalized safety assessment of nanostructured particles in food. Due to the potential impact of toxicological effects, special attention needs to be paid to the possibility that certain nanoparticles can cross the barriers (e.g. gastrointestinal barrier, cellular barrier, blood–brain barrier, placenta barrier, blood–milk barrier).

15.5 FUTURE DEVELOPMENTS AND CHALLENGES

At the first International Food Nanotechnology Conference organized by the Institute of Food Technologists (IFT) in 2006, participants agreed that nanotechnology is still in its infancy, with food applications being rather in a pre-infancy state, but also recognized a great amount of enthusiasm and anticipation surrounding this technology (Bugusu *et al.*, 2006). Consumer acceptance and the regulatory issues will dominate and dictate its growth. In the absence of mandatory product labeling anywhere in the world, it is not easy to pinpoint exactly how many commercial products now contain nano ingredients. It is clear that applications of nanotechnology such as sensors or process innovations have very different risk profiles than those where nanostructures are added to food products and are ingested by the consumer. Likewise, applications where nanotechnology is used to improve certain properties of the packaging material of food products should be considered differently. The nanomaterial first has to migrate from the packaging material into the foodstuff and in the absences of migration consumers will not be affected. Of course also these applications need to be assessed for possible unexpected effects, but the impact will be different than in the case of nanomaterials directly added to food products. The type of governance of applications of nanotechnologies in food and food industry should be dependent on the type of application of nanotechnologies.

Although potential beneficial effects of nanotechnologies are generally well described, the potential (eco)toxicological effects and impacts of nanoparticles have so far received little attention. The high speed of introduction of nanoparticle-based consumer products observed nowadays urges the need to generate a better understanding of the potential negative impacts that nanoparticles may have on biological systems. The main concerns stem from the lack of knowledge about the potential effects and impacts of nano-sized materials on human health and the environment (Bouwmeester et al., 2009). In addition to the scientific risk assessment related concerns, the consumers concerns regarding nanotechnology application in food products are mainly related to safety issues. It is recognized that the public concerns about the safety of products derived from new technologies may differ from those using established technologies (Siegrist, Stampfei, Kastenholz, & Keller, 2008).

Nanotechnologies used to improve certain properties of food products can range from the use of so called soft nanomaterials like micelles and vesicles to encapsulate nutrients and deliver them to specific locations in the gastrointestinal tract, to the use of nano formulated substances to improve the flow-behavior of powdered foodstuffs. It is generally agreed among toxicologists that the supramolecular structures that are designed to break down within the gastrointestinal tract constitute relatively low risks, assuming that the molecules used to make these structures are safe. Also, nanoparticles that easily dissolve in water or are biodegradable will most likely not be very hazardous. Most of the concerns of applications of nanotechnologies in food are focused on non-soluble free and persistent nanoparticles that potentially can pass certain barriers and enter the body, and subsequently enter certain tissues or even individual cells. Because of their persistent nature they can stay there for prolonged periods and induce harmful effects. A special cause of concern is represented by nanoformulations designed to increase the bioavailability of the bulk equivalent. This might impact on the toxic profile of these compounds and needs to be assessed. To ensure that consumers are not subjected to unacceptable risks and that foods that incorporate nanotechnology products are as safe as those foods that do not contain nanomaterials, governance should focus on non-soluble free manmade nanomaterials that

have functional characteristics different from their bulk equivalents in food products.

The general public strongly associates nanotechnology with nanoparticles and therefore assumes that the risks of all applications of nanotechnologies are comparable with the risks of non-soluble free nanoparticles. Since nanotechnology is an enabling technology, the actual form in which the consumer is exposed to the products of nanotechnology can be wide ranging. It is therefore important to educate the public and help it distinguish between the various forms and uses of nanotechnology, as well as the differences in risks between these applications. Unfortunately, the application of other state-of-the-art technologies in the past has shown that it takes time for this type of information to become widely accepted in society.

Proper regulation and monitoring of nanotechnology can help this process, since it would help build trust among users. Regulation implies that at least one impartial and objective body has reviewed and analyzed the specific application of the technology and has concluded that it is safe.

Globally, the scientific and industry communities need to come together to resolve the key issues of safety and public perception of nanotechnology. To fully exploit the benefits of nanomaterials without exposing the public to harm would require a judicious risk analysis and management. For the benefit of the humanity at large there can be no expedient and efficient way of doing it than through global harmonization of necessary regulations on nanomaterials.

References

Balbus, J. M., Maynard, A. D., Colvin, V. L., et al. (2007). Meeting report: Hazard assessment for nanoparticles—report from an interdisciplinary workshop. *Environmental Health Perspectives*, 115(11), 1654–1659.

Ballou, B., Lagerholm, B. C., Ernst, L. A., et al. (2004). Noninvasive imaging of quantum dots in mice. *Bioconjugate Chemistry*, 15(1), 79–86.

Barlow, P. G., Clouter-Baker, A. C., Donaldson, K., et al. (2005). Carbon black nanoparticles induce type II epithelial cells to release chemotaxins for alveolar macrophages. *Particle and Fibre Toxicology, 2*, 11–24.

Boskovic, S., Chon, J. W. M., Mulvaney, P., & Sader, J. E. (2002). Rheological measurements using cantilevers. *The Journal of Rheology, 46*(4), 891–899.

Bouwmeester, H., Dekkers, S., Noordamm, M. Y., et al. (2009). Review of health safety aspects of nanotechnologies in food production. *Regulatory Toxicology and Pharmacology, 53*(1), 52–62.

Bugusu, B., Bryant, C., Cartwright, T. T. et al. (2006). *Report on the First IFT International Food Nanotechnology Conference.* June 28–29, 2006, Orlando, Fla. Available online at http://members.ift.org/IFT/Research/ConferencePapers/firstfoodnano.htm (accessed March 2008).

CDC/NIOSH. (2006). *Centers for Disease Control and Prevention/National Institute for Occupational Safety and Health. Approaches to Safe Nanotechnology: An Information Exchange with NIOSH.* Available at www.cdc.gov/niosh (accessed February 2009).

Chau, C. F., Wu, S. H., & Yen, G. C. (2007). The development of regulations for food nanotechnology. *Trends in Food Science and Technology, 19*(3), 269–280.

Chaudhry, Q., Scotter, M., Blackburn, J., et al. (2008). Applications and implications of nanotechnologies for the food sector. *Food Additives and Contaminants, 25*(3), 241–258.

Chen, H., Weiss, J., & Shahidi, F. (2006). Nanotechnology in nutraceuticals and functional foods. *Food Technology, 60*(3), 30–36.

Das, M., Saxena, N., & Dwivedi, P. D. (2008). Emerging trends of nanoparticles application in food technology: Safety paradigms. *Nanotoxicology, 3*(1), 10–18.

Davies, C. J. (2008). *Nanotechnology Oversight: An Agenda for the Next Administration. Woodrow Wilson International Center for Scholars. Project on Emerging Nanotechnologies (PEN).* Available online at: http://www.nanotechproject.org (accessed February 2009).

De Jong, W. H., Hagens, W. I., Krystek, P., et al. (2008). Particle size-dependent organ distribution of gold nanoparticles after intravenous administration. *Biomaterials, 29*(12), 1912–1919.

des Rieux, A., Fievez, V., Garinot, M., et al. (2006). Nanoparticles as potential oral delivery systems of proteins and vaccines: A mechanistic approach. *Journal of Controlled Release, 116*(1), 1–27.

Donaldson, K., Aitken, R., Tran, L., Stone, V., Duffin, R., Forrest, G., & Alexander, A. (2006). Carbon Nanotubes: a review of their properties in relation to pulmonary toxicology and workplace safety. *Toxicol. Sci., 92*(1), 5–22.

Donaldson, K., Stone, V., Clouter, A., et al. (2001). Ultrafine particles 199. *Occupational and Environmental Medicine, 58*(3), 211–216.

Duffin, R., Tran, C. L., Clouter, A., et al. (2002). The importance of surface area and specific reactivity in the acute pulmonary inflammatory response to particles. *The Annals of Occupational Hygiene, 46*, 242–245.

EPA. (2009). Nanoscale Materials Stewardship Program (NMSP). Interim report. US Environmental Protection Agency. The Office of Pollution Prevention and Toxics. Available online at www.epa.gov (accessed February 2009).

EU. (2002). EC/178/2002. Regulation (EC) No 178/2002 of the European Parliament and of the Council of 28 January 2002 laying down the general principles and the requirements of food law, establishing the European Food Safety Authority and laying down procedures in matters of food safety. Official Journal of the European Union L 31, 1.2.2002.

European Commission. (2008). Commission Recommendation of 07 February 2008 on a Code of Conduct for Responsible Nanoscience and Nanotechnologies Research. Available online at http://ec.europa.eu/nanotechnology/index-en.html.

Fellman, M. (2001). *Nanoparticle Prism could Serve as Bioterror Detector.* Available online at http://unisci.com/stories/20014/1204011.htm (accessed 28 May 2002).

Florence, A. T. (2005). Nanoparticle uptake by the oral route: Fulfilling its potential?. *Drug Discovery Today: Technologies, 2*(1), 75–81.

Franco, A., Hansen, S. F., Olsen, S. I., & Butti, L. (2007). Limits and prospects of the 'incremental approach' and the European legislation on the management of risks related to nanomaterials. *Regulatory Toxicology and Pharmacology, 48*(2), 171–183.

Gajraj, A., & Ofoli, R. (2000). Quantitative technique for investigating macromolecular adsorption and interactions at the liquid–liquid interface. *Langmuir, 16*, 4279–4285.

Gorman, J. (2003). Fracture protection: Nanotubes toughen up ceramics 1, 3. *Science News, 163*.

Gould-Fogerite, S., Mannino, R. J., & Margolis, D. (2003). Cochleate delivery vehicles: Applications to gene therapy. *Drug Delivery Technology, 3*(2), 40–47.

Hagens, W. I., Oomen, A. G., de Jong, W. H., et al. (2007). What do we (need to) know about the kinetic properties of nanoparticles in the body? *Regulatory Toxicology and Pharmacology, 49*(3), 217–229.

Hassellov, M., Readman, J. W., Ranville, J. F., & Tiede, K. (2008). Nanoparticle analysis and characterization methodologies in environmental risk assessment of engineered nanoparticles. *Ecotoxicology, 17*(5), 344–361.

Health Council Netherlands. (2006). *Health significance of nanotechnologies.* The Hague: Health Council of the Netherlands publication no. 2006/06.

Heintz, M. E. (2009). *National Nanotechnology Regulation in Canada?* Posted online at www.nanolawreport.com. 28 January, 2009 (accessed March 2009).

Hillery, A. M., Jani, P. U., & Florence, A. T. (1994). Comparative, quantitative study of lymphoid and non-lymphoid uptake of 60 nm polystyrene particles. *Journal of Drug Targeting*, 2(2), 151–156.

Hillyer, J. F., & Albrecht, R. M. (2001). Gastrointestinal persorption and tissue distribution of differently sized colloidal gold nanoparticles. *Journal of Pharmaceutical Sciences*, 90(12), 1927–1936.

Hodge, G., Bowman, D., & Ludlow, K. (Eds.), (2007). *New global frontiers in regulation: The age of nanotechnology*. Cheltenham UK: Edward Elgar Publishing Ltd.

Hoet, P., Bruske-Hohlfeld, I., & Salata, O. (2004). Nanoparticles, known and unknown health risks. *Journal of Nanobiotechnology*, 2(1), 12.

Huang, W., Taylor, S., Fu, K., et al. (2002). Attaching proteins to carbon nanotubes via diimide-activated amidation. *Nano Letters*, 2(4), 311–314.

Ikeda, S., Morris, V., & Nishinari, K. (2001). Microstructure of Aggregated and Non-Aggregated k-Carrageenan Helices visualized by Atomic Force Microscopy. *Biomacromolecules*, 2, 1331–1337.

International Risk Governance Council (IRCG). (2008). A report for IRGC Risk Governance of Nanotechnology Applications in Food and Cosmetics. International Risk Governance Council, Geneva, September 2008. Available online at: http://www.irgc.org/IMG/pdf/IRGC-PB nano-food-WEB.pdf.

Jani, P., Halbert, G. W., Langridge, J., & Florence, A. T. (1990). Nanoparticle uptake by the rat gastrointestinal mucosa: Quantitation and particle size dependency. *The Journal of Pharmacy and Pharmacology*, 42(12), 821–826.

Jelinski, L. (1999). Biologically related aspects of nanoparticles, nanostructured materials and nanodevices. Available online at http://www.wtec.org (accessed May 2002). In R. W. Siegel, E. Hu, & M. C. Roco (Eds.), *Nanostructure science and technology. A worldwide study. Prepared under the guidance of the National Science and Technology Council and the Interagency Working Group on NanoScience, Engineering and Technology*.

Jin, Z. T., Zhang, H. Q., Sun, D., et al. (2009). Antimicrobial efficacy of zinc oxide quantum dots against *listeria monocytogenes*, *Salmonella enteritidis* and *Escherichia coli* O157: H7. *Journal of Food Science*, 74(1), M46–M52.

John, T. A., Vogel, S. M., Minshall, R. D., et al. (2001). Evidence for the role of alveolar epithelial gp60 in active transalveolar albumin transport in the rat lung. *The Journal of Physiology*, 533(Pt 2), 547–559.

John, T. A., Vogel, S. M., Tiruppathi, C., et al. (2003). Quantitative analysis of albumin uptake and transport in the rat microvessel endothelial monolayer. *American Journal of Physiology Lung Cellular and Molecular Physiology*, 284(1), L187–L196.

Khopade, A. J., & Caruso, F. (2002). Electrostatically assembled polyelectrolyte/dendrimer multilayer films as ultrathin nanoreservoirs. *Nano Letters*, 2(4), 415–418.

Kingsley, D. (2002). *Membranes Show Pure Promise*. ABC Science Online, May 1, 2002. Available online at www.abc.net.au (accessed 22 August 2003).

Kroes, R., Muller, D., Lambe, J., et al. (2002). Assessment of intake from the diet. *Food and Chemical Toxicology*, 40(2–3), 327–385.

Kuo, Y. C., Wang, Q., Ruengruglikit, C., & Huang, Q. R. (2008). Antibody-conjugated CdTe quantum dots for *E. coli* detection. *The Journal of Physical Chemistry C*, 112(13), 4818–4824.

Kuzma, J., & VerHage, P. (2006). *New Report on Nanotechnology in Agriculture and Food Looks at Potential Applications, Benefits and Risks*. Available online at http://www.nanotechproject.org/news/archive/new_report_on_nanotechnology_in/ (accessed April 2008).

Latour, R. A., Stutzenberger, F. J., Sun, Y. P. et al. (2003). *Adhesion-Specific Nanoparticles for Removal of Campylobacter Jejuni from Poultry*. CSREES Grant (2000–2003), Clemson University (SC). http://www.clemson.edu (Accessed June 2003).

Lee, S. B., & Martin, C. R. (2002). Electromodulated molecular transport in gold-nanotube membranes. *Journal of the American Chemical Society*, 124(40), 11850–11851.

Lewinski, N., Colvin, V., & Drezek, R. (2008). Cytotoxicity of nanoparticles. *Small*, 4(1), 6–49.

Linse, S., Cabaleiro-Lago, C., Xue, W. F., et al. (2007). Nucleation of protein fibrillation by nanoparticles. *Proceedings of the National Academy of Sciences of the United States of America*, 104(21), 8691–8696.

Lison, D., Lardot, C., Huaux, F., et al. (1997). Influence of particle surface area on the toxicity of insoluble manganese dioxide dusts. *Archives of Toxicology*, 71(12), 725–729.

Luykx, D. M. A. M., Peters, R. J. B., van Ruth, S. M., & Bouwmeester, H. (2008). A review of analytical methods for the identification and characterization of nano delivery systems in food. *Journal of Agricultural and Food Chemistry*, 56(18), 8231–8247.

Lynch, I., & Dawson, K. A. (2008). Protein-nanoparticle interactions. *Nano Today*, 3(1–2), 40–47.

Lynch, I., Dawson, K. A., & Linse, S. (2006). Detecting cryptic epitopes created by nanoparticles. *Science's STKE*, 2006(327), pe14.

Mathew, A. P., & Dufresne, A. (2002). Morphological investigation of nanocomposites from sorbitol plasticized starch and tunicin whiskers. *Biomacromolecules*, 3(3), 609–617.

Maynard, A. D., Baron, P. A., Foley, M., et al. (2004). Exposure to carbon nanotube material: Aerosol release during the handling of unrefined single walled carbon nanotube material. *Journal of Toxicology and Environmental Health A*, 67(1), 87–107.

McClements, D. J., & Decker, E. A. (2000). Lipid oxidation in oil-in-water emulsions: Impact of molecular environment on chemical reactions in heterogeneous food systems. *Journal of Food Science*, 65(8), 1270–1282.

McNeil, S. E. (2009). Nanoparticle therapeutics: A personal perspective. Wiley Interdisciplinary Reviews: Nanomedicine and Nanobiotechnology DOI: 10.1002/wnan.006.

Monteiro-Riviere, N. A., Nemanich, R. J., Inman, A. O., Wang, Y. Y., & Riviere, J. E. (2005). Multi-walled carbon nanotube interactions with human epidermal keratinocytes. *Toxicol. Lett.*, *155*(3), 377–384.

Moore, S. (1999). Nanocomposite achieves exceptional barrier in films. *Modern Plastics*, *76*(2), 31–32.

Moraru, C. I., Huang, Q., Takhistov, P., et al. (2009). Food nanotechnology: Current developments and future prospects. IUFFoST Handbook. Gustavo Barbosa Canovas (Ed.), *In press*.

Moraru, C. I., Panchapakesan, C. P., Huang, Q., et al. (2003). Nanotechnology: A new frontier in food science. *Food Technology*, *57*(12), 24–29.

Morris, V., Mackie, A., Wilde, P., et al. (2001). Atomic force microscopy as a tool for interpreting the rheology of food biopolymers at the molecular level. *Lebensmittel-Wissenschaft u-Technology*, *34*, 3–10.

Nakajima, K., Mitsui, K., Ikai, A., & Hara, M. (2001). Nanorheology of single protein molecules. *Riken Review*, *37*, 58–62.

National Research Council. (2008). *Review of the federal strategy for nanotechnology-related environmental, health and safety research*. National Academies Press ISBN-10: 0309116996.

Nemmar, A., Hoet, P. H. M., Vanquickenborne, B., Dinsdale, D., Thomeer, M., Hoylaerts, M. F., Vanbilloen, H., Mortelmans, L., & Nemery, B. (2002). Passage of inhaled particles into the blood circulation in humans.. *Circulation*, *105*, 411–414.

Nel, A., Xia, T., Madler, L., & Li, N. (2006). Toxic potential of materials at the nanolevel 622–227. *Science*, *311*(5761).

Oberdörster, G., Ferin, J., Gelein, R., Soderholm, S. C., & Finkelstein, J. (1992). Role of the alveolar macrophage in lung injury—studies with ultrafine particles. *Environ. Health Perspect.*, *97*, 193–199.

Oberdörster, G., Ferin, J., & Lehnert, B. E. (1994). Correlation between particle-size, *in-vivo* particle persistence, and lung injury. *Environmental Health Perspectives Supplement*, *102*(S5), 173–179.

Oberdörster, G., Sharp, Z., Atudorei, V., Elder, A., Gelein, R., Lunts, A., Kreyling, W., & Cox, C. (2002). Extrapulmonary translocation of ultrafine carbon particles following whole-body inhalation exposure of rats. *Journal of Toxicology and Environmental Health, Part A*, *65*(20), 1531–1543.

Oberdörster, G., Maynard, A., Donaldson, K., et al. (2005a). Principles for characterizing the potential human health effects from exposure to nanomaterials: Elements of a screening strategy. *Particle and Fibre Toxicology*, *2*, 8.

Oberdörster, G., Oberdörster, E., & Oberdörster, J. (2005b). Nanotoxicology: An emerging discipline evolving from studies of ultrafine particles. *Environ Health Perspect*, *113*(7), 823–839.

Oberdörster, G., Oberdörster, E., & Oberdörster, J. (2007a). Concepts of nanoparticle dose metric and response metric. *Environmental Health Perspectives*, *115*(6), A290.

Oberdörster, G., Stone, V., & Donaldson, K. (2007b). Toxicology of nanoparticles: A historical perspective. *Nanotoxicology*, *1*(1), 2–25.

Pante, N., & Kann, M. (2002). Nuclear pore complex is able to transport macromolecules with diameters of about 39 nm. *Molecular Biology of the Cell*, *13*(2), 425–434.

Park, H. M., Lee, W. K., Park, C. Y., et al. (2003). Environmentally friendly polymer hybrids. Part I: Mechanical, thermal, and barrier properties of the thermoplastic starch/clay nanocomposites. *Journal of Materials Science*, *38*, 909–915.

PEN (2009). *Consumer Products. An Inventory of Nanotechnology-based Consumer Products Currently on the Market*. Available online at http://www.nanotechproject.org (accessed March 2009).

Powers, K. W., Brown, S. C., Krishna, V. B., et al. (2006). Research strategies for safety evaluation of nanomaterials. Part VI. Characterization of nanoscale particles for toxicological evaluation. *Toxicological Sciences*, *90*(2), 296–303.

Pritchard, D. K. (2004). *Literature Review, Explosion Hazards Associated with Nanopowders*. United Kingdom: Health and Safety Laboratory, HSL/2004/12. Available online at http://www.hse.gov.uk (accessed February 2009).

Quarmley, J., & Rossi, A. (2001). Nanoclays. Opportunities in polymer compounds 52–53. *Industrial Mineral*, *400*, 47–49.

Riley, T., Govender, T., Stolnik, S., et al. (1999). Colloidal stability and drug incorporation aspects of micellar-like PLA-PEG nanoparticles. *Colloids and Surfaces*, *B16*, 147–159.

Roszek, B., de Jong, W., & Geertsma, R. (2005). *Nanotechnology in medical applications: State-of-the-art in materials and devices*. RIVM report 265001001/2005.

Rouhi, M. (2002). Novel chiral separation tool. *Chemical and Engineering News*, *80*(25), 13.

Ryman-Rasmussen, J. P., Riviere, J. E., & Monteiro-Riviere, N. A. (2006). Penetration of intact skin by quantum dots with diverse physiochemical properties. *Toxicological Sciences*, *91*(1), 159–165.

Santangelo, R., Paderu, P., Delmas, G., et al. (2000). Efficacy of oral cochleate-amphotericin B in a mouse model of systemic candidiasis. *Antimicrob Agents Chemother*, *44*(9), 2356–2360.

SCENIHR. (2007a). Scientific Committee on Emerging and Newly Identified Health Risks. Opinion on: The appropriateness of the risk assessment methodology in accordance with the technical guidance documents for new and existing substances for assessing the risks of nanomaterials. European Commission Health & Consumer Protection Directorate-General. Directorate C, Public Health and Risk Assessment; C7, Risk Assessment.

SCENIHR. (2007b). Scientific Committee on Emerging and Newly Identified Health Risks. Opinion on: The scientific aspects of the existing and proposed definitions relating to products of nanoscience and nanotechnologies. European Commission Health & Consumer Protection Directorate-General. Directorate C, Public Health and Risk Assessment; C7, Risk Assessment.

ScienceDaily. (2007). Project on Emerging Nanotechnology (2007, May 23). Nanotechnology Now Used In Nearly 500 Everyday Products. (http://www.sciencedaily.com/releases/2007/05/070523075416.htm).

Shipley, H. J., Yean, S., Kan, A. T., & Tomson, M. B. (2008). Adsorption of arsenic to magnetite nanoparticles: Effect of particle concentration, pH, ionic strenght and, temperature. Environmental Toxicology and Chemistry, 1.

Shvedova, A. A., Kisin, E. R., Mercer, R., et al. (2005). Unusual inflammatory and fibrogenic pulmonary responses to single walled carbon nanotubes in mice. American Journal of Physiology. Lung Cellular and Molecular Physiology, 289, L698–L708.

Siegrist, M., Stampfli, N., Kastenholz, H., & Keller, C. (2008). Perceived risks and perceived benefits of different nanotechnology foods and nanotechnology food packaging. Appetite, 51(2), 283–290.

Singh, R., Pantarotto, D., Lacerda, L., et al. (2006). Tissue biodistribution and blood clearance rates of intravenously administered carbon nanotube radiotracers. Proceedings of the National Academy of Sciences of the United States of America, 103(9), 3357–3362.

Strick, T., Allemand, J., Croquette, V., & Bensimon, D. (2000). Stress-induced structural transitions in DNA and proteins. Annual Review of Biophysics and Biomolecular Structure, 29, 523–543.

Stucky, G. D. (1997). Oral presentation at the WTEC Workshop on R&D status and trends in nanoparticles, nanostructured materials, and nanodevices in the United States, May 8–9, Rosslyn, VA.

Takenaka, S., Karg, D., Roth, C., Schulz, H., Ziesenis, A., Heinzmann, U., Chramel, P., & Heyder, J. (2001). Pulmonary and systemic distribution of inhaled ultrafine silver particles in rats. Environ. Health Perspect., 109(suppl. 4), 547–551.

Terada, Y., Harada, M., & Ikehara, T. (2000). Nanotribology of polymer blends. Journal of Applied Physics, 87(6), 2803–2807.

The Royal Society and the Royal Academy of Engineering. (2004). The Royal Society and the Royal Academy of Engineering. Nanoscience and nanotechnologies: opportunities and uncertainties. London, UK.

Tiede, K., Boxall, A. B., Tear, S. P., et al. (2008). Detection and characterization of engineered nanoparticles in food and the environment. Food Additives and Contaminants, 25(7), 795–821.

Tran, C. L., Buchanan, D., Cullen, R. T., Searl, A., Jones, A. D., & Donaldson, K. (2000). Inhalation of poorly soluble particles. II. Influence of particle surface area on inflammation and clearance. Inhalation Toxicology, 12(12), 1113–1126.

Weiss, J., Takhistov, P., & McClements, J. (2006). Functional materials in food nanotechnology. Journal of Food Science, 71(9), R107–R116.

Zhan, G. D., Kuntz, J., Wan, J., & Mukherjee, A. K. (2003). Single-wall carbon nanotubes as attractive toughening agents in alumina-based nanocomposites. Nature Materials, 2, 38–42.

16

Novel Food Processing Technologies and Regulatory Hurdles

Gustavo V. Barbosa-Canovas and Daniela Bermúdez-Aguirre

Center for Nonthermal Processing of Food, Washington State University, Pullman, WA, USA

16.1 INTRODUCTION

The search for new food processing and preservation technologies is really more than 100 years old (Lelieveld & Keener, 2007), but in the last 20 years food scientists have accelerated this development to newer technologies capable of producing and maintaining a final food product with fresh-like characteristics. Moreover, the goal has been to achieve higher quality products while also ensuring the microbiological safety of the food. A number of novel food processing technologies are still under development, some of which have been recognized and approved by regulatory agencies for use in food processing. High hydrostatic pressure (HHP)* is currently used worldwide for the pasteurization of specific products; its approval in the USA for use as a processing alternative in combination with thermal processing for sterilization has been announced (NCFST: National Center for Food

*Also known as High pressure processing (HPP).

Safety and Technology, 2009). The non-thermal and thermal novel technologies, pulsed electric fields (PEF) and microwave, respectively, are now in the pre-approval phase. Most of the requirements for acceptance as alternative technologies for food processing have now been set up; however, a series of validation experiments must be conducted first. Because of their fast development, including other technologies under progress in the lab, there is a lack of valuable information related to the process (for example, standardization of process variables) and these should all be addressed worldwide. The urgent need for global harmonization of food regulations and legislation on novel technologies is a matter of concern for not only food scientists, but also regulatory agencies, because of the importance of providing consumers with safe food regardless of the processing technology used. Initial attempts have been made to address the above mentioned issue with the establishment of the Global Harmonization Initiative (Lelieveld & Keener, 2007).

This chapter focuses on some of the novel food processing technologies (such as HHP, PEF, irradiation and microwave) and on how the required standardization process and reporting of processing parameters are subjects that must be addressed.

16.2 NOVEL TECHNOLOGIES

The search for alternative methods for food pasteurization and sterilization which would generate a safer product with higher quality nutrient content and sensorial properties prompted food scientists to explore other inactivation factors—those other than heat or heat applied in a different way compared to traditional sterilization (conduction and convection). Two very broad fields of food processing technologies are currently under research (Table 16.1): non-thermal technologies, in which the inactivation factor is different from heat using physical

TABLE 16.1 Examples of novel food processing and preservation technologies around the world

Non-thermal technologies	Thermal technologies
High hydrostatic pressure[*]	Microwave
Pulsed electric fields	Radio frequency
Irradiation[*]	Ohmic heating
Ultraviolet[*]	Inductive heating
Ultrasound	
Cold plasma	
Ozone[*]	
Dense phase carbon dioxide[*]	
Supercritical water	

[*]Currently for commercial use.

hurdles such as pressure, electromagnetic fields, and sound waves, among others; and novel thermal processing technologies, which mainly use energy generated by microwave and radio frequency. However, using such novel technologies to inactivate microorganisms and enzymes in food is not enough. A safe product should also be free of toxic substances and contact of food with certain materials during processing should be avoided (Lelieveld & Keener, 2007). Thus, evaluation of the overall quality of food products processed by emerging technologies is an essential requirement before a product can be commercialized.

It is worth mentioning that most novel technologies were first studied as prospective microbial inactivation technologies to improve the safety of food. However, important results in the final characteristics of many food items were also observed: such as intact nutrient content in most of the novel food products; unique sensorial properties like color, texture, and appearance; and formation of new aroma compounds. Thus, the search for microbial inactivation technologies not only yielded the possibility of a safer product, but also improved overall product quality, and provided new ingredients for the development of other novel food products.

Another point worthy of note relates to the connection that novel technologies have with environmental concerns; most of the developed emerging technologies are environmentally friendly and may even offer significant energy savings. These savings are due, in part, to much shorter processing times.

16.3 NON-THERMAL TECHNOLOGIES

The list of non-thermal technologies under research is quite long, the most popular being HHP, which 20 years ago was under research in very few research centers worldwide. Today, HHP application is extensively scattered around the world, not only for use in research, but in industry as well, as a lot of food industries now process specific products with high acceptance by consumers. HHP was initially used to pasteurize high-acid foods such as juices and smoothies, with successful results. Another use that followed was microbial inactivation in some packaged foods, as demonstrated in ready-to-eat and deli-meat products, considerably extending shelf life. Today, the list of commercially pressurized products includes guacamole, sauces, oysters, jellies, jams, fruit products, and more. The big challenge for food scientists in the past was to use HHP for processing shelf-stable, low-acid foods (i.e. for spore inactivation); many attempts were thus conducted using extremely elevated high pressures (up to 1 GPa). However, this focus has since changed with the ruling in February 2009 in which Pressure Assisted Thermal Processing PATP* was accepted by FDA (USA) for processing and preserving food as an alternative sterilization technology (NCFST, 2009). PATP does not require extremely elevated high pressures;

*PATP (Pressure Assisted Thermal Processing) and PATS (Pressure Assisted Thermal Sterilization) have the same meaning, but we prefer to use PATP in this chapter.

it works within the standard high pressure range already established for food pasteurization (600 MPa), but adds the intelligent combination of thermal treatment and fixed processing times. With the approval of PATP, a new era in food science has begun. The possibility of PATP processed shelf-stable foods, such as breakfast items, meats, stews, soups, dairy desserts, high quality fruits and vegetables, pasta sauces, or even ready-to-drink teas and coffee, has indeed opened new niches in the global commercialization of PATP—a novel technology that offers important improvements in food quality and safety, while also being environmentally friendly.

High pressure and PEF are probably the two most intensively researched non-thermal technologies evaluated over the last few decades. This fact is based on their potential use in various industrial activities such as pasteurization, sterilization or extraction; available information for food processors on the benefits of HHP and PEF for food processing has been published and delivered in many ways (Ramaswamy, Balasubramaniam, & Kaletunc, 2004a; Jin, Balasubramaniam, & Zhang, 2004b), informing both the industrial community and consumers.

Irradiation is another non-thermal technology that has been approved for specific uses; in 1990, more than 40 countries used this technology for commercial purposes (Molins, 2001). The first use of irradiation dates back to 1958 when it was recognized by the FDA as more of an additive than a process, even though irradiation is really just energy applied to food (HPS, 2009). Currently, irradiation facilities are regulated by federal and/or state licensing agencies, and according to the actual dose applied, its effect on inactivating microorganisms, extending product shelf life, or inhibiting post-harvest changes in certain food products can vary quite significantly. The list of irradiated food products is very comprehensive; a few examples are flour, potatoes, spices, pork, fruit, fresh vegetables, poultry, meat, pet food, and specific food items for NASA's Space Program and immune-compromised patients. Several 'fact sheets' have been published on irradiation (FDA, 1997a, 1997b; HPS, 2009; Keener, 2009) to show the advantages of this technology and to probe the erroneous belief about radioactivity in foods following irradiation. Even the use of other terms instead of irradiation, such as cold pasteurization, has been suggested (Ehlermann, 2009).

Other non-thermal technologies under research are PEF, ultrasound, ultraviolet, cold plasma, ozone and dense phase carbon dioxide. Pulsed electric fields technology is probably the most explored on this list, as evidenced by the number of products and microorganisms tested under this technology, and the important advances and encouraging results with PEF as an alternative for liquid food pasteurization. Further non-thermal examples include the use of ultraviolet and ozone for water disinfection; however, they are still under research for opaque liquids (e.g. milk) and liquids with small particulates, representing new challenges for food scientists.

16.4 THERMAL TECHNOLOGIES

In the search for new alternatives to conventional thermal processing of food, the application of heat generated inside the food seems to be a viable option for preserving the quality of products and inactivating microorganisms. The microwave energy moves the water and charged food molecules, which aligns them with a specific electric field, producing a movement and friction between them, and subsequently generating heat inside the food. Because the heat transfer time from a heating source to the food is short, food quality is excellent after this process. Washington State University participates in an important academic-industry-government consortium in the development and implementation of this technology; a formal petition to use microwave as a sterilization technology (at

45 kW, 915 MHz; semi-continuous system) was submitted to the FDA in October 2008 and has made important headway (Tang, 2009). Other novel thermal technologies under research and that could be viable options for food processing in the coming years, are radio frequency, inductive heating, and ohmic heating.

16.5 LEGISLATIVE ISSUES CONCERNING NOVEL TECHNOLOGIES

The world of food regulations is huge. There is a significant number of regulations concerning farming and agricultural activities, food formulation and labeling, and of course food production and processing technologies. The pressing need for a global regulation of all food processing activities has been ongoing for some time (Rogers, 1999).

A new process or product must meet a series of standards and regulations before it can be used commercially. Depending on the type of product, there is a list of safety regulations that a food item must meet: these are related to the guidelines established in the HACCP (Hazard Analysis Critical Control Point) and GMPs (Good Manufacturing Practices) documents, and must be implemented during processing. A number of international regulations and guidelines must be followed, such as the recommendations of the World Trade Organization (WTO) to ensure the safety of novel products or processes. With the creation of WTO in 1995, the search for global harmonization in food safety regulations became an important issue needing to be addressed by many countries. Agreements, such as the Agreement on the Application of Sanitary and Phytosanitary Measures (SPS), together with the Codex Alimentarius Commission, encouraged countries to work toward international legislation on food standards, regulations, and guidelines

(Motarjemi, van Schothorst, & Käferstein, 2001). The WTO is not in charge of developing food safety standards, but it does have the authority to limit and control some food safety actions by using the SPS Agreement and Technical Barriers to Trade (TBT) Agreement, which covers other food safety and food quality issues (Mansour, 2004). The *Codex Alimentarius* definitely plays a significant role in global harmonization, together with other non-governmental institutions, not only for novel technologies, but also for other food science issues that require globalization (Newsome, 2007).

16.6 GLOBAL HARMONIZATION CONCERNING NOVEL TECHNOLOGIES

There are many regulations concerning food safety around the world; in most cases each country has established their own standards for specific food products. These regulations are established to show that a specific food product or ingredient is safe for human consumption or food formulation. However, showing that the same product is also safe in other countries usually requires compliance with different legislations. This is often time-consuming and costly, not to mention delays in the food processing chain (Lelieveld & Keener, 2007; Rogers, 1999; Sawyer, Kerr, & Hobbs, 2008). On the other hand, many foodborne outbreaks have been generated because of imported food that has served as a vehicle for pathogens from one country to another, even in countries with strict and modern control systems at borders (Motarjemi *et al.*, 2001). Nevertheless, without international trade of foodstuffs, many products would not be commercialized in specific and remote markets. In addition, travelers are also a source of widespread pathogenic bacteria, as shown by Notermans and Lelieveld (2001); the probability of contracting a foodborne disease is very high in specific countries because of poor general hygiene practices when handling food (e.g. 63% in Egypt).

The main priority at present is to establish regulations and legislation for food safety that would declare that a particular food product is safe regardless of where it is processed (Lelieveld & Keener, 2007; Motarjemi *et al.*, 2001). Global harmonization of these regulations and protocols should be addressed, including a system that monitors and assures that this legislation is followed (Lelieveld & Keener, 2007). Harmonization, as defined by Horton (1997) *'exists when two or more countries have a common set of requirements in place.'* According to Horton, global harmonization of food issues is important but will be difficult. With harmonization, however, the consumer will benefit greatly in the assurance that a product is of equal quality worldwide; competition between countries in terms of trade will also be more fairly balanced (Motarjemi *et al.*, 2001). From an economic point of view, food that is regulated under international harmonization protocols would be more economical because of the costs avoided in having to comply with standards that differ between countries (Horton, 1997).

There is a number of internationally recognized institutions that advise on regulation and legislation of foods, such as the *Codex Alimentarius* (a joint FAO/WHO Commission), World Trade Organization (WTO), or the European Food Safety Authority (EFSA).

Nevertheless, some countries either do not participate in these organizations (Lelieveld & Keener, 2007) or do not apply the international agreements even if they have been officially accepted by that country (Joppen, 2005). In the United States, the Food and Drug Administration (FDA) is the main regulatory agency established for the approval of novel food processing technologies and novel products. In the European Union Regulation EC 258/97 is similarly used to regulate novel foods and novel ingredients (EU, 1997). The European list of novel foods includes many different cases; for example, one is related to food and food ingredients processed under non-current technologies. Some examples of food items in the European Union that have been approved under this regulation include fruit preparations using HHP (approved in 2001), which are processed by an important multi-national company.

There are many reported attempts to regulate food in other nations by various organizations with specific standards for food products (Motarjemi et al., 2001), but these are in small geographical zones related to specific foodstuffs. Some of the hurdles in global harmonization encountered in the past by the United States and European Union involve economic factors, mainly due to small producers who are afraid of losses in competing with multi-national brands, or who fear that the process would lead to Americanization (Horton, 1996).

A Global Harmonization Initiative (GHI) was launched in 2004 by the International Division of the Institute of Food Technologists (IFT) and the European Federation of Food Science and Technology (EFFoST) to eliminate differences in regulations and legislation (Lelieveld & Keener, 2007) and set up a basis for food safety regulation (Joppen, 2005). The Global Harmonization Initiative (GHI) has shown important progress as portrayed by Lelieveld (2009); during a workshop organized by GHI in 2007 in Lisbon, Portugal, four working groups discussed global harmonization. One of these, the food preservation group, focused on high pressure processing of foods (Lelieveld, 2009) because of the impact that this novel technology could have on food processing around the world. However, without regulations and standards, producing a safe food product using this method would be difficult. For example, the time–temperature criteria that are followed for thermal pasteurization and sterilization do not exist for high pressure processing. In 2004, there was an attempt conducted by the International Commission on Microbiological

Specifications for Foods (ICMSF) to find and establish equivalency between the high pressure processing parameters (Balasubramaniam, Ting, Stewart, & Robbins, 2004). Even though it was found that equivalence could not be identical in two or more countries, there should be enough similarity to be considered equal (Sawyer et al., 2008) for any purpose (processing, commercialization, experimentation, etc.). Many industries are interested in novel food processing technologies, but with the lack of global regulations to monitor them, investors have doubts about their acceptance by consumers (Joppen, 2005).

In 2006, a group of scientists in academia and industry from 32 organizations (mainly in Europe) met together to establish a research consortium, NovelQ, based on the use of novel technologies (De Vries, Lelieveld, & Knorr, 2007). Their research was mainly focused on HHP and PEF for food pasteurization and sterilization, and the use of cold plasma for surface disinfection, but they also addressed issues related to other novel thermal technologies such as microwave, ohmic heating, and radio frequency. The consortium planned a series of interconnected projects in stages for each technology, from basic food science and kinetics, packaging, consumer perception, development of techniques, to technology transfer and management, which would allow a comprehensive overview of each technology. Preliminary results were reported for the first year of the NovelQ consortium (De Vries et al., 2007), but ambitious plans were stipulated for the next 5 years, closely following the Global Harmonization Initiative (GHI).

Progress in HHP research in the last 20 years has been remarkable. Hundreds of references can be found on HHP pertaining to not only microbial inactivation, but to food components within a large number of food products, and studies of packaging materials for these products. However, the lack of uniformity in reporting processing conditions continues to be a problem. Reported come-up times (CUT) in HHP technology, for example, is something noticeably absent in many references, which makes the comparison between treatments difficult. Moreover, the thermal effects during high pressure were not reported by many researchers in early studies (Balasubramaniam *et al.*, 2004) because of the unknown effects of compression heating at the beginning of the technology. Most studies conducted in the first years of HHP research showed important results, but without knowledge of the thermal effects, it is difficult to compare these with recent studies. Other obstacles in comparing past and present HHP treatments are differences in equipment design, configuration and operation, effect of natural differences in food composition, and process variables; but lack of definitions and ambiguousness in reporting data are probably more likely (Balasubramaniam *et al.*, 2004). Although most information reported during HHP experimentation is similar to other science experiments and follows scientific format for publication, there are a number of additional considerations that should be taken into account and reported at the time of publication. According to Balasubramaniam *et al.* (2004), some of the process engineering aspects that should be reported in HHP studies are: process time (including come-up time, holding time, decompression time), process pressure, initial temperature, product temperature at process pressure (during adiabatic compression heating), pressure-transmitting fluid, and packaging material. A standardization process is currently being conducted in most research centers, universities and industries around the world using HHP technology. The process underway has been positively pushed forward by GHI; for food scientists the mission will be to spread the information related to this standardization and HHP, and other novel technologies in the coming years. This effort will establish the basis of global legislation, making safe food products a reality in every aspect, and taking advantage of all the unique effects gained from novel food processing technologies.

16.7 CONCLUDING REMARKS

Global harmonization of all novel technologies is indeed a requirement that must be addressed in the coming years. It has been shown that there are still many barriers between countries in commercializing novel products. Regulatory agencies must work diligently with research centers and non-governmental agencies in following the Global Harmonization Iniative, and help develop the basis of food safety regulations that are the main concerns for emerging technologies. A standardization process from equipment manufacturers would be an important starting point which can be addressed according to the type of product and major ingredients in product formulation. The identification of benchmarks for each product according to key characteristics would help set up the basis for process standardization, which could lead to a barrier-free international commercialization of novel food products and technologies.

References

Balasubramaniam, B., Ting, E. Y., Stewart, C. M., & Robbins, J. A. (2004). Recommended laboratory practices for conducting high-pressure microbial inactivation experiments. *Innovation of Food Science Emerging*, 5, 299–306.

De Vries, H., Lelieveld, H., & Knorr, D. (2007). Consortium researches novel processing methods. *Food Technology*, 61(11), 34–39.

Ehlermann, D. A. E. (2009). The RADURA-terminology and food irradiation. *Food Control*, 20, 526–528.

EU. (1997). Regulation (EC) No 258/97 of the European Parliament and of the Council of 27 January 1997 concerning novel foods and novel food ingredients. *Official Journal of the European Communities*, L43, 1–7.

FDA. (1997a). Irradiation in the production, processing and handling of food. Food and Drug Administration. *Federal Register*, 62(232), 64107–64121.

FDA. (1997b). Irradiation in the production, processing and handling of food, Final rule. Food and Drug Administration. *Federal Register*, 62(232), 64101–64107.

Horton, L. (1997). The United States Food and Drug Administration: Its role, authority, history, harmonization activities, and cooperation with the European Union.

In *European Union Studies Association (EUSA), Biennial Conference*, 5th, 29 May–June 1, Seattle, WA, 36 pp.

HPS. (2009). Food Irradiation, Health Physics Society Fact Sheet. Health Physics Society. http://www.hps.org/ (accessed 30 March 2009).

Joppen, L. (2005). Global harmonization of food safety regulations: Putting science first. *Food Engineering & Ingredients*, (December), 22–26.

Keener, K. M. (2009). Food irradiation. Fact Sheet (FSR 98-13). Raleigh, NC: North Carolina State University, Department of Food Science.

Lelieveld, H. (2009). Progress with the global harmonization initiative. *Trends in Food Science Technology*, 20, S82–S84.

Lelieveld, H., & Keener, L. (2007). Global harmonization of food regulations and legislation—the Global Harmonization Initiative. *Trends in Food Science Technology*, 18, S15–S19.

Mansour, M. (2004). One world for all: International harmonization of food regulations. *Journal of Food Science*, 69(4), 127–129.

Molins, R. A. (2001). Introduction. In R. A. Molins (Ed.), *Food irradiation: Principles and applications* (pp. 1–21). New York: John Wiley & Sons, Inc.

Motarjemi, Y., van Schothorst, M., & Käferstein, F. (2001). Future challenges in global harmonization of food safety legislation. *Food Control*, 12, 339–346.

NCFST. (2009). National Center for Food Safety and Technology receives regulatory acceptance of novel food sterilization process. Press release, 27 February, 2009. Summit-Argo, IL.

Newsome, R. (2007). Codex vital in global harmonization. *Food Technology*, 10, 100.

Notermans, S., & Lelieveld, H. (2001). Food Safety: A burning issue in the past, present and future. *Food Engineering & Ingredients*, (May), 33–38.

Ramaswamy, R., Balasubramaniam, B., & Kaletunç, G. (2004a). *High Pressure Processing. Extension Fact Sheet*. Columbus, OH: Ohio State University.

Ramaswamy, R., Jin, T., Balasubramaniam, B., & Zhang, H. (2004b). *Pulsed Electric Field Processing. Extension Fact Sheet*. Columbus, OH: Ohio State University.

Rogers, P. (1999). Pending regulations for Canada, Mexico bring closeness in NAFTA. *Candy Industry*, 50, 56.

Sawyer, E. N., Kerr, W. A., & Hobbs, J. E. (2008). Consumer preferences and international harmonization of organic standards. *Food Policy*, 33, 607–615.

Tang, J. (2009). *Personal communication*. Pullman, WA: Washington State University.

Nutrition and Bioavailability: Sense and Nonsense of Nutrition Labeling

Adelia C. Bovell-Benjamin and Elaine Bromfield

Department of Food and Nutritional Sciences, Tuskegee University, Tuskegee, AL, USA

17.1 INTRODUCTION

Chronic diseases are a leading cause of preventable deaths in the United States (US) and the rest of the world (HHS, 2001). It is recognized that chronic diseases are often diet-related and therefore may be managed or prevented through appropriate diet and lifestyle practices. Changes in dietary patterns require that

sufficient information be provided at the point of food purchase. This information can be provided in a number of ways, of which food labeling is one of the most immediate and direct sources of information, which can be supported with education and advertising. The section of information on the food label that declares nutrient content is termed 'nutrition labeling', 'nutrition panel', 'nutrition facts' or 'nutrition facts panel'. The current Nutrition Facts Panel

289

(NFP) that appears on food labels was conceived as an important public health tool to reduce diet-related disease. It includes the percent daily value (%DV), and is a critical tool for the consumer to make informed food choices.

Since 1941, nutrition labeling in the US has reflected the current scientific knowledge on the relationship between diet and health. For example, the changes in nutrition labeling regulations promulgated by the Food and Drug Administration (FDA) in 1973 required that both positive and negative aspects of the nutrient content of food appear on the label to emphasize the relationship between diet and health (Hutt, 1981). The Nutrition Facts Panel and the related nutrition information on the label continued this effort to encourage healthier food choices. To achieve this health goal, the 1993 US version of nutrition labeling included a new tool, the %DV, which enables consumers to rapidly and efficiently understand how a particular food fits in the context of a healthy diet.

Nutrition labeling is a population-based approach, which provides information to consumers on the nutrient content of a food; its intent is to make the food selection environment more conducive to healthy choices (Cowburn & Stockley, 2005). The US, Canada, Australia and New Zealand have implemented mandatory nutrition labeling, although the format and content of the labels differ between these countries (Sibbald, 2003; Curran, 2002). In the European Union (EU), nutrition labeling is currently not mandatory unless a nutrition claim is made (Cowburn & Stockley, 2005). Nutrition labeling can be used to help prevent the progress of poor nutrition, obesity and other chronic diseases. However, it is crucial that nutrition labeling is combined with education on healthy lifestyles; including clear advice about the contribution that all foods make to a healthy diet, and the importance of physical activity. Table 17.1 shows that in general, countries can be characterized as having one of four types of nutrition labeling regulatory environment: i) mandatory

nutrition labeling on all prepackaged food products; ii) voluntary nutrition labeling, which becomes mandatory on foods where a nutrition claim is made; iii) voluntary nutrition labeling, which becomes mandatory on foods with special dietary uses; and iv) no regulations on nutrition labeling (Hawkes, 2004).

One of the intents of nutrition labeling is to make the food selection environment more conducive to healthy choices. An ultimate outcome of healthier food choices in populations is savings through increased productivity; lower health care costs associated with cancer, diabetes, cardiovascular disease and other chronic diseases; and overall improved health over time. The increase in prepackaged and processed foods means that the nature of food is not always clear from visual inspection and information is required about contents, storage and preparation. The food label provides information for consumer protection. For example, the increased use of additives in the food system over the past few decades requires governmental regulatory activities. Consumers who are allergic to certain product ingredients could be protected if the food label is read. Many food label regulations prohibit the use of misleading advertising or health claims, putting the burden of proof of nutritive or any other health benefit on the manufacturer while protecting the consumer.

Epidemiological evidence on the relationships between changing dietary patterns and disease has underscored the importance between nutrition and health. Many countries have suggested reductions in the mean intake of nutrients such as sugar, salt, total and saturated fat. On the other hand, increased consumption of whole-grain cereals, vegetables and fruits are being encouraged. Nutrition labels are meant to educate consumers regarding the extent of salt, sugar, fat, cholesterol, minerals, some vitamins and protein in processed foods.

Currently absorption and bioavailability rates do not have to be tested under any of the nutrition labeling requirements worldwide. A main

TABLE 17.1 Nutrition labeling regulations in 74 countries and areas, by category (Hawkes, 2004)

Mandatory (date implemented)	Voluntary, unless a nutrition claim is made[a]	Voluntary, except certain foods with special dietary uses[b]	No regulations
Argentina (will have as of 08/2006, currently voluntary)	Austria[EC]	Bahrain	Bahamas
Australia (12/2002)	Belgium[EC]	China[d]	Bangladesh
Brazil (9/2001)	Brunei Darussalam	Costa Rica	Barbados
Canada (1/2003)	Chile	Croatia	Belize
Israel (1993)	Denmark[EC]	India	Bermuda
Malaysia (on a wide range of foods) (9/2003)	Ecuador[Codex]	Kuwait[GCC]	Bosnia and Herzegovina
New Zealand (12/2002)	Finland[EC]	Republic of Korea[e]	Botswana
Paraguay (will have as of 08/2006, currently voluntary)	France[EC]	Mauritius[Codex]	Dominican Republic
United States (1994)	Germany[EC]	Morocco	Egypt
Uruguay (will have as of 08/2006, currently voluntary)	Greece[EC]	Nigeria	El Salvador
	Hungary (2001, only for energy)	Oman[GCC]	Guatemala
	Indonesia[c]	Peru	Honduras
	Italy[EC]	Philippines	Hong Kong, SAR[g]
	Japan	Poland[f]	Jordan
	Luthuania[EC]	Qatar[GCC]	Kenya
	Luxembourg[EC]	Saudi Arabia[GCC]	Nepal
	Mexico	United Arab Emirates[GCC]	Netherlands Antilles
	Netherlands[EC]	Venezuela	Pakistan
	Portugal[EC]		Turkmenistan
	Singapore		
	South Africa		
	Spain[EC]		
	Sweden[EC]		
	Switzerland		
	Thailand[d]		
	United Kingdom[EC]		
	Viet Nam[d]		

EC = regulations based on the European Commission Regulation on Nutrition Labeling (Council Directive 90/496/EEC).

GCC = regulations based on the Gulf Cooperation Council Standard (GS) 9/1995 on Nutrition Labeling.

Codex = regulations developed taking guidance from the Codex Guidelines on Nutrition Labeling.

[a]Countries that require labeling when a nutrition claim is made often also require nutrition labeling on foods with special dietary uses.

[b]Specific foods vary, but may include diabetic food, low-sodium food, gluten-free food, infant formula, milk products and/or fortified foods.

[c]and on foods with health claims.

[d]and on food targeted at special groups, such as the elderly and children.

[e]also on bread, noodles and retort foods or of any nutrient emphasized on the label (retort: foods such as dried packaged sauce mixes, to be mixed with water and then eaten).

[f]including all dairy foods, and all dairy foods must be labeled with fat content.

[g]currently developing regulations mandating nutrition labels on all prepackaged foods, which will be preceded by voluntary requirements.

drawback with nutrition labeling is that the nutrient content is not supported by information regarding its bioavailability. Knowledge of the quantity of nutrients in a food product is of very limited use when assessing its nutritional adequacy. For example, two food products could have nutrients in the same quantities, but very different levels of bioavailability as is clearly demonstrated with calcium. Calcium in milk is more easily absorbed by the intestine than the calcium from vegetables and cereals. Phytates and oxalates present in cereals, beans and pulses, and in leafy vegetables, respectively, and long-chain saturated fatty acids and dietary fiber can reduce the bioavailability of calcium by forming insoluble calcium complexes (Fairweather-Tait *et al.*, 1989).

Furthermore, there are a large number of dietary and host-related factors, which affect the absorption of nutrients, especially minerals (Fairweather-Tait, 1992). Added information regarding the bioavailability of nutrients in the Nutrition Facts will be much more useful to consumers in their quest for healthier food choices. Information about bioavailability of the nutrients that they are consuming will be important to consumers because of the direct relationship between dietary consumption and chronic diseases. It is against this background that the present objective for this chapter was formulated. Therefore, this chapter will briefly review the current state of knowledge on nutrition and bioavailability with respect to nutrition labeling.

17.2 SCOPE

This chapter is limited to a discussion of the Nutrition Facts Panel (a portion of the food label) and not the entire food label. It focuses briefly on the information on the basic Nutrition Facts Panel and the inclusion of nutrient bioavailability on the panel. Discussion regarding dietary supplements, health and nutrition claims are beyond the scope of this chapter. Details about methods to assess

bioavailability and the mechanism of absorption are also beyond the scope of this chapter.

17.3 METHODOLOGY

A review of the existing literature was conducted. The literature surveyed covered scientific journals, trade journals, magazines, market reports, conference proceedings, books and other published materials. Web page content was used, as necessary. Literature was collected using numerous search engines and databases (for example, EBSCOhost, Ingenta, ScienceDirect, Google, Google Scholar, PubMed) in addition to library databases and Internet libraries of international organizations.

17.4 STRUCTURE OF THE REVIEW

In this review, Sections 17.1 to 17.4 justify the topic, present the objective, outline the scope and structure of the review. Section 17.5 presents an overview of the history of nutrition labeling focusing on the US, Canada, Australia and New Zealand, and developing countries. Section 17.6 is a more in-depth discussion regarding similarities and differences of nutrition labeling between countries. Section 17.7 reviews the consumers' understanding and use of nutrition labels while Section 17.8 covers bioavailability and nutrition labeling. Section 17.9 consists of conclusion and future scope. Acknowledgements and a references section complete the chapter.

17.5 OVERVIEW OF NUTRITION LABELING

17.5.1 United States

In the US, the regulatory agency for food nutrition labels on certain foods is the US FDA. In 1972, nutrition labeling which would allow some nutrients to be listed as a percent of a daily dietary intake standard per serving was proposed by the FDA (Pennington & Hubbard, 1997). The US has experienced three major phases of nutrition labeling revisions during which various reference values were used on the label. Between 1941 and 1972, Minimum Daily Requirements were used and from 1973 to 1993, US Recommended Daily Allowances (US RDAs) were used. A further modification in 1993 required %DVs to be used. The objective was to allow consumers to understand the relative significance of food in the context of total daily intake of nutrients, and use the label information to plan a healthy overall diet (Pennington & Hubbard, 1997). The FDA proposed a set of values called US Recommended Daily Allowances (US RDAs) for proteins, vitamins and minerals based on the 1968 Recommended Dietary Allowances (RDAs) issued by the National Academy of Sciences. The RDAs suggested levels of intake adequate to meet the nutrient needs of all healthy persons. In 1973, FDA issued a final rule and established nutrition labeling of a single set of daily intake standards called US RDAs for protein, 12 vitamins and 7 minerals (Table 17.2).

The FDA proposed regulations to update and expand the daily intake standards for nutrition labeling of foods in 1990. The Nutrition Labeling and Education Act (NLEA), which required foods and dietary supplements to bear nutrition labeling, became law in 1990 (Pray, 2003). The FDA issued proposed rules to implement NLEA, stating that vitamins would be held to the same standards as other medications, and that any claims would be required to withstand scientific scrutiny because companies were making fraudulent claims (Pray, 2003). NLEA allows a format for pre-approved health claims that make a nutrient or diet–disease. Only a limited number of such health claims are approved in the US after the FDA conducts a thorough review of the scientific studies documenting the nutrient or diet–disease link. Outside the US, the inclusion of a disease in a health claim classifies the product as intended for medical uses. In such instances, classification and approval as a drug and not as a food product is required.

FDA summarized and reviewed the 1990 NLEA requiring that food labels provide nutrient information for 10 food components in terms of %DV per serving portion. These new regulations were published and implemented in 1993 and 1994, respectively. Mandatory food components included total fat, saturated fat, cholesterol, sodium, total carbohydrate, dietary fiber, calcium, iron, vitamins A and C (Pennington & Hubbard, 1997). A sample US Nutrition Facts Panel is shown in Figure 17.1. The reference daily intakes (RDIs) for vitamin K, selenium, manganese, chromium, molybdenum and chloride were established in 1995 (Pennington & Hubbard, 1997). In the 1995 final rule, the units of measure for biotin and folate were changed from mg to μg, and calcium and phosphorus from g to mg (Pennington & Hubbard, 1997). Inclusion on the label of *trans* fat content became effective in 2006.

17.5.2 Canada

The Food and Drugs Act is the primary federal decree governing the labeling of all foods sold in Canada (Canada, 2003). Regulations made under the Act include ingredient listing, nutrition labeling, and all types of claims. Health Canada and the Canadian Food Inspection Agency (CFIA) oversee the regulatory process of food labeling in Canada (CFIA, 2001). Health Canada is responsible for setting health and safety standards and for developing food labeling policies related to health and nutrition under the Food and Drugs Act. CFIA is responsible for administering other food labeling policies and enforcing all food labeling regulations.

Nutrition labeling guidelines were introduced in Canada in 1988, along with amendments to the Food and Drug Regulations, which was voluntary, with a few exceptions (Canada, 2003). *The Guidelines on Nutrition Labeling* regulated format, nutrient content information and a declaration of

TABLE 17.2   US Recommended Daily Allowances (US RDAs) established by the Food and Drug Administration in 1973 for nutrition labeling

Nutrient	US RDA	Basis for US RDA
Mandatory		
Protein[a]	65 g[b]	1968 Recommended Dietary Allowance (RDA) for men
Vitamin A[a]	5000 IU	1968 RDA for men
Vitamin C[a,c]	60 mg	1968 RDA for men
Thiamin(e)[a,c]	1.5 mg	1968 RDA for teenage boys; RDA for men was 1.4 mg
Riboflavin[a,c]	1.7 mg	1968 RDA for men
Niacin[a]	20 mg	1968 RDA for teenage boys; RDA for men was 18 mg
Calcium[a]	1.0 mg	1968 RDA; higher than RDA for adults (800 mg) and lower than the RDA for teenagers (1.2 g)
Iron[a]	18 mg	1968 RDA for women
Optional		
Vitamin D	400 IU	1968 RDA for children and adults
Vitamin E	30 IU	1968 RDA for men
Vitamin B-6	2.0 mg	1968 RDA for men and women
Folic acid[c]	0.4 mg	1968 RDA for men and women
Vitamin B-12	6.0 μg	1968 RDA for men and women
Biotin	0.3 mg	Text in the 1968 RDA book
Pantothenic acid	10 mg	Text in the 1968 RDA book
Phosphorus	1.0 g	1968 RDA; higher than the RDA for adults (800 mg) and lower than the RDA for teenagers (1.2 g)
Iodine	150 μg	1968 RDA for men aged 14 to 18 years; 1968 RDA was 140 μg for men aged 18 to 35 years; 125 μg for men aged 35 to 55 years, and 110 μg for men older than 55 years
Magnesium	400 mg	1968 RDA for teenage boys; RDA for men was 350 mg
Zinc	15 mg	Text in the 1968 RDA book
Copper	2 mg	Text in the 1968 RDA book

[a]Required component for the nutrition label in 1973; others were voluntary unless claims were made about them or they were added to foods.
[b]The protein US RDA was 45 g if the protein efficiency ratio of the total protein in the product was equal to or greater than that of casein; the protein US RDA was 65 g if the protein efficiency ratio was less than that of casein.
[c]Permitted synonyms for nutrition labeling were ascorbic acid for vitamin C, vitamin B-1 for thiamin, vitamin B-2 for riboflavin, and folacin for folic acid.
Taken from Pennington & Hubbard (1997).

serving size (Canada, 1989). The nutrition information panel was required to list amounts of vitamins and minerals as a percentage of a single set of nutrient reference values, Recommended Daily Intakes, per serving of stated size (Canada, 1986). In 2003, Canada published and implemented new food labeling regulations (Canada, 2003).

The new regulations established nutrition labeling on most prepackaged food, updated and consolidated permitted nutrient content claims, and introduced a new regulatory framework and process for diet-related health claims (Canada, 2003). Samples of the Canadian nutrition label are shown in Figure 17.2.

Nutrition Facts

Serving Size 1 oz. (28g/About 21 pieces)
Servings Per Container About 2

Amount Per Serving

Calories 170   Calories from Fat 110

	% Daily Value*
Total Fat 11g	**17%**
Saturated Fat 1.5g	**8%**
Trans Fat 0g	
Cholesterol 0mg	**0%**
Sodium 250mg	**10%**
Total Carbohydrate 14g	**5%**
Dietary Fiber less than 1g	**2%**
Sugars 0g	
Protein 2g	

Vitamin A 2%	•	Vitamin C 0%
Calcium 0%	•	Iron 4%
Vitamin E 6%	•	Thiamin 4%
Riboflavin 2%	•	Niacin 4%
Vitamin B$_6$ 2%	•	Phosphorus 2%

* Percent Daily Values are based on a 2,000 calorie diet. Your daily values may be higher or lower depending on your calorie needs:

		Calories:	2,000	2,500
Total Fat	Less than		65g	80g
Sat Fat	Less than		20g	25g
Cholesterol	Less than		300mg	800mg
Sodium	Less than		2,400mg	2,400mg
Total Carbohydrate			300g	375g
Dietary Fiber			25g	80g

Calories per gram:
Fat 9 • Carbohydrate 4 • Protein 4

FIGURE 17.1 Sample, United States Nutrition Facts Panel. (Source: *Guidance on How to Understand and Use the Nutrition Facts Panel on Food Labels.* Washington DC, Food and Drug Administration, Center for Food Safety and Applied Nutrition, 2003. http://www.cfsan.fda.gov/~dms/foodlab.html).

In 2007, nutrition labeling for all prepackaged foods became mandatory in Canada. These labeling regulations, updated from 2003, revised the requirements for nutrient content claims and allowed health claims on diet–health relationships to be used on food labels. Such claims include: sodium and potassium and their association with blood pressure; calcium and vitamin D and their association with osteoporosis; saturated fat and *trans* fat and their association with heart disease; and vegetables and fruits and their association with some types of cancer (Canada, 2003). The regulations stipulate the prescribed wording for the permitted claims.

The Canadian regulations require *trans* fat to be incorporated with saturated fat with the %DV for the sum of saturated and *trans* fats being 20 g based on 10% of energy with a 2000-calorie dietary energy reference value. Expression of a %DV was considered important to assist consumers in understanding the relative significance of the amount of these nutrients in a food. The %DV for cholesterol is optional. There is no %DV for protein because protein intakes in Canada were not considered to be a public health concern. Explanatory footnotes related to the DV are similar to those used in the US and may be included in the Nutrition Facts Panel. The graphic elements of the Nutrition Facts Panel are tightly regulated to ensure the use of a consistent and legible format. The Canadian regulations, unlike those of the US, do not include specific regulations to define the serving size except in the case of single-serving containers.

17.5.3 Australia and New Zealand

Australia and New Zealand share joint food labeling standards developed by Food Standards Australia New Zealand (FSANZ). FSANZ was established by the Food Standards Australia New Zealand Act 1991. Figure 17.3 shows the Organization Chart of FSANZ. FSANZ, which was formerly the Australia New Zealand Food Authority (ANZFA), develops food standards and joint codes of practice with industry, covering the content and labeling of food sold in Australia and New Zealand. The joint arrangement led to a joint Australia New Zealand Food Standards Code (the Code), which replaced the New Zealand Food Regulations made under the New Zealand Food Act 1981, and the Australian Food Standards Code. The Code is the law that applies in Australia and New Zealand.

Nutrition Facts 1

Per 4 crackers (20g) 2   3

Amount	% Daily Value
Calories 90	
Fat 3g	5%
Saturated Fat 0.5g	8%
+Trans Fat 1g	
Cholesterol 0mg	
Sodium 132mg	6%
Carbohydrate 14g	5%
Fibre 2g	8%
Sugars 2g	
Protein 2g	
Vitamin A 0% Vitamin C 0%	
Calcium 0% Iron 4%	

4

6   **Ingredients:** Whole wheat, vegetable oil shortening, salt.

5   **Low fat, cholesterol-free, source of fibre**

Nutrition Facts
Valeur nutritive

Per 125 mL (87g) / par 125 mL (87g)

Amount Teneur	% Daily Value % valeur quotidienne
Calories/Calories 80	
Fat/Lipides 0.5g	1%
Saturated/saturés 0g	0%
+Trans/trans 0g	
Cholesterol/Cholestérol 0mg	
Sodium/Sodium 0mg	0%
Carbohydrate/Glucides 18g	6%
Fibre/Fibres 2g	8%
Sugars/Sucres 2g	
Protein/Protéines 3g	
Vitamin A/Vitamine A	2%
Vitamin C/Vitamine C	10%
Calcium/Calcium	0%
Iron/Fer	2%

1   Nutrition Facts Table   4   Core Nutrients
2   Specific amount of Food   5   Nutrition Claims
3   % Daily Value   6   List of Ingredients

FIGURE 17.2   Samples, Canada Nutrition Label (Source: *Interactive Nutrition Label: Get the Facts*, Health Canada. http://www.hc-sc.gc.ca/fn-an/label-etiquet/nutrition/cons/inl_main-eng.php; *Guide to Food Labelling and Advertising*, CFIA. http://www.inspection.gc.ca/english/fssa/labeti/guide/ch5e.shtml#5_4).

The main responsibility of FSANZ is to develop and administer the Code. The Code lists requirements for foods such as additives, food safety, labeling and genetically modified (GM) foods. FSANZ's ultimate goals are a safe food supply and well-informed consumers. The harmonization of food standards between the two countries is obvious because of the considerable amount of food trade between them. According to FSANZ, the nutrition information panel must be presented in a standard format which shows the amount per serving or 100 g or 100 mL of the food. Figure 17.4 shows an example of a nutrition information panel and the nutrients which should be listed. Some exceptions to products requiring a nutrition information panel include: i) very small packages which are about the size of a larger chewing gum packet; ii) foods with no significant nutritional value, such as a single herb or spice; iii) tea and coffee; iv) foods sold unpackaged (unless a nutrition claim is made); and v) foods made and packaged at the point of sale, for example, bread made in a local bakery.

17.5.4 Developing Countries—*Codex Alimentarius*

Several developing countries have adopted the *Codex Alimentarius* guidelines for nutrition labeling. The Codex Alimentarius Commission[1]

---

[1]Codex Alimentarius Commission. *Codex Alimentarius*, http://www.codexalimentarius.net.

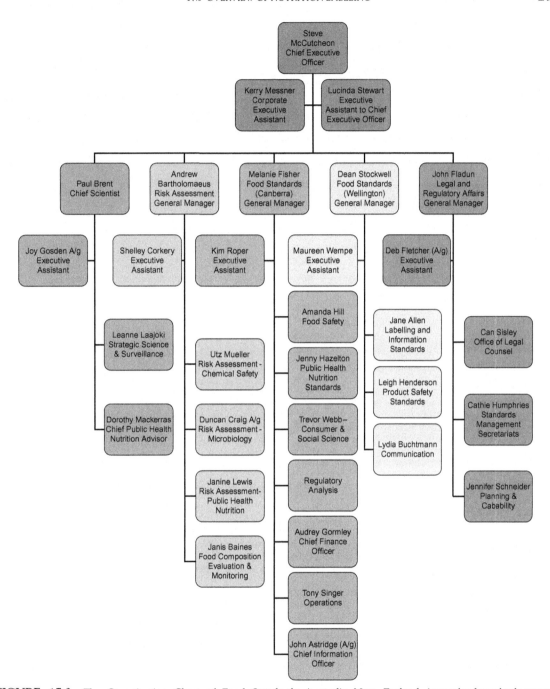

FIGURE 17.3 The Organization Chart of Food Standards Australia New Zealand (www.foodstandards.gov.au/aboutfsanz/organizationchart.cfm).

NUTRITION INFORMATION (AVERAGE)

average serving size - 30g (2/3 metric cup †)

	quantity per serving	%daily intake▲ per serving	per serve with 1/2 cup skim milk	quantity per 100g
ENERGY	450 kJ	5%	650 kJ	1500 kJ
PROTEIN	3.0 g	6%	7.6 g	9.9 g
FAT, TOTAL	0.5 g	0.6%	0.6 g	1.5 g
- SATURATED	< 0.1 g	0.4%	0.2 g	0.3 g
CARBOHYDRATE	20.7 g	7%	27.2 g	68.9 g
- SUGARS	4.9 g	5%	11.4 g	16.3 g
DIETARY FIBRE	4.1 g	14%	4.1 g	13.5 g
- SOLUBLE	0.7 g	-	0.7 g	2.3 g
- INSOLUBLE	3.6 g	-	3.6 g	11.9 g
SODIUM ^	99 mg	4%	156 mg	330 mg
POTASSIUM	137 mg	-	342 mg	455 mg
		%RDI*		
THIAMIN (VIT B1)	0.28 mg	25%	0.33 mg	0.92 mg
RIBOFLAVIN (VIT B2)	0.4 mg	25%	0.7 mg	1.4 mg
NIACIN	2.5 mg	25%	2.6 mg	8.3 mg
VITAMIN B6	0.4 mg	25%	0.4 mg	1.3 mg
FOLATE	100 μg	50%	106 μg	333 μg
IRON	3 mg	25%	3.1 mg	10 mg
MAGNESIUM	38 mg	12%	54 mg	128 mg
ZINC	1.8 mg	15%	2.3 mg	6 mg

† Cup measurement is approximate and is only to be used as a guide. If you have any specific dietary requirements please weigh your serving.
▲ %Daily Intakes are based on an average adult diet of 8700kJ. Your daily intakes may be higher or lower depending on your energy needs.
 * % Recommended Dietary Intake (Aust/NZ) per serving
 ^ 12% wheat bran and 8% wheat bran from whole wheat

INGREDIENTS: Whole wheat (67%), sugar, wheat bran (12%), barley malt extract, salt, minerals (iron, zinc oxide), vitamins (niacin, riboflavin, thiamin, folate).
Contains gluten containing cereals.
May contain traces of peanuts and/or tree nuts.
Blé entier (67%), sucre, son de blé (12%), extrait de malt d'orge, sel, minéraux (fer, oxyde de zinc), vitamines (niacine, riboflavine, thiamine, folate).
Contient gluten contenir les céréales.
Peut contenir des traces de cacahuètes et/ou noix d'arbres.

Contains 20% wheatbran*
*from wheatbran (12%) and whole wheat (8%)

FIGURE 17.4   Nutrition Information (Average). Example of a Food Standards Australia New Zealand (FSANZ) nutrition information panel and the nutrients which should be listed (http://www.kelloggs.com.au/Home/tabid/36/Default.aspx).

is an intergovernmental body with over 170 members. The Commission resides within the framework of the Joint Food and Agriculture Organization (FAO)/World Health Organization (WHO) Food Standards Programme. It was established by the FAO/WHO of the United Nations (UN) in 1963.

The Commission compiles internationally adopted food standards, guidelines, codes of practice and other recommendations called *Codex*

Alimentarius (FAO/WHO, 2007). The objective of *Codex Alimentarius* is to protect the health of consumers and ensure fair practices in the food trade. The Codex *Guidelines on Nutrition Labelling* were adopted by the Codex Alimentarius Commission at its 16th Session, 1985. The 'Nutrient Reference Values for Food Labeling Purposes'; 'Listing of Nutrients'; 'Presentation of Nutrient Contents'; and 'Definitions' were amended by the 20th, 26th and 29th Sessions of the Commission in 1993, 2003 and 2006, respectively (FAO/WHO, 2007). The *Guidelines on Nutrition Labelling* (CAC/GL 2-1985) in *Food Labelling* (5th edition) include text adopted by *Codex Alimentarius* up to 2007 (FAO/WHO, 2007).

The purpose of the *Codex Alimentarius* guidelines is to ensure that nutrition labeling is effective in: i) providing the consumer with information about a food so that wise food choices can be made; ii) providing a means for conveying information of the nutrient content of foods on the label; iii) encouraging the use of sound nutrition principles in the formulation of foods which would benefit public health; and iv) providing the opportunity to include supplementary nutrition information on the label. Their purpose is also to ensure that nutrition labeling does not present product information which is false, misleading or deceptive, and that nutrition claims are appropriately labeled (FAO/WHO, 2007).

The Codex Alimentarius Commission has also defined several terms for the purpose of the guidelines including nutrition labeling, nutrition declaration, nutrition claim, nutrient and sugars, dietary fiber, polyunsaturated fatty acids and *trans* fatty acids. Extensive details regarding calculation of energy and protein, presentation of nutrient content and format of presentation and periodic review are also included in the guidelines. For example, numerical information on vitamins and minerals should be expressed in metric units and/or as a percentage of the Nutrient Reference Value (NRV) per 100 g, 100 mL or per package if the package has a single portion (FAO/WHO, 2007). A sample NRV for nutrition labeling, which

Nutrient	Amount
Protein (g)	50
Vitamin A (µg)	800
Vitamin D (µg)	5
Vitamin C (mg)	60
Thiamin (mg)	1.4
Riboflavin (mg)	1.6
Niacin (mg)	18
Vitamin B6 (mg)	2
Folic acid (µg)	200
Vitamin B12 (µg)	1
Calcium (mg)	800
Magnesium (mg)	300
Iron (mg)	14
Zinc (mg)	15
Iodine (µg)	150
Selenium	Value to be established
Copper	Value to be established

FIGURE 17.5 *Codex Alimentarius* Nutrient Reference Values (NRV) for nutrition labeling (FAO/WHO, 2007).

should be used for labeling purposes in the interests of international standardization and harmonization is shown in Figure 17.5.

The 37th Session of the Codex Alimentarius Commission on Food Labeling will be held on 4–8 May, 2009 in Calgary, Canada. A draft revision of the guidelines on Nutrition Labeling (CAC/GL 2-1985) concerning list of nutrients usually declared on a voluntary or mandatory basis has been proposed. Also, listed on the provisional agenda are labeling of foods and food ingredients obtained through certain techniques of genetic modification/genetic engineering[2].

Codex Alimentarius has also outlined principles for nutrition labeling, which consists of nutrient declaration and supplementary nutrition information. According to FAO and WHO (2007), the nutrient declaration should give consumers an accurate summation of the nutritionally important

[2]http://www.codexalimentarius.net/web/current.jsp.

constituents of the product. The information should be truthful and convey only the quantity of nutrients contained in the product. Nutrient declaration should be mandatory for foods which have nutrition claims and voluntary for all other foods. Energy value, amounts of protein, available carbohydrate (excluding dietary fiber) and fat should be mandatory in the nutrient declaration (FAO/WHO, 2007). An extensive description regarding listing of nutrients can be obtained elsewhere (FAO/WHO, 2007).

Supplementary nutrition information on food labels should be optional and given in addition to the nutrient declaration. Furthermore, supplementary nutrition information on labels should be accompanied by consumer education programs to increase understanding and use of the information. The content of supplementary nutrition information will vary from one country to another and within countries from one target group to another based on the country's educational policy, and the needs of the target groups. In situations where the target populations have high illiteracy rate and/or limited nutrition knowledge, food group symbols or other pictorial or color presentations may be used without the nutrient declaration (FAO/WHO, 2007).

Nigeria and South Africa require nutrition labeling only on foods with special dietary uses and on foods for which a nutrition claim is made, respectively (Hawkes, 2004). The Food Regulations of 1999, made under the Food Act 1998, allowed Mauritius to introduce nutrition labeling. The regulations set out the specific nutrients that must be labeled for a series of selected nutrition claims (Ministry of Health and Quality of Life, 1998). It also mandates the labeling of protein, fat, carbohydrate, vitamin and mineral content on infant foods, per 100 g of the packaged food. Botswana and Kenya are in the process of developing nutrition labeling standards, drawing on the Codex *Guidelines on Nutrition Labelling*.

Regulations in Latin America range from no regulations on nutrition labeling as in El Salvador and Guatemala, to mandatory labeling

in Brazil (Hawkes, 2004). Brazil passed legislation mandating labeling on all prepackaged foods in 2001 (Hawkes, 2004). Argentina, Paraguay and Uruguay currently require prepackaged food to be labeled when a nutrition claim is made (Hawkes, 2004). In Venezuela and Chile, nutrition labels are required only on foods with special dietary uses and nutrition labeling is voluntary unless a nutrition claim is made, respectively. Mexico instituted new regulations in 1999 requiring nutrition labeling when a nutrition claim is made. No Caribbean country was identified with regulations on nutrition labeling (Hawkes, 2004). A sample nutrition label from Brazil is shown in Figure 17.6. India requires labeling of foods with special dietary uses (Hawkes, 2004). Labeling is voluntary unless a nutrition claim is made in Indonesia and Thailand. In Thailand, labeling is required if the food is targeted at

INFORMAÇÃO NUTRICIONAL Porção ___ g ou ml (medida caseira)		
Quantidade por porção		%VD (*)
Valor energético	....kcal =....kJ	
Carboidratos	g	
Proteínas	g	
Gorduras totais	g	
Gorduras saturadas	g	
Gorduras trans	g	(Não declarar)
Fibra alimentar	g	
Sódio	mg	
"Não contém quantidade significativa de ......(valor energético e ou nome dos nutrientes)" (Esta frase pode ser empregada quando se utiliza a declaração nutricional simplificada)		
*% Valores Diários com base em uma dieta de 2.000 kcal, ou 8400 KJ. Seus valores diários podem ser maior ou menor dependendo de suas necessidades energéticas.		

FIGURE 17.6   Sample, Mandatory Nutrition Label from Brazil. Also applies to Argentina, Paraguay and Uruguay as of 2006 (Hawkes, 2004).

special groups, such as the elderly or children. There is no evidence of nutrition labeling in Bangladesh, Nepal and Pakistan (Hawkes, 2004). Bahrain, Kuwait, Oman, Qatar, Saudi Arabia and the United Arab Emirates regulate nutrition labeling of foods for special dietary uses (Hawkes, 2004).

17.6 SIMILARITIES AND DIFFERENCES BETWEEN COUNTRIES

In the current global and economic framework, the need exists for a common framework of nutrition labeling so that products can be sold competitively worldwide. Harmonization of labeling regulations is desirable, although this should not supersede national standards. For example, in some instances, countries may not be able to uphold the global standard because of economic reasons; maintaining standards requires financial resources, which may be unaffordable. In such situations the national standards which are specific to the country should prevail. Such harmonization will make a positive contribution to global movements of foods, and prevent the exploitation of different national labeling regulations (Marks, 1984). Even though there is variation among countries in the extent of labeling, most developed countries have evolved a similar minimum set of regulations.

For example, within the EU and in various countries with regular trade links, there are eight types of information which should appear on all prepackaged foods: i) the customary, legal or descriptive name under which the product is sold, what condition the food is in, and if it is treated in any way; ii) the complete list of ingredients, listed in descending order of weight, and including the chemical names or serial numbers of additives; certain prepackaged foods such as fresh fruit and vegetables are exempted; iii) the net quantity; iv) the date of minimum durability; v) any special storage conditions or conditions of sale; vi) name and address of manufacturer; vii) place of origin; and viii) instructions for use (Marks, 1984). In general, similar labeling regulations are in force in Australia/New Zealand, Austria, Canada, Finland, Norway, Sweden and the US (Marks, 1984).

The following points demonstrate some of the similarities and minor differences between the nutrition labeling systems in Canada and the US (Canada, 2003).

- *Trans* **Fat**: The *trans* fatty acid declaration is mandatory on Canadian and US labels. Both countries require food manufacturers to list *trans* fatty acids, or *trans* fat, on the Nutrition Facts Panel. However, the US did not establish a reference standard for the sum of saturated and *trans* fats or for *trans* fats on their own, thus no %DV is declared in their table.
- **Percent DV for Mandatory Vitamins and Minerals**: In both countries, vitamins and minerals must be declared as %DV. However, the %DV is based on the 1968 US Reference Daily Intakes and 1983 Recommended Daily Intakes for Canadians, respectively. There are differences in the DVs for 14 vitamins and minerals.
- **Protein**: The US requires a DV for protein when a food is destined for children less than four years of age or when the protein is of low value, while this is not essential in Canada.
- **Rounding to Zero**: In Canada, total fat may be rounded to '0' only when the product contains ≤0.5 g fat and ≤0.2 g saturated and *trans* fats per serving and per reference amount.
- **Servings per container**: This is mandatory and optional in US and Canada, respectively. In Canada, a declaration of servings per container on the basis of 'cups' or 'tablespoons' is prohibited. The measuring systems in Canada (1 cup = 250 ml) and the US (1 cup = 240 ml) are different.

17.7 CONSUMER UNDERSTANDING AND USE OF NUTRITION LABELS

The Nutrition Facts Panel provides one of the most readily available sources of food choice information for identification of the relative healthfulness of packaged foods available to consumers (Blitstein & Evans, 2006; Hawthorne, Moreland, Griffin, & Abrams, 2006). Generally, the Nutrition Facts Panel, which often includes amounts of protein, carbohydrate and fat, is presented in tabular form on a food product's package (Visschers & Siegrist, 2009). The Nutrition Facts Panel defines a serving size and describes the weights of macronutrients (fat, carbohydrate, protein) in a serving. Figure 17.7 demonstrates the details of the nutrition labeling information.

The intent of the Nutrition Facts Panel is for people to use and understand the information on the panel to assist in making decisions about their dietary choices in order to reduce the risk for some types of cancer, diabetes, obesity and cardiovascular disease (Visschers & Siegrist, 2009). However, nutrition information is often misinterpreted (Pelletier, Chang, Delzell, & McCall, 2004; Hogbin & Hess, 1999). The European Heart Network (2003) Higginson, Kirk, Rayner, and Draper (2002) and Higginson, Rayner, Draper, and Kirk (2002) also noted that consumers pay

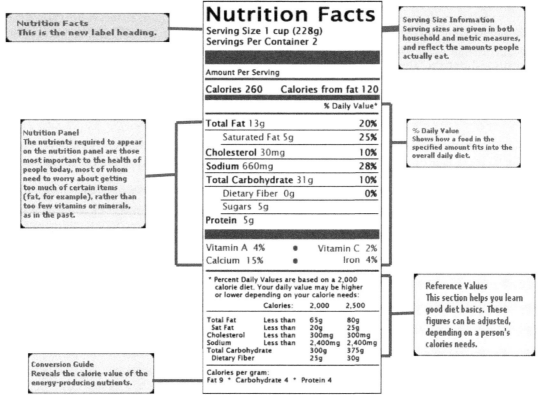

FIGURE 17.7   Details of the Nutrition Facts Panel of a Typical Label (Source: *Guidance on How to Understand and Use the Nutrition Facts Panel on Food Labels*. Washington DC, Food and Drug Administration, Center for Food Safety and Applied Nutrition, 2003. http://www.cfsan.fda.gov/~dms/foodlab.html).

little attention to nutrition labeling, although they frequently indicate doing so. One reason consumers have given for not reading the nutrition label is 'poor comprehension'. In one study, 70% of adults desired easier to understand food labels (Kristal *et al.*, 1998; European Heart Network, 2003; Grunert & Wills, 2007).

In a systematic review of 100 studies, Cowburn and Stockley (2005) reported that nutrition labeling was confusing, with many consumers having difficulty interpreting serving size information. The European Heart Network (2003) reported that consumers were able to correctly use nutrition panel information for simple calculations and comparisons; however, calculating the total nutritional value of a product was more challenging for them. According to the Institute of Medicine (IOM, 2003), consumers are expected to understand that calculation of sugar content must include the sugar listed on the snack food label as well as the fructose and corn syrup.

Furthermore, it was reported by Scheibehenne, Miesler, and Todd (2007) that consumers' choices of food products were based on a single attribute rather than a multi-attribute comparison of these products. Rothman *et al.* (2006) examined patient comprehension of food labels and the relationship of comprehension to their underlying literacy and numeracy skills. Respondents (89%) reported using food labels and 69% answered the food label questions correctly. Some reasons for inaccurate responses included misapplication of the serving size, confusion due to extraneous material on the food label, and incorrect calculations.

Huang *et al.* (2004) studied the relationship between reading nutrition labels and percent calorie intake from fat. In adolescent boys and girls, reading nutrition labels was associated with higher fat intake, but this does not necessarily translate into healthier diets. Likewise, McCullum and Achterberg (1997) found that nutrition labels, compared with taste, habit, and price, ranked very low in how adolescents determine their food choices. This may reflect a lack

of understanding of label information or inability to translate it into practical use.

Eight consumer focus groups in four US cities were utilized to understand consumer interest in nutrition information on food labels and fast food restaurant menu boards (Lando & Labiner-Wolfe, 2007). The results indicated that although participants were interested in having nutrition information available, they would not use it at every eating occasion. Respondents thought that food products typically consumed at one eating occasion should be labeled as a single serving; and they also indicated that more healthful options should be highlighted on labels and menu boards (Lando & Labiner-Wolfe, 2007).

In some instances, the nutrition label has been viewed as a useful educational tool, which helps consumers plan their diets. For example, Crane, Hubbard, and Lewis (1999) stated that 48 and 30% of survey respondents reported changing their minds about buying or using a food product after reading the nutrition label. Jay *et al.* (2009) studied a multimedia intervention to improve food label comprehension in a sample of low income patients in New York City. They concluded that a multimedia intervention is an effective way to improve short-term food label comprehension in patients with adequate health literacy. Further research is necessary to improve understanding of food labels in patients with limited health literacy.

Hawthorne *et al.* (2006) assessed the understanding and response of young adolescents to an educational program about Nutrition Facts Panels (NFP). Initially, 55% of pre-test questions were answered correctly, but scores increased to 70% in the post-test after the educational intervention. The researchers concluded that young adolescents can learn how to read and understand the Nutrition Facts Panels through educational sessions. Sociodemographic variables and beliefs about the causes of obesity associated with reported use of Nutrition Facts Panel information were examined by Blitstein and Evans (2006). Fifty-three percent of the sample reported using NFP information on a consistent basis. Females, those with more education, and those currently married were more likely to use NFP labels. The importance of knowledge in order to maintain healthy body weight was the only belief variable associated with use of nutrition labeling information.

Byrd-Bredbenner, Wong, and Cottee (2000) evaluated and compared the abilities of 50 women residing in the United Kingdom (UK) to locate and manipulate information and to assess the accuracy of nutrient content claims on Nutrition Facts Panels prepared in accordance with US regulations, EU Directive and UK food labeling Regulations 1996. The findings indicated that the women could locate and manipulate information on all three labels equally well. However, they were significantly more able to assess nutrient content claims using the US Nutrition Facts Panel. The researchers concluded that EU labeling changes, which may facilitate consumer use of labels in making dietary planning decisions, were warranted. Gorton, Ni Mhurchu, Chen, and Dixon (2008) investigated understanding and preferences regarding nutrition labels among ethnically diverse shoppers at 25 supermarkets in New Zealand. The survey instrument assessed nutrition label use, understanding of the mandatory Nutrition Information Panel (NIP), and preference for and understanding of four nutrition label formats. Sixty six to 87% of the respondents reported reading food labels always, regularly or sometimes. There were ethnic differences in ability to use the NIP to determine if a food was healthy.

Scott and Worsley (1997) determined the effectiveness of nutrition panel regulations using a nationwide postal survey in New Zealand to examine consumers' opinions and search behaviors relating to nutrition labeling. Of the 300 respondents, 60% claimed to have read food package labels for nutrition information in the last 10 days; most people sought information about nutrients which are generally regarded as being present in excess in Western diets. Respondents also had good knowledge of the recommendations for those nutrients but poor understanding of, and interest in, other nutrient terms. Most respondents were in favor of compulsory nutrition labeling on packaged foods. The researchers concluded that many consumers felt the information supplied in the nutrition panel was irrelevant and suggested further research to test how appealing and understandable the basic nutrition panel format is compared to other information on labels.

17.8 BIOAVAILABILITY AND NUTRITION LABELING

Effective nutrition labels are part of a supportive environment, which encourages healthier food choices. However, globally, nutrition labels often focus on the total amount of nutrients in the particular product, giving no indication on the bioavailability of these nutrients once they are ingested. The bioavailability of the nutrients ingested in a product completes the whole picture about how nutritionally sound the product is. Nutrient content on a nutrition label does not guarantee its nutritional value. Nutrients in foods and food products can exist in different forms, which result in diverse levels of bioavailability, therefore food manufacturers should be encouraged to provide information on the bioavailability of the nutrient. Additional information about bioavailability on nutrition labels would be more beneficial to consumers and enable them to make healthier food choices.

There is no consensus in the literature regarding a definition of bioavailability. However, researchers have coined several definitions of the term. Reeves and Chaney (2008) have defined bioavailability as the extent to which a nutrient, toxin, or any other substance becomes available for body use or deposition after intake, oral or otherwise. They further stated that in the instances of oral exposure to the nutrient, bioavailability usually involves absorption, body utilization, and/or deposition. Similarly, Welch and House (1984) defined bioavailability as the proportion of the total amount of a mineral element present in a nutrient medium, which is potentially absorbable in a metabolically active form. Southgate (1989) argued that bioavailability represents the response of the human, animal, or cells in culture to the diet or food, and is not an inherent property of the food as such. For example, in rats, zinc bioavailability from bread was variable and dependent on the zinc status of the body (Hallmans *et al.*, 1987). House (1999) has indicated that the bioavailability of a trace mineral in a specific food is not static.

Bioavailability has no universally accepted definition; it has been defined in many ways. The FDA has defined bioavailability as the rate and extent to which the active substances or therapeutic moieties contained in a drug are absorbed and become available at the site of action (Shi & Le Maguer, 2000). Jackson (1997) described bioavailability as the 'fraction of an ingested nutrient that is available for utilization in normal physiological functions and for storage,' although it should be recognized that there is no true storage of a water-soluble vitamin such as folate. Gregory, Quinlivan, and Davis (2005) described bioavailability as the product of absorption efficiency (that is, fractional absorption, F1) and post-absorptive events involved in metabolic utilization (F2).

According to Fairweather-Tait (1992), bioavailability is the proportion of the total nutrient in a food, meal or diet that is utilized for normal body functions, which involves various stages, each of which is affected by different dietary and physiological factors (Figure 17.8). Briefly, factors which impact upon the bioavailability of nutrients include the quantity consumed, including the chemical forms, dietary composition and gastrointestinal (GI) secretions; the quantity available for absorption, which is affected by factors such as nutritional status and gut microflora;

food preparation or processing; host factors and the quantity absorbed. However, bioavailability still remains an important, but often vague notion linked to the effectiveness of absorption and metabolic utilization of consumed nutrients (Gregory *et al.*, 2005; Solomons, 2001).

Minerals, which are crucial for optimal health, are the most well researched example when discussing bioavailability. Microminerals, which have been established to be either essential or beneficial for humans or animals include iodine, iron, selenium and zinc (House, 1999). This section discusses calcium and iron bioavailability issues to highlight the importance of disclosing nutrient bioavailability information on nutrition labels. Heaney, Rafferty, Dowell, and Bierman (2005) have demonstrated that calcium in products is absorbed with different efficiencies. The researchers fed women commercially marketed calcium-fortified orange juice and compared the bioavailability of calcium from calcium citrate malate and a combination of tricalcium phosphate and calcium lactate. The increase in calcium in the serum was measured up to nine hours after ingestion of the test drink. Their results indicated that calcium citrate malate was better absorbed (more bioavailable to the body) than tricalcium phosphate/calcium lactate (Heaney *et al.*, 2005). Heaney, Dowell, Rafferty, and Bierman (2000) have also reported that tricalcium phosphate in soy beverage was 25% less bioavailable than calcium in cow's milk.

Human diets contain two basic forms of iron: Fe(II) and Fe(III) and heme where iron is complexed to protoporphyrin IX (Bleackley *et al.*, 2009; Benito & Miller, 1998). However, iron exists in oxidation states ranging from −II, as in the $Fe(CO)_4^{2-}$ anion, to +VI, as in the ferrate ion FeO_4^{2-}. Biochemically, Fe(II) and Fe(III) are the most relevant oxidation states (Bleackley *et al.*, 2009). In an average diet, inorganic iron accounts for approximately 90% of total dietary iron content, whereas heme makes up the remaining 10% (Sharp & Srai, 2007; Anderson

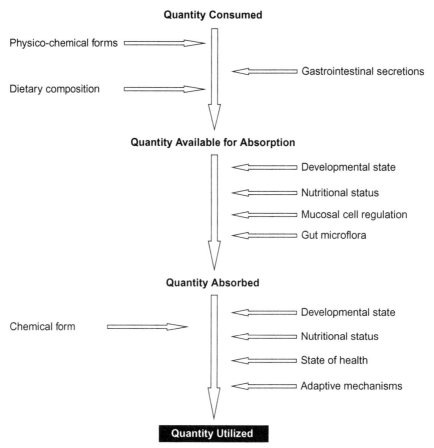

FIGURE 17.8   The different stages of bioavailability (Fairweather-Tait, 1992).

et al., 2005). Iron absorption varies significantly with diet composition, iron status of the individual, and, most importantly, bioavailability of the different iron forms. Bioavailability of inorganic iron is dependent on other dietary components. Enhancers, such as ascorbic acid, increase inorganic iron bioavailability by promoting the reduction of Fe(III) to soluble Fe(II). Inhibitors such as phytates in cereal and polyphenols in plants form insoluble complexes with inorganic iron and thereby reduce its absorption (Sharp & Srai, 2007). Additionally, inorganic iron absorption is influenced by the level of gastric acid secretion in the stomach with acidity increasing the solubility of inorganic iron. Dietary iron

absorption occurs in the proximal small intestine by specialized epithelial cells called duodenal enterocytes.

Several researchers have shown that iron is absorbed with different efficiencies. Iron is only poorly absorbed from high-extraction flours because of the presence of phytate and other inhibitory factors (Hurrell *et al.*, 2002, 2004). Findings from an efficacy trial in Thailand suggest that two forms of elemental iron, electrolytic iron and hydrogen-reduced iron have bioavailability which is 50–79% that of ferrous sulfate (Zimmermann *et al.*, 2005). Two other forms of reduced iron, carbon-monoxide-reduced and atomized iron, are poorly absorbed

(Zimmerman & Hurrell, 2007). Sodium iron ethylenediaminetetraacetic acid (NaFeEDTA) has shown effectiveness as a fortificant in soy sauce in China (Huo *et al.*, 2002), fish sauce in Vietnam (van Thuy *et al.*, 2003) and maize flour in Kenya (Andang'o *et al.*, 2007). NaFeEDTA is absorbed twice to three times more than ferrous sulfate from diets high in phytic acid (Bothwell & MacPhail, 2004).

17.9 CONCLUSION

Nutrition labels are intended to educate consumers regarding the extent of salt, sugar, fat, cholesterol, minerals, some vitamins and protein in processed foods.

The intent is that people use and understand the information in the Nutrition Facts Panel to assist them in making decisions about their dietary choices to reduce risk for chronic diseases such as some types of cancer, diabetes, obesity and cardiovascular disease. It is crucial that nutrition labeling is combined with education on healthy lifestyles; including clear advice about the contribution that all foods make to a healthy diet, and the importance of physical activity.

When consumers read nutrition labels, it is assumed that the amount listed in the %DV is the amount that is utilized by the body; however, this is not always the case. The US FDA and other global regulatory institutions should open discussions regarding the inclusion of bioavailability information of nutrients, especially minerals on nutrition labels. Harmonization of labeling regulations is desirable especially in the current global and economic framework. A common framework of nutrition labeling, complete with bioavailability information, will contribute to products being sold more competitively worldwide. Harmonization will make a positive contribution to global movements of foods, and help to minimize the exploitation of different national labeling regulations. Further

research is needed to determine how appealing and understandable the basic nutrition panel format is compared to other information on labels. Research is also needed to provide additional information about the inclusion of nutrient bioavailability information on nutrition labels and its benefit to consumers in terms of making healthier food choices.

ACKNOWLEDGEMENTS

The authors wish to thank Mr. Larry Keener for the pivotal role he played in making this chapter a reality. Also, the Food and Nutritional Sciences Advisory Board, Department of Food and Nutritional Sciences, Tuskegee University for their role in making the chapter possible.

References

Andang'o, P. E., Osendarp, S. J., Ayah, R., et al. (2007). Efficacy of iron-fortified whole maize flour on iron status of schoolchildren in Kenya: A randomised controlled trial. *Lancet, 369*, 1799–1806.

Anderson, G. J., Frazer, D. M., McKie, A. T., et al. (2005). Mechanisms of haem and non-haem iron absorption: Lessons from inherited disorders of iron metabolism. *Biometals, 18*, 339–348.

Benito, P., & Miller, D. (1998). Iron absorption and bioavailability: An updated review. *Nutrition Research, 18*, 581–603.

Bleackley, M. R., Wong, A. Y. K., Hudson, D. M., et al. (2009). Blood iron homeostasis: Newly discovered proteins and iron imbalance. *Transfusion Medicine Reviews, 23*, 103–123.

Blitstein, J. L., & Evans, D. W. (2006). Use of nutrition facts panels among adults who make household food purchasing decisions. *Journal of Nutrition Education and Behavior, 38*, 360–364.

Bothwell, T. H., & MacPhail, A. P. (2004). The potential role of NaFeEDTA as an iron fortificant. *International Journal for Vitamin and Nutrition Research, 74*, 421–434.

Byrd-Bredbenner, C., Wong, A., & Cottee, P. (2000). Consumer understanding of US and EU nutrition labels. *British Medical Journal, 102*, 615–629.

Canada. (1986). *Nutrition labelling* Information Letter No. 713, July 24. Ottawa: Food Directorate, Health Protection Branch.

Canada. (1989). *Guidelines on Nutrition Labelling*. Food Directorate Guideline No. 2, 30 November. Ottawa: Food Directorate, Health Protection Branch.

Canada. (2003). SOR/2003–11. Regulations amending the Food and Drug Regulations (Nutrition labeling, nutrient content claims and health claims). *Canada Gazette, Part II, 137*, 154–405.

CFIA. (2001). *Guide to Food Labelling and Advertising*. Online. Canadian Food Inspection Agency. http://www.inspection.gc.ca/english/fssa/labeti/guide/toce.shtml.

Cowburn, G., & Stockley, L. (2005). Consumer understanding and use of nutrition labeling: A systematic review. *Public Health Nutrition, 8*, 21–28.

Crane, N. T., Hubbard, V. S., & Lewis, C. J. (1999). American diets and year 2000 goals. Agriculture Information Bulletin No. 750. In E. Frazao (Ed.), *America's eating habits: Changes and consequences* (pp. 111–133). Washington, DC: US Department of Agriculture.

Curran, M. A. (2002). Nutrition labeling perspectives of a bi-national agency for Australia and New Zealand. Asia Pacific. *The Journal of Clinical Nutrition, 11*, S72–S76.

European Heart Network. (2003). *A systematic review on the research on consumer understanding of nutrition labeling*. Brussels: European Heart Network.

Fairweather-Tait, S. J. (1992). Bioavailability of trace elements. *Food Chemistry, 43*, 213–217.

Fairweather-Tait, S. J., Johnson, A., Eagles, J., et al. (1989). Studies on calcium absorption from milk using a double-label stable isotope technique. *The British Journal of Nutrition, 62*, 379–388.

FAO/WHO. (2007). Guidelines on nutrition labelling CAC/GL 2–1985. In *Food labelling* (5th ed.). *Codex Alimentarius*, FAO and WHO of the United Nations, Rome, Italy. ftp://ftp.fao.org/docrep/fao/010/a1390e/a1390e00.pdf.

Gorton, D., Ni Mhurchu, C., Chen, M.-H., & Dixon, R. (2008). Nutrition labels: A survey of use, understanding and preferences among ethnically diverse shoppers in New Zealand. *Public Health Nutrition, 17*, 1–7.

Gregory, J. F., Quinlivan, E. P., & Davis, S. R. (2005). Integrated the issues of folate bioavailability, intake and metabolism in the era of fortification. *Trends in Food Science and Technology, 20*, 229–240.

Grunert, K., & Wills, J. (2007). A review of European research on consumer response to nutrition information on food labels. *Journal of Public Health, 15*, 385–399.

Hallmans, G., Nilsson, U., Sjoèstroèm, R., et al. (1987). The importance of the body's need for zinc in determining Zn availability in food: A principle demonstrated in the rat. *The British Journal of Nutrition, 58*, 59–64.

Hawkes, C. (2004). *Nutrition labels and health claims: The global regulatory environment*. Geneva, Switzerland: World Health Organization.

Hawthorne, K., Moreland, K., Griffin, I. J., & Abrams, S. A. (2006). An educational program enhances food label understanding of young adolescents. *Journal of the American Dietetic Association, 106*, 913–916.

Heaney, R. P., Dowell, M. S., Rafferty, K., & Bierman, J. (2000). Bioavailability of the calcium in fortified soy imitation milk, with some observations on method. *The American Journal of Clinical Nutrition, 71*, 1166–1169.

Heaney, R. P., Rafferty, K., Dowell, M. S., & Bierman, J. (2005). Calcium fortification systems differ in bioavailability. *Journal of the American Dietetic Association, 105*, 807–809.

HHS. (2001). *The Surgeon General's call to action to prevent and decrease overweight and obesity*. Washington, DC: U.S. Government Printing Office.

Higginson, C. S., Kirk, T. R., Rayner, M. J., & Draper, S. (2002). How do consumers use nutrition label information? *Nutrition Food Science, 32*, 145–152.

Higginson, C. S., Rayner, M. J., Draper, S., & Kirk, T. R. (2002). The nutrition label: Which information is looked at? *Nutrition Food Science, 32*, 92–99.

Hogbin, M. B., & Hess, M. A. (1999). Public confusion over food portions and servings. *Journal of the American Dietetic Association, 99*, 21209–21211.

House, W. A. (1999). Trace element bioavailability as exemplified by iron and zinc. *Field Crops Research, 60*, 115–141.

Huang, T., Kaur, H., Mccarter, K. S., et al. (2004). Reading nutrition labels and fat consumption in adolescents. *Journal of Adolescent Health, 35*, 399–401.

Huo, J., Sun, J., Miao, H., et al. (2002). Therapeutic effects of NaFeEDTA-fortified soy sauce in anaemic children in China. *Asia Pacific Journal of Clinical Nutrition, 11*, 123–127.

Hurrell, R., Bothwell, T., Cook, J. D., et al. (2002). SUSTAIN Task Force. The usefulness of elemental iron for cereal flour fortification: A SUSTAIN task force report. *Nutrition Reviews, 60*, 391–406.

Hurrell, R. F., Lynch, S., Bothwell, T., et al. (2004). Enhancing the absorption of fortification iron. *International Journal for Vitamin and Nutrition Research, 74*, 387–401.

IOM. (2003). Report. *Health literacy: A prescription to end confusion*. Institute of Medicine.

Jackson, M.J. (1997). The assessment of bioavailability of micronutrients. *European Journal of Clinical Nutrition, 51*, S1–S2.

Jay, M., Adams, J., Herring, S. J., et al. (2009). A randomized trial of a brief multimedia intervention to improve comprehension of food labels. *Preventive Medicine, 48*, 25–31.

Kristal, A. R., Levy, L., Patterson, R. E., et al. (1998). Trends in food label use associated with new nutrition labeling regulations. *American Journal of Public Health, 88*, 1212–1215.

Lando, A. M., & Labiner-Wolfe, J. (2007). Helping consumers make more healthful food choices: Consumer views on modifying food labels and providing point-of-purchase nutrition information at quick-service restaurants. *Journal of Nutrition Education and Behavior, 39*, 157–163.

Marks, L. (1984). What's in a label? Consumers, public policy and food labels. *Food Policy, 9*, 252–258.

McCullum, C., & Achterberg, C. L. (1997). Food shopping and label use behavior among high school-aged adolescents. *Adolescence, 32*, 181–197.

Ministry of Health and Quality of Life. (1998). *Food Regulations made under the Food Act 1998: Part I. Food composition and labeling.* Republic of Mauritius http://ncb.intnet.mu/moh/foodreg.htm.

Pelletier, A. L., Chang, W. W., Delzell, J. E., & McCall, J. W. (2004). Patients' understanding and use of snack food package nutrition labels. *The Journal of the American Board of Family Practice, 17*, 319–323.

Pennington, J.A.T., & Hubbard, V.S. (1997). Derivation of Daily Values used for nutrition labeling. *Journal of the American Dietetic Association, 97*, 1407-1412.

Pray, W. S. (2003). *A history of nonprescription product regulation.* Binghamton, NY: The Haworth Press Inc. pp. 205–238.

Reeves, P. G., & Chaney, R. L. (2008). Bioavailability as an issue in risk assessment and management of food cadmium: A Review. *The Science of the Total Environment, 398*, 13–19.

Rothman, R. L., Housam, R., Hilary Weiss, H., et al. (2006). Patient understanding of food labels the role of literacy and numeracy. *American Journal of Preventive Medicine, 31*, 391–398.

Scheibehenne, B., Miesler, L., & Todd, P. M. (2007). Fast and frugal food choices: Uncovering individual decision heuristics. *Appetite, 49*, 578–589.

Scott, V., & Worsley, A. (1997). Consumer views on nutrition labels in New Zealand. *The Australian Journal of Nutrition and Dietetics, 54*, 6–13.

Sharp, P., & Srai, S. K. (2007). Molecular mechanisms involved in intestinal iron absorption. *World Journal of Gastroenterology, 13*, 4716–4724.

Shi, J., & Le Maguer, M. (2000). Lycopene in tomatoes: chemical and physical properties affected by food processing. *Critical Reviews in Biotechnology, 20*, 293–334.

Sibbald, B. (2003). Canada's nutrition labels: a new world standard? 887. *Canadian Medical Association Journal, 168.*

Solomons, N. (2001). Bioavailability of nutrients and other bioactive components from dietary supplements. *The Journal of Nutrition, 131*, 1392S–1395S.

Southgate, D. A. T. (1989). Conceptual issues concerning the assessment of nutrient bioavailability. In D. A. T. Southgate, I. T. Johnson & G. R. Fenwick (Eds.), *Nutrient availability: Chemical and biological aspects* (pp. 10–12). Special Publication No. 72, Cambridge: Royal Society of Chemistry.

van Thuy, P. V., Berger, J., Davidsson, L., et al. (2003). Regular consumption of NaFeEDTA-fortified fish sauce improves iron status and reduces the prevalence of anemia in anemic Vietnamese women. *The American Journal of Clinical Nutrition, 78*, 284–290.

Visschers, V. H. M., & Siegrist, M. (2009). Applying the evaluability principle to nutrition table information. How reference information changes people's perception of food products. *Appetite, 52*, 505–512.

Welch, R. M., & House, W. A. (1984). Factors affecting the bioavailability of mineral nutrients in plant foods. Special Publication No. 48. In R. M. Welch & W. H. Gabelman (Eds.), *Crops as sources of nutrients for humans* (pp. 37–54). Madison, WI: American Society of Agronomy.

Zimmerman, M. B., & Hurrell, R. F. (2007). Nutritional iron deficiency. *Lancet, 370*, 511–520.

Zimmermann, M. B., Winichagoon, P., Gowachirapant, S., et al. (2005). Comparison of the efficacy of wheat-based snacks fortified with ferrous sulphate, electrolytic iron, or hydrogen-reduced elemental iron: randomized, double-blind, controlled trial in Thai women. *The American Journal of Clinical Nutrition, 82*, 1276–1282.

CHAPTER

18

New RDAs and Intended Normal Use (Part II)—Efficient Tools in the Universal Management of Risks and Benefits of Micronutrients

Jaap C. Hanekamp[1] and Bert Schwitters[2]

[1]Roosevelt Academy, Middelburg, The Netherlands; HAN-Research, Zoetermeer, The Netherlands
[2]International Nutrition Company, The Netherlands

OUTLINE

18.1 INTRODUCTION

Food and drink are *sine qua non* to the maintenance, development, functioning, and reproduction of human life. During his or her lifetime an individual consumes on average, 30 tons of food, in seemingly endless dietary varieties. The digestive system splits all the foods found in all these different diets into the same basic categories of nutrients (De Vries, 1997).

Food is chemistry, and the mixture of chemicals that food represents is usually divided into four basic categories: 1) nutrients; 2) non-nutritive naturally occurring components (including anti-nutritives[1] and natural toxins; 3) man-made contaminants and; 4) additives. Nutrients account for more than 99% of the food content. The main classes of nutrients are carbohydrates, proteins, fats, and vitamins and minerals. The former three constituents of food are called macronutrients and are the major sources of energy and building materials for humans. The latter are called micronutrients, as these are only found and required in relatively small amounts.

Micronutrients differ from all other chemical substances in foods in that they are essential for the human physiology. Adverse (toxicological) effects can result from intakes that are too low (the typical deficiency diseases). Nevertheless, adverse effects can also arise as a result of intakes that are too high. Food products as a whole are estimated to consist of many hundreds of thousands of different chemicals. All of these food-content chemicals have their own specific toxicological profile, showing, both individually and interactively the adverse effects of under as well as overexposure.

Dietary imbalance is a high-risk aspect of food consumption. Two types of risks are *grosso modo* associated with repetitive and unbalanced diets. On the one hand they increase the risk of deficiencies, resulting in acute (e.g. scurvy in the case of vitamin C deficiency) and chronic (e.g. cancer in the case of a shortage in fruits and vegetables) diseases. On the other hand, chronic (over)exposure to detrimental loads (by load we simply refer to the total intake of certain bio-available food-endogenous compounds, resulting in a certain concentration within the organism) of food compounds (e.g. triglycerides and carbohydrates causing obesity) over longer periods of time might be harmful.

In this chapter we will focus on the science of micronutrients and health, and the accompanying risk assessments and regulatory policies. Apart from the well-known vitamins and minerals we will also incorporate in the discussion 'other substances' such as polyphenols (a group of antioxidants), for reasons we will consider anonymous. Deficiency and overexposure of micronutrients are the two physiological aspects we will consider in terms of toxicology. Although, as we will see, European regulatory preoccupation lies with the overexposure of vitamins and minerals through supplementary and fortified food-products; from the viewpoint of public health, micronutrients require a more nuanced, symmetrical approach as James *et al.*, (1999) showed in their report on the then projected, but never established, European Food and Public Health Authority:

'To have scientific analysis on a European basis is important because currently many policy makers simply consider that the answer to tobacco problems is to "educate" the individual consumer not to start smoking. This naïve approach is evident in many other dimensions of public health, e.g. those relating to inappropriate diets in pregnancy; the substantial problems of low birth weight babies; the continuing challenge of iodine deficiency within the EU; the widespread anaemia in children and adult women; the major issues relating to

---

[1]Anti-nutritives are food components that induce toxic effects by causing nutritional deficiencies by interference with the functioning and utilization of nutrients. Examples are lectins, phytic acid, and oxalic acid. See later in this chapter.

the health of Asians and other immigrant communities within the EU; the challenge of coping with escalating rates of adult chronic diseases and the huge and growing impact of the poor health of Europe's elderly. In societal terms the health impact of societal deprivation, social exclusion and poverty is now becoming a major European issue which requires much more objective scientific analyses than are currently available...'

James *et al.* (1999), in line with the focus of this book, converge on the interminable questions of public health and diet that go beyond worries about the safety of food and drink, and the potential for overconsumption of micronutrients in food supplements and fortified foods. But, we are getting ahead of ourselves. Therefore, in this chapter, we will first briefly describe the governing principles of European policies in relation to micronutrient regulation and the general assessment methodology of micronutrients in terms of benefits and risks. Second, we will explain, concisely, the state-of-art concerning micronutrients and health issues. Third, we assess the viability of the current European policies and concomitant assessments. Finally, we will propose a simple and transparent common basis for a global harmonized approach to *ex post* managing of the risks and benefits of micronutrients. We contend that this approach entails the least interventionist effort to create economic, regulatory and scientific level-playing fields, opening the door to the highest possible potential for micronutrients to make a contribution to human health; i.e. in all intents and purposes to the benefit of a healthy lifespan for everybody. We will place our approach against the backdrops of the predominantly interventionist experience we now have in Europe in approximating health-related policies of Member States and the equally interventionist supranational guidelines evolving in the context of the *Codex Alimentarius*.

18.2 STANDARDIZING FOOD— EUROPEAN FOOD STANDARDS LEGISLATION

Setting scientific, nutritional and policy standards that benchmark the benefits and risks of foods is of great consequence for industry, health professionals and, last but not least, consumers. In Europe, the core regulatory framework in food law is Regulation 178/2002/EC (General Food Law; GFL) (EU, 2002a). According to this Regulation, 'food' (or 'foodstuff') denotes 'any substance or product, whether processed, partially processed or unprocessed, intended to be, or reasonably expected to be ingested by humans.' The scope of Regulation 178/2002/EC concerns 'all stages of the production, processing and distribution of food ...' and its general objective is to provide 'a high level of protection of human life and health and the protection of consumers' interests...' This Regulation thus sets general rules for all products, including dietary supplements and fortified foods that are brought to market. To that effect, the general requirements of this Regulation deal with food safety, presentation, traceability and related responsibilities of food business operators. Importantly, the Regulation also constitutes the European Food Safety Authority (EFSA) and defines the Authority's task and fields of competence and authority.

Within this context, setting minimum and maximum levels for micronutrients (vitamins and minerals), but also for 'other substances', in view of the growing market for food supplements, is now a foremost regulatory topic in Europe. 'Other substances' are defined as food-endogenous substances with a nutritional or physiological effect other than the forms of vitamins and minerals approved for use in food supplementation and food fortification. Examples are amino- and fatty acids, carotenoids, and polyphenols (Scalbert *et al.*, 2005). The European Food Supplements Directive (Directive 2002/46/EC; FSD) regulates food supplements marketed as foodstuffs and presented as such for the purpose of supplementing the human diet (EU, 2002b). The FSD was implemented in order to safeguard human health in view of the potential toxicity of excess intake of micronutrient food supplements that have become increasingly available and are consumed in increasing amounts. Regulation 1925/2006/EC (Food Fortification Regulation, FFR) sets requirements for 'the addition of vitamins and minerals and of certain other substances to foods' (EU, 2006a).

These two laws complement the principles of general food law laid down in Regulation 178/2002/EC. In combination, the FSD and FFR positively list vitamins and minerals (admitted only when listed); and negatively list 'other substances' (forbidden or restricted when listed). The rules for positively listed vitamins and minerals have been fully approximated, while the 'other substances'—when not negatively listed—are governed by the principle of free movement under Mutual Recognition.

Obviously, it must not be overlooked that all regulatory measures within the Eurozone have as their legal basis one or more articles of the Treaty Establishing the European Community. In the case of the GFL, FSD and FFR, Article 95(3) is one of the articles forming their legal basis. Article 95(3) sets two overarching 'endpoints' for the aforementioned regulatory measures: principally, the approximation of the laws of Member States in order to remove barriers to trade, and, subsidiarily, a high level of protection of consumers. In our approach proposed in this chapter, we will fully adhere to Article 95(3) of the EU Treaty, which states that (EU, 2006b):

'The Commission, in its proposals envisaged in paragraph 1 (measures for the approximation of the provisions laid down by law, regulation or administrative action in Member States which have as their object the establishment and functioning of the internal market; authors)

concerning health, safety, environmental protection and consumer protection, will take as a base a high level of protection, taking account in particular of any new development based on scientific facts. Within their respective powers, the European Parliament and the Council will also seek to achieve this objective.'

18.3 THE SCIENCE OF MICRONUTRIENT SAFETY— HAZARDS, RISKS, BENEFITS, AND PRECAUTION

Within the context of food, risks and benefits can have multiple meanings, as previously noted. The GFL defines 'risk' as 'a function of the probability of an adverse health effect and the severity of that effect, consequential to a hazard.' The term 'hazard' is defined in the GFL as 'a biological, chemical or physical agent in, or condition of, food or feed with the potential to cause an adverse health effect, (EU, 2002a).

The Codex Alimentarius Committee on Nutrition and Foods for Special Dietary Uses (CCFNSDU) defined that '[n]utritional risk analysis considers the risk of adverse health effects from inadequate and/or excessive intakes of nutrients and related substances, and the predicted reduction in risk from proposed management strategies. In situations that address inadequate intake such a reduction in risk might be referred to as [one form of] a nutritional benefit' (CAC, 2008). In the same report of the CCFNSDU a 'nutritional risk' is defined as 'a function of the probability of an adverse health effect associated with inadequate or excessive intake of a nutrient or related substance and the severity of that effect, consequential to a nutrient-related hazard(s) in food' (CAC, 2008, p. 75).

Safety in the FSD and the FFR is roughly defined in terms of trying to prevent, by way of risk management, overexposure to micronutrients and 'other substances' by taking into consideration Safe Upper Limits (SULs) previously established by way of risk assessment. The setting of EU-wide maximum levels intends to provide an approximated framework in which consumers can make informed decisions about intake, having confidence that harm will not ensue (Hanekamp & Bast, 2007).

SULs are doses of vitamins and minerals that potentially susceptible individuals could take daily on a life-long basis in reasonable safety, without medical supervision. The European Food Safety Authority (EFSA) defines the SUL as the 'Tolerable Upper Intake Level.' In EFSA terminology, this means 'the maximum level of total chronic daily intake of a nutrient (from all sources) judged to be unlikely to pose a risk of adverse health effects to humans.' 'Tolerable intake' in this context connotes what is physiologically tolerable and is a scientific judgment as determined by assessment of risk, i.e. the probability of an adverse effect occurring at some specified level of exposure. It is an estimate of the highest level of intake which carries no appreciable risk of adverse health effects' (EFSA, 2006).

Risks of food and its assessments have been given a specific embedment by the European legislature, namely the precautionary principle. The GFL defines the contours thereof as follows: 'In those specific circumstances where a risk to life or health exists but scientific uncertainty persists, the precautionary principle provides a mechanism for determining risk management measures or other actions in order to ensure the high level of health protection chosen in the Community' (EU, 2002b). Micronutrients and the supplemental and fortified food-products that are produced therewith require, within the context of European Food Law, risk assessments and, if so deemed necessary, precautionary management.

The customary model to assess micronutrient in general and SULs (Safe Upper Limits), in particular, is the Deficiency–Excess (D–E) model[2] (Figure 18.1) derived from the underlying physiological model which we will come across later in this chapter. On the left part of this model's scale, where the levels of exposure decrease and the levels of deficiency increase, the organism will become exposed to increasing risks of adverse effects. Here we find the well-known Recommended Dietary (Daily) Allowances (RDAs) that are principally advisory tools aimed at preventing deficiencies. The Recommended Daily Allowance (RDA) is the average daily dietary intake level that is regarded as sufficient to meet the nutrient requirement of nearly all (97 to 98%) healthy individuals in a particular life stage and gender group. The Estimated Average Requirement (EAR) is the daily nutrient intake value that is estimated to meet the requirement of half the healthy individuals in a group.[3]

On the right of the model's scale, where the levels of exposure increase, the organism incurs an increasing risk of adverse effects, caused by excess intake. Here we find the SULs (or ULs).

---

[2]*Verwendung von Vitaminen in Lebensmitteln Toxikologische und ernährungsphysiologische Aspekte, Teil I* 2004. Bundesinstitut für Risikobewertung. This report can be downloaded from: http://www.bfr.bund.de/cm/238/verwendung_von_vitaminen_in_lebensmitteln.pdf (accessed 17 February, 2009). *Verwendung von Mineralstoffen in Lebensmitteln. Toxikologische und ernährungsphysiologische Aspekte. Teil II.* 2004. Bundesinstitut für Risikobewertung. This report can be downloaded from: http://www.bfr.bund.de/cm/238/verwendung_von_mineralstoffen_in_lebensmitteln_bfr_wissenschaft_4_2004.pdf (accessed 17 February, 2009).

[3]See for instance: IOM, 1998, Dietary Reference intakes for thiamin, riboflavin, niacin, vitamin B6, folate, vitamin B12, pantothenic acid, biotin, and choline. A Report of the Standing Committee on the Scientific Evaluation of Dietary Reference Intakes and its Panel on Folate, Other B Vitamins, and Choline and Subcommittee on Upper Reference Levels of Nutrients, Food and Nutrition Board, Institute of Medicine, National Academies Press, USA.

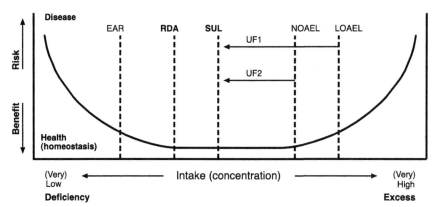

FIGURE 18.1   Deficiency–Excess model for micronutrients.

SULs operate as a basis for regulatory tools implemented at the level of the food industry to ensure safety. Per definition, within the bandwidth between deficiency (lack of function) and toxicity (lack of safety), the optimum level of exposure is coterminous with the point of RDA on the x-axis, where the micronutritional needs of practically everybody are fulfilled, and health, as expressed on the y-axis, ensues. In other words, the x-axis of the model forms the baseline that crosses the y-axis at the level of homeostasis implying health and thus absence of adverse effects. Evidently, the model may vary for different micronutrients, individuals and populations. It must be noted that the model is usually presented in a theoretical, general and non-substance-specific manner. This allows the designer to artistically and elegantly draw the curves as symmetrical, where in fact, were the model to express values for an actual real life substance, no symmetry exists as such. This we will discuss later.

In order to establish a SUL (in the customary toxicology jargon this translates into Tolerable Daily Intake), the NOAEL (No-Observed Adverse Effect Level) and LOAEL (Lowest-Observed Adverse Effect Level) levels for micronutrient exposure are divided by an uncertainty factor (UF). Safety or uncertainty factors (UFs) are applied to allow for uncertainties in the use of data obtained from human or animal studies in order to establish the amount of a particular substance that can be consumed without harm. Applying UFs to a NOAEL (or LOAEL) will result in a value for the derived UL that is less than the experimentally demonstrated NOAEL. The larger the uncertainty, the larger the UF and the lower the UL, which represents a lower estimate of the threshold, beyond which risks of exposure to the specific micronutrient may increase.

Generally, values for uncertainty factors of 10 for inter-human variations, 10 for animal to human (inter-species) extrapolations, and less than 10 for LOAEL to NOAEL extrapolations (usually 3) are used when dealing with non-carcinogens. These separate factors allow for differences in sensitivity between individuals and between species that may result from differences in, for example, absorption, metabolism or biological effect of the substance under consideration. The separate factors are multiplied assuming that they are independent variables; the standard factor between a NOAEL and an ADI is 100 (10×10). The above-described methodology is also used for micronutrients, as, in this case, the under and overdose makes the poison.

The UK Expert Group on Vitamins and Minerals (EVM) in 2003 produced a report in which the normative methodology is described for assessing the safety of vitamins and minerals.[4] They remark that 'the use of more refined values requires data specific to the chemical under consideration to support the use of a smaller or larger chemical-specific factor.' Although the EVM model is quite liberal in its approach, it is nevertheless exemplary in the sense that this and other approaches characteristically do not consider health-related data (the functional benefits) of micronutrients in setting regulatory safety standards for micronutrients in food-products.

Whether or not supplemental and/or fortified micronutrient products could make a contribution to a healthy lifespan is never discussed in the context of the Deficiency–Excess model and this issue also falls outside the scope of the legislature. The x-axis of the Deficiency-Excess model is spiked on the y-axis at the point of homeostasis of currently healthy people, not at 'health in the future.' As for the legislature, safety, not function, is central. Nevertheless, European Food Law repeatedly emphasizes that a 'varied and balanced diet' is adequate in terms of micronutrients content and that, in principle, it takes care of the nutritional needs of European consumers, or any other consumer in the world for that matter. As a consequence, a 'varied and balanced diet' as the source of a micronutrient or 'other substance' is coterminous with the RDA on the x-axis of the model. Whether or not that is a valid approach we will discuss subsequently.

18.4 ASSESSING EUROPEAN MICRONUTRIENT POLICIES— THE ADEQUATE, VARIED AND BALANCED DIET

At the center of this book stands the observation that '[m]ost food safety legislation and regulations have been devised in the first decades after the Second World War…More recent legislation and regulations often have been developed in response to media hypes. Today's reality is that there are differences between countries that too often lead to draconic measures such as the destruction of huge quantities of food to protect consumers, lacking any scientific justification, while a large part of the human population suffers from undernourishment…' This translates unreservedly into questions about adequate and varied diet, the technological potential to enhance diet under less than ideal conditions, and such.

According to the EU legislature, an 'adequate and varied diet' produced under conditions of safety as specified by the legislature stands firmly at the basis of a healthy European population. As the FSD states (EU, 2002b):

'(3) An adequate and varied diet could, under normal circumstances, provide all necessary nutrients for normal development and maintenance of a healthy life in quantities, which meet those established and recommended by generally acceptable scientific data. However, surveys show that this ideal situation is not being achieved for all nutrients and by all groups of the population across the Community.

(5) In order to ensure a high level of protection for consumers and facilitate their choice, the products that will be put on to the market must be safe and bear adequate and appropriate labelling.

(9) Only vitamins and minerals normally found in, and consumed as part of, the diet should be allowed to be present in food supplements although this does not mean that their presence therein is necessary. Controversy as to the identity of those nutrients that could potentially

---

[4]Expert Group on Vitamins and Minerals. *Safe Upper Levels for vitamins and minerals*, 2003. This report can be downloaded from: www.food.gov.uk/multimedia/pdfs/vitmin2003.pdf (accessed 17 February 2009).

arise should be avoided. Therefore, it is appropriate to establish a positive list of those vitamins and minerals.

(13) Excessive intake of vitamins and minerals may result in adverse effects and therefore necessitate the setting of maximum safe levels for them in food supplements, as appropriate. Those levels must ensure that the normal use of the products under the instructions of use provided by the manufacturer will be safe for the consumer.

(14) When maximum levels are set, therefore, account should be taken of the upper safe levels of the vitamins and minerals, as established by scientific risk assessment based on generally acceptable scientific data, and of intakes of those nutrients from the normal diet. Due account should also be taken of reference intake amounts when setting maximum levels.'

The reference to an adequate and varied diet as a primary source of 'all necessary nutrients' in (3) is intriguing. The truism that we can obtain everything that we need from a balanced diet only holds if people in fact eat such a balanced diet consistently and moreover have accurate knowledge (if at all available) to put together such a varied diet. The perspective here expounded by the EC is tautological: adequate is by default adequate. How this adequacy can be achieved, and what that adequate diet would actually be like remains unresolved. Importantly, factors impinging on the individual nutritional status are only partly related to actual dietary intake. Malabsorption (genetic or otherwise) and increased nutritional requirements (e.g. during a disease period) also greatly affect the nutritional status and requirements of individuals. This, the FSD and the FFR cannot address.

Conversely, (3) implies that even this adequate and varied diet nevertheless could be an insufficient source for all necessary nutrients.

The question then is whether the adequate and varied diet is or is not a sufficient source of all necessary nutrients. In this context, the FFR is noteworthy in its following conclusive statements (EU, 2006a):

'Recital (7) (FFR)

An adequate and varied diet can, under normal circumstances, provide all necessary nutrients for normal development and maintenance of a healthy life in quantities as those established and recommended by generally acceptable scientific data. However, surveys show that this ideal situation is not being achieved for all vitamins and minerals and by all groups of the population across the Community. Foods to which vitamins and minerals have been added appear to make an appreciable contribution to the intake of these nutrients and as such may be considered to make a positive contribution to overall intakes.

(8) Some nutrient deficiencies, although not very frequent, can be demonstrated to exist at present in the Community. Changes in the socio-economic situation prevailing in the Community and the life styles of different groups of the population have led to different nutritional requirements and to changing dietary habits. This in turn has led to changes in the energy and nutrient requirements of various groups of the population and to intakes of certain vitamins and minerals for these groups that would be below those recommended in different Member States. In addition, progress in scientific knowledge indicates that intakes of some nutrients for maintaining optimal health and well-being could be higher than those currently recommended.'

The closing line of (7) states that addition of micronutrients to food rendered a positive contribution to overall intakes, which thus seem to be lower than required when considering an 'adequate and varied diet' lacking this fortification (Lucock, 2004; MRC Vitamin Study Group, 1991). What's more, dietary habits of the lower socio-economic classes are known to be of a lower nutritional standard than on average would be required for a diet intended to provide the basis for a healthy life (Shohaimi *et al.*, 2004). Food selection is determined by economic, lifestyle and other socio-cultural considerations and conditions, whereby healthy eating patterns are frequently compromised, resulting in nutritional inadequacies. In particular, for most micronutrients, amplification of the cost-constraint results in a progressive decrease in nutrient density of the diet (James, Nelson, Ralph, & Leather, 1997; Darmon, Ferguson, & Briend 2002).

As James *et al.* (1997) already remarked for the EU, in the US '[n]utrients identified as potential (deficiency) problems for most gender/age groups based on comparisons to Estimated Average Requirements include vitamins A, E, C, and magnesium. Other nutrients that may be problems only for certain segments of the population are vitamin B_6 for older adult females; zinc for older adult males, females, and teenage females; and phosphorus for pre-teen and teenage females. Vitamin K, calcium, potassium, and dietary fiber, nutrients for which no Estimated Average Requirements have been established, may also be of concern' (Moshfeg, Goldman, & Cleveland, 2005). In 2008, the Dutch Health Council remarked on a similar trend in relation to at least two micronutrients. Data on vitamin A intake reveals that 20 to 30% of the Dutch population may have an excessively low vitamin A intake (Health Council of the Netherlands, 2008a). The vitamin D status of the Dutch population seems to be inadequate in all sections thereof (Health Council of the Netherlands, 2008b). Indeed, as another survey in the Netherlands shows, under-nourishment in hospitals and other care institutions is not uncommon, suggesting that even in professional

environments, the maintenance of an 'adequate and varied diet' is not without its problems, to say the least (Meijers *et al.*, 2005).

Summarizing, AD 2009 significant sections of the American and European population live on a sub-RDA diet. A modest way forward to deal with this micronutrient undernourishment is proposed by, among others, Ames (2005), requiring, however, a maturation of global regulation, which we tackle in the closing part of this chapter:

'A metabolic tune-up through an improved supply of micronutrients is likely to have great health benefits, particularly for those with inadequate diets, such as many of the poor, young, obese and elderly. The issues discussed here highlight the need to educate the public about the crucial importance of nutrition and the potential health benefits of a simple and affordable daily multivitamin/mineral supplement. Tuning up metabolism to maximize human health and lifespan will require scientists, clinicians and educators to abandon outdated models and explore more meaningful ways to prevent chronic disease and achieve optimum health. It is becoming clear that unbalanced diets will soon become the largest contributor to ill health, with smoking following close behind.'

18.5 PRECAUTIONARY IMPEDIMENTS

Ames unwittingly directs our attention to the precautionary aspect of current European micronutrient regulation. With the installation of the European Food Safety Authority the precautionary principle is specifically embedded in Article 7 of the GFL, and hence it takes prime position in the development of European regulation within the food area (EU, 2002a). A common characterization of the precautionary principle holds that it seeks to impose timely protective measures to prevent uncertain risks, i.e. risks as to which there is little or no data on their probability and magnitude (Wiener, 2001). Uncertainty is the key here. Indeed, the precautionary perspective on—or lack of—knowledge is that scientific research needs to be focused on guaranteeing safety, which has become a strategic requirement for basically all new products and processes. As the European Commission states in its communication on the precautionary principle (Commission of the European Communities, 2000): 'Countries that impose a prior approval (marketing authorization) requirement on products that they deem dangerous *a priori* reverse the burden of proving injury, by treating them as dangerous unless and until businesses do the scientific work necessary to demonstrate that they are safe.' Within the context of micronutrients regulation, precautionary measures are focused on the avoidance of excess exposure. The reference to an adequate and varied diet as a primary source of all necessary nutrients underlines this perspective as it suggests (quite implicitly) that food supplements and fortification are for all intents and purposes superfluous.

The aspiration to prevent uncertain risks is, however, unachievable due to a problem common to virtually all formulations of the precautionary principle: 'The real problem with the Precautionary Principle … is that it is incoherent; it purports to give guidance, but it fails to do so, because it condemns the very steps that it requires. The regulation that the principle requires always give rise to risks of its own—and hence the principle bans what it simultaneously mandates' (Sunstein, 2005). The logical difficulty of precaution is the fact that any true node in a decision tree must at the very least have two branches (McKinney & Hammer, 2000): we may either undertake the action or we may refrain from undertaking it. Each of these choices—action and inaction—entails consequences, both foreseen and unforeseen.

However, it is crucial to remember that a decision *not* to undertake an action is every bit of an action as is undertaking it. In other words, risks are on all sides of the societal and regulatory equations to which precaution alone cannot give any guidance.

This is abundantly clear when reviewing micronutrients and their effects on human health. Micronutrients cannot be characterized other than by way of a 2-sided benefits–risks profile (the U-shaped dose–response curve that marks benefits and risks; see Figure 18.2), in which the benefits of exposure to micronutrients may not be left to the legislature's admonishments to follow an 'adequate and varied diet', but must be an integral factor in the (symmetrical) regulatory equation. Incontrovertibly then, the most critical and most volatile problems cannot be solved without the effective marshalling of expert scientific knowledge and judgment. Food safety is no different. Securing objective knowledge about safety, health, and the like, despite the inherent and attendant value judgments, pre-eminently remains a scientific task and a challenge for the future. This then leaves us with the state-of-art of science in the field of nutrition to which we will now turn.

18.6 MICRONUTRIENTS, HUMAN HEALTH, AND SCIENCE—THE STATE-OF-ART AND BEYOND

The D–E model we touched on above is derived from the generalized physiological U-shape dose–response curve of micronutrients. Obviously, this U-shape does not have any regulatory objective, yet it underlines the issue of 'nutritional risk' as captured by the CCFNSDU. Thus risk within the confines of food is not only related to exposure to an excess of a certain micronutrient, which we denote in the scheme as 'E-risk'. In a situation of deficient intake it means risk of loss of benefits of essential

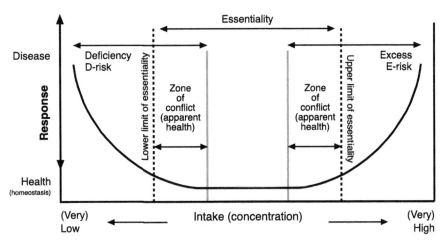

FIGURE 18.2 Classic physiological dose–response model for micronutrients.

nutrients, denoted as 'D-risk'. The scheme presented below centers on the organism as such as it is exposed across a certain range of loads of a micronutrient or an 'other substance.'

In the history of food standards, the upper limits of exposure—which at the time of writing need to be taken as a basis for 'maximum levels' in supplemental and fortified food-products within the context of European Food Law—did not become 'en vogue' until quite recently, as undernourishment was dominant, and of course still is in many parts of the world including Europe. The 1930s, the time of the Great Depression in which food security was the foremost issue, is effectively captured by Boudreau: 'delegates to the League of Nations, together with League officials, launched what came to be known as the world food movement, designed to release the economic jam by emphasizing that adequate diets were essential to human health…' (Boudreau, 1947).

Avoiding the classic micronutrient deficiency diseases through adequate diet was the twentieth-century driver to gain factual scientific knowledge about food requirements. Focusing on micronutrients, the overarching research efforts have, among other things, culminated in RDAs for micronutrients. The original concept

of RDA was a 'goal' or 'baseline' for intake below which risks of inadequacy begin to significantly increase. RDAs, based on a specific criterion of adequacy, were designed to serve as dietary standards for the planning of food supplies for population groups. They were originally formulated as reference standards for use by qualified individuals who have the responsibility for assuring that food, distributed to large groups of people, would be nutritionally adequate (Harper, 1987). Subsequent policies based on the scientific findings that spawned the RDAs were aimed at preventing the major health problems that affect the majority of the population from *early on* in life, and quite successfully so (Hanekamp & Bast, 2008).

RDAs, however, do not take into account the needs arising from infections, metabolic disorders, or degenerative diseases that take a long time to become established, originating when an individual is still apparently healthy, and thereby do not define an optimal level of any nutrient. In view of the developing science of nutrition the latter has become an important research focus. The focal point therefore has shifted from current and apparent, to long-term and enduring health. This not only affects the way we view and understand the physiological workings of vitamins and minerals but also brings into view 'other substances' that might add to human health (Ferguson, 2001), although classical deficiencies have not been demonstrated for these classes of food-endogenous compounds.

Long-term health and degenerative diseases related to micronutrients and 'other substances' have come to the fore over the last three decades or so. The US Food and Nutrition Board (FNB) for instance, 'believes that the science of nutrition has advanced significantly, and the next edition of the RDAs will need to reflect this progress. One consideration is expanding the RDA concept to include reducing the risk of chronic disease' (IOM, 1994). Despite advancing knowledge concerning the role of food components in the prevention of more subtle, subclinical metabolic changes resulting over time in noticeable symptoms of degenerative diseases, current RDAs do not yet reflect this progress (Ames, 2003).

Nevertheless, diet and dietary ingredients are now regarded as a key factor in reducing risk of disease especially by maintaining genomic integrity, i.e. protecting DNA from deleterious damage through cellular mechanisms such as prevention, repair or apoptosis (Fenech, 2002). Degenerative diseases such as cancer, as well as the process of aging, are partly related to DNA damage (Ames, 1983; Ames, Gold, & Willett, 1995; Ames, Atamna, & Killilea, 2005; Kirkwood, 2008; Willett, 1994). There is accumulating scientific evidence that higher levels of some micronutrients and 'other substances' may be necessary for various DNA maintenance reactions, and that the current RDAs for some micronutrients seem inadequate to protect against genomic instability (Fenech & Ferguson, 2001). The need to set micronutrient requirements to minimize DNA damage seems a way forward (Ames, 2005). As stated above, this would also include 'other substances' for which there is accumulating evidence that they add to a healthy lifespan, such as the polyphenolic antioxidants that have, in scientific studies, been implicated to contribute notably to healthy ageing (Hanekamp & Bast, 2007).

Expanding RDAs beyond their original intent, both in terms of degenerative diseases and the range of food components, highlights the issue of uncertainty in the existing RDAs, currently offered in single numbers as a seemingly conclusive expression of comprehensive scientific insight. An all-inclusive RDA, a newRDA (nRDA) so to speak, from the viewpoint of optimal intake related to short and long-term health, underscores the potential to expand the RDA beyond its original borders (Fenech, 2003). Vitamin D might serve here as a good example. The basic effect of vitamin D on human health is generally regarded as the maintenance of a healthy skeleton. For adults, bone mineral content (BMC), bone mineral density (BMD), and fracture risk, in combination with serum 25(OH)D and PTH (parathyroid hormone) concentrations, are considered to be the most useful indicators of optimal vitamin D status (IOM, 1997). Over a range of life stages a suitable RDA has been derived based on these markers.

However, in the 1970s and 1980s, nuclear receptors for the active metabolite of vitamin D, $1\alpha,25(OH)_2D_3$, were discovered in a variety of tissues *not* directly involved in calcium homeostasis. Numerous proteins are now known to be regulated by $1\alpha,25(OH)_2D_3$, including several oncogenes that are inhibited by $1\alpha,25(OH)_2D_3$ (Bijlsma *et al.*, 2006; Bijlsma, Peppelenbosch, & Spek, 2007; Giovannucci *et al.*, 2006). The classical limits of vitamin D regulated calcium homeostasis are thus far exceeded (Rucker, Suttie, McCormirck, & Machlin, 2001). It has been suggested that a daily intake of $25\,\mu g$ of vitamin D_3, which is substantially higher than the current RDA, may well lower the risk of developing different cancers substantially (Garland *et al.*, 2006; Mehta & Mehta, 2002). This is open to further scientific scrutiny, yet underscores the current limitations of RDAs in light of scientific developments in relation to chronic disease.

As an example of 'other substances' that positively influence health, we mention here certain polyphenols, such as flavonoids. Unlike micronutrients such as selenium and folate, plant polyphenols are a large group of chemicals some of which may play a beneficial role in human nutrition. They are not regarded as essential for human health, because no deficiency diseases have been demonstrated. Nevertheless, the group as a whole is characterized by a wide range of biological effects including antioxidant, anti-mutagenic and anti-inflammatory properties (Bagchi *et al.*, 2002; Bartel & Matsuda, 2003; Ferguson, 2001; Philpott *et al.*, 2003). Polyphenols are the most abundantly present antioxidants in the diet and are widespread constituents of fruits, vegetables, cereals, dry legumes, chocolate, and beverages, such as tea, coffee, and red wine. Apart from vitamins and minerals, certain types of polyphenols are probably the widest marketed groups of dietary supplements. This class of plant chemicals contains more than 8000 known compounds (Bravo, 1998). The total dietary intake of polyphenols is roughly estimated to be in the range of 1 g per day, although this intake may differ as a result of varying dietary habits (Scalbert & Williamson, 2000).

Epidemiological studies associating the intake of various dietary sources of polyphenols (e.g. flavanols from green tea and red wine) have been, in the main, indicative of protection against a variety of diseases (Li *et al.*, 2006; Manach *et al.*, 2005; Mattivi, Zulian, Nicolini, & Valenti, 2002; Soleas *et al.*, 2002; Williamson & Manach, 2005). Experimental studies on animals and cultured human cell lines corroborate a role of polyphenols in the prevention of cardiovascular diseases, cancers, neurodegenerative diseases, etc. (Bagchi *et al.*, 2003; Lambert *et al.*, 2005). Indeed, there is evidence from many different scientific fields supporting the argument that frequent consumption of, for instance, green tea is inversely associated with the risk of degenerative human diseases. The chemopreventive

and chemoprotective effects of green tea have been largely attributed to anti-oxidative and anti-inflammatory activities of its polyphenolic compounds (Lee *et al.*, 2005). Equally, polyphenols from red wine, for instance, inhibit the process of colon carcinogenesis (induced by chemicals) in rodents, and reduce colonic mucosa DNA oxidation (Dolara *et al.*, 2005).

18.7 THE nRDA-GENOMIC INTEGRITY HOMEOSTASIS U-SHAPE CURVE

This developing perspective on micronutrients, including 'other substances', might be portrayed in the subsequent scheme (Figure 18.3). Here we basically modified the micronutrients' U-shape curve into two curves that overlap, the new-deficiency curve adapted to the incorporation of the long-term perspective and the known excess curve.

Figure 18.3 barely differs from Figure 18.2. We merely propose, in line with Article 95(3) of the European Treaty, a new way to present 'new developments based on scientific facts' in relation to the function of micronutrients. The 'new' deficiency (nD-risk) encompasses the long-term perspective of degenerative diseases related to micronutrients intake. Now, the curve hits the x-axis beyond the RDA as it precipitates into the deliberate expansive portrayal of the nRDA. Concomitantly, the x-axis now spikes the y-axis at the point of what we propose as enduring or 'genomic integrity homeostasis'.

Figure 18.3 by and large covers the inherent uncertainty in the erstwhile RDAs in terms of an expression of scientific progress, considering the growing knowledge-base of micronutrients vis-à-vis long-term health issues. At what nRDA-point the genomic integrity homeostasis level is reached is not clear and, moreover, differs from micronutrient to micronutrient and micronutrients interactions. Uncertainty

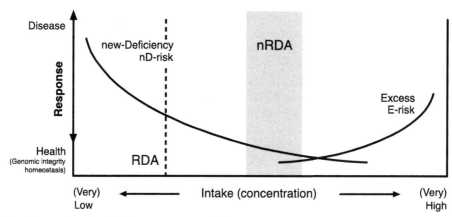

FIGURE 18.3   A new physiological dose–response model for micronutrients.

also relates to the point where E-risks overlap with the potential benefits of certain nRDA-dosages of micronutrients. This brings to light the symmetrical and integral regulatory approach micronutrient compounds in fact require (Hanekamp & Bast, 2008). European food-safety legislation has as its goal 'a high level of protection for human life and health' whereby *mutatis mutandis* the potential benefits side of micronutrients cannot be ignored. Precaution demands this integral approach in conformity with Article 7 of the EU's GFL: '...provisional risk management measures necessary to ensure the high level of health protection chosen in the Community...pending further scientific information for a more comprehensive risk assessment.'

Summarizing, the scientific evidence generated hitherto is as of yet deemed to be insufficient to upgrade RDAs to nRDAs that incorporate long-term effects *in casu* genomic integrity and thereby could cover 'other substances' as well. Evidently, disagreement abounds within this scientific (and any other) discourse, but if that is the case, the dispute is about whether some information truly provides a ground for everyone to believe that RDAs can in fact incorporate long-term perspectives evolving into nRDAs (See for a discussion

thereon: Snyder, 1998). This issue brings us to the current scientific assessments and regulation of micronutrients and 'other substances'. The following, however, will be more than just a summing up of the current regulatory status (EFSA, 2006). It will probe its strengths and weaknesses and we will subsequently propose a route towards regulatory maturation and global harmonization.

18.8 INTEGRATING nRDAs IN THE MODEL OF INTENDED NORMAL USE—TOWARDS REGULATORY MATURATION (SCHWITTERS *et al.*, 2007)

In the previous sections, we have proposed that micronutrients are essential not only in short-term apparent health, but also in long-term enduring human health. With the latter, 'other substances' have become 'en vogue' as well. We have proposed, in a tentative fashion, the nRDA as a tool to incorporate long-term health issues. However, we are still confronted by the regulatory demands, within and outside the Eurozone, for product safety. The SULs and the derivative maximum levels in supplements and fortification are an expression thereof.

Conversely, we know that even in relation to the RDAs, undernourishment is still rather the rule than the exception, even in modern, developed regions of the world. For instance, the intake of iodine in the Netherlands is mainly related to the consumption of iodized salt, as Dutch food does not naturally contain enough iodine. Iodized salt used for baking bread and other baked products contains more iodine (up to 65 milligrams per kilogram of salt) than iodized salt destined for other foods (up to 25 milligrams per kilogram of salt). Roughly 50% of iodine intake is from bread (Health Council of the Netherlands, 2008c). The maximum permitted level for iodine may turn out to be below the current baker's salt fortification level. This would lead to a decline in the iodine intake of the Dutch population, which would lead to a greater risk of iodine deficiency and goiter.

The micronutrients' regulation, whether European or otherwise, with a focus on safety related to the minimization of excessive intake has opportunity costs: striving to guarantee public safety in relation to excess toxicity, the foregone opportunity is the cost-effective reduction of micronutrient deficiencies and its concomitant short and long-term health effects. To counter this development of maximum levels that only cover the minimum requirements related to RDAs, we propose a distinctive approach with global implications *and* the flexibility with respect to regional diets that, in some instances, cannot deliver sufficient micronutrients. As food supplements and fortified foods could be a relatively safe and cost-effective addition to the human diet (Ames, 2003), how then should micronutrients best be regulated?

When the 'high level of protection for human life and health' is taken seriously, firstly the breadth and depth (in other words integrity) of new developments based on emerging scientific knowledge in this field also need to be taken seriously. There should be no room for skepticism, nor any room for scientism (Stenmark, 2001—Religion, here, is referred to

in the wider context as world views). This is in line with a 'full-weight-of-evidence' approach ideally expounded in risk assessment procedures (Barnard, 1994). Secondly, therefore, a realistic regulatory approach of micronutrients cannot be founded on preclusive precautionary thinking. Thirdly, any rational regulatory approach has to decide on which level public intervention is justified. This in effect addresses the trade-off between market failure and government failure.

To be sure, individual freedom and responsibility and the governmental prerogative to intervene for the benefit of the people is a complicated dilemma in any democracy. We like to put this dilemma in the following way. On the one hand, democratic governments are obliged to take their citizens seriously in their personal freedom. However, on the other hand democratic governments have a duty—often inscribed in law—to provide as much good for society as it can generate from the public means. The duty of wealth and health distribution is a strong driver of numerous public policies in diverse fields. These two duties in not a few instances do not match up. It therefore may be prudent to recapitulate the words of John Stuart Mill (1859):

'Nevertheless, when there is not a certainty, but only a danger of mischief, no one but the person himself can judge of the sufficiency of the motive which may prompt him to incur the risk: in this case, therefore, (unless he is a child, or delirious, or in some state of excitement or absorption incompatible with the full use of the reflecting faculty,) he ought, I conceive, to be only warned of the danger; not forcibly prevented from exposing himself to it.'

For instance, applying both cost-benefit and cost-effectiveness analytic techniques, it is estimated that folic acid fortification is associated with annual economic benefit of US$312 to

US$425 million. The cost savings (net reduction in direct costs) were estimated to be in the range of US$88 million to US$145 million per year (Grosse, Waitzman, Romano, & Mulinare, 2005). Another example relates to vitamin D. The US economic burden due to vitamin D insufficiency from inadequate exposure to solar UVB irradiance, diet, and supplements was estimated in 2004 at US$40–56 billion, whereas the economic burden for excess UV irradiance was estimated at US$6–7 billion. These results suggest that increased vitamin D through UVB irradiance, fortification of food, and supplementation could reduce the health care burden in the United States, UK, and most likely elsewhere (Grant *et al.*, 2005).

Keeping in mind the above, and placing interventionist influence in the strict confines of a symmetrical approach to the risks and (emerging) benefits of micronutrients, we propose the following tenets to compose a realistic and efficient model for managing marketable food supplements: (i) risk-benefit context; (ii) *ex post* oriented; (iii) innovation oriented; and (iv) market oriented (level-playing field). In particular, the latter tenet leads, in our view, to the inevitable acceptance of Intended Normal Use (INU) as the guiding principle for the flow-chart that is descriptive for the policy-direction we envision (Figure 18.4).

INU in terms of, for example, safe consumption levels of daily portions, as unambiguously clarified and presented by the manufacturer on a product's packaging and accompanying information, should be the core regulatory and market ordering principle. *A priori*, the scheme places all micronutrients, including 'other substances', in an *ex post* approach. Depending on the ingredient(s) used, manufacturers need to make specific indications concerning a product's conditions of use. Because products define markets, a product's INU will automatically and without further ado or consideration place a product in a certain market as that market is defined by law. So it is that fortified foods and food supplements shall make up different

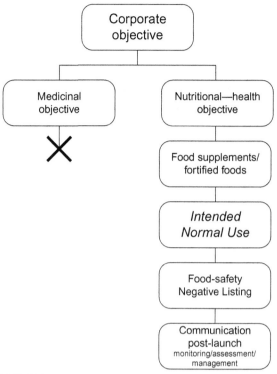

FIGURE 18.4 Flow-chart for managing risks and benefits of micronutrients.

markets, not on the basis of their composition or technical/nutritional characteristics, but simply on the basis of their intended use.

This *de facto* state of affairs has been noted by the EFSA as well, when they observe in their Discussion Paper on 'botanicals' that 'this heterogeneous group of commodities…mainly depending on their intended uses and presentations, fall under different Community regulatory frameworks' (EFSA, 2004). Similarly, the definition of the term 'botanical' provided by the US Food and Drug Administration (FDA) states that: 'a finished, labeled product that contains vegetable matter, which may include plant materials (a plant or plant part (e.g. bark, wood, leaves, stems, roots, flowers, fruits, seeds, or parts thereof) as well as exudates thereof), algae, macroscopic fungi, or combinations of these. Depending in part on its intended use, a botanical product may be a food, drug, medical device, or cosmetic' (EFSA, 2004).

Although approximation is the European legislature's preferred way of intervening, approximation is, almost by definition, redundant in the supra-national legal system that is founded on the principle of the free movement of goods between Member States. Likewise, *Codex Alimentarius* sets rules by indirectly approximating rules and laws of otherwise sovereign states. Our approach rests on the premise of free movement of goods and services between sovereign nations and between equally sovereign food business operators and consumers. In European case-law this is expressed as the principle of Mutual Recognition. In a Mutual Recognition situation, the threshold for a level playing field is set by the market participants who are allowed to operate under the greatest amount of freedom and related private—as opposed to public—responsibilities.

Our choice for applying Mutual Recognition is sustained by the EU legislature in the Commission's Report of 5 December 2008 to the Council and the European Parliament, in which the Commission admitted that, when faced with the complexities of regulating 'other substances' and their role in human health, this is best done by letting things take their natural national courses under the open system of Mutual Recognition (Commission of the European Communities, 2008).

18.9 SAFETY, GOOD MANUFACTURING PRACTICE AND INITIAL TYPE TESTING

The INU as presented on a finished micronutrient food product shall determine in which market it will have its place. Evidently, in determining INUs, safety rules, as laid down in GFL, must be taken into account by the food business operator. In this respect, the role of science and a history of safety that has been established as a result of long-term widespread use (tacit knowledge[5]) are different yet complementary and need to be internalized and/or explicated by the manufacturer, whether through experimental scientific research, literature desk-top studies, or both (Ocké, Buurma-Rethans, & Fransen, 2005). We envision a product's quality, purity (when applicable), strength, consistency and stability guaranteed through applicable and appropriate standards of good manufacturing practice (GMP) and/or other industry standards that match today's safety requirements and concerns. This is an important aspect in the safety-guarantee that producers need to assess, manage and communicate. This could be defined as the Initial Type-Testing for food supplements and/or fortified foods. When it comes to food supplements, individuals consciously and voluntarily make a choice to consume these supplements, contrary to being unconsciously and involuntarily exposed to food-endogenous compounds such as acrylamide. Therefore, individuals making a conscious purchase of food supplements, and to a lesser degree of fortified foods, expect those products to be safe, and rightly so (Starr, 1969).

Food supplements and fortified foods that come to market need to be safe (e.g. in terms of carrying clear and simple indications for normal recommended intake). Even without the present regulatory context this is a crucial exigency that food business operators and other economic parties must take seriously in view of issues of trust, liability, product safety and consumer protection. Additionally, compounds with a

[5]Tacit knowledge, opposite to codified (usually scientific) knowledge, is part and parcel of our daily lives and is transmitted through interpersonal contact, not through schoolbooks or scientific publications. Skills and traditions that have formed in laboratories, for instance, are utilized extensively, yet are not part of the codified output, such as journal publications and books. Therefore, even scientific knowledge in the public domain needs to be found, interpreted by specialists, and reprocessed for actual use.

long-standing use, whether within or outside the EU (EU, 1997)[6] could, in principal, be generally regarded as safe (GRAS) (Wheeler & Wheeler, 2004). Tea, as an example, has been consumed literally for thousands of years, and it is this long safety record of tea consumption that makes the potentially beneficial compounds, present in tea, an attractive target for research and marketing.

In order to stimulate a level-playing field and innovative developments within the field of food, we propose that this approach to micronutrient compounds shall be *ex post*, whereby the aspect of safety is not tackled on the basis of politically dominated precautionary thinking but rather on the basis of prevention, i.e. on the basis of objective, verifiable scientific data concerning safety, placing the responsibility squarely on the shoulders of the manufacturer. Contrary to the precautionary approach, such an approach to safety would support and sustain innovative industry and thus, eventually, public health and the global economy. Positive listing through the no-data-no-market strategy will counteract innovation (Kaput *et al.*, 2005), as increasing regulatory demands, fuelled by precautionary deliberations, will hinder market-entrance, and—continuance (Burgess, 2001). This is illustrated in the EC communication on the precautionary principle, which states that the provisional nature of precautionary measures, which is usually a ban, 'is not bound up with a time limit but with the development of scientific knowledge' (Commission of the European Communities, 2000). As mistrust in science is widespread, scientific knowledge is hardly deemed to be sufficient to overcome the knowledge-barrier, so any precautionary ban will have an 'enduring temporality' (Forrester & Hanekamp, 2006; Hottois, 2000).

An effective opposite therefore would comprise of a preventive negative list of compounds proven to be damaging to public health (Hanekamp,

Frapporti, & Olieman, 2003; Hanekamp & Kwakman, 2004; Hanekamp & Wijnands, 2004). This is the way chosen in the FFR to regulate the use of 'other substances' in food supplements and fortified foods. There are evidently good reasons to take a preventive regulatory approach with regard to safety, when confronted with products with only a very limited local or traditional use, and of which limited if any (scientific) knowledge is available. This reflects the overall approach that manufacturers need to be sure of their product food-safety, amongst other things in relation to the recommended dosage, that is, INU.

Overall, as is shown in our scheme, the primary responsibility, we believe, lies most (cost-) effectively with the food business operator and his/her objectives, the reason being that there is considerable evidence—as we have shown above—for health benefits of micronutrients at intake levels beyond the RDA, paralleled by the fact that few, if any, risks at intakes within or to some extent above dietary bounds have come or will come to the fore. It is likely that, in the future, the effects of nutrients on risk reduction of diseases will be used increasingly to establish novel nutrient requirements (Renwick *et al.*, 2004). In principle, INU recommendations for the intake of nutrients to achieve such benefits could be based on a similar approach to that for establishing the RDA, taken into account long-term benefits like cancer and aging prevention (Ames & Wakimoto, 2002).

In view of the fact that nRDAs or certain recommended levels of 'other substances' might overlap with an ingredient's SUL, monitoring of public health in relation to the intake of micronutrient food supplements (a post-launch system analogous to the pharmaco-vigilance system for medicinal products) is a further part of the proposed scheme. This is both of interest to governments as to food business operators, as it will reveal patterns of intake and associated potential risks and benefits. Assessment and management

---

[6]In fact, this regulation defines a novel food or ingredient as novel when it is without a history of use in the EU (sic).

options remain open to governments (but also producers), when monitoring studies revealing potential risks associated with intake of micronutrient food supplements. Communicating benefits and risks within this context is a viable and efficient strategy.[7] Disproportionate claims on health and consumption of certain food supplements can, within the context of proper communication, be scrutinized and publicly commented on with reference to the state-of-scientific-art. This, we believe, will generate a global and harmonized market that is sustainable in view of safety, innovation and last, but most importantly, optimum human health.

References

Ames, B. N. (1983). Dietary carcinogens and anticarcinogens. Oxygen radicals and degenerative diseases. *Science, 221,* 1256–1264.

Ames, B. N., Gold, L. S., & Willett, W. C. (1995). The causes and prevention of cancer. *Proceedings of the National Academy of Sciences of the United States of America, 92,* 5258–5265.

Ames, B. N. (2003). The metabolic tune-up: Metabolic harmony and disease prevention. *Journal of Nutrition,* 1544S–1548S.

Ames, B. N. (2005). Increasing longevity by tuning up metabolism. *EMBO Reports, 6,* S20–S24.

Ames, B. N., & Wakimoto, P. (2002). Are vitamin and mineral deficiencies a major cancer risk? *Nature, 2,* 694–704.

Ames, B. N., Atamna, H., & Killilea, D. W. (2005). Mineral and vitamin deficiencies can accelerate the mitochondrial decay of aging. *Molecular aspects of medicine, 26,* 363–378.

Bagchi, D., Bagchi, M., Stohs, S. J., et al. (2002). Cellular protection with proanthocyanidins derived from grape seeds. *Annals of the New York Academy of Sciences, 957,* 260–270.

Bagchi, D., Sen, C. K., Ray, S. D., et al. (2003). Molecular mechanism of cardioprotection by a novel grape seed proanthocyanidin extract. *Mutation research, 523–524,* 87–97.

Barnard, R. C. (1994). Scientific method and risk assessment. *Regulation Toxicology Pharmacy, 19,* 211–218.

Bartel, B., & Matsuda, S. P. T. (2003). Seeing red. *Science, 299,* 352–353.

Bijlsma, M. F., Peppelenbosch, M. P., & Spek, C. A. (2007). Pro-vitamin D as treatment option for hedgehog-related malignancies. *Medicine Hypotheses, 70*(1), 202–203.

Bijlsma, M. F., Spek, C. A., Zivkovic, D., et al. (2006). Repression of smoothened by patched-dependent (pro-) vitamin D3 secretion. *PLoS Biology, 4*(8), 1397–1410.

Boudreau, F. G. (1947). Nutrition in war and peace. *The Milbank Quarterly, 25*(3), 231–246.

Bravo, L. (1998). Polyphenols: Chemistry, dietary sources, metabolism and nutritional significance. *Nutrition Reviews, 56,* 317–333.

Burgess, A. (2001). Flattering consumption. Creating a Europe of the consumer. *Journal of Consumer Culture, 1*(1), 93–117.

CAC. (2008). Joint FAO/WHO Food Standard Programme. Codex Alimentarius Commission. *Report on the 29th Session of the Codex Commission on Nutrition and Foods for Special Dietary Uses.* Alinorm 08/31/26, pp. 74–75.

Commission of the European Communities. (2000). *Communication from the Commission on the Precautionary Principle.* Brussels, p. 5.

Commission of the European Communities. (2008). *Report from the Commission to the Council and the European Parliament on the use of substances other than vitamins and minerals in food supplements,* Brussels.

Darmon, N., Ferguson, E. L., & Briend, A. (2002). A cost constrained alone has adverse effects on food selection and nutrient density: An analysis of human diets by linear programming. *Journal of Nutrition, 132,* 3764–3771.

De Vries, J. (Ed.). (1997). *Food safety and toxicity.* New York: CRC Press.

Dolara, P., Luceri, C., De Filippo, C., et al. (2005). Red wine polyphenols influence carcinogenesis, intestinal microflora, oxidative damage and gene expression profiles of colonic mucosa in F344 rats. *Mutation research, 591,* 237–246.

EFSA. (2004). *Discussion paper on botanicals and botanical preparations widely used as food supplements and related products: Coherent and comprehensive risk assessment and consumer information approaches,* Brussels.

EFSA. (2006). European Food Safety Authority, *Tolerable Upper Intake Levels for Vitamins and Minerals.* Scientific Committee on Food Scientific Panel on Dietetic Products, Nutrition and Allergies, p. 9.

EU. (1997). Regulation (EC) No 258/97 of the European Parliament and the Council of 27 January 1997 concerning novel foods and novel ingredients. *Official Journal of the European Communities, L43,* 1–7.

EU. (2002a). Regulation (EC) No 178/2002 of the European Parliament and of the Council of 28 January 2002 laying down the general principles and requirements of food law, establishing the European Food Safety Authority and laying down procedures in matters of food safety. *Official Journal of the European Communities, L31,* 1–24.

---

[7]See, for example: *Making sense of chemical stories. A briefing for the lifestyle sector on misconceptions about chemicals,* 2006. Sense about Science, London, UK. The report can be downloaded from http://www.senseaboutscience.org (last visited on the 17 February, 2009).

EU. (2002b). Directive 2002/46/EC of the European Parliament and of the Council of 10 June 2002 on the approximation of the laws of the Member States relating to food supplements. *Official Journal of the European Communities, L183*, 51–57.

EU. (2006a). Regulation (EC) No 1925/2006 of the European Parliament and of the Council of 20 December 2006 on the addition of vitamins and minerals and of certain other substances to foods. *Official Journal of the European Communities, L404*, 26–38.

EU. (2006b). Consolidated versions of the treaty on European Union and of the treaty establishing the European Community. *Official Journal of the European Union, C321*, 1–331.

Fenech, M. (2002). Micronutrients and genomic stability: A new paradigm for recommended dietary allowances (RDAs). *Food and chemical toxicology, 40*, 1113–1117.

Fenech, M. (2003). Nutritional treatment of genome instability: A paradigm shift in disease prevention and in the setting of recommended dietary allowances. *Nutrition Research Reviews, 16*, 109–122.

Fenech, M., & Ferguson, L. R. (2001). Vitamins/minerals and genomic stability in humans. *Mutation research, 475*, 1–6.

Ferguson, L. R. (2001). Role of plant polyphenols in genomic stability. *Mutation research, 475*, 89–111.

Forrester, I., & Hanekamp, J. C. (2006). Precaution, science and jurisprudence: A test case. *Journal of risk research, 9*(4), 297–311.

Garland, C. F., Garland, F. C., Gorham, E. D., et al. (2006). The role of vitamin D in cancer prevention. *American Journal of Public Health, 96*, 252–261.

Giovannucci, E., Liu, Y., Rimm, E. B., et al. (2006). Prospective study of predictors of vitamin D status and cancer incidence and mortality in men. *Journal of the National Cancer Institute, 98*, 451–459.

Grant, W. B., Cedric, F., Garland, C. F., et al. (2005). Comparisons of estimated economic burdens due to insufficient solar ultraviolet irradiance and vitamin D and excess solar UV irradiance for the United States. *Photochemistry and photobiology, 81*, 1276–1286.

Grosse, S. D., Waitzman, N. J., Romano, P. S., & Mulinare, J. (2005). Re-evaluating the benefits of folic acid fortification in the United States: Economic analysis, regulation, and public health. *American journal of public health, 95*(11), 1917–1922.

Hanekamp, J. C., Frapporti, G., & Olieman, K. (2003). Chloramphenicol, food safety and precautionary thinking in Europe. *Environmental Liab, 6*, 209–221.

Hanekamp, J. C., & Kwakman, J. (2004). Beyond zero-tolerance: A novel and global outlook on food-safety and residues of pharmacological active substances in foodstuffs of animal origin. *Environmental Liab, 1*, 33–39.

Hanekamp, J. C., & Wijnands, R. J. (2004). Analytical technology, risk analysis and residues of veterinary substances: A précis and a proposal for coherent and logical clinical residue legislation. In: *Joint FAO/WHO Technical Workshop on Residues of Veterinary Drugs without ADI/MRL*. 24–26 August, Bangkok, Thailand, pp. 81–86.

Hanekamp, J. C., & Bast, A. (2008). Why RDA's and UL's are incompatible standards in the U-Shape Micronutrient Model. A philosophically orientated analysis of micronutrients standardisations. *Risk Analysis, 28*(6), 1639–1652.

Hanekamp, J. C., & Bast, A. (2007). Food supplements and European regulation within a precautionary context: A critique and implications for nutritional, toxicological and regulatory consistency. *Critical Reviews in Food Science and Nutrition, 47*, 267–285.

Harper, A. E. (1987). Evolution of recommended dietary allowances—new directions? *Annual review of nutrition, 7*, 509–537.

Health Council of the Netherlands. 2008a. *Towards an adequate intake of vitamin D*. The Hague, publication no. 2008/26.

Health Council of the Netherlands. 2008b. *Towards an adequate intake of vitamin D*. The Hague, publication no. 2008/15E.

Health Council of the Netherlands. (2008c). *Towards maintaining an optimum iodine intake*. The Hague, publication no. 2008/14E.

Hottois, G. (2000). A philosophical and critical analysis of the European convention of bioethics. *The Journal of medicine and philosophy, 25*(2), 133–146.

IOM. (1994). *How should the recommended dietary allowances be revised? 1994*. Washington DC: Food and Nutrition Board, Institute of Medicine. National Academies Press.

IOM. (1997). *Dietary reference intakes for calcium, phosphorus, magnesium, vitamin D, and fluoride*. Washington DC: Standing Committee on the Scientific Evaluation of Dietary Reference Intakes, Food and Nutrition Board, Institute of Medicine. National Academies Press.

James, P., Kemper, F., & Pascal, G. (1999). *A European Food and Public Health Authority. The future of scientific advice in the EU*, p. 42, http://ec.europa.eu/food/fs/sc/future_food_en.pdf.

James, W. P. T., Nelson, M., Ralph, A., & Leather, S. (1997). Socioeconomic determinants of health: The contribution of nutrition to inequalities in health. *British medical journal, 314*, 1545–1549.

Kaput, J., Ordovas, J. M., Ferguson, L., et al. (2005). The case for strategic international alliances to harness nutritional genomics for public and personal health. *The British journal of nutrition, 94*, 623–632.

Kirkwood, T. B. L. (2008). A systematic look at an old problem. *Nature, 451*, 644–647.

Lambert, J. D., Hong, J., Yang, G., et al. (2005). Inhibition of carcinogenesis by polyphenols: Evidence from laboratory investigations. *The American journal of clinical nutrition, 81*(suppl), 284S–291S.

Lee, J.-S., Oh, T.-Y., Young-Kyung Kim., et al. (2005). Protective effects of green tea polyphenol extracts against ethanol-induced gastric mucosal damages in rats: Stress-responsive transcription factors and MAP kinases as potential targets. *Mutation research, 579*, 214–224.

Li, H.-L., Huang, Y., Zhang, C.-N., et al. (2006). Epigallocatechin-3 gallate inhibits cardiac hypertrophy through blocking reactive oxidative species-dependent and independent signal pathways. *Free Radical Biological Medicine, 40*, 1756–1775.

Lucock, M. (2004). Is folic acid the ultimate functional food component for disease prevention? *British medical journal, 328*, 211–214.

Manach, C., Williamson, G., Morand, C., et al. (2005). Bioavailability and bioefficacy of polyphenols in humans, I. Review of 97 bioavailability studies. *The American journal of clinical nutrition, 81*(Suppl), 230S–242S.

Mattivi, F., Zulian, C., Nicolini, G., & Valenti, L. (2002). Wine, biodiversity, technology, and antioxidants. *Annals of the New York Academy of Sciences, 957*, 37–56.

Mckinney, W. J., & Hammer Hill, H. (2000). Of sustainability and precaution: The logical, epistemological, and moral problems of the precautionary principle and their implications for sustainable development. *Ethics and the Environment, 5*(1), 77–87.

Mehta, R. G., & Mehta, R. R. (2002). Vitamin D and cancer. *The Journal of nutritional biochemistry, 13*, 252–264.

Meijers, J., Janssen, M. A. P., Van de Boekhorst-van der Schueren, M., et al. (2005). Prevalentie van Ondervoeding: de Landelijke Prevalentiemeting Zorgproblemen ['Prevalence of Under-nourishment: the National Prevalence Survey Care Problems']. *Nederlands Tijdschrift voor Diëtisten, 60*(1), 12–15.

Mill, J. S. (1859). *On Liberty*. Cited from http://www.utilitarianism.com/ol/five.html (accessed 17 February 2009).

Moshfeg, A., Goldman, J., & Cleveland, L. (2005). What we eat in America. NHANES 2001–2002: Usual Nutrient Intakes from Food Compared to Dietary Reference Intakes. USDA, Agricultural Research Service.

MRC Vitamin Study Group. (1991). Prevention of neural tube defects: Results of the medical research council vitamin study. *Lancet, 338*, 131–137.

Ocké, M. C., Buurma-Rethans, E. J. M., & Fransen, H. P. (2005). *Dietary supplement use in the Netherlands. Current data and recommendations for future assessment*. RIVM report 350100001/2005, Bilthoven, The Netherlands.

Philpott, M., Gould, K. S., Markham, K. R., et al. (2003). Enhanced coloration reveals high antioxidant potential in new sweet potato cultivars. *Journal of the science of food and agriculture, 83*, 1076–1082.

Renwick, A. G., Flynn, A., Fletcher, R. J., et al. (2004). Risk-benefit analysis of micronutrients. *Food Chemistry Toxicology, 42*, 1903–1922.

Rucker, R. B., Suttie, J. W., McCormick, D. B., & Machlin, L. J. (Eds.), (2001). *Handbook of vitamins*. New York, Basel: Marcel Dekker Inc.

Scalbert, A., Manach, C., Morand, C., et al. (2005). Dietary polyphenols and the prevention of diseases. *Critical Reviews in Food Science and Nutrition, 45*, 287–306.

Scalbert, A., & Williamson, G. (2000). Dietary intake and bioavailability of polyphenols. *Journal of Nutrition, 130*, 2073S–2085S.

Schwitters, B., Achanta, G., Van der Vlies, D., et al. (2007). The European regulation of food supplements and food fortification. Intended Normal Use—the ultimate tool in organising level playing field markets and regulations or how to break the fairy ring around 'other substances'. *Environmental law of Management, 19*, 19–29.

Shohaimi, S., Welch, A., Bingham, S., et al. (2004). Residential area deprivation predicts fruit and vegetable consumption independently of individual educational level and occupational social class: A cross-sectional population study in the Norfolk cohort of the European Prospective Investigation into Cancer (EPIC–Norfolk). *Journal of Epidemiology and community health, 58*, 686–691.

Snyder, L. J. (1998). Is evidence historical? In M. Curd & J. A. Cover (Eds.), *Philosophy of science. The central issues* (pp. 460–480). New York: W.W. Norton & Company.

Soleas, G. J., Grass, L., Josephy, P. D., et al. (2002). A comparison of the anticarcinogenic properties of four red wine polyphenols. *Clinical biochemistry, 35*, 119–124.

Starr, C. (1969). Social benefit versus technological risk. *Science, 165*, 1232–1238.

Stenmark, M. (2001). *Scientism. Science, ethics and religion*. Burlington: Ashgate Publishing Limited.

Sunstein, C. R. (2005). *Laws of Fear: Beyond the precautionary principle*. Cambridge, UK: Cambridge University Press.

Wheeler, D. S., & Wheeler, W. J. (2004). The medicinal chemistry of tea. *Drug development research, 61*, 45–65.

Wiener, J. B. (2001). *Precaution in a Multi-Risk World*. Duke Law School Public Law and Legal Theory Working Paper Series, Working Paper No. 23.

Willett, W. C. (1994). Diet and health: What should we eat? *Science, 264*, 532–537.

Williamson, G., & Manach, C. (2005). Bioavailability and bioefficacy of polyphenols in humans II. Review of 93 Intervention Studies. *The American journal of clinical nutrition, 81*(Suppl), 243S–2552S.

Nutraceuticals: Possible Future Ingredients and Food Safety Aspects

V. Prakash[1] and Martinus A. J. S. van Boekel[2]

[1]Central Food Technological Research Institute, Mysore, India

[2]Product Design and Quality Management Group, Wageningen University & Research Centre, Wageningen, The Netherlands

19.1 INTRODUCTION

The importance and role of basic nutrients in the growth, maintenance, and wellness of the body are well established. Food supplies energy, nutrients (fats, carbohydrates, proteins, vitamins, minerals) and non-nutrients (fiber, antioxidants, inducers of beneficial enzyme activities, prebiotics and probiotics); and the human body is well capable of utilizing all these molecules from the food. It is, however, a very complex process that is far from being understood completely. Recently, a newer array of molecules, such as antioxidants, carotenoids,

flavonoids, glucosinolates and the like (the above-mentioned non-nutrients), have been the focus of research. When such compounds are isolated from a food matrix they are called 'nutraceuticals', a term coined by DeFelice in 1979 and defined as 'food or parts of food that provide medical or health benefits, including the prevention and treatment of disease.'

The traditional foods of China, South East Asia, the Mediterranean and Europe are a treasure of information on nutrition and wellness and may perhaps play a major role for future markets. Often, the impact of such traditional foods has been confirmed by scientific nutritional research and with the aid of such information such foods have been improved by adjusting processing and preparation methods. There are various regions in the world where local ethnic knowledge is of potential interest, usually passed on from generation to generation over hundreds of years. In this way, data could be captured for documentation so that the benefits reach society as a whole.

One example is that of the loss of nutritional value of rice bran resulting from the rice polishing process. This rice bran contains good quality proteins, edible dietary fiber, triacontanol, rice bran oil, lecithin, oryzanol, fatty acids, vitamin E and sterols; it is important to consider each one of these components as a dietary supplement when we look at value addition. Therefore, food fortification by dietary supplements is nothing new when we see the broader perspective of ethnic and traditional foods which have used these concepts many times. The value of such traditional supplements, however, depends on how they are used and processed, to be certain of both the nutritional value and the safety of the products ultimately.

There are several forces that shape health effects and nutritional food formulations and their role in prevention of diseases and promoting well-being. Bioactive molecules reach the target organ through various ways. Predigestion in the mouth, biochemical effects in the digestive tract and in organs, indirect effects of prebiotics and probiotics, may modify such molecules. Whether or not molecules are present in a food matrix may have a considerable effect on the eventual biological effect. In this chapter, nutraceuticals are defined as bioactive compounds that are extracted from their original food matrix.

19.2 CHALLENGES FACING NUTRACEUTICALS

The question that needs to be discussed is whether nutraceuticals can indeed significantly contribute to health. According to the present authors this is not at all clear. What is definitely needed is a thorough risk–benefit analysis. It may seem at first sight that such isolated bioactive compounds are almost by definition 'healthy' but this is not always true. The prime example that corroborates this is the Finland study in which carotenoids were supplied to a group of people (smokers and non-smokers) based on the presumed antioxidant activity of these compounds in foods. However, the experiment had to be stopped prematurely because of the damage done by carotenoids to the smokers. The carotenoids were supposed to act as antioxidants but they did not function as such. This shows that bioactive compounds may act completely differently when they are taken out of their natural environment. While we cannot generalize—based upon this one example—it definitely indicates that synergistic effects that occur in the food matrix can be of great importance.

Nevertheless, new nutritional products may be very important, from a technological as well as a nutritional point of view and new nutraceutical products from agro-based raw materials may provide opportunities for value addition to the informal, organized and unorganized agrofood sector.

As the production of food and the realization of balanced nutrition in the urban world are changing and challenging tasks, food from rural to urban areas must benefit the farmer and grower as well as the local environment; especially for nutraceuticals, it must be clear what the purpose of the value addition is and who is actually benefitting. These days, there is a paradigm shift of production to processing and technology because of shifting consumer demand from quantity to quality. In addition, sustainable production and consumption involving the entire chain of nutritionals and dietary supplements has become of importance. It is also important that processing of plant material, especially to prevent loss of value added products in it, means increasing the availability of both nutritionals and nutraceuticals in the system. This is, or should be, part of a mega agenda of a greater reach out of nutrition and health foods and it is also important to ultimately link the basic nutrition and micronutrients from infant nutrition up to and including that of elderly people .

The diets of humans consist of many foods, and health effects should indeed be ascribed to diets and not to individual foods; it is the combination of all the components that end up in the digestive tract that will have an effect. With functional foods, a specific effect is targeted, such as calcium supplementation, vitamin supplementation, reduction of cholesterol levels, prebiotics, probiotics, but all within a food matrix. Nutraceuticals go one step beyond functional foods by taking out the bioactive compounds from a food matrix. The danger then becomes that an 'overdose' of bioactive molecules is ingested. With functional foods, this is less likely because of the very fact that the intake is limited to the food and there will be a limit of what people eat.

We can observe a paradigm shift from the 'Food Guide Pyramid' to today's 'Phytochemical complex ladder' of nutrients and bioactives such as those from garlic, cabbage, licorice, soybean, ginger, carrot, celery, onions, turmeric, whole wheat, flax seeds, brown rice, tomatoes, eggplants, peppers, broccoli, cauliflower, brussels sprouts, oats, mints, oregano, cucumber, rosemary, sage, potato, thyme, chives, cantaloupe, basil, curry leaves, cloves, coriander leaves, chilies, bay leaves, moringa leaves, garcinia fruit, tamarind fruit, pomegranate, asafetida, tarragon, and barley to name a few. These raw materials contain phytochemicals that have been fairly well related to possible preventive properties of diseases and could perhaps be ranked into different scales of importance based on their content of bioactive molecules on the one hand and bioavailability on the other.

Many questions arise in the area of nutraceuticals especially when looked at from a food safety angle and the claims that one makes for a product in the market. Some of these are: How should our policies approach health management? How dynamic should it be for regular updating? What are the significant challenges that must be overcome as we try to maximize health, based on a food approach? Aren't our current food safety policies based on science? Is it a fair enough level playing field for all the small and large-scale industries? How could the policy makers determine what is an appropriate level of risk? How well is industry responding to new incentives for food safety improvement and self regulation? Are we building enough centers of excellence so that we are continuously on the cutting edge technology to guarantee food safety? Are we able to deliver safe and healthy food in which the levels of any chemical contaminant are well below the toxicity level and where the concentration of potentially harmful microorganisms is so low as to present no significant risk to the consumer?

One of the global pandemics is the obesity problem and the quickening of change of, especially, the lifestyle and habits leading to circulatory related diseases, which is rapidly emerging as a cause of death in many developing countries. Therefore, when we look at such a situation as this pandemic, perhaps we should also look at the nutritional solutions for overall better health and wellness. In other words, the nutritional knowledge reaching society must also pay attention to the translation of nutrition as a solution to health problems by making it accessible to society and by identifying obstacles that prevent implementation of new scientific insights.

Often the basic primary processing of an herb, condiment, or spice from whichever source the nutraceutical molecule is coming from, decides the final activity of the compound that is liberated in the body. If it is possible to achieve value addition by extracting nutraceuticals from these products, and if these nutraceuticals are proven to be safe, both the grower and the micro-industries may become linked as one market.

In a wider sense for quality nutraceuticals, good agricultural practice, good harvesting practice, good transport practice, good manufacturing practice, and many of the accredited procedures for health and safety regulations must operate together and in coherence. Before offering these products to consumers, the positive effects must be clear and there must be no ill effects. The Codex specifications, as well as the local regulatory systems, need to be followed when validating to the customer and consumer in the ultimate market. All this requires very good chain coordination and governance, which is not always easy.

19.3 THE MOLECULE–GENE INTERACTION

When we talk of nutraceuticals, we have to keep in mind the 'molecule–gene interaction.' The relatively new scientific discipline of nutrigenomics plays a major role in clearly identifying the benefits that the nutraceuticals are supposed to bring about. Nutrigenomics may thus provide evidence-based effects of nutraceuticals. The way molecules interact at a cellular level among the individual genotype or phenotype, either with a single gene polymorphism or with a multi-gene polymorphic interaction, is going to be important information to design new foods and to study the impact of nutraceuticals. Several parameters need to be considered here, including the metabolic profile, structure of the molecule, function, pathway, metabolic pool, and phyto-genetic relations.

Ultimately, when we look at nutraceuticals, dietary supplements, and bioactive molecules, a holistic approach to food, medicine, health, wellness, exercise and age is perhaps more important than looking at any one of them in isolation. The disparity in the world with respect to expenditure on nutrition, let alone nutraceuticals and buying capacity, is huge! Firstly, it is vital that in the area of nutraceuticals, as we get better nutritional products with a pathway to work towards sustaining health, we need to ensure that the

claims are truthful and based on scientific evidence; and have verifiable documentation. Secondly, the level in which they are present in the foods must also reflect the level in which they are being substituted and/or fortified, otherwise a toxic level may be reached upon ingestion of a single component rather than micro-doses of multiple components that may otherwise have synergy. Thirdly, we cannot overlook the synergistic effect of one component with another. In that sense, the food-based approach is always an easier way than a component-based approach.

Lastly, it is important that we have a clear understanding of the chemistry of a molecule or a group of molecules, before we recommend it as part of a food after isolating and injecting it back in as an ingredient. Until we perfect this— maybe even after proving generation effects— some of the components will still baffle us and are bound to create a certain amount of disbelief with the consumer on whether it is safe or not. Therefore, scientists, food technologists, manufacturers, academia, institutions, policy makers, regulators, marketers and health care providers have a great responsibility in ensuring that the nutraceuticals that one recommends, either through an enriched form or through a food form, are not toxic to the individual and do not create more complex problems than when eating 'normal' food.

The subjects of immunity, disease prevention, weight management, heart and bone health, as well as mental health, are nowadays connected to ingestion of bioactive compounds and it is discussed whether or not they have remediating effects, both as dietary supplement and functional food. When we talk of functional foods, there are several terms that come to mind—such as foods for special dietary use, fortified or enriched food, medical foods, etc. This may contribute to the consumer's confusion, but from a scientific standpoint, it is supposed to work as a functional ingredient in the body to promote health and wellbeing. Today nutraceuticals, nutritional substitutes, and nutritional supplements have reached worldwide acceptance and demand; and consumers assume they are safe when they are marketed. Therefore, safety of these substances is a very important issue. These bioactives have to comply with basic claims, and we need to address the question as to whether the quality and safety of the phytochemicals used in conjunction with global food comply with the safety standards.

Whether it is allergies treated with seed extract, gut health and probiotics, the gall bladder and vitamin C, breast cancer and cranberry products, eye health and carotenoids, bone health and calcium and vitamin B, or even some bioactive peptides, it needs to be investigated by modern science whether or not the organs can benefit from being targeted by a food-based approach. This is where nanotechnology's impact on food, nutrition and health may make a difference. The question is: can nanotechnology change the total industrial scenario of bioactives or nutritionals, for instance, by using spice extracts, which are highly valued, in nanoparticles? Are the R&D institutions or industries ready for such a transformation? The power of nanotechnology may be to enhance some of the physical properties —such as solubility and controlled release— to improve bioavailability and stability of the micronutrients; even to stabilize them during processing, storage and distribution is already a challenge. Ultimately, with targeted delivery, food manufacturers could in principle realize smart food systems capable of ensuring optimal health through nanotechnology with a clear innovation.

Tomorrow's demand for nutritionals, dietary supplements and nutraceuticals will be one of a personalized diet, which is already emerging based on individual genetic codes. Such a diet can lessen the risk of some diseases that an individual may be susceptible to. Studies that focus on the health benefits of ingredients may ultimately pave the way for identification and understanding of individuals, population differences, and similarities in gene expression in response to the diet that can lead to newer food products customized for an individual's nutrition needs.

It is of utmost importance that analytical methods to detect and quantify nutraceuticals become very reliable when we define their safe and accepted levels. Currently, new methods are emerging, especially those on how to avoid interfering materials, and the analytical procedures are becoming more stringent for the claims that are attributed.

19.4 CONCLUSION

In a global context of health, in most countries governments lay down policies and guidelines. Research and development institutions and academia conduct a large amount of research along with industrial R&D houses. These generate technologies, training, and also quality standards that come together in a production system involving small industries on the cottage and village level, as well as medium and large local ones, and finally large industries on the global level. They will all try to reach the market, interfacing with governments in many welfare and food safety measures.

It is this responsibility that is complex and the consumer must be involved whether or not this huge area of nutraceuticals should expand. However, it does have enormous potential provided science supports the claims with a mandate of quality. Such an approach requires a thorough risk–benefit analysis that may be different from that used for foods today; since we talk about very bioactive compounds, the presently available methodologies may not be sufficient. It should ensure adequate scientific evidence for the benefits and claims that are going to be made. A global harmonization approach needs to be developed to make a sustainable solution possible for the beneficial use of nutraceuticals in society.

Further Reading[*]

Biesalski, H. K. (2002). Nutraceuticals: the link between nutrition and medicine. *Cutaneous and Ocular Toxicology*, *21*, 9–30.

Chen, H., Weiss, J., & Shahidi, F. (2006). Nanotechnology in nutraceuticals and functional foods. *Food Technology*, *60*(3), 30–36.

DeFelice, S. L. (1992). Nutraceuticals: Opportunities in an emerging market, Scrip Mag 9.

Dillard, C., & German, J. B. (2000). Review—Phytochemicals: Nutraceuticals and human health. *Journal of the Science of Food and Agriculture*, *80*, 1744–1756.

Dureja, H., Kaushik, D., & Kumar, V. (2003). Developments in nutraceuticals. *Indian Journal of Pharmacology*, *35*, 363–372.

Espin, C. J., Garcia-Conesa, M. T., & Tomas-Barberan, F. A. (2007). Review. Nutraceuticals: Facts and fiction. *Phytochemistry*, *68*, 2986–3008.

Fahey, J. W., & Kensler, T. W. (2007). Role of dietary supplements/nutraceuticals in chemoprevention through induction of cytoprotective enzymes. *Chemical Research in Toxicology*, *20*, 572–576.

FAO. (2004). Report of the Regional Expert Consultation of the Asia–Pacific Network for Food and Nutrition on functional foods and their implications in the daily diet.

Kottke, M. K. (1998). Scientific and regulatory aspects of nutraceutical products in the United States. *Drug Development and Industrial Pharmacy*, *24*, 1177–1195.

Kratz, A. M., & Pharm, D. (1998). Nutraceuticals: New opportunities for pharmacists. *JANA*, *68*, 27–28.

Ohr, L. M. (2005). Nutraceuticals and functional foods. *Food Technology*, *59*(4), 84–100.

Omenn, G. S., Goodman, G. E., Thornquist, M. D., et al. (1996). Risk factors for lung cancer and for intervention effects in CARET, the Beta-Carotene and Retinol Efficacy Trial. *Journal of the National Cancer Institute*, *88*, 1550–1559.

Satia, J. A., Littman, A., Slatore, C. G., et al. (2009). Long-term use of β-carotene, retinol, lycopene, and lutein supplements and lung cancer risk: Results from the VITamins And Lifestyle (VITAL) study. *American Journal of Epidemiology*, *169*(7), 815–828.

The Alpha-Tocopherol, Beta-Carotene Cancer Prevention Study Group. (1994). The effect of vitamin E and beta carotene on the incidence of lung cancer and other cancers in male smokers. *The New England Journal of Medicine*, *330*, 1029–1035.

[*]The source of information for this chapter stems from the information in this list and also the authors' experience in the field of research and development spanning over 35 years in the area of food science and food technology underpinning food safety. The information is also the distilled knowledge of several talks that the authors have delivered in many national and international conferences focusing on Nutraceuticals and Phytochemicals.

Harmonization of International Standards

John G. Surak

Surak and Associates, Clemson, SC, USA

OUTLINE

20.1 INTRODUCTION

Harmonization of international standards is critical if countries and food processors want to benefit from globalization. Globalization and liberalized trade bring growth and prosperity to both the exporting and importing countries. The process creates new markets for both nations, thus, increasing the demand for high-value goods and services. In developing countries, one of the first uses of an increase in discretionary spending is the purchase of high value-added food products. Many of these products are imported. As one walks through grocery stores in developing nations, products labeled as 'Made in the USA' convey high quality and high value. In addition, liberalized trade provides benefits for the citizens of industrialized nations. For example, international trade allows us to eat fresh fruits and vegetables nearly 12 months in the year, rather than waiting for the product to be sold in-season.

International food trade is not without its critics. There are political issues such as dealing with subsidies to farmers who cannot profitably produce food at international prices. Another is trying to maintain the resource capability of being able to completely feed its citizens.[1] As a result, nations may take actions to limit the amount of trade. In addition to subsidizing food production, the country may enact other barriers to trade such as tariffs, import quotas, or barriers that are disguised as food safety regulations.

In mature free market economies, food safety issues are being separated from quality issues. Food safety issues are regulated by the government to protect the consumers. However, quality issues can be regulated by market forces.

From the food processors' perspective, shipping to global markets is not easy. International markets increase the length of the supply chain, which brings additional complexity. These new challenges must be met while accomplishing the following opportunities for repeat sales:

- The product meets or exceeds the regulatory food safety requirements of the importing country;
- The product meets or exceeds the needs of the customer.

Understanding government regulations is not simple. The regulations between the exporting and importing countries may not be equivalent. This can add needless cost to the company trying to develop products for export markets, since new systems must be developed that do not add any level of food safety to the product. This highlights the need to harmonize standards and regulations at the international level.

The harmonization of standards and regulations presents a number of benefits for international trade. All food processing companies can understand the basic rules that must be followed. This allows the companies to invest into the food safety systems that will be accepted internationally. Knowing the basic requirements allows the food processor to enter into negotiations, and determine what requirements may be added to meet the specific needs of the customer.

A number of organizations have focused technical efforts on harmonizing both regulatory and customer requirements. These organizations include the World Trade Organization (WTO), the Codex Alimentarius Commission (Codex), the International Organization for Standardization (ISO), and the Global Food Safety Initiative (GFSI). Two of these organizations develop international standards using a consensus process. Codex develops standards that can be used by nations to harmonize their

---

[1]This chapter is not intended to go into the political reasons for trade barriers, or the economic benefits from trade liberalization. Table 20.1 presents some of the benefits and cost of international trade. For further information, the author suggests that the reader explore the WTO website (www.wto.org), and consider viewing some of their webcasts.

food regulations, and ISO develops standards that meet marketplace needs.

20.2 WORLD TRADE ORGANIZATION

The WTO is a government-to-government organization headquartered in Geneva, Switzerland and is composed of 153 member nations. The WTO was formed on 1 January 1995 as an outcome of the Uruguay Round of multi-lateral trade talks.[2]

The WTO is the only global organization that deals with the trading rules between nations. The Organization gives the same rights to both small and large countries.[3] Thus, if trade disputes occur between member nations, these can be brought before the WTO (WTO, 2009a).

The WTO accomplishes its work by negotiating trading rules between nations. The agreements that are developed must be ratified by congresses or parliaments of the member nations. The ultimate goal of the WTO is to help producers, exporters, and importers of goods and services and other forms of intellectual property conduct their business; its overarching objective being to help trade to flow as freely as possible, as long as there are no undesirable side effects. By having a set of trading rules, trade becomes predictable (Table 20.1).

If there is a trade dispute between member nations, the WTO provides a forum where member nations can work out trade problems and settle trade disputes. The objective is to first negotiate a resolution to the dispute. If a resolution cannot be achieved, the dispute can ultimately lead to trade sanctions, which are allowed by the WTO. These trade sanctions cannot be punitive. They must not exceed the loss that was presented in the formal dispute document.

The WTO's objective is to develop liberalized trade. Liberalized trade is not free trade. There are areas where the WTO supports trade barriers. These include the need to protect consumers, or prevent the spread of disease between humans, animals, or plants (SPS measures) and to allow certain technical barriers to trade (TBT measures), such as labeling requirements.

20.2.1 SPS Measures

The WTO permits countries to develop food safety regulations known as the sanitary and phytosanitary or SPS measures. The SPS measures are composed of two parts:

- Sanitary (human and animal health);
- Phytosanitary (plant health) measures.

The SPS measures must be applied to domestically produced food or local animal and plant diseases, as well as to products coming from other countries.

---

[2]Prior to the formation of the WTO, the General Agreement on Tariffs and Trade (GATT) managed the rules that governed world trade. The GATT was developed as a provisional organization with a limited scope of action (manufactured goods). It had positive results in starting the process to liberalize trade. However, there were also numerous problems such as loopholes in the trade of agricultural products, and an increase in trade of services and intellectual property; the latter were not covered by GATT.

[3]One of the major benefits that small nations, and nations that are classified either as developing economies or emerging economies have in belonging to the WTO, is that they have the same power as the industrialized nations when it comes to defending their position with regard to trade disputes. In addition, the WTO provides for a structure and system for a relatively rapid resolution to trade disputes. If a country does not comply with a ruling, it can be subjected to trade sanctions.

TABLE 20.1   Is trade fair to everyone?

Trade is not fair to all of the citizens. In general, the countries' economies benefit with an increase in international trade. One measure that can be used to measure the success of international trade is an increase in the gross domestic product (GDP).

There are two sides to international trade. On any specific trade issue there will be companies that prosper because of international trade. This is accomplished by taking advantage of the expanded market potential and producing products that meet the customer needs of the new market. On the other side, there will be those companies that will not prosper and can lose market share in their domestic markets because of foreign imports. Unfortunately, this leads to layoffs of employees and increased unemployment.

From a macro economic perspective, this should force businesses that are not doing well to look at new ways to reallocate resources so they can be competitive in both the domestic and international markets.

'For the purposes of the SPS Agreement, sanitary and phytosanitary measures are defined as any measures applied:

- 'to protect human or animal life from risks arising from additives, contaminants, toxins or disease-causing organisms in their food,
- 'to protect human life from plant- or animal-carried diseases,
- 'to protect animal or plant life from pests, diseases, or disease-causing organisms,
- 'to prevent or limit other damage to a country from the entry, establishment or spread of pests' (WTO, 2009b).

The SPS agreement allows countries to set their own health standards. The WTO agreement states that the regulations must be science-based and encourages the use of a risk-based approach. The SPS agreement encourages governments to harmonize or develop their national regulations using international standards, guidelines and recommendations. WTO specifically recognizes the FAO/WHO Codex Alimentarius Commission for food safety; the World Organization for Animal Health (OIE) for animal health; and the International Plant Protection Convention (IPPC) for plant health.[4]

In addition, WTO states that the national regulations should apply to the extent necessary to protect human, animal or plant life and health. They should not arbitrarily discriminate between countries. When national regulations are based on international standards, this automatically provides a measure of due diligence in arbitrating a WTO trade dispute.

The WTO permits the establishment of more stringent regulations than existing international standards, if there is scientific justification. However, when this is done and it leads to a trade dispute, the WTO will determine if the SPS issue is being used as a means to protect domestic suppliers.

20.2.2 TBT Measures

TBT measures cover all technical regulations and voluntary standards that are not sanitary or phytosanitary measures. Thus, they cover a wide variety of issues. WTO states 'labeling requirements, nutrition claims and concerns, quality and packaging regulations are generally not considered to be sanitary or phytosanitary measures and hence are normally subject to the TBT Agreement' (WTO, 2009c).

[4]International standards are encouraged because they are developed by international experts using the consensus process. In addition, the standard development process incorporates international scrutiny and review.

TABLE 20.2 Codex standards by subject matter as of July 2008

Type of standard	Number of standards
Commodity standards	186
Commodity related texts	46
Food labeling	9
Food hygiene	5
Food safety risk assessment	3
Sampling and analysis	15
Inspection and certification procedures	8
Animal food production	6
Contaminants in foods (maximum levels, detection and prevention)	12
Food additive provisions that cover 292 additives	1112
Food additives related texts	7
Maximum limits for pesticide residues covering 218 pesticides	2930
Maximum limits for veterinary drugs in food covering 49 veterinary drugs	441
Regional guidelines	3

Source: Codex, 2006.

Under the TBT agreement, member nations may decide that international standards are not appropriate for reasons including fundamental technological problems or geographical factors.

Labeling of food products can be both an SPS and a TBT issue. If the labeling requirements deal with food safety issues, the specific requirements fall under the SPS agreement. All other labeling requirements fall under the TBT agreement.

20.3 THE CODEX ALIMENTARIUS COMMISSION AND OTHER UNITED NATIONS AGENCIES

20.3.1 The Codex Alimentarius Commission

The Codex Alimentarius Commission (Codex) is an international organization under two United Nations agencies, the Food and Agriculture Organization (FAO) and the World Health Organization (WHO). Codex was established in 1963 and is headquartered in Rome, Italy. There are currently 180 member nations. Codex contact point in the member nations is their national or federal agency that regulates food safety. In the United States, the Codex office is located within the USDA Food Safety Inspection Service (Codex, 2006).

Codex develops standards that protect the health of consumers and ensures fair practices in food trade. One of its goals is to harmonize national regulations to reduce barriers to trade and increase the free movement of food products among countries. As a result, developing and emerging economies can use the Codex standards to develop regulations and deal with issues of trade facilitation.

Since 1963, the organization has published over 4700 standards, guidelines or codes of practice covering a wide variety of food safety issues (Table 20.2). These standards are developed using an eight-step process. Prior to publication, consensus must be reached by the member nations.

The following principles are used for developing its standards, guidelines or codes:

- **Excellence**: Codex uses internationally recognized expertise. The work of the Commission is connected to a forum for global scientific discussion.
- **Independence**: Experts contribute in their own capacity and not on behalf of a government or institution. In addition, Codex requires that all experts declare possible conflicts of interest.
- **Transparency**: All stakeholders have access to all the necessary reports, safety assessments, and evaluations during the development process.
- **Universality**: Codex uses a broad base of scientific data in setting standards. All interested parties throughout the world are invited to make data available (FAO, 2009a).

Codex achieves it mission by collaborating with a number of other organizations including: the Joint FAO/WHO Expert Committee on Food Additives (JECFA), the Joint FAO/WHO Expert Meetings on Microbiological Risk Assessment (JEMRA), the Joint FAO/WHO Meetings on Pesticide Residues (JMPR), and the World Organisation for Animal Health (OIE) (Codex, 2009).

Two Codex standards have direct effect on any food processor. These standards are: The *Food Hygiene—Basic Texts*, and the *Guideline for the Validation of Food Safety Control Measures* (CAC/GL 69-2008) (Codex, 2006).

The food hygiene basic texts consist of four parts:

- *Recommended International Code of Practice— General Principles of Food Hygiene* (CAC/RCP 1-1969, revision 2003);

- Hazard Analysis and Critical Control Point (HACCP) System and Guidelines for its Application (which is an annex to the *General Principles of Food Hygiene*);
- *Principles for the Establishment and Application of Microbiological Criteria for Foods* (CAC/GL 21-1997);
- *Principles and Guidelines for the Conduct of Microbiological Risk Assessment* (CAC/GL 30-1999).

The food hygiene principles provide internationally accepted good manufacturing practices (Table 20.3). This provides the basic foundation for the implementation of HACCP. In addition the document provides the international definition for HACCP. This consists of the 5 preliminary steps and 7 principles of HACCP. Sometimes this will be referred to as the 12 steps of Codex HACCP (Table 20.4). At the time of writing, the implementation of HACCP may or may not be an SPS requirement by an importing nation. For example, in the European Union, HACCP is required by law for any food processor. However at the time of writing, in the United States, HACCP is required by law for meat and poultry processors, seafood processors, and the juice industry. The US low-acid canned foods and acidified foods regulations are also HACCP-based. Many customers of the food processing industry require that their suppliers implement and maintain effective HACCP plans as part of the contractual requirements.

The Codex standard on the validation of food safety control measures is a significant change in the practice of HACCP (Codex, 2008).

This standard makes a distinction between validation and verification activities.[5] In addition, the standard presents guidance on the following issues:

- Concept of validation;
- Nature of validation;

[5]Many times there is confusion between the concepts of validation, verification and monitoring. Validation: Collection of information that the HACCP plan is capable of being effective. This is an assessment conducted prior to starting operations; Verification: Confirmation that specific requirements of the HACCP plan have been fulfilled. This is an assessment that can be made during or after operations; Monitoring: Collection of planned sequence of observations or measurements to assess whether control measures are operating as intended. This is an activity taken during operations.

TABLE 20.3   The major elements of the Codex general principles of food hygiene

Primary production	Pest control systems
Environmental hygiene	Waste management
Hygienic production of food sources	Monitoring effectiveness
Handling, storage and transport	Establishment: Personal hygiene
Cleaning, maintenance and personal hygiene at primary production	Health status
	Illness and injuries
Establishment: Design and facilities	Personal cleanliness
Location	Personal behavior
Premises and rooms	Visitors
Equipment	Transportation
Facilities	General
Control of operations	Requirements
Control of food hazards	Use and maintenance
Key aspects of hygiene control systems	Product information and consumer awareness
Incoming material requirements	Lot identification
Packaging	Product information
Water	Labeling
Management and supervision	Consumer education
Documentation and records	Training
Recall procedures	Awareness and responsibilities
Establishment: Maintenance and sanitation	Training programs
Maintenance and cleaning	Instruction and supervision
Cleaning programs	Refresher training

Source: Codex, 2003.

- Tasks to be completed prior to a validation study;
- Validation process;
- Need for re-validation.

The standard recognizes the following approaches to validation:

- 'Reference to scientific or technical literature, previous validation studies or historical knowledge of performance of control measures;
- Scientifically valid experimental data that demonstrate the adequacy of control measures;
- Collection of data during operating conditions in the whole food operation;
- Mathematical modeling;
- Surveys' (Codex, 2008).

The necessity of validating control measures is a major requirement in a number of the food safety management standards, such as ISO 22000.

20.3.2 Joint FAO/WHO Expert Committee on Food Additives

The Joint FAO/WHO Expert Committee on Food Additives (JECFA) was established in 1956 and is headquartered in Rome, Italy. The

TABLE 20.4   HACCP principles as defined by Codex

Traditional numbering	Alternative Codex numbering	HACCP principle
Preliminary step 1	Step 1	Assemble HACCP team
Preliminary step 2	Step 2	Describe product
Preliminary step 3	Step 3	Identify intended use
Preliminary step 4	Step 4	Construct flow diagram
Preliminary step 5	Step 5	On-site confirmation of flow diagram
Principle 1	Step 6	Conduct a hazard analysis
Principle 2	Step 7	Determine the Critical Control Points (CCPs)
Principle 3	Step 8	Establish critical limit(s)
Principle 4	Step 9	Establish a system to monitor the CCP
Principle 5	Step 10	Establish the corrective action to be taken when monitoring indicates that a particular CCP is not under control
Principle 6	Step 11	Establish procedures tor verification to confirm that the HACCP system is working effectively
Principle 7	Step 12	Establish documentation concerning all procedures and records appropriate to these principles and their application

Source: Codex, 2003.

committee performs risk assessments and provides advice to the FAO, WHO and member countries. In addition, the committee provides independent scientific advice to Codex. This advice is used in the development of standards and guidelines (FAO, 2006). Since its inception, JECFA has evaluated over 1500 food additives, over 40 contaminants and naturally occurring toxins, and over 90 residues of veterinary drugs.

20.3.3 Joint FAO/WHO Expert Meetings on Microbiological Risk Assessment

The Joint FAO/WHO Expert Meetings on Microbiological Risk Assessment (JEMRA) was founded in 2000 and is headquartered in Rome, Italy. It undertakes activities in the following areas (FAO, 2009b):

- Generates risk assessments;
- Develops guidelines on the different steps of risk assessment;
- Collects and generates data for risk assessment;
- Uses the risk assessment process within the framework of risk management;
- Provides information and technology transfer on risk assessment.

The committee provides advice on microbiological aspects of food safety, and risk assessment. It develops guidelines in related areas such as data collection and the application of risk assessment to Codex and other UN health-related agencies.

20.3.4 Joint FAO/WHO Meetings on Pesticide Residues

The Joint FAO/WHO Meetings on Pesticide Residues (JMPR) was founded in 1963 and provides independent scientific expert advice to Codex on pesticide residues (FAO, 2009c). This advice serves as the input for the establishment of the Maximum Residue Levels (MRLs) for pesticides and other environmental contaminants in food. In addition, the committee also recommends methods for sampling and analysis of pesticides and other environmental contaminants.

20.4 WORLD ORGANISATION FOR ANIMAL HEALTH

The World Organisation for Animal Health was founded in 1924 as the Office International des Epizooties (OIE) (OIE, 2009). In 2003, the OIE was renamed the World Organisation for Animal Health; however, it retains the historical acronym. The OIE is headquartered in Paris, France and has 167 member nations.

The OIE collects, analyzes and disseminates veterinary scientific information on animal disease control. In addition, the organization provides assistance to developing, and least developed nations on animal disease control and eradication operations. The OIE rules are recognized by the WTO as international sanitary rules regarding animal health.

20.5 INTERNATIONAL ORGANIZATION FOR STANDARDIZATION

The International Organization for Standardization (ISO) was formed in 1947 to develop product and process standards in all areas except electrotechnical and telecommunication standards.[6] ISO has developed over 17,500 standards and guides (ISO, 2009a).

ISO has over 150 member nations. The point of contact for ISO is a country's national standards organization. For the United States, this is the American National Standards Institute or ANSI. The standards are voluntary standards, and are developed because of marketplace needs. Therefore, they describe state of the art requirements for products and processes.

The ISO standards are developed using a transparent consensus process at the international level with strong support at the national level. The international team tends to be small since each nation can send a maximum of three international experts. In addition, at the international level, the experts do not represent the national position but are to serve as international experts. Any comment or suggestion on the specific standard that is received from the national level must be addressed. If the comment or suggestion is not adopted, either the national or international committee must provide justification of why the comment was not adopted. These meeting notes are then available to anyone who makes a request to see them.

At the national level there is a mirror group of national experts. This mirror group develops a national response of comments and suggestions to aid in the development of the standard. These comments are then submitted to the international committee for action.

A standard must be developed within a 5-year timeframe once ISO approves its development. If this is not done, ISO can stop the standard development process. Once a standard is developed, the standard will first be reviewed 3 years after publication and then at 5-year intervals. During the review process, the committee determines whether the standard is retained,

---

[6]Electrotechnical standards are developed by the International Electrotechnical Commission (IEC). And telecommunication standards are developed by the International Telecommunication Union (ITU).

TABLE 20.5   The ISO 22000 family of standards

ISO 15161:2001	Guidelines on the application of ISO 9001:2000 for the food and drink industry
ISO 22000:2005	Food safety management systems—Requirements for any organization in the food chain
ISO/TS 22003:2007	Food safety management systems—Requirements for bodies providing audit and certification of food safety management systems
ISO/TS 22004:2005	Food safety management systems—Guidance on the application of ISO 22000:2005
ISO/DIS 22006	Quality management systems—Guidelines for the application of ISO 9001:2000 in crop production
ISO 22005:2007	Traceability in the feed and food chain—General principles and basic requirements for system design and implementation
ISO/CD 22008	Food irradiation—Requirements for the development, validation and routine control of the ionizing radiation process used for the treatment of food for human consumption

Source: ISO, 2009d.

revised or withdrawn. This review process is critical to ensure that the standard is timely and does not create a barrier to trade (ISO, 2009b).

ISO has no legal authority to enforce its standards. Conformance to the standards is handled by the private sector. ISO develops conformity assessment standards and guides through CASCO (Committee on Conformity Assessment), an ISO policy development committee.

Conformity assessment is a process that determines if products or processes meet the requirements of standards, specifications or regulations. It can be accomplished by one of three different types of audits or assessments:

- **First party**—or the company ensuring that their products meet customer requirements or their processes conform to stated procedures.
- **Second party**—or the customer ensuring that their supplier's products or processes conform to the stated requirements.
- **Third party**—or an independent third party ensuring that a company's products and/or processes conform to stated requirements. Many times third party audits are performed for a customer.

CASCO defines the requirements to ensure effective assessments (ISO, 2009c).

ISO is organized into technical committees (TCs). These individual technical committees are responsible for the development of the standards. TC 34 is responsible for developing food products standards. This committee has developed over 730 standards on products or analytical techniques. In addition, the committee has an additional 120 standards under development. This Committee is responsible for the ISO 22000 series of standards (Table 20.5). The hallmark of these standards is ISO 22000 and 22003. ISO 22000 describes requirements of a food safety management system which is based on three parts (Table 20.6).

- HACCP as defined by Codex HACCP;
- Prerequisite programs that are based on Codex good hygiene practices;
- Other management system components to ensure that food safety management systems operate effectively and efficiently.

ISO 22003 is a standard that provides the requirements for accreditation bodies, certification bodies, and auditors to effectively audit a

TABLE 20.6   The major elements of ISO 22000:2005—Food safety management systems—Requirements for any organization in the food chain

Food safety management system	Planning and realization of safe products
Documentation	General
General requirements	Prerequisite programs
Documentation requirements	Preliminary steps to hazard analysis
Management responsibility	Hazard analysis
Management commitment	Establishing operational prerequisite programs
Food safety policy	Establishing the HACCP plan
Food safety management system planning	Updating of preliminary information and documents specifying PRPs and the HACCP plan
Responsibility and authority	
Food safety team leader	Verification planning
Communication	Traceability system
Emergency preparedness and response	Control of nonconformity
Management review	Validation verification and improvement of the food safety management system
Resource management	
Provision of resources	General
Human resources	Validation of control measure combinations
Infrastructure	Control of monitoring and measuring
Work environment	Food safety management system verification
	Improvement

Source: ISO, 2005a.

food safety management system. This standard addresses issues such as auditor competencies in areas such as food safety, knowledge of the specific processing systems being audited and auditing techniques.

20.6 PAS 220

PAS stands for a Publicly Available Specification. This is a document based on the British Standard model and is used to standardize best practices on a specific subject for the benefit of an industry (BSI, 2009).

PAS 220:2008 (BSI, 2008) (Table 20.7) is a standard that is to be used with ISO 22000 certifications of food safety management programs. The standard is intended to be used by food processors, and provides detail for element 7.2 (Prerequisite programs).

20.7 GLOBAL FOOD SAFETY INITIATIVE

In 2000, CIES—The Food Business Forum—launched the Global Food Safety Initiative (GFSI). Initially, membership was limited to European food retailers. However, over the years, membership has been extended to other associations, service providers to retailers, food manufacturing suppliers and cooperatives (GFSI, 2009).

The GFSI original objective was to have a common set of requirements for the European food safety schemes. This has expanded to 'Continuous improvement in food safety management systems to ensure confidence in the delivery of safe food to consumers' (GFSI, 2009). In response to these objectives, the organization developed a series of guidelines to benchmark certification schemes for food safety management

TABLE 20.7   Major elements of PAS 220:2008

The standard addresses the following prerequisite programs

    Construction and layout of buildings

    Layout of premises and workspace

    Utilities—air water energy

    Waste disposal

    Equipment suitability, cleaning and maintenance

    Management of purchased materials

    Measures for prevention of cross-contamination

    Cleaning and sanitizing

    Pest control

    Personal hygiene and employee facilities

    Product recall procedures

    Rework

    Warehousing

    Product information and consumer awareness

    Food defense

Source: BSI, 2008.

system standards. The certification scheme consists of the following components:

• The food safety management system standard which consists of HACCP based on Codex HACCP, good practices,[7] and management system components;
• A clearly defined scope;
• A certification system that consists of requirements for auditors, a statement of the approximate duration and frequency of the audits, and the minimum content of the audit report.

At the time of writing, five standards developed by private organizations have met all of the benchmarking requirements. These standards are British Retail Consortium (BRC) Global Standard for Food Safety, version 5; Foundation for Food Safety Certification, FSSC 22000; International Food Standard (IFS)—Standard for Auditing Retailer and Wholesaler Branded Food Products,

version 5; Dutch HACCP (option B); Safe Quality Foods 2000 version 5.

In February 2008, the Foundation for Food Safety Certification, presented an audit scheme to the GFSI for benchmarking. The scheme uses as a basis the following standards: ISO 22000, PAS 220 and ISO 22003. The certification scheme is designed to meet all of the GFSI benchmarking requirements for food safety management systems (Groenveld, 2009). In May 2009, GFSI announced that the FSSC 22000 met its benchmarking requirements.

20.8 CONCLUSION

Harmonization of standards, specifications and regulations is critical to international trade. Harmonization allows companies to understand the minimum regulatory and customer requirements of international markets. This in turn allows companies to produce goods for those markets.

There are a number of public, private and government-to-government organizations that are involved in harmonization of standards. The primary objective of these efforts is to reduce the barriers to trade thus increasing a freer movement of food products among countries. These efforts bring financial benefits to the companies that take advantage of new markets, and to the countries that reap the benefit of an increase in their gross domestic product.

20.9 INTERNATIONAL TRADE RELATED WEBSITES

Codex Alimentarius Commission (Codex): www.codexalimentarius.net

The Joint FAO/WHO Committee on Food Additives (JEFCA): http://www.fao.org/ag/agn/agns/jecfa_index_en.asp

---

[7]Good practices include: Good Manufacturing Practices, Good Agricultural Practices, Good Distribution Practices.

The Joint FAO/WHO Expert Meetings on Microbiological Risk assessment (JEMRA): http://www.fao.org/ag/agn/agns/jemra_index_en.asp

The Joint FAO/WHO Meetings on Pesticide Residues (JMPR): http://www.fao.org/agriculture/crops/core-themes/theme/pests/pm/en/

Global Food Safety Initiative (GFSI): http://www.ciesnet.com/2-wwedo/2.2-programmes/2.2.foodsafety.gfsi.asp

International Organization for Standardization (ISO): www.iso.org

World Organisation for Animal Health (OIE): www.oie.int

World Trade Organization (WTO): www.wto.org

References

BSI. (2008). *PAS 220:2008, Prerequisite programmes on food safety food manufacturing*. London UK: British Standards Institution.

BSI. (2009). *What is a PAS (Publicly Available Specification)?* London, UK: British Standards Institution www.bsi-global.com (accessed 12 March 2009).

Codex. (2003). Recommended international code of practice, General principles of food hygiene. CAC/RCP 1-1969, Revision 4 Rome, Italy: Codex Alimentarius Commission. http://www.codexalimentarius.net/web/publications.jsp?lang=en (accessed 13 March 2009).

Codex. (2006). *Understanding the Codex Alimentarius* (Third edition). Rome, Italy: Codex Alimentarius Commission.

Codex. (2008). Guideline for the validation of food safety control measures. CAC/GL 69 2008.

Codex. (2009). *Codex Alimentarius*. Rome, Italy: Codex Alimentarius Commission http://www.codexalimentarius.net/web/index_en.jsp (accessed 12 March 2009).

FAO. (2006). *What is JEFCA, WHO*. Rome, Italy: Food and Agricultural Organization.

FAO. (2009a). *Codex and science*. Rome, Italy: Food and Agriculture Organization http://www.fao.org/docrep/008/y7867e/y7867e06.htm (accessed 12 March 2009).

FAO. (2009b). *Food safety and quality FAO*. Rome, Italy: Food and Agriculture Organization http://www.fao.org/ag/agn/agns/jemra_index_en.asp (accessed 12 March 2009).

FAO. (2009c). *APG-Pesticide management*. Rome, Italy: Food and Agriculture Organization http://www.fao.org/agriculture/crops/core-themes/theme/pests/pm/en/ (accessed 12 March 2009).

GFSI. (2009). Global Food Safety Initiative, Paris, France, http://www.ciesnet.com/2-wwedo/2.2-programmes/2.2.foodsafety.gfsi.asp (accessed 12 March 2009).

Groenveld, C. (2009). FSSC 22000—Food safety system certification scheme—ISO 22000, and PAS 220. CIES Food Safety Conference, Barcelona, Spain. http://www.ciesfoodsafety.com/.

ISO. (2009a). *Discover ISO*, Geneva, Switzerland: International Organization for Standardization. http://www.iso.org/iso/about/discover-iso_the-scope-of-isos-work.htm (accessed 12 March 2009).

ISO. (2009b). *Stages of the development of International Standards*. Geneva, Switzerland: International Organization for Standardization http://www.iso.org/iso/standards_development/processes_and_procedures/stages_description.htm (accessed 12 March 2009).

ISO. (2009c). *What is conformity assessment?* Geneva, Switzerland: International Organization for Standardization http://www.iso.org/iso/resources/conformity_assessment/what_is_conformity_assessment.htm (accessed 12 March 2009).

ISO. (2009d). *TC 34 – Food products*. Geneva, Switzerland: International Organization for Standardization http://www.iso.org/iso/standards_development/technical_committees/list_of_iso_technical_committees/iso_technical_committee.htm?commid=47858 (accessed 12 March 2009).

OIE. (2009). *About us OIE*. Paris, France: World Organisation for Animal Health http://www.oie.int/eng/OIE/en_about.htm?e1d1 (accessed 12 March 2009).

WTO. (2009a). *Understanding the WTO: The agreements. Agriculture: Fairer markets for farmers*. Geneva, Switzerland: World Trade Organization http://www.wto.org/english/thewto_e/whatis_e/tif_e/agrm3_e.htm (accessed 12 March 2009).

WTO. (2009b). *Understanding the WTO Agreement on Sanitary and Phytosanitary Measures*. Geneva, Switzerland: World Trade Organization http://www.wto.org/english/tratop_e/sps_e/spsund_e.htm (accessed 12 March 2009).

WTO. (2009c). *Understanding the WTO Agreement on Technical Barriers to Trade*. Geneva, Switzerland: World Trade Organization http://www.wto.org/english/tratop_e/sps_e/spsund_e.htm (accessed 12 March 2009).

21

The First Legislation for Foods with Health Claims in Korea

Ji Yeon Kim[1], Oran Kwon[2] and Sangsuk Oh[3]

[1]Division of Nutrition and Functional Food, Bureau of Nutrition and Functional Food, Korea Food and Drug Administration, Seoul, Korea

[2]Department of Nutritional Science and Food Management, Ewha Womans University, Seoul, Korea

[3]Department of Food Science and Technology, Ewha Womans University, Seoul, Korea

21.1 INTRODUCTION

The aging population is growing exponentially throughout the world and facing financial difficulties in medical care costs due to the increase in chronic diseases, such as diabetes, cardiovascular disease, and cancer. These trends have compelled scientists to identify physiologically active components in foods. This increasing knowledge supporting the vital role of foods in health and disease stimulates the food industry to match consumers' desire for health benefits through the food products, such as functional foods or food supplements. Information regarding the health benefits of foods is considered important for both consumers and manufacturers. Consumers can use the information to make purchasing decisions, and the manufacturers can use the information to promote sales by emphasizing the health benefits of their products. Therefore, labeling and advertising should be clear and correct to avoid any misunderstanding or exaggeration.

The requirement to protect consumers and ensure their right to accurate information on the physiological value of foods prompted governments to establish a regulatory framework for approval of foods with health claims in many nations. The Ministry of Health, Labour and Welfare (MHLW) of Japan first established a regulatory system to review and approve label statements regarding health benefits of foods in 1991 under the Health Promotion Law (Ohama, Ikeda, & Moriyama 2006; Shimizu, 2003). The Food and Drug Administration (FDA) of the United States promulgated new regulations implementing the provision authorizing disease prevention claims of foods in 1993 under the Nutrition Labelling and Education Act (NLEA) of 1990. However, the Dietary Supplement Health and Education Act (DSHEA) of 1994 established substantial limitations on the FDA's authority over dietary supplements by exempting dietary ingredients of dietary supplement products from the food additive requirements of the Food, Drug and Cosmetic (FD&C) Act; and substituted more flexible food safety provisions and exempted literature reprints from the labeling provisions of the FD&C Act (Hutt, 2000). The National Assembly of Korea enacted the Health/Functional Food Act (HFFA) in 2002, and instructed the Korea Food and Drug Administration (KFDA) to promulgate new regulations for the approval of food supplements. These new regulations were promulgated in January 2004. This chapter reviews the regulatory framework for health/functional foods (HFFs) under HFFA, focusing on the evaluation of new functional ingredients for health/functional foods.

21.2 HEALTH/FUNCTIONAL FOOD ACT

The most important accomplishment in HFFA is the statutory definition of HFFs as one of food products; and the introduction of new considerations for reviewing the safety and efficacy of functional ingredients.

Article 3 of the Act defines HFFs as the foods containing health-benefit ingredients or components that are intended to be used for enhancing or preserving human health. This Article also limits the form of HFFs only to tablet, capsule, powder, granule, pill or liquid. Therefore, the term 'HFF' was originally the synonym of food supplements, dietary supplements, or nutraceuticals. However, the scope of HFFs has been extended to conventional foods according to the revision of HFFA in 2008.[1]

Article 15 of the Act provides the concept that all HFFs are subject to be reviewed in terms of the safety and substantiation for claims on the basis of their ingredients or physiologically active components before marketing. Authorization would be granted in two different ways: 1) Provision 1 shows the way to list the authorized ingredients in the Code of HFFs by regulatory amendments, which is for wide use, although time-consuming; and 2) Provision 2 shows the other way to issue a certificate for each ingredient without regulatory amendments. Manufacturers or distributors have the responsibility to provide all evidence for backing up the claims of their products by developing substantiation for claims or relying on existing information. The Act does not define what health

---

[1]See the Amendment of the Health/Functional Food Act on 21 March 2008.

claims are and what constitutes 'substantiation' for a health claim made for an HFF. Instead, it gives KFDA the exclusive authority to define the health claims and to review the data.

Besides reviewing for new functional ingredients, this Act has important articles for the validity of the health functional food market in Korea. According to Article 16, any label and advertisement for the efficacy of health functional food shall be approved before marketing by the advisory committee. Moreover, for the purpose of manufacturing and quality control of good health functional food, KFDA may also designate Good Manufacturing Practices.

21.3 HEALTH CLAIMS ALLOWED FOR HFFS

The KFDA Regulation on the Labeling of HFFs describes the health claims allowed for. Only categories of claims—such as nutrient function claims, other function claims and disease risk reduction claims—are allowed for labeling and advertising of HFFs. Any claims that state or imply properties for the prevention, treatment or curve of human disease are prohibited. These definitions of health claims are compatible with those adopted by the Codex Alimentarius Commission (CAC) in 2004 and summarized as follows (CCFL, 2004):

- Nutrient function claims—these claims describe the physiological role of the nutrient in the growth, development, and normal functions of the body. Such claims should be applied to the nutrients, which have their own RDAs and be based on current, university-level nutrition texts as a possible source of evidence.
- Other function claims—these claims concern specific beneficial effects of HFFs in the context of total diet on normal functions or biological activities of the body. Such claims relate to a positive contribution to health,

to the improvement of a function, or to modifying or preserving health.

- Reduction-of-disease-risk claims—these claims describe the relationship between the consumption of HFFs (in the context of the total diet) and the reduced risk of developing a disease or health-related condition.

21.4 SCIENTIFIC SUBSTANTIATION OF HEALTH CLAIMS FOR HFFS

This brings up two issues which should take precedence over the substantiation of health claims: 1) the identification and stability of ingredients or components shall be evaluated by reviewing the origin, nature, composition, and processing methods; and 2) the safety evaluation shall be done within the risk analysis frameworks.

21.4.1 Identification and Stability of Functional Ingredients or Components

Functional ingredients can be obtained through processes such as extraction, centrifugation, filtration and/or fractionation. These are formulated as dietary supplements or added to conventional foods. In order to get a good quality product, standardization is necessary. Standardization is the process that optimizes the batch-to-batch consistency using index materials however, there are many factors to affect the standardization from handling of raw materials to the processing for final products. In order to assure the quality of active ingredients of HFFs, KFDA requires manufacturers to submit data on the contents and the analytical method of the index material. It is important that the index material is the active compound. As there are many chemicals that have similar activities in natural ingredients, it can be very difficult to find out what is the exact active compound.

Instead of active compounds, marker compounds could be used as the index material. Marker compounds should be representative and have characteristics such as specificity, stability and generality in the analytical method. In order to develop the analytical method, it must be verified by method validation. The petitioner should establish selectivity, accuracy, ranges for limit of detection and quantification, and reproducibility. Finding out the index material and validating the analytical method are key components in assuring the quality of product and protecting consumers from misleading label information.

21.4.2 Safety Evaluation of Functional Ingredients or Components

All scientific information regarding history of safe use, the manufacturing process, exposure assessment, nutritional evaluation, bioavailability and toxicological data are useful for the safety evaluation of functional ingredients or components. Safety evaluation shall be done within the risk analysis framework. Once safety is assured, there is the need to review the efficacy. No benefit–risk analysis is allowed under the Act. The basic principle of the safety assessment is confirmation of the novelty. If the active ingredient in the food is consumed traditionally, it might be safe without further documentation. However, if it is a fraction of the plant consumed as food, it should not be treated the same as a raw plant. The fraction should be substantiated as to its safety by using all available methods.

To make a transparent and consistent evaluation when preparing the safety documents, KFDA guidelines were provided using the decision tree approach as presented in Figure 21.1. The three major factors considered are the information regarding: 1) the raw materials (first column); 2) the processing methods (second column); and 3) the intake level (third column). According to materials, manufacturing process,

and intake level, there are four categories in the degree of scientific substantiation for safety. First is the category that covers components that are not allowed as functional ingredients. These are the ingredients or components that are listed in the 'Regulations of prohibited ingredients as health/functional food.' Second is the category of necessary documentation for history of use, safety information and intake assessment. These are ingredients that have been traditionally consumed as food and there is no increase in the intake amount compared to average intake level. Third is the category of ingredients that need other safety documentations because the intake amounts are considered to be increased although they have been consumed as food traditionally. Fourth might require toxicological data, including all available documents such as history of use, intake assessment, etc.

21.4.3 Review of Scientific Substantiation of Health Claims

KFDA applies a standard of 'competent and reliable scientific evidence', not only to provide manufacturers or distributors flexibility in the precise amount and type of evidence, but also to help maintain consumer confidence in HFFs. Although no formula exists as to how many or what types of studies are needed to substantiate a claim, review articles, meta-analyses, and abstracts would be excluded. This is because these do not contain sufficient information on the individual studies that were reviewed and therefore scientific conclusions cannot be drawn from this information.

Firstly, the studies included would be reviewed independently in terms of the design type and scientific quality of the study. Competent and reliable scientific evidence adequate to substantiate a claim would generally consist of information derived primarily from human studies. Especially a randomized, double-blind, parallel-group, placebo-controlled intervention study is considered

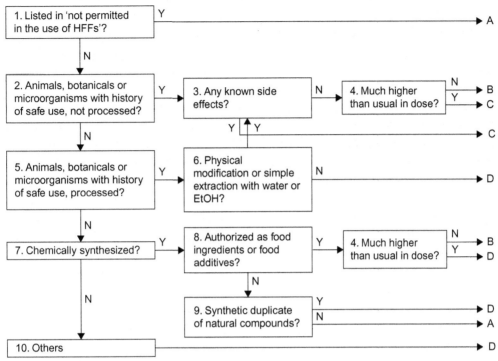

FIGURE 21.1   Decision tree for the preparation of safety data. Documents required to support safety of the functional ingredients: A, Not permitted to use; B, History of safe use, Estimates of intake; C, History of safe use, Estimates of intake, Toxicity/safety information, Nutritional information; D, History of safe use, Estimates of intake, Toxicity/safety information, Nutritional information, Toxicological assessment.

the 'gold' standard. Other types of scientific evidence such as animal studies, *in vitro* studies, anecdotal evidence, meta-analysis and review articles would generally be considered background information, but alone may not be adequate to substantiate a claim. However, animal studies and *in vitro* studies which are relevant and sufficient enough to explain the biochemical and physiological mechanisms, or to show dose-response relationships, would be strong supportive data for the health claims (CAC, 2006; Health Canada, 2001; US FDA, 2007).

Next, the scientific quality of each study would be reviewed based on several factors including study design and conduct, study population, data collection, outcome measures, statistical analysis, and confounding variables

(AHRQ, 2002). If the scientific study adequately addressed all or most of these factors, it would be considered of high quality. To identify the proposed relationship between an ingredient or a component and a health endpoint, relevant biomarkers or clinical endpoint may be used. Biomarkers can be classified according to whether they relate to: 1) the exposure to the food component (can give some indication, but not absolute proof); 2) the target function or biological response; or 3) an appropriate intermediate endpoint (Aggett *et al.*, 2005; Asp & Contor, 2003; Cummings, Pannemars, & Persin 2003; Howlett & Shortt, 2004; Richardson *et al.*, 2003; US FDA, 2005).

Lastly, the review of the totality of studies would be followed to evaluate the strength of evidence. Although the type and quality of individual studies are important, each piece of data therefrom should be considered in the context of all available information. The strength of the entire body of scientific evidence can be considered based on several criteria including quantity, consistency, and relevance (USA FDA, 2003; WHO, 2004). The more data from independently conducted studies are developed or collected, the more persuasive the evidence becomes. If the evidence used to substantiate a claim agrees with the background information, it would be ideal. Conflicting or inconsistent results raise questions as to whether a particular claim is substantiated (Aggett *et al.*, 2005; Asp & Contor, 2003; Cummings *et al.*, 2003; Howlett & Shortt, 2004; Richardson *et al.*, 2003; US FDA, 2005).

21.4.4 Grading of Scientific Evidence

Because new evidence is constantly emerging in the scientific literature, there is a need to accommodate emerging science and to develop a system to make a continuum from the emerging science to the consensus science. As mentioned above, the strength of the entire body of scientific evidence can be considered based on several criteria including quantity, consistency and relevance.

There are concerns that consumer information on health benefits of foods may be too limited if only claims reaching the consensus of significant scientific agreement are allowed to be used for labeling and advertising of HFFs. Therefore, KFDA introduced the concept of an 'evidence-based rating system' according to the four categories to grade the evidence created by WHO (2004): convincing, probable, possible and insufficient. The rank is determined, taking into account the type and quality of individual studies, and the quantity, consistency, and relevance of the aggregated studies.

Claims related to the reduction of disease require the highest level of evidence, primarily based on well-designed human intervention studies that are sufficient to reach 'convincing' levels. In contrast a wider range of scientific evidence can be used for other function claims. Although human intervention studies may be most preferable, other studies such as animal studies and *in vitro* studies alone may usefully demonstrate other function claims of HFFs, if those are relevant or sufficiently close to the human metabolism. Considering these variations in scientific evidence, KFDA defined three levels of other function claims, namely 'probable', 'possible' and 'insufficient'.

21.4.5 Kinds of Functional Ingredients

There are about 140 ingredients, including 76 product-specific and 74 generic ingredients. There are two types of generic ingredients. One is for nutrients, including 14 vitamins, 11 minerals, protein, essential fatty acids, and dietary fiber; and the other is for functional ingredients having other function claims. Dietary fiber and protein could be considered both nutrients and functional ingredients. Nutrients can be any source of fiber or protein; whereas, functional ingredients need to have the appropriate ingredients listed. There are 14 fibers, such as guar gum/guar gum hydrolysates, indigestible dextrin, polydextrose, soy fiber, oat fiber, etc. Each fiber has its own claims and intake amounts. For example, guar gum or guar gum hydrolysates have claims for maintaining healthy cholesterol levels, postprandial glucose levels, and gastrointestinal health; whereas, psyllium husk could have claims only for maintaining good gastrointestinal health. As of December 2008, 77 ingredients have been approved as product-specific functional ingredients. However, among those ingredients, 11 were approved despite limited scientific evidence claiming them as a health/functional food. As shown in Figure 21.2, there are various kinds of efficacies in health/functional foods. About 17% of health/functional foods claim that they are 'maintaining good gastrointestinal conditions.'

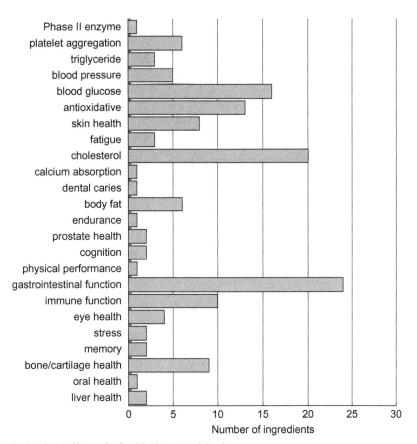

FIGURE 21.2   The kinds of efficacy for health/functional foods.

Oligosaccharides, probiotics and dietary fibers are the major active ingredients in this category. The other category, representing 14% of health/functional foods, makes health claims that they are 'good for maintaining healthy cholesterol levels' Dietary fiber, phytosterol, soybean protein, etc. are the major active ingredients in this category.

There have been two claims for the reduction-of-disease risk: one is the relationship between calcium and osteoporosis and the other is for xylitol and dental caries.

21.4.5.1 Calcium

Based on the Korean Dietary Reference Intake, calcium is the nutrient that Koreans need

more consumption of. Daily intake of calcium from health/functional food should be in the range of 210–800 mg. Labeling should include the following: the product contains adequate calcium, and that the intake of a proper amount of calcium contained in healthy meals with appropriate exercise may support bone health in young women and reduce the risk of osteoporosis later in life.

21.4.5.2 Xylitol

Daily intake of xylitol from health/functional food should be 10–25 g. The claim shall not imply that consuming non-cariogenic carbohydrate sweetener-containing foods is the only recognized means of achieving a reduced risk of dental caries. The other sweetener shall be included below 50% in health/functional food bearing claims for xylitol and dental caries. Moreover, when carbohydrates other than xylitol are present in the health/functional food, the food shall not produce acid after consumption.

21.4.6 Connection of Scientific Evaluation to Consumer Expression

The evidence-based ranking system linked the grading of scientific evidence to the wording of relevant claims, where different levels of evidence would result in different appropriate statements. However, because there was concern of consumer confusion, KFDA conducted a survey of consumer-response to the qualified wordings. KFDA evaluated a range of product label formats and message language. About 2000 consumers were presented with several kinds of labels. According to the results, consumers could not distinguish the level of strength for scientific evidence. In order to help consumers to understand labeling, the translation from scientific terms to consumer terms should be developed by both government and industry.

21.5 FUTURE DIRECTION

The consumer's understanding of the claims is of paramount importance. The ultimate goals of HFFA are to reduce consumer confusion regarding health claims made by food manufacturers, and to ensure that such claims are truthful and do not mislead consumers. To achieve these objectives, research in korea should focus on consumer perception of health claims, and development of appropriate and meaningful language and methods of expression.

In early 2008, the HFFA was amended to extend the scope of HFFs as supplements only to all types of foods, including conventional foods. To prevent an overflow of claims to all of the foods, the regulation on the evaluation of HFFs is under revision. Nutrient profiling to describe the disqualifying criteria, as well as the minimum requirements for health claims in conventional foods, will be considered. The exposure assessment of functional ingredients will also be addressed to assure safety.

References

Aggett, P. J., Antoine, J. M., Asp, N. G., et al. (2005). Process for the assessment of scientific support for claims on foods (PASSCLAIM): Concensus on criteria. *Eur J Nutr (Suppl)*, *44*, I/5–I/30.

AHRQ. (2002). Systems to rate the strength of scientific evidence. http://www.ahrq.gov/clinic/epcsums/strength-sum.pdf.

Asp, N. G., & Contor, L. (2003). Process for the assessment of scientific support for claims on foods (PASSCLAIM): overall introduction. *Eur J Nutr(Suppl)*, *42*, I/3–I/5.

CAC. (2006). Proposed Draft recommendations on the scientific basis of health claims at step 3, ftp://ftp.fao.org/codex/ccnfsdu28/nf28_07e.pdf.

CCFL. (2004). Codex guidelines for use of nutritional and health claims. ALINORM 04/27/41. Codex Committee on Food Labeling.

Cummings, J. H., Pannemans, D., & Persin, C. (2003). PASSCLAIM, Report of the first plenary meeting including a set of interim criteria to scientifically substantiate claims on foods. *Eur J Nutr (Suppl)*, *42*, I/112–I/119.

Health Canada. (2001). Product-specific authorization of health claims for foods. http://www.hc-sc.gc.ca/fn-an/label-etiquet/claims-reclam/final_proposal-proposition_final01-eng.php.

Howlett, J., & Shortt, C. (2004). PASSCLAIM, Report of the second plenary meeting: Review of a wider set of interim criteria for the scientific substantiation of health claims. *Eur J Nutr (Suppl)*, *43*, II/174–II/183.

Hutt, P. B. (2000). US Government regulation of food with claims for special physiological value. In M. K. Schmidl & T. P. Labuza (Eds.), *Essentials of functional foods* (pp. 339–352). Gaithersburg, MD: Aspen Publishers, Inc.

Ohama, H., Ikeda, H., & Moriyama, H. (2006). Health foods and with health claims in Japan. *Toxicology*, *221*, 95–111.

Richardson, D. P., Affertshol, T., Asp, N. G., et al. (2003). PASSCLAIM, Synthesis and review of existing processes. *Eur J Nutr (Suppl)*, 42, I/96–I/111.

Shimizu, T. (2003). Health claims on functional foods: the Japanese regulations and an international comparison. *Nutr Res Rev*, 16, 241–252.

US FDA. (2005). *Substantiation for dietary supplement claims made under section* 403(r)(6) of the Federal Food, Drug, and Cosmetic Act. http://www.fda.gov/Food/GuidanceComplianceRegulatoryInformation/GuidanceDocuments/DietarySupplements/ucm073200.htm.

US FDA. (2007). Guidance for Industry: Evidence-based review system for the scientific evaluation of health claims. http://www.fda.gov/Food/GuidanceComplianceRegulatoryInformation/GuidanceDocuments/FoodLabelingNutrition/ucm053850.htm (accessed 11 March 2008).

WHO. (2004). Global strategy on diet, physical activities, and health. http://apps.who.int/gb/ebwha/pdf_files/EB113/eeb113r7.pdf.

22

Bioactivity, Benefits and Safety of Traditional and Ethnic Foods

Adelia C. Bovell-Benjamin

Department of Food and Nutritional Sciences, Tuskegee University, Tuskegee, AL, USA

22.1 INTRODUCTION

Globally, there is growing research and consumer interest regarding diet-related (chronic) diseases and their influence on the health and well-being of communities (Day *et al.*, 2008; Urquiaga & Leighton, 2000). Several factors have contributed to this interest. Firstly, industrialization, urbanization and market globalization have impacted lifestyles, diets and nutritional status of populations worldwide. For example, in developing countries, while urbanization has reduced under-nutrition in metropolitan areas, it has increased physical inactivity and inadequate dietary patterns. Therefore, in many developing countries, under-nutrition may coexist with a high prevalence of chronic diseases such as certain types of cancer, obesity, hypertension, cardiovascular diseases and non-insulin dependent diabetes mellitus. Secondly, consumers in developing countries are experiencing escalating food prices, land scarcity and population growth. As a result, interest in food composition has broadened beyond nutrients to include bio-active compounds in traditionally consumed foods, which may help to prevent malnutrition and chronic diseases.

Thirdly, in the developed world, growing environmental awareness and concerns about safer foods have resulted in increased demand for natural or organic foods, which are perceived to be healthier than conventionally grown or genetically modified foods (Saba & Messina, 2003). Another reason is the impact of global emerging ethnic food markets on dietary intake and ultimately on chronic diseases. The evidence indicates that total sales for ethnic foods in the United Kingdom (UK) have doubled between 2003 and 2006 (Leatherhead Food International, 2004, 2007). Leatherhead Food International (2007) has estimated that from 2007 to 2011, ethnic food markets will have annual growths of up to 10% in Ireland, and between 6 and 8% in Spain, the Netherlands, Denmark, Belgium and Italy Khokhar *et al.*, (2009) have reported that increased consumption of traditional/ethnic foods will impact on nutrient intake.

These phenomena have led to increased consumer demands for nutritious foods with additional health-promoting activities, and also point to the need for foods to address the chronic diseases, which have become public health problems in various populations throughout the world. Foods contain nutrients which are essential for growth, maintenance and repair of the body. More recently, scientists have reported that foods also contain non-essential bioactive compounds, which have proven or potential beneficial effects on human health. A growing number of studies have linked traditional/ethnic foods to bioactive compounds, which have the capacity to prevent various chronic diseases, and confer other putative health benefits in humans. Therefore, the notion of traditional/ethnic foods appears to be one approach to meet the worldwide challenge of chronic diseases. However, there are significant gaps in the data regarding the nutrient and non-nutrient composition of traditional/ethnic foods, especially those from developing countries. This shortage of information slows down effective health and disease prevention efforts. It is apparent that more information and better understanding of the composition of traditional/ethnic foods, which enable them to promote human health and prevent disease, are needed.

22.2 OBJECTIVE

This chapter aims to review the available scientific literature related to the bioactivity, potential health benefits and safety of traditional and ethnic foods from selected countries in different regions of the world, namely, Latin America, Africa and Asia.

22.3 SCOPE

For the purposes of this chapter, bioactive food compounds are defined as naturally occurring non-essential constituents in or derived from plant, animal or marine sources, which have the ability to modulate biochemical, physiological and metabolic processes in the human body while exerting beneficial effects beyond basic nutritional functions (ADA, 2004; Denny & Buttriss, 2008; Gry *et al.*, 2007; Health Canada, 2004; Tejasari, 2007). Bioactive compounds can be produced either *in vivo* or by industrial enzymatic digestion (food processing activities). In plant and animal-derived foods, bioactive compounds are usually found in multiple forms such as glycosylated, esterified, thiolated, or hydroxylated. Bioactive compounds in plants are usually found in the leaves, stems, roots, tubers, buds, fruits, seeds and flowers; they influence the color, flavor, structure, function and defense system of plants (Cushnie & Lamb, 2005). The major classes of plant bioactives include: flavonoids and other phenolic compounds, carotenoids, plant sterols, glucosinolates and other sulfur compounds (Denny & Buttriss, 2008).

Traditional and ethnic foods (the two terms are used interchangeably) are defined as those that have been consumed as part of a usual diet locally or regionally for an extensive time period by specific group(s) of people. In general, *'traditional/ethnic'* foods should: i) be communicated from ancestors to descendants; ii) have a long history of consumption; and iii) be usually part of the history and culture of the population concerned. Traditional foods are valued for more than their sustenance role and are linked with cultural identity and civilization. Most traditional food processes have stemmed from the need to preserve food for the off season or to make it safe for consumption. Traditional food products are produced from indigenous crops and raw materials and are therefore typical to a certain region or area. Increased consumer awareness and demands about the role of diet and nutrition in chronic disease prevention have led to more research regarding the benefits and safety of traditional/ethnic foods.

Foods or food ingredients consumed as part of traditional/ethnic diets, eaten for health-promoting properties or not, are included, even when the existing scientific evidence for these benefits may not yet be substantial. In many instances, there is little documented information about the content and concentration of bioactive compounds of several traditional/ethnic foods. The scope is limited to mainly plant foods or drink, but animal-source foods may be included. The review focuses on traditional/ethnic foods in the context of developing countries. The target developing regions are: Latin America, Africa and Asia. They were selected to represent different traditional/ethnic foods from varying parts of the world.

22.4 METHODOLOGY

A review of the existing literature was conducted. The literature surveyed covered scientific journals, trade journals, magazines, market reports, conference proceedings, books and other published materials. Web page content was used, as necessary. Literature was collected using numerous search engines and databases (for example, EBSCOhost, Ingenta, ScienceDirect, Google, Google Scholar, PubMed) in addition to library databases and Internet libraries of international organizations.

22.5 STRUCTURE OF THE REVIEW

In this review, Sections 1 to 5 justify the topic, present the objective, and outline the scope and structure of the review. Sections 6 and 7 discuss the relationship between food and chronic diseases and summarize the biological mechanism of bioactive food compounds. Section 8 discusses the bioactive compounds and beneficial effects and safety of traditional/ethnic foods from Latin America in general and Mexico in particular; Africa (South Africa and Uganda); and Asia (India and Japan). Sections 9 and 10 consist of conclusion, future scope. Acknowledgements and a references section complete the chapter.

22.6 FOOD AND CHRONIC DISEASES

It has been well established that certain types of foods, including fruits and vegetables are associated with a decrease in chronic diseases. For example, a meta-analysis of 26 studies found an association between the risk of breast cancer and intake of fruits and vegetables (Gandini, Merzenich, Robertson, & Boyle 2000). In another multi-ethnic (Japanese, African American, Chinese and Caucasian) case-control study consisting of 1619 and 1618 men as prostate cancer cases and controls, respectively, Kolonel *et al.* (2000) evaluated the protective effects of fruit and vegetable intake.

Cruciferous and yellow-orange vegetable intake was inversely related to prostate cancer.

Bazzano *et al.* (2002) reported that the incidences of stroke were decreased for individuals consuming more than three servings of fruits and vegetables daily. Similarly, participants who consumed less than one serving daily of fruits and vegetables had a higher incidence of stroke than those who consumed more than three servings. Kim and Kwon (2009) concluded that there is limited evidence to support a relationship between garlic consumption and reduced risk of colon, prostate, esophageal, larynx, oral, ovary or renal cell cancers. Wen *et al.* (2009) prospectively evaluated the association of dietary carbohydrates, glycemic index and glycemic load and dietary fiber with breast cancer risk to determine whether the effect of these dietary intakes is modified by age and selected insulin- or estrogen-related risk factors. It was concluded that a high carbohydrate diet with a high glycemic load may be associated with breast cancer risk in pre-menopausal women or women less than 50 years of age. In general, these studies suggest a relationship between certain components in food and chronic diseases. The following sections discuss some bioactive compounds in traditional/ethnic foods.

22.7 BIOLOGICAL MECHANISM OF BIOACTIVE FOOD COMPOUNDS

Polyphenols or phenolic compounds are present in a variety of plants utilized as important components of human food systems (Crozier *et al.*, 2000). Polyphenols, products of the secondary metabolism of plants are the most abundant and widely distributed group of bioactive compounds (Crozier *et al.*, 2000). Polyphenols constitute a range of substances with an aromatic ring and one or more hydroxyl substituents. In biological systems, polyphenols serve as free radical scavengers, metal chelators and prevent inhibition of cell communication; all of which are precursors to chronic diseases (Fraga, 2007; Sigler & Ruch, 1993; Masibo & He, 2008). The presence of the phenolic groups confers their antioxidant capacity. These characteristics are due to the hydrogen of the phenoxyl groups, which is prone to be donated to a radical, and by the ensuing structure that is chemically stabilized by resonance (Fraga, 2007). The schematic in Figure 22.1 relates polyphenols to potential health benefits.

As shown in Figure 22.2, the basic structure of flavonoid compounds, the most common subgroup of plant phenolic compounds, is the 2-phenyl-benzo[α]pyrane or flavane nucleus,

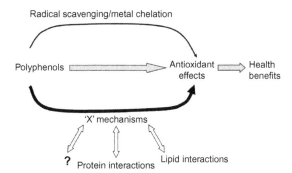

FIGURE 22.1   Scheme relating polyphenols with health benefits, through their observed antioxidant effects. The body of the black arrows indicates the 'X' mechanism with free radical scavenging or metal chelating capacity of polyphenols (Fraga, 2007).

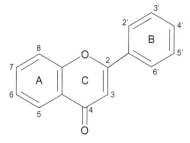

FIGURE 22.2   The skeleton structure of the flavones (a class of flavonoids) with rings named and positions numbered (Harborne & Baxter, 1999).

which consists of two benzene rings (A and B), each containing at least one hydroxyl, which are connected through a three-carbon 'bridge' and become part of a six-member heterocyclic ring (C) (Beecher, 2003; Brown, 1980). Flavonoids can be classified according to biosynthetic origin. For example, flavanones and flavan-3-ols are intermediates in biosynthesis as well as end products, which have the ability to accumulate in plant tissues. Others such as anthocyanidins, flavones and flavonols are end products of biosynthesis only (Crozier, Jaganath, & Clifford, 2006); and the isoflavones and isoflavonoids in which the 2-phenyl side chain of flavanone isomerizes to the 3-position. Figure 22.3 shows the categories of flavonoids.

Most of the beneficial health effects of flavonoids are attributed to their antioxidant and chelating capacities (Heim, Tagliaferro, & Bobilya,

2002). Antioxidants are substances, which inhibit oxidation and protect the body against the damaging effects of free radicals. Briefly, flavonoids protect the body against reactive oxygen species (ROS) by preventing injury caused by free radicals (Masibo & He, 2008; Pietta, 2000). Free radicals are species which contain unpaired electrons, making them highly unstable and reactive. Free radicals cause cellular membrane damage, which is associated with chronic diseases such as cancer, diabetes and coronary heart disease morbidity (Halliwell, 1994).

Flavonoids directly scavenge free radicals by stabilizing the ROS by reacting with the reactive compound of the radical as shown (Pietta, 2000):

$$FOH + R^\cdot \rightarrow FO^\cdot + RH$$

Where FOH is a flavonoid; $R^\cdot$ is a free radical; and $FO^\cdot$ is the less reactive flavonoid phenoxyl radical. Flavonoids may also suppress lipid oxidation by recycling other antioxidants by donating a hydrogen atom (McAnlis McEneny, Pearce, & Young, 1999). The chemistry, metabolism and structure-activity relationships of flavonoids have been extensively reviewed by Heim *et al.* (2002). Bioactive food compounds such as polyphenols and flavonoids have the capacity to prevent cellular membrane damage and suppress lipid oxidation, which all play a role in chronic disease prevention.

22.8 BIOACTIVE FOOD COMPOUNDS IN TRADITIONAL/ ETHNIC FOODS

22.8.1 Latin America

22.8.1.1 *Beneficial Effects of yerba mate*

Latin American cultures have a tradition of using many native plants, for specific functional food purposes. Mate or yerba mate (*Ilex paraguariensis*), an indigenous plant, is used for the preparation of the most commonly consumed

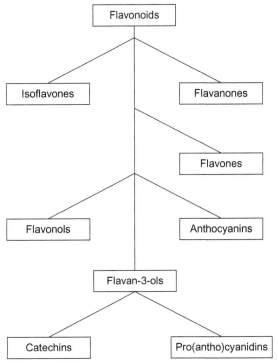

FIGURE 22.3 Categories of Flavonoids (Source: Denny & Buttriss, 2008).

traditional tea-like beverage in South American countries (Filip *et al.*, 2001). It is traditionally consumed by millions of South Americans as a tonic, a healthful alternative to coffee, a stimulant to reduce fatigue, and as an appetite suppressant (Cardozo *et al.*, 2007; Di Gregorio *et al.*, 2004). *I. paraguariensis* grows naturally in northeastern Argentina, southern Brazil and eastern Paraguay where it is also cultivated (Gorzalczany *et al.*, 2001). The habit of drinking yerba mate has remained unchanged, and it is widely consumed in Argentina, Paraguay, Uruguay and Brazil, with a reportedly 30% of the population drinking more than one liter of mate infusions daily (Dellacassa & Bandoni, 2001; Filip, Lotito, Ferraro, & Fraga, 2000; Filip *et al.*, 2001). Yerba mate (Figure 22.4) is usually prepared by pouring hot water unto a high concentration of the dried and minced leaves (50 g/L).

Yerba mate might be considered one of the main antioxidant-rich beverages consumed in various South American countries. The leaves contain many bioactive compounds, such as chlorogenic acid and phenolic acids, which appear to be responsible for the antioxidant activity of the tea, both *in vivo* and *in vitro* (Chandra & Gonzalez de Mejia, 2004; Bracesco *et al.*, 2003; Schinella *et al.*, 2000; Filip *et al.*, 2000). Bastos *et al.* (2006) reported comparable antioxidant efficacy in green mate and mate tea infusions and BHT (a well-known phenolic antioxidant). da Silva *et al.* (2008) described yerba mate extract as a source of phenolic compounds, which contain *in vitro* antioxidant activities that may reduce cardiovascular disease risk. According to da Silva *et al.* (2008), yerba mate contains practically all of the vitamins and minerals necessary to sustain life. Additionally, Bixby, Spieler, Menini, & Gugliucci (2005) and Bracesco *et al.* (2003) have demonstrated that *I. paraguariensis* is a more potent antioxidant than red wine or green and black tea.

da Silva *et al.* (2008) examined the acute effects of the consumption of mate infusion on *ex vivo* plasma and low-density lipoprotein (LDL) oxidation, plasma antioxidant capacity, and platelet aggregation. Their results indicated that phenolic compounds from yerba mate infusion promoted plasma and LDL protection against *ex vivo* lipid peroxidation and also impacted significantly on the antioxidant capacity of plasma. Bravo, Luis, & Lecumberri (2007) compared the total polyphenols and antioxidant activity of mate infusions with commonly consumed commercial beverages (orange juice, green and black teas and red, rosé and white wines). The total polyphenol content of mate was comparable to tea and orange juice. The antioxidant activity of mate was slightly higher than wines, orange juice and black tea, but lower than green tea. Using rat models, Prediger *et al.* (2008) concluded that acute administration of hydroalcoholic extract of *I. paraguariensis* improved cognition by differentially modulating short- and long-term learning and memory. Overall, da Silva *et al.* (2008) indicated that, besides its stimulant and nutritional proprieties, yerba mate might be considered an important source of antioxidants to humans.

22.8.1.2 Safety of yerba mate

Literature regarding the safety of yerba mate is scarce, but consumption of yerba mate has been suggested as a risk factor for development of cancers of the oral cavity and upper aerodigestive tract, partly due to the very hot temperature at which this beverage is usually consumed (Goldberg & Brinckmann, 2000; Sewram, De Stefani, Brennan, & Boffetta, 2003). Di Gregorio *et al.* (2004) reported that yerba mate, yerba mate leaves and tea manufactured in Apóstoles, Argentina showed the presence of ^{137}Cs (radioactive contaminants from the Chernobyl nuclear fallout) contamination in concentrations of 7–10 Bq/kg. However, it was stated that these levels do not represent a public health risk. While it is recognized that this traditional food has excellent bioactive compounds, the presence of contaminants or its safety has not been extensively documented. However, it can be argued that the long history of use of traditional foods is in itself evidence of their safety; evidently their use would have been discontinued if they were inexplicably unsafe. Furthermore, it can be argued that it is inappropriate to apply only scientific parameters to safety assessments of traditional foods without considering the traditional precautions, which are integral parts of their safe preparation and use.

22.8.1.3 Beneficial Effects of Pulque (Mexico)

Pulque, which is the most important traditional non-distilled alcoholic beverage of Mexico was inherited from the Aztecs, and remains an essential part of the contemporary diet (Escalante *et al.*, 2004). It is obtained by fermentation of the sap (*aguamiel*) from several species of the maguey plant such as *Agave atrovirens* and *Agave americana* (Figure 22.4). The sap of the Agave plant consists of calcium oxalate crystals, an acrid volatile oil, Agave gum, and other compounds. Pulque processing is a complex succession of yeast and bacteria that produce ethanol, a diversity of chemical compounds, and some polymers that give a distinctive viscous consistency to the final product (Peña-Alvarez, 2004).

Pulque is viewed as healthy, and is usually consumed as a low-alcohol beverage and as a nutritional supplement. Backstrand, Allen, Martinez, & Pelto (2001) have postulated that alcoholic beverages, such as Pulque could provide substantial amounts of vitamins and minerals to diets if they are not distilled or overly processed, and consumed in moderation. Pulque can provide important quantities of ascorbic acid, non-heme iron, riboflavin, folate, several other B vitamins and some bioactive compounds (Backstrand *et al.* 2001). Overall, modest Pulque consumption has the potential to enhance iron status, increase intakes of key micronutrients and improve nutritional status (Backstrand *et al.*, 2001). Medicinal qualities have also been attributed to Pulque, and it is consumed for ailments such as renal infections, anorexia and gastrointestinal disorders.

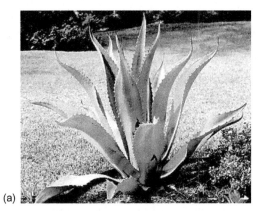
(a)

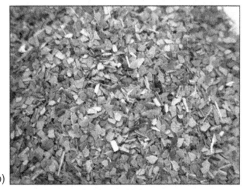
(b)

FIGURE 22.4 (a) *Agave americana* plant (b) Dried leaves of yerba mate (http://www.florahealth.com/flora/home/Canada/HealthInformation/Encyclopedias/Mate.htm).

Saponins are natural glycosides of steroid or triterpene, which exhibit many different biological and pharmacological actions (Lacaille-Dubois, 2005; Sparg, Light, & Van Staden, 2004). Pulque contains significant quantities of steroidal saponins, many of which are bioactive. Several Agave species produce steroidal sapogenins and saponins, the raw materials for steroid hormone synthesis (Tinto, Simmons-Boyce, McLean, & Reynolds, 2005). Saponins are being studied for their medicinal uses, including antispasmodic activity, and toxicity to cancer cells. The biological activities of saponins have been extensively reviewed elsewhere (Sparg *et al.*, 2004; Lacaille-Dubois, 2005). Steroidal saponins have been described as the most important bioactive

TABLE 22.1   Biological activity of steroidal saponins

Biological Activity	Reference
Anti-cancer	Ravikumar, Hammesfahr, & Sih (1979); Sung, Kendall, & Rao (1995)
Anti-thrombotic	Peng et al. (1996); Zhang et al. (1999)
Anti-viral	Aquino et al. (1991)
Hemolytic	Zhang et al. (1999); Santos et al. (1997)
Hypercholesterolemic	Sauvaire, Ribes, Baccuo, & Loubatierés-Mariani (1991); Malinow (1985)
Hypoglycemic	Kato, Miura, & Fukunaga (1995)

compounds in yam (Yang, Lu, & Hwang, 2009) and several biological activities, such as anti-cancer have been documented (Table 22.1). Saponins are said to make up the active major constituents of ginseng (*Panax ginseng*) (Sparg *et al.*, 2004). The saponins present in Agave species have shown hypocholesterolemic, anti-inflammatory and antibiotic activity, but the functional effects of those in Pulque have not been detailed in the literature. Backstrand, Allen, and Black (2002) concluded that consumption of Pulque predicted less risk of low ferritin and hemoglobin values for pregnant women in Solís Valley, Mexico.

22.8.1.4 Safety of Pulque

Some γ-Proteobacteria have been identified in Pulque; although these are ubiquitous in fresh water, soil, vegetable surfaces, etc., some are also considered opportunistic human pathogens (Escalante *et al.*, 2008; Waleron, Waleron, Podhajsa, & Lojkowska, 2002). Escalante *et al.* (2008) speculated that some of the γ-Proteobacteria detected in Pulque could have come from the natural bacterial diversity of the sap, whereas others could have been incorporated during its extraction, handling and storage under non-aseptic

conditions. Backstrand *et al.* (2001) reported that high consumption of Pulque was associated with poor infant outcomes among women in Solís Valley, Mexico. Consumption of Pulque by pregnant women was also linked to increased risk of the negative effects of fetal exposure to alcohol (Backstrand *et al.*, 2001).

In summary, it has been shown that Pulque contains steroidal saponins and various other micronutrients. Although the biological activities of saponins have been extensively reviewed, their functional effect in Pulque has not been clearly elucidated; this warrants further research. The possibility of bacterial contamination during the processing of Pulque also needs to be addressed in future research studies.

22.8.2 Africa

22.8.2.1 Beneficial Effects of Rooibos (South Africa)

Traditionally, a number of plants such as *Aspalathus linearis* (Rooibos) and *Cyclopia intermedia* (Honeybush) have been used as teas in South Africa. This review discusses Rooibos. Rooibos tea originates from the leaves and fine stems of the indigenous South African plant *A. linearis* (Figure 22.5). About three centuries ago, the indigenous Khoi-Khoi tribe of the Western Cape Province, South Africa used the leaves of the Rooibos plant as a tea, with an exceptional taste and aroma (Morton, 1983). It was consumed as a strong, hot brew with milk and sugar (Joubert, Gelderblom, Louw, & de Beer, 2008). The leaves and stems of the plant were boiled in water and kept hot at low heat. Water, leaves or stems were added to the pot after each serving. Surveys conducted by Oldewage-Theron, Dicks, Napier, & Rutengwe (2005) revealed that Rooibos tea was one of the 10 most frequently consumed foods in an informal settlement in the Vaal Triangle, South Africa. More recently, however, Rooibos is consumed as an herbal tea with or without milk and sugar, and is also used cold or hot.

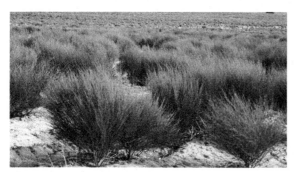

FIGURE 22.5 Mature Rooibos plants (*Aspalathus linearis*). Rooibos Ltd/SunnRooibos (2003) (www.rooibosltd.co.za).

Rooibos is naturally caffeine-free with a low tannin content, which decreases the risk of poor iron bioavailability, a phenomenon frequently found in tea drinkers due to the formation of nonheme iron-tannin complexes (Erickson, 2003; Morton, 1983). The leaves and stems of *A. linearis* could be used as fermented or unfermented. The unfermented type is called green Rooibos; fermentation changes the Rooibos leaves from green to red due to oxidation of the constituent polyphenols; it is called red Rooibos or red tea (McKay & Blumberg, 2007). Today, the traditional fermented tea is processed in the same way it was done by the indigenous people centuries ago and also on a commercial basis.

Rooibos has been associated with antioxidant capacity, chemopreventive potential, modulated immune effect and anti-allergenic actions (Hesseling & Joubert, 1982; Kunishiro, Tai, & Yamamoto, 2001; Lamosova *et al.*, 1997; Nakano *et al.*, 1997a; Nakano, Nakashima, & Itoh, 1997b; Schulz, Joubert, & Schutze, 2003). Free radicals (unstable molecules that have lost an electron) can damage the DNA in cells and increase the risk for chronic and other diseases. Antioxidants, such as polyphenols, are capable of binding free radicals before they become harmful to the body. Polyphenols have subgroups such as flavonoids and phenolic acids, which are potent free radical scavengers (Erickson, 2003). Brewed green and red Rooibos teas are rich sources of different phenolic compounds (McKay & Blumberg, 2007; Dos, Ayhan, & Sumnu, 2005). Red Rooibos is known to contain the following phenolic acids: caffeic, ferulic, *p*-coumaric, *p*-hydroxybenzoic, vanillic and protocatechuic (Rabe *et al.*, 1994). The major flavonoids found in Rooibos tea are aspalathin, iso-orientin, orientin, isovitexin, vitexin, isoquercitrin, hyperoside, quercetin, luteolin, chrysoeriol and rutin (McKay & Blumberg, 2007; Shimamura *et al.*, 2006). Aspalathin, a naturally occurring C-glycosyldihydrochalcone is found exclusively in *A. linearis* (Koeppen, & Roux, 1965; Koeppen, 1970; Shimamura *et al.*, 2006).

Generally, green Rooibos contains higher levels of total polyphenols. These differences are attributed to the enzymatic and chemical changes, which occur during the fermentation process (Joubert, 1996). For example, aspalathin is oxidized to dihydro-iso-orientin during fermentation, and its concentration was shown to reduce from 49.9 to 1.2 mg/g for green and red Rooibos, respectively (Bramati, Aquilano, & Pietta 2003). Standley *et al.* (2001) also reported more total polyphenols in green than red Rooibos (41.0 versus 35.0%). In 2% (w/v) solutions of Rooibos tea, green had more total polyphenols than red (41.2 versus 29.7%), more flavonoids (28.1 versus 18.8%) and 13.1 versus 10.9% non-flavonoids (Marnewick, Gelderblom, & Joubert 2000). Other flavonoids such as iso-orientin, orientin, isovitexin and vitexin are also degraded during fermentation of *A. linearis*.

Several studies, mostly animal and *in vitro*, have investigated the potential health benefits of *A. linearis*. Shindo and Kato (1991) reported that weekly consumption of 1500 mL fermented red tea (0.2 g leaves/100 mL water, boiled for 20 minutes) was beneficial to patients with a wide range of dermatological diseases. It was also reported to decrease the incidence of *herpes simplex*, and the incurable human papilloma virus infection. In an animal model, Uličná *et al.* (2006) fed male Wistar rats a water extract (0.25g leaves/100mL water, boiled for 10 minutes, steeped for 20 minutes); an alkaline extract (10g water-extracted leaves/100 mL 1% Na_2CO_3 extracted for 3 hours at 45°C); *ad libitum* and a gavage of 5mL/kg body weight. They reported that the extracts (red tea) significantly decreased plasma creatinine, lowered advanced glycation end-products and lipid peroxidation in the plasma and lens. The water extract also decreased lipid peroxidation in the liver. Male Fischer rats were fed extracts of 2.0 g leaves/100mL freshly boiled water, steeped for 30 minutes; freeze-dried (fermented and unfermented) by Sissing (2008). It was demonstrated that the extract reduced the number and size of methylbenzylnitrosamine-induced esophageal papillomas. In a recent study conducted by Juráni *et al.* (2008) using red tea, aged Japanese quails were fed 0.175g leaves/100mL water, boiled for 10 minutes and steeped for 20 minutes, *ad libitum* or as supplemented feed with milled plant material (3.5g/kg). They concluded that the extract prolonged productive life of the quails. Other potential health benefits of Rooibos are extensively discussed by Joubert *et al.* (2008).

22.8.2.2 Safety of Rooibos

The general assumption is that Rooibos is safe because of its long history of traditional consumption by the South African population without documented adverse reports. It has been reported that chronic ingestion of green and red Rooibos extracts by rats for 10 weeks did not adversely affect the liver, body weight and kidney parameters (Marnewick *et al.*, 2003). Quality control of commercially produced Rooibos is limited to pesticide residues and microbial contamination (Joubert *et al.*, 2008). Commercial producers are less reliant on traditional use as an indicator of safety and toxicity. Several manufacturers use varying standards to predict quality of the tea, for example, objective color measures, total polyphenol (TP), total antioxidant activity (TAA) and aspalathin content

(Joubert, 1995). Much more scientific evidence is needed to conclusively establish the safety of Rooibos.

In summary, it has been shown that Rooibos contains bioactive compounds, which may help protect against free radical damage that can lead to cancer, heart attack, and stroke. However, it should be borne in mind that the evidence presented is primarily from animal models; human studies are very limited. Unfermented (green) Rooibos has a higher amount of polyphenols than traditionally fermented Rooibos, and generally demonstrates higher antioxidant and antimutagenic capabilities *in vitro*. The bioavailability, tissue distribution and biological activities of the bioactive compounds in Rooibos need to be further researched. Further research is also needed to determine whether the bioactivity of Rooibos observed *in vitro* and in animals translate into health benefits for humans.

22.8.2.3 Beneficial Effects of Java plum (Uganda)

In Central Uganda, the dried and powdered seeds of Java plum (*Syzygium cumini*) are traditionally consumed as herbal medicine to treat asthma and the fruit is also eaten, especially by young children (Stangeland *et al.*, 2009). The Java plum was brought to Uganda in the early 1900s by the Indians who mainly ate the juicy pulp as ordinary fruit or used it in jam production (Figure 22.6). In their examination of the bioactivity of several commonly eaten Ugandan fruits and vegetables, Stangeland *et al.* (2009) revealed that Java plum seeds and fruits have high antioxidant activity. In a preliminary study, Ndyomugyenyi (2008) demonstrated that the bioactive compounds in Java plum included sterols, triterpenes, coumarins, tannins, glycosides (cardiac and steroids), alkaloids, reducing compounds, anthocyanin pigments and saponins.

Banerjee, Dasgupta, & De (2005) concluded that the fruit skin of *S. cumini* has significant

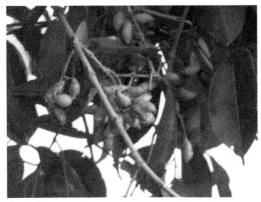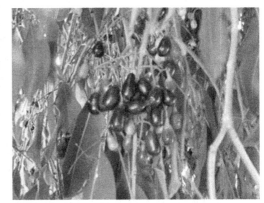

FIGURE 22.6   The tree and fruit of Java plum (*Syzygium cuminii*) (http://www.daleysfruit.com.au/forum/bugagali1/).

antioxidant activity, which may come in part from antioxidant vitamins, phenolics or tannins and/ or anthocyanins. In their study, Veigas, Narayan, Laxman, & Neelwarne (2007) characterized and evaluated anthocyanin pigments from *S. cumini* fruit peels for their antioxidant efficacy and stability. Total anthocyanin content was 216mg/100 mL of extract, equivalent to 230mg/100 g fruit on a dry weight basis. Three anthocyanins were identified as glucoglucosides of delphinidin, and the researchers concluded that *S. cumini* extract was a more efficient free radical-scavenger than BHA. Consumption of *S. cumini* fruit may supply substantial antioxidants, which may provide health promoting and disease preventing effects.

22.8.2.4 Safety of Java plum

Literature regarding the safety of Java plum is not forthcoming. In general, the traditionally-eaten fruits are considered safe even though they may contain microorganisms, anti-nutrients, toxins or allergens. Very often, special preparation or processing techniques have been associated with traditional foods to minimize any risks associated with them. The knowledge required to manage the risks associated with traditional foods has been acquired in the

course of their long history of use. Much more research is needed to determine the safety of Java plum.

22.8.3 Asia

22.8.3.1 Beneficial Effects of the Mango (India)

Fruits from tropical and subtropical climates contain various bioactive compounds (Ribeiro *et al.*, 2007). Mango (*Mangifera indica* L.) is a commonly eaten, traditional fruit in many tropical and subtropical countries throughout the world (Kim, Lounds-Singleton, & Talcott, 2009). *M. indica* has been cultivated in the Indian subcontinent for thousands of years; cultivation spread to East Asia and East Africa between the 5th–4th century BC and 10th century AD, respectively. Mangoes were subsequently introduced to Brazil, West Indies and Mexico (Kim *et al.*, 2009). Brazil, Mexico, the Philippines, India, China, Nigeria and Pakistan are among the world's major mango producing countries (Kim *et al.*, 2009; Ribeiro *et al.*, 2007; FAO, 2007). The ripe fruit is variable in size and color (Figure 22.7). In the center of the fruit is a single flat oblong seed that can be fibrous or hairy on the surface,

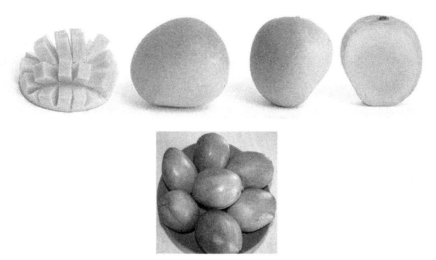

FIGURE 22.7   Mature ripe and green mango (*Mangifera indica* L.) (http://www.spicegrenada.com/).

depending on the cultivar. The ripe fruits are usually eaten uncooked while the unripe fruits or green mangoes can be made into pickles or chutneys. Table 22.2 shows some traditional dietary uses of mangoes in selected developing countries.

Mango is a rich source of bioactive compounds including phenols and carotenoids (Kim, Brecht, & Talcott, 2007; Berardini *et al.*, 2005; Godoy & Rodriguez-Amaya, 1989). Ribeiro *et al.* (2008) identified the following flavonoids and xanthone glycosides in the pulp of Brazilian Ubá mango: mangiferin, mangiferin gallate, iso-mangiferin gallate, kaempferol and quercetin. It was noted that the bioactive compound varied with variety of mango. Ribeiro *et al.* (2007) identified mango pulp as a rich source of antioxidants. Kim *et al.* (2009) reported free gallic acid and four gallotannins as the major polyphenols in mango. *p*-OH-benzoic acid, *p*-coumaric acid, ferulic acid and catechin were also identified in mango at low concentrations by Kim *et al.* (2009). Other polyphenolic compounds which have been identified in mango include: isoquercetin, ellagic acid and β-glucogallin (Schieber, Ullrich, & Carle, 2000).

The main bioactive compound in mango is mangiferin or C-glucosyl xanthone (xanthones are some of the most potent antioxidants). Using cultured human peripheral blood lymphocytes, Jagetia and Baliga (2005) reported that mangiferin was protective against radiation-induced sickness and bone marrow mortality. Mangiferin has also been associated with anti-diabetic, anti-atherogenic, anti-hyperlipidemic activities in rats (Yoshikawa *et al.*, 2001; Muruganandan *et al.*, 2002; Randle, Garland, Hales, & Newsholme, 1963). It has also been reported that mangiferin has antibacterial and antifungal effects (Stoilova, Gargova, Stoyanova, & Ho, 2005).

22.8.3.2 *Safety of the Mango*

Human intake studies have indicated that consumption of 1g total polyphenols daily has not resulted in any adverse effect or lethal toxicity (Scalbert & Williamson, 2000). Although this widely used traditional fruit has been reported to have excellent bioactive compounds, the question of its safety has not been extensively studied. In summary, mango and possibly its derived products, traditionally used in developing countries are

TABLE 22.2 Traditional dietary uses of mango (*Mangifera indica* L.) in selected developing countries

Food	Country	Description
Chutney	Indian subcontinent	Unripe mangoes with chili or limes
Aampadi	India	Ripe mango cut into thin layers, dessicated, folded then cut
Ayurvedic mango lassi	India	Sweet drink, which uses yogurt and milk as the base
Ras	India	Squeezed mango juice used on a variety of bread items
Unripe or green mangoes	India	Eaten with salt and chili
	Philippines	Eaten with bagoong, a salty paste made with fermented fish or shrimp
	Indonesia	
	Thailand	Sugar and salt and/or chili
Panha or Panna	India	Raw ripe mango drink
Mango	Mexico	Sliced mango with chili powder, juices, smoothies, fruit bars etc.; whole in chili-salt mixture
Pickled mangoes	Southeast Asia	Pickled with fish sauce and wine vinegar
Amchur	Trinidad and Tobago, India, Southeast Asia	Dried unripe mango used as a condiment
Rujak or rojak	Malaysia, Singapore, Indonesia	Green mangoes in a sour salad

rich sources of bioactive compounds; however, the safety aspects and the effect of processing on the bioactive compounds have not been very well studied. Kim *et al.* (2009) studied the polyphenolic and antioxidant changes to mature green mangoes following different hot water treatment times and during storage. They indicated that gallic acid, gallotannins and total soluble phenolics decreased as the length of hot water treatment increased. Further research is needed in this area to determine the safety and whether the bioactive compounds in the mango fruit are still intact in the derived products (Table 22.2).

22.8.3.3 Beneficial Effects of Edible Algae (Japan)

In Asian countries, Japanese are the main consumers of seaweed with an average annual consumption of 1.6 kg (dry weight) per capita (Fujiwara-Arasaki, Mino, & Kuroda, 1984). A wide variety of sea algae such as wakame (*Undaria pinnatifida*) and hizikia (*Hizikia fusiforme*) are a part of staple diet in Japan from time immemorial (Dawczynski, Schubert, & Jahreis, 2007; Nagai & Yukimoto, 2003). Wakame is the dominant alga in Japan accounting for more than 50% consumption (Davidson, 1999). It is consumed in soups, salads, sweetened vinegar, cooked food and ingredients. Wakame is rich in fucoxanthin, which is a xanthophyll characteristic of brown sea algae, and accounts for more than 10% of estimated total natural production of carotenoids (Miyashita & Hosokawa, 2006, 2008; Shiratori *et al.*, 2005). Fucoxanthin and its metabolites have been reported to possess anti-oxidative, anti-cancerous, anti-obesity and anti-inflammatory properties (Miyashita & Hosokawa, 2008). Hizikia (*Hizikia fusiforme*), also called Hijiki, is eaten as fried food, sea lettuce, in sweetened vinegar and green laver. It could be eaten fresh, but is mostly dried and rehydrated before use (Davidson, 1999). Data regarding the bioactive compounds of edible algae consumed in Japan are sparse.

Brown sea algae are known to contain more bioactive compounds than either green or red sea algae (Seafoodplus, 2008). Some of the bioactive compounds identified in brown sea algae include phylopheophylin, phlorotannins, fucoxanthin and various other metabolites (Hosokawa,

Bhaskar, Sashima, & Miyashita, 2006). Nagai and Yukimoto (2003) investigated the preparation and functional properties of beverages made from brown sea algae. Four beverages were prepared from four sea algae (wakame, sea trumpet, hizikia, sea lettuce). The phenolic compounds in one of the beverages (48.3 mg/g dry matter) were similar to those in green tea (50.7 mg/g dry matter) of equivalent amounts. The antioxidant activity of the algae correlated with their polyphenol contents; the researchers concluded that the algae had high antioxidant properties. From their evaluation of three brown seaweeds from India, Chandini, Ganesan, & Bhaskar (2008) concluded that sea algae can be utilized as a source of natural antioxidant compounds as their crude extracts and fractions exhibit antioxidant activity.

Another brown alga haba-nori (*Petalonia binghamiae* (J. Agaradh) Vinogradova) is consumed as a traditional food along the fisheries town areas in Japan (Kuda, Hishi, & Maekawa, 2006). It is usually dried then lightly roasted for consumption. There are limited reports regarding the bioactivity of dried algae plants (Kuda, Tsunekawa, Hishi, & Araki, 2005). Kuda *et al.* (2006) examined the beneficial properties of *P. binghamiae* for human food, and found that the water extract was a rich source of phenolic compounds with reducing power and radical scavenging activity. The radical scavenging activity was described as being promoted by heat treatment such as retorting and the antioxidant activities were dependent on the phenolic compounds (Kuda *et al.*, 2006).

Kuda *et al.* (2005) also investigated another brown alga, *Scytosiphon lomentaria*. The dried product of *Scytosiphon lomentaria* (*Scytosiphonales, Phaeophyceae*) called kayamo-nori in Japan, is consumed as a traditional food in the Noto, Ishikawa area of Japan (Kuda *et al.*, 2005). It is eaten after drying and roasting lightly. Kuda *et al.* (2005) pointed out that *S. lomentaria* is not usually soaked before eating as is the case with other dried algae, which are usually eaten after swelling with 20 to 40 volumes of water. The researchers demonstrated that *S. lomentaria* contained total

phenols and showed strong antioxidant properties. Jiménez-Escrig, Jiménez-Jiménez, Pulido and Sauro-Calixto. (2001) reported that the radical scavenging activity of a brown alga *Fucus* was decreased by 98% after drying at 50°C for 48 hours.

22.8.3.4 Safety of Edible Algae

It has been reported that the arsenic content of *H. fusiforme* extract is high (Nagai & Yukimoto, 2003). According to Araki (1983), drying and storage reduce the bioactive compounds in algal products. Prabhasankar *et al.* (2009) reported that fucoxanthin was not affected when pasta was prepared with wakame as well as an additional cooking step.

Bioactive compounds found in edible sea algae have great potential for increased use in diets and chronic disease prevention if further researched.

22.9 CONCLUSION

In most developing and developed countries traditional foods are included in the daily diets; therefore they could play an important role in the prevention of chronic diseases. This chapter supports the idea that some traditional/ethnic foods are good sources of bioactive compounds. Indeed, the foods discussed in this chapter have been reported to contain bioactive compounds in high levels. While it is recognized that yerba mate has excellent bioactive compounds, the presence of contaminants or its safety has not been extensively documented. Pulque contains steroidal saponins and various other micronutrients, while Rooibos contains bioactive compounds, which may help protect against free radical damage that can lead to cancer, heart attack, and stroke. Unfermented (green) Rooibos has higher amounts of polyphenols than traditionally fermented Rooibos, and generally demonstrates higher antioxidant and antimutagenic capabilities *in vitro*. The bioactive compounds reported for Java plum included: sterols, triterpenes, coumarins, tannins, glycosides, alkaloids, reducing compounds, anthocyanin pigments and saponins. Mango and possibly its derived products are rich sources of bioactive compounds; however, the safety aspects and effect of processing on these have not yet been very well studied. Bioactive compounds identified in brown sea algae, *Scytosiphon lomentaria* (*Scytosiphonales, Phaeophyceae*) and *Petalonia binghamiae* (J. Agaradh) Vinogradova include: phylopheophylin, phlorotannins, fucoxanthin and various other metabolites.

Even though the evidence is accumulating for the beneficial effects of bioactive compounds, the database remains incomplete and fragmented. Much of the evidence for the beneficial effects of bioactive compounds in traditional foods come primarily from *in vitro* and animal models with short duration, which frequently use pharmacological doses; much more than is consumed in the diet. Furthermore, little is known about absorption, bioavailability and safety of bioactive compounds in human cells. Bioavailability from different kinds of bioactive compounds will probably vary greatly, given the current variations in concentrations reported from food to food.

22.10 FUTURE SCOPE

The current chapter is a small effort in the direction of highlighting the benefits and safety of traditional/ethnic foods and their role in the prevention of chronic diseases. Although research has been done to evaluate the composition, beneficial effect and safety of traditional/ethnic foods, much more work needs to be done to develop a comprehensive, globalized database. National and local governments, health agencies, scientists, international organizations, community-based organizations (CBOs) and non-governmental organizations (NGOs)

should come forward to ensure the research is conducted to meet this urgent need. Such a database will have the potential to meet increasing consumer demand for foods to address and prevent chronic diseases.

In general, there is an urgent need for long term systematic studies involving humans to evaluate the benefits, safety and bioavailability of traditional/ethnic foods. Also, food preparation methods of traditional/ethnic foods need to be researched with emphasis on the best methods to preserve the bioactive compounds, without impacting on sensory, nutritional and consumer properties. Further research is needed to establish the safety of these foods and their potential as possible natural substitutes for the prevention of chronic disease.

Specifically, the functional effect of saponins in Pulque has not been clearly elucidated; this warrants further research. The possibility of bacterial contamination during the processing of Pulque also needs to be addressed in future research studies. The bioavailability, tissue distribution and biological activities of the bioactive compounds in Rooibos need to be further researched. Further research is also needed to determine whether the bioactive compounds of Rooibos observed *in vitro* and in animals translate into health benefits for humans. Much more research is needed to determine the safety of Java plum and mango, and to determine whether the bioactive compounds in the mango are still intact in the derived products. Bioactive compounds found in edible sea algae have great potential for increased use in diets and chronic disease prevention if further researched.

Much more research and information campaigns on bioactive compounds in these traditional/ethnic foods might have the potential to improve the health situation globally in a reasonable and sustainable way. As the food system becomes more globalized and harmonized, traditional/ethnic foods, which have many health benefits, may be able to alleviate the development of chronic diseases. The notion of the bioactivity, benefits and safety of traditional/ethnic foods constitutes a very interesting topic, which requires further research.

ACKNOWLEDGEMENTS

The author wishes to thank Mr. Larry Keener for the pivotal role he played in making this chapter a reality. Also, the Food and Nutritional Sciences Advisory Board, Department of Food and Nutritional Sciences, Tuskegee University for their role in making the chapter possible.

References

ADA. (2004). American Dietetic Association. Position paper of the American Dietetic Association: Functional foods. *Journal of the American Dietetic Association, 104*, 814–826.

Araki, S. (1983). Processing of dried porphyra (nori). In: The Japanese Society of Scientific Fisheries (Ed.), *Biochemistry and utilization of marine algae*. Tokyo: Koseisha Koseikaku (in Japanese).

Aquino, R., Conti, C., deSimone, F., et al. (1991). Antiviral activity of constituents of *Tamus communis*. *Journal of Chemotherapy, 3*, 305–309.

Backstrand, J. R., Allen, L. H., Black, A. K., et al. (2002). Diet and iron status of nonpregnant women in rural Central Mexico. *The American Journal of Clinical Nutrition, 76*, 156–164.

Backstrand, J. R., Allen, L. H., Martinez, E., & Pelto, G. H. (2001). Maternal consumption of Pulque, a traditional central Mexican alcoholic beverage: Relationships to infant growth and development. *Public health nutrition, 4*, 883–891.

Banerjee, A., Dasgupta, N., & De, B. (2005). *In vitro* study of antioxidant activity of *Syzygium cumini* fruit. *Food Chemistry, 90*, 727–733.

Bastos, D. H. M., Ishimoto, E. Y., Marques, M. O. M., et al. (2006). Essential oil and antioxidant activity of green mate and mate tea (*Ilex paraguariensis*) infusions. *Journal of Food Composition and Analysis, 19*, 538–543.

Bazzano, L. A., He, J., Ogden, L. G., et al. (2002). Fruit and vegetable intake and risk of cardiovascular disease in US adults: The first National Health and Nutrition Examination Survey Epidemiologic Follow-up Study. *The American Journal of Clinical Nutrition, 76*, 93–99.

Beecher, G. R. (2003). Overview of dietary flavonoids: Nomenclature, occurrence and intake. *Journal of Nutrition, 133*, 3248S–3254S.

Berardini, N., Fezer, R., Conrad, J., et al. (2005). Screening of mango (*Mangifera indica* L.) cultivars for their contents of flavonol O- and xanthone C-glycosides, anthocyanins, and pectin. *Journal of Agricultural and Food Chemistry, 53*, 1563–1570.

Bixby, M., Spieler, L., Menini, T., & Gugliucci, A. (2005). *Ilex paraguariensis* extracts are potent inhibitors of nitrosative stress: A comparative study with green tea and wines using a protein nitration model and mammalian cell cytotoxicity. *Life Science, 77*, 345–358.

Bracesco, N., Dell, M. R. A., Behtash, S., et al. (2003). Antioxidant activity of a botanical extract preparation of *Ilex paraguariensis*: Prevention of DNA doublestrand breaks in *Saccharomyces cerevisiae* and human low-density lipoprotein oxidation. *Journal of Alternative and Complementary Medicine, 9*, 379–387.

Bramati, L., Aquilano, F., & Pietta, P. (2003). Unfermented Rooibos tea: Quantitative characterization of flavonoids by HPLC-UV and determination of the total antioxidant activity. *Journal of agricultural and food chemistry, 50*, 7472–7474.

Bravo, L., Luis, G., & Lecumberri, E. (2007). LC/MS characterization of phenolic constituents of mate (*Ilex paraguariensis*, St. Hil.) and its antioxidant activity compared to commonly consumed beverages. *Food research international, 40*, 393–405.

Brown, J. P. (1980). A review of the genetic effects of naturally occurring flavonoids, anthraquinones and related compounds. *Mutation Research, 75*, 243–277.

Cardozo, E. L., Ferrarese-Filho, O., Filho, L. C., et al. (2007). Methylxanthines and phenolic compounds in mate (Ilex paraguariensis St. Hil.) progenies grown in Brazil. *Journal of Food Composition and Analysis, 20*, 553–558.

Chandini, S. K., Ganesan, P., & Bhaskar, N. (2008). *In vitro* antioxidant activities of three selected brown seaweeds of India. *Food Chemistry, 107*, 707–713.

Chandra, S., & Gonzalez de Mejia, E. (2004). Polyphenolic compounds, antioxidant capacity, and quinone reductase activity of aqueous extract of *Ardisia compressa* in comparison to mate (*Ilex paraguariensis*) and green (*Camellia sinensis*) teas. *Journal of Agricultural and Food Chemistry, 52*, 3583–3589.

Crozier, A., Burns, J., Aziz, A., et al. (2000). Antioxidant flavonols from fruits, vegetables and beverages: Measurements and bioavailability. *Biological Research, 33*, 79–88.

Crozier, A., Jaganath, I. B., & Clifford, M. N. (2006). Phenols, polyphenols and tannins: An overview. In A. Crozier, M. N. Clifford, & H. Ashihara (Eds.), *Plant secondary metabolites* (pp. 1–24). Oxford: Blackwell Publishing Ltd.

Cushnie, T. P. T., & Lamb, A. J. (2005). Antimicrobial activity of flavonoids. *International Journal of Antimicrobial Agents, 26*, 343–356.

da Silva, E. L., Neiva, T. J. C., Shirai, M., et al. (2008). Acute ingestion of yerba mate infusion (*Ilex paraguariensis*) inhibits plasma and lipoprotein oxidation. *Food Research International*, 41, 973–979.

Davidson, A. (1999). *The oxford companion to food.* Frome, Somerset, Great Britain: Butler and Tanner Ltd pp. 831–832.

Dawczynski, C., Schubert, R., & Jahreis, G. (2007). Amino acids, fatty acids, and dietary fibre in edible seaweed products. *Food Chemistry*, 103, 891–899.

Day, L., Seymour, R. B., Pitts, K. F., et al. (2008). Incorporation of functional ingredients into foods 10.1016/j.tifs.2008.05.002. *Trends Food Science and Technology.*

Dellacassa, E., & Bandoni, A. L. (2001). El mate. *Revista de Fitoterapia*, 1, 269–278.

Denny, A., & Buttriss, J. (2008). Synthesis Report No. 4: Plant foods and health: focus on plant bioactives. EuroFIR Project Management Office/British Nutrition Foundation.

Di Gregorio, D. E., Huck, H., Aristegui, R., et al. (2004). [137]Cs contamination in tea and yerba mate in South America. *Journal of Environmental Radioactivity*, 76, 273–281.

Dos, A., Ayhan, Z., & Sumnu, G. (2005). Effects of different factors on sensory attributes, overall acceptance and preference of Rooibos (*Aspalathus linearis*) tea. *Journal of Sensory Studies*, 20, 228–242.

Erickson, L. (2003). Rooibos tea: Research into antioxidant and antimutagenic properties. *Journal of American Botanical Council*, 59, 34–45.

Escalante, A., Giles-Gómez, M., Hernández, G., et al. (2008). Analysis of bacterial community during the fermentation of Pulque, a traditional Mexican alcoholic beverage, using a polyphasic approach. *International Journal of Food Microbiology*, 14, 126–134.

Escalante, A., Rodríguez, M. E., Martínez, A., et al. (2004). Characterization of bacterial diversity in Pulque, a traditional Mexican alcoholic beverage, as determined by 16S rDNA analysis. *FEMS Microbiology Letters*, 235, 273–279.

FAO. (2007). *FAO Statistical Database, Agriculture.* http://apps.fao.org (accessed 11 February 2009).

Filip, R., López, P., Giberti, P. G., et al. (2001). Phenolic compounds in seven South American *Ilex* species. *Fitoterapia*, 72, 774–778.

Filip, R., Lotito, S. B., Ferraro, G., & Fraga, C. G. (2000). Antioxidant activity of *Ilex paraguariensis* and related species. *Nutrition Research*, 20, 1437–1446.

Fraga, C. G. (2007). Plant polyphenols: How to translate their *in vitro* antioxidant actions to *in vivo* conditions. *IUBMB Life*, 59, 308–315.

Fujiwara-Arasaki, T., Mino, N., & Kuroda, M. (1984). The protein value in human nutrition of edible marine algae in Japan. *Hydrobiologia*, 116/117, 513–516.

Gandini, S., Merzenich, H., Robertson, C., & Boyle, P. (2000). Meta analysis of studies on breast cancer risk and diet: The role of fruit and vegetable consumption and the intake of associated micronutrients. *European Journal of Cancer*, 36, 636–646.

Godoy, H., & Rodriguez-Amaya, D. B. (1989). Carotenoid composition of commercial mangoes from Brazil. *Lebensmittel-Wissenschaft und-Technologie*, 22, 100–103.

Goldberg, B. M., & Brinckmann, A. (2000). *Herbal medicine: Expanded commission E monographs.* Newton, MA: Integrative Medicine Communications pp. 249–252.

Gorzalczany, S., Filip, R., Alonso, M.-R., et al. (2001). Choleretic effect and intestinal propulsion of 'mate' (*Ilex paraguariensis*) and its substitutes or adulterants. *Journal of Ethnopharmacol*, 75, 291–294.

Gry, J., Eriksen, F. D., Pilegaard, K., et al. (2007). EuroFIR-BASIS: A combined composition and biological activity database for bioactive compounds in plant-based food. *Trends Food Science and Technology*, 18, 434–444.

Halliwell, B. (1994). Free radicals, antioxidants and human disease: Curiosity cause or consequence. *Lancet*, 344, 721–724.

Harborne, J. B., & Baxter, H. (1999). *The Handbook of Natural Flavonoids* (Vols 1–2). Chichester, UK: John Wiley and Sons.

Health Canada. (2004). Final policy paper on nutraceuticals/functional foods and health claims on foods.

Heim, K. E., Tagliaferro, A. R., & Bobilya, D. J. (2002). Flavonoid antioxidants: Chemistry, metabolism and structure-activity relationships. *The Journal of Nutritional Biochemistry*, 13, 572–584.

Hesseling, P. B., & Joubert, J. R. (1982). The effect of rooibos tea on the type I allergic reaction. *South African Medical Journal*, 62, 1037–1038.

Hosokawa, M., Bhaskar, N., Sashima, T., & Miyashita, K. (2006). Fucoxanthin as a bioactive and nutritionally beneficial marine carotenoid, A review. *Carotenoid Science*, 10, 15–28.

Jagetia, G. C., & Baliga, M. S. (2005). Radioprotection by mangiferin in Dbaxc57bl mice: A preliminary study. *Phytomedicin*, 12, 209–215.

Jiménez-Escrig, A., Jiménez-Jiménez, I., Pulido, R., & Saura-Calixto, F. (2001). Antioxidant activity of fresh and processed edible seaweeds. *Journal of the Science of Food and Agriculture*, 81, 530–534.

Joubert, E. (1996). HPLC quantification of the dihydro-chalcones, aspalathin and nothogagin in rooibos tea (*Aspalathus linearis*) as affected by processing. *Food Chemistry*, 55, 403–411.

Joubert, E., Gelderblom, W. C. A., Louw, A., & de Beer, D. (2008). South African herbal teas: *Aspalathus linearis*, *Cyclopia* spp. and *Athrixia phylicoides*, A review. *Journal of Ethnopharmacol*, 119, 376–412.

Juráni, M., Lamošová, D., Máčajová, M., et al. (2008). Effect of rooibos tea (*Aspalathus linearis*) on Japanese quail growth, egg production and plasma metabolites. *British Poultry Science*, 49, 55–64.

Kato, A., Miura, T., & Fukunaga, T. (1995). Effects of steroidal glycosides on blood glucose in normal and diabetic mice. *Biological and Pharmaceutical Bulletin*, *18*, 167–168.

Khokhar, S., Gilbert, P. A., Moyle, C. W. A., et al. (2009). Harmonised procedures for producing new data on the nutritional composition of ethnic foods. *Food Chemistry*, *113*, 816–824.

Kim, J.-Y., & Kwon, O. (2009). Garlic intake and cancer risk: An analysis using the food and drug administration's evidence-based review system for the scientific evaluation of health claims. *The American Journal of Clinical Nutrition*, *89*, 257–264.

Kim, Y., Brecht, J. K., & Talcott, S. T. (2007). Antioxidant phytochemical and fruit quality changes in mango (*Mangifera indica* L.) following hot water immersion and controlled atmosphere storage. *Food Chemistry*, *105*, 1327–1334.

Kim, Y., Lounds-Singleton, A. J., & Talcott, S. T. (2009). Antioxidant phytochemical and quality changes associated with hot water immersion treatment of mangoes (*Mangifera indica* L.). *Food Chemistry*, *15*(3), 989–993.

Koeppen, B. H. (1970). C-glycosyl compounds in Rooibos tea. *Food Industries of South Africa*, *49*(April).

Koeppen, B. H., & Roux, D. G. (1965). Aspalathin: A novel C-glycosylflavonoid from Aspalathin linearis. *Tetrahedron Letters*, *39*, 3497–3503.

Kolonel, L. N., Hankin, J. H., Whittemore, A. S., et al. (2000). Vegetables, fruits, legumes and prostate cancer: A multiethnic case-control study. *Cancer Epidemiol Biomark Prevention*, *9*, 795–804.

Kuda, T., Hishi, T., & Maekawa, S. (2006). Antioxidant properties of dried product 'haba-nori', an edible brown alga, *Petalonia binghamiae* (J. Agaradh) Vinogradova. *Food Chemistry*, *98*, 545–550.

Kuda, T., Tsunekawa, M., Hishi, T., & Araki, Y. (2005). Antioxidant properties of dried 'kayamo-nori', a brown alga *Scytosiphon lomentaria* (*Scytosiphonales, Phaeophyceae*). *Food Chemistry*, *89*, 617–622.

Kunishiro, K., Tai, A., & Yamamoto, I. (2001). Effects of rooibos extract on antigen-specific antibody production and cytokine generation *in vitro* and *in vivo*. *Bioscience, biotechnology, and biochemistry*, *65*, 2137–2145.

Lacaille-Dubois, M.-A. (2005). Bioactive saponins with cancer related and immunomodulatory activity: Recent developments. *Studies in Natural Products Chemistry* Elsevier, *32*, pp. 209–246.

Lamosova, D., Jurani, M., Greksak, M., et al. (1997). Effect of Rooibos tea (*Aspalathus linearis*) on chick skeletal muscle cell growth in culture. *Comparative Biochemistry and Physiology. Part C, Pharmacology, toxicology & endocrinology*, *116*, 39–45.

Leatherhead Food International. (2004). *The European ethnic foods market report* (2nd ed.). Leatherhead: LFI.

Leatherhead Food International. (2007). *The European ethnic foods market report* (3rd ed.). Leatherhead: LFI.

Malinow, M. R. (1985). Effects of synthetic glycosides on cholesterol absorption. *Annals of the New York Academy of Sciences*, *454*, 23–27.

Marnewick, J. L., Gelderblom, W. C. A., & Joubert, E. (2000). An investigation on the antimutagenic properties of South African herbal teas. *Mutation research*, *471*, 157–166.

Marnewick, J. L., Joubert, E., Swart, P., et al. (2003). Modulation of hepatic drug metabolizing enzymes and oxidative status by green and black (*Camellia sinensis*), rooibos (*Aspalathus linearis*) and honeybush (*Cyclopia intermedia*) teas in rats. *Journal of agricultural and food chemistry*, *51*, 8113–8119.

Masibo, M., & He, Q. (2008). Major mango polyphenols and their potential significance to human health. *Compr Rev Food Sci Food Safety*, *7*, 309–319.

McAnlis, G. T., McEneny, J., Pearce, J., & Young, I. S. (1999). Absorption and antioxidant effects of quercetin from onions, in man. *European Journal of Clinical Nutrition*, *53*, 92–96.

McKay, D. L., & Blumberg, J. B. (2007). A review of the bioactivity of South African herbal teas: Rooibos (*Aspalathus linearis*) and Honeybush (*Cyclopia intermedia*). *Phytotherapy research*, *21*, 1–16.

Miyashita, K., & Hosokawa, M. (2008). Beneficial health effects of seaweed carotenoid, fucoxanthin. In C. Barrow & F. Shahidi (Eds.), *Marine nutraceuticals and functional foods* (pp. 297–320). Boca Raton, USA: CRC Press.

Morton, J. F. (1983). Rooibos tea, *Aspalathus linearis*, a caffeineless, low-tannin beverage. *Economic Botany*, *37*, 164–173.

Muruganandan, S., Gupta, S., Kataria, M., et al. (2005). Mangiferin protects the streptozotocin-induced oxidative damage to cardiac and renal tissues in rats. *Toxicology and pharmacology*, *176*, 165–173.

Nagai, T., & Yukimoto, T. (2003). Preparation and functional properties of beverages made from sea algae. *Food Chemistry*, *81*, 327–332.

Nakano, M., Itoh, Y., Mizuno, T., et al. (1997a). Polysaccharide from *Aspalathus linearis* with strong anti-HIV activity. *Bioscience, biotechnology, and biochemistry*, *61*, 267–271.

Nakano, M., Nakashima, H., & Itoh, Y. (1997b). Anti-human immunodeficiency virus activity of oligosaccharides from rooibos tea (*Aspalathus linearis*) extracts *in vitro*. *Leukemia*, *11*, 128–130.

Ndyomugyenyi, K.E. (2008). *Nutritional evaluation of Java plum (Syzygium cumini) beans in broiler diets. MSc. Thesis*. Available at Makerere University Library, pp. 35–39.

Oldewage-Theron, W. H., Dicks, E. G., Napier, C. E., & Rutengwe, R. (2005). Situation analysis of an informal settlement in the Vaal Triangle. *Development Southern Africa*, *22*, 13–26.

Peña-Alvarez, A., Díaz, L., Medina, A., et al. (2004). Characterization of three *Agave* species by gas chromatography and solid-phase microextraction–gas chromatography–mass spectrometry. *Journal of Chromatography. A*, *1027*, 131–136.

Peng, J. P., Chen, H., Qiao, Y. Q., et al. (1996). Two new steroidal saponins from Allium sativum and their inhibitory effects on blood coagulability. *Acta Pharmacol Sinica*, *31*, 613–616.

Pietta, P. G. (2000). Flavonoids as antioxidants. *Journal of Natural Products*, *63*, 1035–1042.

Prabhasankar, P., Ganesan, P., Bhaskar, N., et al. (2009). Edible Japanese seaweed, wakame (*Undaria pinnatifida*) as an ingredient in pasta: Chemical, functional and structural evaluation. *Food Chemistry*, *15*(2), 501–508.

Prediger, R. D. S., Fernandes, M. S., Rial, D., et al. (2008). Effects of acute administration of the hydroalcoholic extract of mate tea leaves (*Ilex paraguariensis*) in animal models of learning and memory. *Journal of Ethnopharmacology*, *120*, 465–473.

Rabe, C., Steenkamp, J. A., Joubert, E., et al. (1994). Phenolic metabolites from Rooibos tea (*Aspalathus linearis*). *Phytochem*, *35*, 1559–1565.

Randle, P. J., Garland, P. B., Hales, C. N., & Newsholme, E. A. (1963). The glucose-fatty acid cycle, its role in insulin sensitivity and metabolic disturbances in diabetes mellitus. *Lancet*, *1*, 785–789.

Ravikumar, P. R., Hammesfahr, P., & Sih, C. J. (1979). Cytotoxic saponins form the Chinese herbal drug Yunnan Bai Yao. *Journal of Pharmaceutical Sciences*, *68*, 900–903.

Ribeiro, S. M. R., Barbosa, L. C. A., Queiroz, J. H., et al. (2008). Phenolic compounds and antioxidant of Brazilian mango (*Mangifera indica* L.) varieties. *Food Chemistry*, *110*, 620–626.

Ribeiro, S. M. R., de Queiroz, J. M., Lopes, M. A., et al. (2007). Antioxidant in mango (*Mangifera indica* L.) pulp. *Plant Foods for Human Nutrition*, *62*, 13–17.

Saba, A., & Messina, F. (2003). Attitudes towards organic foods and risk/benefit perception associated with pesticides. *Food Quality and Preference*, *14*, 637–645.

Santos, W. N., Bernardo, R. R., Pecanha, L. M. T., et al. (1997). Haemolytic activities of plant saponins and adjuvants. Effect of Periandra mediterranea saponin on the humoral response to the FML antigen of Leishmania donovani. *Vaccine*, *15*, 1024–1029.

Sauvaire, Y., Ribes, G., Baccou, J. C., & Loubatierés-Mariani, M. M. (1991). Implication of steroid saponins and sapogenins in the hypocholesterolemic effect of fenugreek. *Lipids*, *26*, 191–197.

Scalbert, A., & Williamson, G. (2000). Dietary intake and bioavailability of polyphenols. *The Journal of nutrition*, *130*, 2073–2085.

Schieber, A., Ullrich, W., & Carle, R. (2000). Characterization of polyphenols in mango puree concentrate by HPLC with diode array and mass spectrometric detection. *Innov Food Sci Emerg Technol*, *1*, 161–166.

Schinella, G. R., Troiani, G., Dávila, V., et al. (2000). Antioxidant effects of Na aqueous extract of *Ilex paraguariensis*. *Biochemical and Biophysical Research Communications*, *269*, 357–360.

Schulz, H., Joubert, E., & Schutze, W. (2003). Quantification of quality parameters for reliable evaluation of green rooibos (*Aspalathus linearis*). *European Food Research and Technology*, *216*, 539–543.

Seafoodplus (2008). *Seafoodplus web page*; www.seafoodplus.org/fileadmin/files/news/2004-01-22SFRTD1launchBrussels.pdf (accessed 11 February 2009).

Sewram, V., De Stefani, E., Brennan, P., & Boffetta, P. (2003). Mate consumption and the risk of squamous cell esophageal cancer in Uruguay. *Cancer Epidemiology, Biomarkers and Prevention*, *12*, 508–513.

Shimamura, N., Miyase, T., Umehara, K., et al. (2006). Phytoestrogens from Aspalathus linearis. *Biological and Pharmaceutical Bulletin*, *29*, 1271–1274.

Shiratori, K., Ohgami, I., Ilieva, X., et al. (2005). Effects of fucoxanthin on lipopolysaccharide-induced inflammation *in vitro* and *in vivo*. *Experimental Eye Research*, *81*, 422–428.

Sigler, K., & Ruch, R. J. (1993). Enhancement of gap junctional intercellular communication in tumor promoter-treated cells by components of green tea. *Cancer Letters*, *69*, 5–9.

Sissing, A. (2008). Investigations into the cancer modulating properties of *Aspalathus linearis* (rooibos), *Cyclopia intermedia* (honeybush) and *Sutherlandia frutescens* (cancer bush) in oesophageal carcinogenesis. MSc Thesis. Available at the University of the Western Cape, Bellville, South Africa.

Sparg, S. G., Light, M. E., & van Staden, J. (2004). Biological activities and distribution of plant saponins. *Journal of Ethnopharmacology*, *94*, 219–243.

Stangeland, T., Remberg, S. F., & Lye, K. A. (2009). Total antioxidant activity in 35 Ugandan fruits and vegetables. *Food Chemistry*, *113*, 85–91.

Stoilova, I., Gargova, S., Stoyanova, A., & Ho, L. (2005). Antimicrobial and antioxidant activity of the polyphenol mangiferin. *Haematologica Polonica*, *51*, 37–44.

Sung, M. K., Kendall, C. W. C., & Rao, A. V. (1995). Effect of saponins and gypsophila saponin on morphology of colon carcinoma cells in culture. *Food Chemical Toxicology*, *33*, 357–366.

Tejasari. (2007). Evaluation of ginger (*Zingiber officinale* Roscoe) bioactive compounds in increasing the ratio of T-cell surface molecules of CD3 + CD4:CD3 + CD8 + In-Vitro. *Mal Journal of Nutrition*, *13*, 161–170.

Tinto, W. F., Simmons-Boyce, J. L., McLean, S., & Reynolds, W. F. (2005). Constituents of agave Americana and agave barbadensis. *Fitoterapia*, *76*, 594–597.

Ulicná, O., Vancová, O., Božek, P., et al. (2006). Rooibos tea (*Aspalathus linearis*) partially prevents oxidative stress in streptozotocin-induced diabetic rats. *Physiological Research, 55,* 157–164.

Urquiaga, I., & Leighton, F. (2000). Plant polyphenol antioxidants and oxidative stress. *Biological Research, 33,* 2–11.

Veigas, J. M., Narayan, M. S., Laxman, P. M., & Neelwarne, B. (2007). Chemical nature, stability and bioefficacies of anthocyanins from fruit peel of *Syzygium cumini* Skeels. *Food Chemistry, 105,* 619–627.

Waleron, M., Waleron, K., Podhajska, A. J., & Lojkowska, E. (2002). Genotyping of bacteria belonging to the former *Erwina* genus by PCR-RFLP analysis of a *recA* gene fragment. *Microbiology, 148,* 583–595.

Wen, W., Shu, X.-O., Li, H., et al. (2009). Dietary carbohydrates, fiber, and breast cancer risk in Chinese women. *The American Journal of Clinical Nutrition, 89,* 283–289.

Yang, D.-J., Lu, T.-J., & Hwang, L. S. (2009). Effect of endogenous glycosidase on stability of steroidal saponins in Taiwanese yam (*Dioscorea pseudojaponica yamamoto*) during drying processes. *Food Chemistry, 113,* 155–159.

Yoshikawa, M., Nishida, N., Shimoda, H., et al. (2001). Polyphenol constituents from salacia species: Quantitative analysis of mangiferin with glucosidase and aldose reductase inhibitory activities. *Yakugaku Zasshi, 121,* 371–378.

Zhang, J., Meng, Z., Zhang, M., et al. (1999). Effect of six steroidal saponins isolated from Anemarrhenae rhizoma on platelet aggregation and hemolysis in human blood. *Clinica Chimica Acta, 289,* 79–88.

Further Reading

Charmaine, S. (1998). *Asia food. Encyclopedia of Asian food (Periplus editions).* Australia: New Holland Publishers Pty Ltd.

Henry, M., & Harris, K. S. (2002). *LMH Official dictionary of Jamaican herbs and medicinal plants and their uses.* LMH Publishing Ltd.

Mitchell, S. A., & Ahmad, M. H. (2006). A review of medicinal plant research at the University of the West Indies, Jamaica, 1948–2001. *The West Indian Medical Journal, 55,* 243–269.

Ricks, R. M., Vogel, P. S., Elston, D. M., & Hivnor, C. (1999). Purpuric agave dermatitis. *Journal of the American Academy of Dermatology, 40,* 356–358.

Stangeland, T., Remberg, S. F., & Lye, K. A. (2007). Antioxidants in some Ugandan fruits. *African Journal of Ecology, 45,* 29S–30S.

Vanisree, M., Alexander-Lindo, R. L., DeWitt, D. L., & Nair, M. G. (2008). Functional food components of Antigonon leptopus tea. *Food Chemistry, 106,* 487–492.

Processing Issues: Acrylamide, Furan and *Trans* Fatty Acids

Lauren S. Jackson[1] and Fadwa Al-Taher[2]

[1]US Food and Drug Administration, National Center for Food Safety and Technology,
Summit-Argo, IL, USA

[2]Illinois Institute of Technology, National Center for Food Safety and Technology,
Summit-Argo, IL, USA

23.1 INTRODUCTION

Processed foods have become a way of life in the modern world (Rupp, 2003). Processing allows for a more consistent supply of foods, increasing consumer convenience and variety and in general, increasing food safety and palatability (Rupp, 2003). Processing unit operations such as washing, trimming, milling, leaching and mechanical separation may decrease the natural toxicity of some raw materials by eliminating specific undesirable components (Sikorski, 2005). However, processing can decrease nutrient levels and bioavailability and produce chemical and physical changes that may render a food hazardous (Rupp, 2003). Thermal processing may induce the formation of harmful compounds such as various mutagens, carcinogenic heterocyclic aromatic amines, polycyclic aromatic hydrocarbons, furan, acrylamide and *N*-nitrosamines. Other detrimental chemical changes in food that can occur as the result of processing include the formation of *trans* fatty acids during the hydrogenation of fats and the creation of chloropropanols during the production of hydrolyzed vegetable protein (Hamlet & Sadd, 2009; Hunter, 2005).

Processing-induced food toxicants such as acrylamide, furan and *trans* fatty acids have now gained widespread attention. The precursors and mechanisms of formation of these compounds are different, but they all are formed during processing of food. Acrylamide and furan are formed during thermal processing of carbohydrate-rich foods via Maillard-type reactions. *Trans* fatty acids are formed when liquid oils are partially hydrogenated to improve their plasticity or oxidative stability. There have been concerns about the potential health issues associated with the dietary intake of acrylamide, furan and *trans* fatty acids. Thus, much attention has been focused on finding ways to reduce or prevent the formation of these three process-induced hazards without compromising food safety, sensory properties (e.g. taste,

texture, and color) or nutritional quality. This chapter will provide an overview of the factors affecting the formation of acrylamide, furan and *trans* fatty acids in processed food and will give a perspective on the current tools that are being used to manage these chemical hazards.

23.2 ACRYLAMIDE

23.2.1 Introduction

Acrylamide (2-propenamide) is a colorless and odorless solid at room temperature in its pure form. The compound is an industrial chemical primarily used in the preparation of polyacrylamide, a flocculant used in the treatment of the municipal water supply and for removal of suspended solids from industrial waste water before discharge. Other applications of polyacrylamide are in paper and pulp processing, as cosmetic additives, and in the formulation of grouting agents. Acrylamide is known to be a neurotoxin, a genotoxin and a carcinogen in animals, and a possible carcinogen in humans as defined by the International Agency for Research on Cancer (IARC) (IARC, 1994).

In 2002, researchers at the Swedish National Food Administration and Stockholm University reported finding acrylamide at levels over $1000\mu g/kg$ in a wide range of heated, carbohydrate-rich foods such as fried, baked and roasted potato products, breakfast cereals, breads and crackers (Tareke *et al.*, 2002). This resulted in heightened worldwide interest in determining the mechanisms by which acrylamide is formed, its occurrence and levels in food, and its effects on human health. Acrylamide is generated in foods that are subjected to high-temperature ($>120°C$) processes such as frying, baking, roasting and extrusion and can be found in industrially processed foods as well as those prepared in a food service operation or at home by the consumer. Acrylamide is generated during heat treatment as a result mainly of the Maillard reaction between certain amino acids and reducing sugars in food (Mottram, Wedzicha, & Dodson, 2002; Rydberg *et al.*, 2003; Tareke *et al.*, 2002).

Since the discovery of acrylamide in food, a wealth of information has been gathered on the levels of acrylamide in food, toxicological properties of the compound, mechanisms by which acrylamide is formed and methods for reducing the acrylamide content of food. Several excellent resources are available for obtaining up-to-date information on the status of acrylamide. For example, the FAO/WHO Acrylamide in Food Network (http://www. foodrisk.org/acrylamide/index.cfm) was established as a result of the June 2002 FAO/WHO Consultation on the Health Risks of Acrylamide in Food. This network functions as a global resource and inventory of ongoing research on acrylamide in food and includes formal research, surveillance/monitoring and industry investigations. The HEATOX project, an international multidisciplinary program funded by the European Commission from 2002 to 2007, focused on the health risks associated with hazardous compounds such as acrylamide and other similar compounds formed in heat treated carbohydrate-rich foods. Research topics explored by the HEATOX project included mechanisms of formation, impact of raw material composition, inhibiting factors, and the effects of cooking and processing methods on formation of hazardous compounds such as acrylamide. Reports on the findings from the project are available from the HEATOX website (www.heatox.org). Since this chapter serves only to summarize the current status of the acrylamide issue, the reader is referred to several comprehensive volumes (Friedman & Mottram, 2005; Skog & Alexander, 2006; Stadler & Lineback, 2009) on acrylamide and other heat-induced food toxicants, a status report on acrylamide compiled by the Council for Agricultural Science and Technology (CAST, 2006), and entire issues of *Journal of Agricultural and Food Chemistry* (volume 56, number 15) and *Food Additives and Contaminants* (volume 24, supplement 1) devoted to the topic of acrylamide in food.

23.2.2 Occurrence and Levels of Acrylamide in Food

Since the discovery of acrylamide in food in 2002, there have been considerable efforts from national regulatory agencies such as the US Food and Drug Administration (FDA), and multinational organizations such as the World Health Organization (WHO) and the European Commission's Directorate General Joint Research Center to gather data on the acrylamide content of foods. The FDA has developed a database of acrylamide levels in individually purchased foods (FDA, 2006a) and samples from a Total Diet Study (FDA, 2006b). Initially, food groups were chosen for analysis if they were previously reported to contain acrylamide or if they contributed significantly to the diet of infants or young adults. Most products were analyzed as received, while others were examined before and after cooking. FDA's exploratory data on acrylamide levels in individual foods are summarized in Table 23.1. Wide variations in levels of acrylamide have been observed in different food categories as well as in different brands of the same food category. The variations result from different levels of acrylamide precursors present and cooking or processing conditions such as temperature or time.

One of the most extensive databases on the acrylamide content of food was compiled by the European Commission (2006) and includes acrylamide levels for over 7000 food samples obtained throughout Europe. Overall, the data provided in the European Commission database are in agreement with those cited in FDA's exploratory survey.

In general, foods that contribute most to dietary exposure include processed foods such as potato products (French fries, potato chips, baked

TABLE 23.1   Summary of acrylamide levels in various food categories[1]

Food category	Acrylamide concentration (μg/kg)	Food product with highest concentration of acrylamide
Baby food	ND–130	Teething biscuits
French fries	20–1325	Baked fries
Potato chips	117–2762	Sweet potato chips
Infant formula	ND	–
Protein foods	ND–116	Grilled veggie burgers
Breads and bakery products	ND–364	Dark, rye bread, toasted
Cereals	52–1057	Wheat cereal
Snack food (other than potato chips)	12–1340	Veggie crisps
Gravies and seasonings	ND–151	Pecan liquid smoke
Nuts and nut butters	ND–457	Smokehouse almonds
Crackers	26–1540	Graham crackers
Chocolate products	ND–909	Hershey's cocoa
Canned fruits and vegetables	ND–83	Oven baked beans
Cookies	ND–955	Ginger snap
Coffee	27–609	Blend coffee and chicory; ground, not brewed
Frozen vegetables	<10	–
Dried foods	11–1184	Onion soup and dip mix
Dairy	ND–43	Evaporated milk
Fruits and vegetables	ND–1925	Ripe olives
Hot beverages	93–5399	Instant hot beverage; powdered, not brewed
Juice	267	Prune
Taco, tostada, and tortilla products	29–794	Original tostadas
Miscellaneous	ND–804	Toasted corn

[1]Data from FDA (2006b).
ND = Not Detected (<LOQ of analysis—10 ng/g).

potatoes), bakery and cereal products (bread, cereal, crackers, cookies, cakes), and coffee. Table 23.2 lists the top 20 foods that contribute the most acrylamide to the US diet. The top acrylamide sources differ from country to country due to differences in the national diet and the manner in which foods are prepared (CAST, 2006; Mills, Mottram, & Wedzicha, 2009). Although cereals are a major dietary source of acrylamide, the percentage of total acrylamide that cereals contribute varies for different populations, ranging from ~24% in the diet of Swedish adults to ~44% in the diet of Belgian adolescents, with the American diet at 40%. The contribution of potato products to total acrylamide intake ranges from ~29% for adult Norwegian women to ~69% for Dutch children/adolescents with ~38% for the US population (Bagdonaite, Derler, & Murkovi, 2008; Dybing, *et al.*, 2005; FDA, 2006c).

The contribution of coffee to the dietary intake of acrylamide varies widely demographically and can be high in countries with

TABLE 23.2 Top 20 foods contributing acrylamide to the US diet[1]

Food category	Mean acrylamide intake (μg/kg body weight/day)	Cumulative percentile
French fries (RF)[2]	0.070	0.16
French fries (OB)[3]	0.051	0.28
Potato chips	0.045	0.38
Breakfast cereal	0.040	0.47
Cookies	0.028	0.53
Brewed coffee	0.027	0.60
Toast	0.023	0.65
Pies and cakes	0.018	0.69
Crackers	0.017	0.73
Soft bread	0.014	0.77
Chile con carne	0.014	0.80
Corn snacks	0.011	0.82
Popcorn	0.007	0.84
Pretzels	0.007	0.86
Pizza	0.006	0.87
Burrito/tostada	0.006	0.88
Peanut butter	0.003	0.89
Breaded chicken	0.003	0.90
Bagels	0.003	0.90
Soup mix	0.003	0.91

[1]Data from FDA (2006c).
[2]RF = restaurant fries.
[3]OB = oven baked.

a high coffee consumption. It ranges from ~8% for the United States, to 13% for the Netherlands, to ~28% for Norwegian adults, and to ~39% for Swedish adults (Bagdonaite et al., 2008; Dybing et al., 2005; Friedman & Levin, 2008; FDA, 2006c). These data indicate that the amount of acrylamide that coffee contributes to the diet may be important in some populations.

Estimated dietary acrylamide intake in populations has been determined by national food administrations for several countries (France,

Germany, Norway, The United Kingdom, The Netherlands, Sweden, United States) (Wenzl & Anklam, 2007; Wenzl, Lachenmeier, & Gökmen, 2007). The average dietary intake of acrylamide has been estimated by the Joint FAO/WHO Expert Committee on Food Additives (JECFA) (JECFA, 2005) for the general population as well as by different national organizations for the inhabitants of their respective countries (Wenzl et al., 2007). A daily intake of 1μg/kg body weight/day was estimated by JECFA for the average consumer, and 4μg/kg body weight/day for consumers of food items with higher concentrations of acrylamide (JECFA, 2005). These exposure estimates differ slightly with those estimated by FDA for US consumers; 0.4μg/kg body weight/day for average consumers and 1.0μg/kg body weight/day for high consumers (FDA, 2006c). Intake estimation for different countries may deviate from the above levels due to dissimilarities in the eating habits and food items consumed, and differences in the methods used to model dietary intake (Boon et al., 2005; Fohgelberg, Rosen, Hellenäs, & Abramsson-Zetterberg, 2005). A comprehensive review has been written on exposure assessment for acrylamide and the association of dietary intake with biomarkers (Dybing et al., 2005).

23.2.3 Mechanism of Formation

Research suggests that acrylamide forms in foods mainly through the Maillard reaction between reducing sugars or a source of carbonyl compounds and certain amino acids. Model systems demonstrated that asparagine is the major amino acid precursor (Becalski et al., 2004; Mottram et al., 2002; Stadler et al., 2002; Zyzak et al., 2003). This explains the occurrence of acrylamide in potato- and grain-based foods, which are particularly rich in free asparagine (Mottram et al., 2002). Maillard reaction products are also responsible for the desirable flavors and colors of heat-processed foods. Consequently, methods for preventing acrylamide formation by limiting

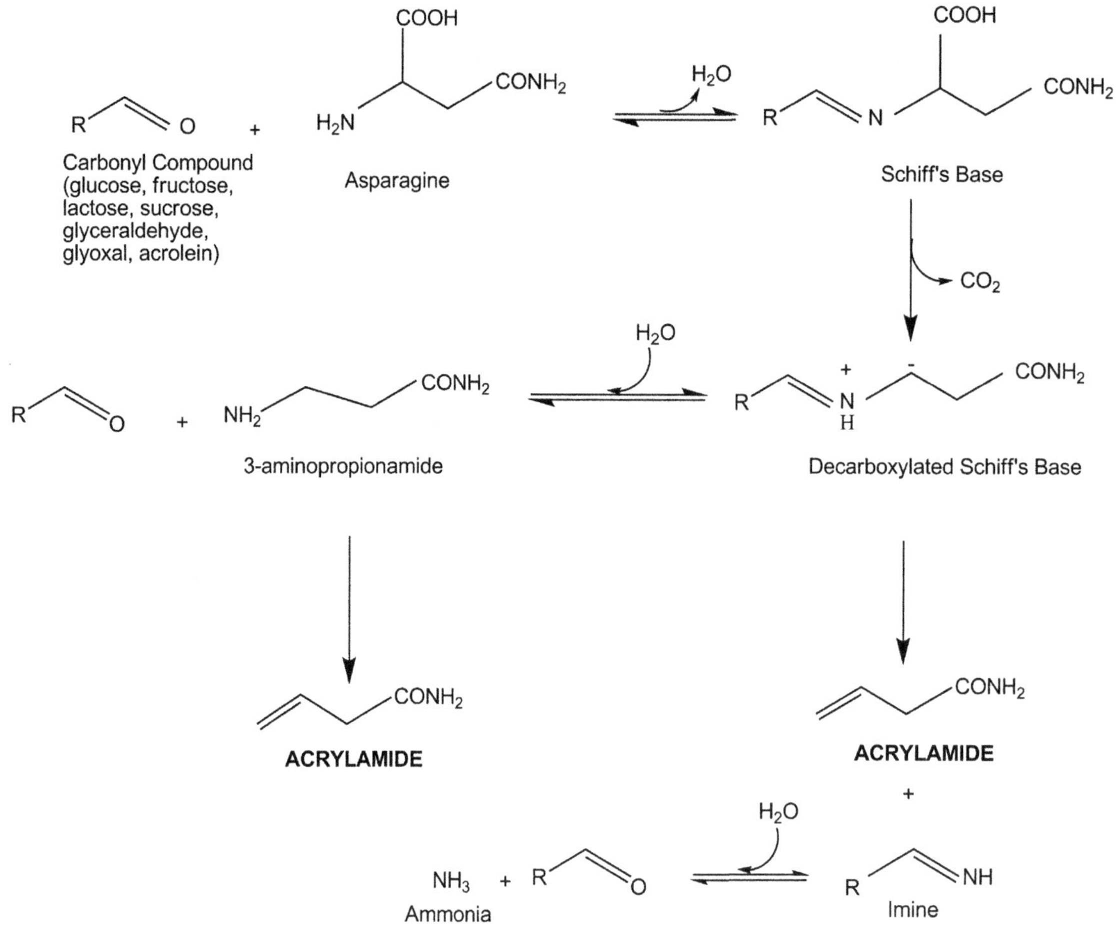

FIGURE 23.1   Mechanisms of formation of acrylamide in thermally processed/cooked food. Adapted from Friedman and Levin (2008), Blank *et al.* (2005), Yaylayan, Locas, Wronowski & O'Brien (2005), Granvogl and Schieberle (2006), Zyzak, Locas, Wronowski, & O'Brien (2003) and Claus, Weisz, Scieber, & Carle (2006).

the Maillard reaction frequently compromise the flavor and color of cooked or processed food.

Figure 23.1 shows the major pathways generating acrylamide from asparagine and a source of carbonyl compounds. Acrylamide in food is derived mainly from heat-induced reactions (temp >120°C) between the amino group of free asparagine and the carbonyl group of reducing sugars such as glucose during baking, frying and other thermal treatments. Studies have shown that the major mechanistic pathway in

the formation of acrylamide in foods involves a Schiff's base where a decarboxylation is necessary, followed by further degradation of the decarboxylated Schiff's base. This degradation step involves cleavage of a nitrogen-carbon bond, which can occur by two different mechanisms. One involves direct degradation of the decarboxylated Schiff's base to form acrylamide via elimination of an imine and the other involves hydrolysis of the decarboxylated Schiff base to yield aminopropionamide and a carbonyl compound (Blank *et al.*, 2005; Claus *et al.*, 2006; Granvogl & Schieberle, 2006; Friedman & Levin, 2008; Stadler *et al.*, 2004; Zyzak *et al.*, 2003). It is important to note that the yield of acrylamide in simple model systems is low, whereby less than 1% of asparagine is converted to acrylamide (Becalski *et al.*, 2003; Stadler *et al.*, 2002; Stadler, 2006; Surdyk, Rosén, Andersson, & Aman, 2004). These yields are even further reduced in more complex systems such as food.

The detailed mechanism at each step in the formation of acrylamide may depend on the species involved (type of carbonyl compound), the chemical environment (water content, pH) and processing or cooking temperature (Mills *et al.*, 2009). Stadler *et al.* (2002) reported equal reactivities of fructose, glucose and sucrose in model systems with asparagine at 180°C. In contrast, Claeys, DeVleeschouwer, & Hendrickx (2005) found sucrose to have roughly half the reactivity of glucose to react with asparagine to form acrylamide in the temperature range of 140 to 200°C. Although acrylamide can form in the presence of water, acrylamide tends to form in dry environments such as the crust of breads and the outer surface of fried potatoes (Friedman & Levin, 2008; Surdyk *et al.*, 2004).

23.2.4 Factors Affecting Formation

23.2.4.1 *Processing Conditions*

Processing and cooking conditions such as temperature and time are important factors affecting the levels of acrylamide in model systems and in foods (potato products, cereal-based foods, roasted almonds, coffee, etc.) (Amrein *et al.*, 2007; Friedman & Levin, 2008; Jackson & Al-Taher, 2005; Mottram *et al.*, 2002; Stadler *et al.*, 2002; Tareke *et al.*, 2002; Taubert *et al.*, 2004). However, the manner in which heat is transferred to a food (e.g. frying, baking, roasting, microwave-heating) does not impact the rate of acrylamide formation (Stadler *et al.*, 2004).

In general, acrylamide content increases in the temperature range of 120–185°C, then decreases when the food is heated at higher temperatures (Mottram *et al.*, 2002; Rydberg *et al.*, 2003; Tareke *et al.*, 2002). The mechanism(s) by which acrylamide degrades at higher temperatures have not been identified, but it has been hypothesized that acrylamide reacts further or that another reaction mechanism occurs that bypasses acrylamide (CAST, 2006).

Acrylamide levels for deep-fat fried French fries ranged from 265 μg/kg for potatoes fried at 150°C for 6 minutes to 2130 μg/kg for French fries prepared at 190°C for 5 minutes (Jackson & Al-Taher, 2005). At frying temperatures of 180–190°C, acrylamide levels in French fries increased exponentially at the end of the frying process (Jackson & Al-Taher, 2005). In potato slices with low surface-to-volume ratios (SVRs), acrylamide levels increased with increasing frying temperatures as well as with frying time, reaching maximum levels of 2500 μg/kg. However, in samples with higher SVRs, acrylamide levels were the greatest at 160–180°C with maximal acrylamide formation of 18,000 μg/kg, then decreased with higher frying temperatures and more prolonged frying times (Taubert *et al.*, 2004).

A study assessing the effects of time and temperature on acrylamide formation in wheat bread (Surdyk *et al.*, 2004) showed that the majority (99%) of acrylamide was formed in the crust layer and that levels increased with baking time and temperature. Studies performed on the effects of baking times and temperature (180°C and 200°C) on acrylamide formation in gingerbread showed that acrylamide formation occurred linearly over a 20 min baking period (Amrein *et al.*, 2004).

Coffee is a complex matrix in terms of acrylamide formation and reduction. It has been shown that roasting time and temperature had an impact on acrylamide formation in coffee beans (Taeymans *et al.*, 2004). Although coffee beans are roasted at very high temperatures

(240–300°C), significant amounts of acrylamide are formed during the first few minutes of roasting, then levels decrease exponentially toward the end of the roasting cycle (Stadler, 2006; Taeymans *et al.*, 2004). Maximum acrylamide levels in Robusta (3800 μg/kg) and Arabica (500 μg/kg) coffee beans were found during the first minutes of the roasting process (Guenther, Anklam, Wenzl, & Stadler, 2007). Kinetic models and spiking experiments with isotope-labeled acrylamide have shown that >95% of acrylamide formed in coffee beans is degraded during roasting (Bagdonaite *et al.*, 2008). These findings may explain why light roasted coffees contain higher amounts of acrylamide than dark roasted coffees (Guenther *et al.*, 2007).

In most cases, acrylamide concentrations are highly correlated to the degree of browning on the surface (crust) of cooked or processed potato- and cereal-based foods (Amrein, Schonbachler, Escher, & Amado, 2004; CAST, 2006; Jackson & Al-Taher, 2005; Surdyk *et al.*, 2004). Since acrylamide and the brown color of cooked foods are formed during the Maillard reaction, it is likely that acrylamide is formed parallel with browning. Thus, the degree of surface browning could be used as a visual indicator of acrylamide formation during cooking. However, the extent of browning may not necessarily indicate the acrylamide content of a food when additives such as ammonium bicarbonate (Amrein *et al.*, 2004) or ingredients that contain asparagine are added (Surdyk *et al.*, 2004).

23.2.4.2 *Raw Material Composition*

The presence and concentration of precursors affect acrylamide formation, but presence of compounds that compete with reducing sugars and/or amino acids in the Maillard reaction are also important compositional factors. In potato products, acrylamide levels are highly correlated with glucose and fructose concentrations in the uncooked potato tubers, whereas asparagine levels do not predict acrylamide levels in cooked potato products (Amrein *et al.*, 2003; Becalski *et al.*,

2004; CAST, 2006; Haase, 2006). When prepared under similar conditions, acrylamide contents of thermally-processed potato products can vary depending on potato cultivar mainly due to the variability in the reducing sugar content of the different cultivars (Amrein *et al.*, 2003; Haase, 2006).

The high variability in reducing sugar content among potatoes of the same cultivar suggest that storage conditions may have a stronger influence on sugar content of raw potato tubers than cultivar (Noti *et al.*, 2003). Short-term storage of potatoes at 4°C (e.g. in the refrigerator of a supermarket) significantly increases the potential for acrylamide formation (Biedermann *et al.*, 2002; Noti *et al.*, 2003). Cooling potatoes to temperatures less than 10°C causes the reducing sugars to increase thus, increasing the potential for acrylamide formation (Biedermann *et al.*, 2002; Jackson & Al-Taher, 2005; Noti *et al.*, 2003). Reconditioning of potatoes at room temperature following cold storage, results in significant reductions in the content of reducing sugars and the acrylamide forming potential (Haase, 2006).

Lowering the amount of nitrogen fertilizer resulted in a 30–65% increase in acrylamide levels in fried potato products. In addition to fertilizer application rate, dry and hot weather seems to increase acrylamide formation by increasing the content of reducing sugars in potato cultivars (De Wilde *et al.*, 2006). These studies indicate that acrylamide content of potato products can be reduced through agricultural practices and by carefully selecting potato cultivars with low levels of reducing sugars.

In cereal-based foods, acrylamide levels are more highly correlated with levels of asparagine rather than reducing sugars (Konings, Ashby, Hamlet, & Thompson, 2007). No correlation was reported between reducing sugar and acrylamide contents of heated flour or breads (Claus *et al.*, 2006). In contrast, asparagine levels of the flour significantly affected acrylamide contents with levels differing by a factor of five due to marked differences in free asparagine and crude protein contents.

Use of nitrogen fertilizers during the growth of cereal crops caused an increase in amino acid and protein contents of the grain, thus increasing acrylamide levels in bread products (Claus et al., 2006). Therefore, to minimize acrylamide levels, nitrogen fertilization should be adjusted to the minimum requirement of the crops.

23.2.5 Prevention and Mitigation

International food monitoring agencies in collaboration with the food industry and academia have put forth strategies for reducing acrylamide levels in food. Food manufacturers in Europe have worked with researchers through the Confederation of the Food and Drink Industries of the EU (CIAA) to produce a series of guidelines known as the 'CIAA Acrylamide Toolbox' for reducing acrylamide levels in different food classes (potato products, cereal-based foods, coffee and coffee mixtures) (CIAA, 2006). Designing mitigation strategies is often a challenge since methods that reduce acrylamide can adversely affect food quality and safety.

Acrylamide mitigation strategies fall into five major categories: methods that interrupt reactions leading to acrylamide formation, treatments that reduce the levels of acrylamide precursors, approaches that reduce the cooking or processing time and/or temperature, procedures that change the product recipe or formulation, and agronomic methods (Amrein et al., 2004; CAST, 2006; Jung, Choi, & Ju, 2003; Mestdagh et al., 2008; Muttucumaru et al., 2008; Taubert et al., 2004). These mitigation strategies are summarized below and described in detail by Friedman and Levin (2008), Konings et al. (2007), Guenther et al. (2007) and Foot, Haase, Grob, & Gondé (2007).

23.2.5.1 Methods that Interrupt Reactions Leading to Acrylamide Formation

Several approaches have been somewhat successful at inhibiting acrylamide formation by preventing the key reactions responsible for generating the compound. Lowering the pH of foods blocks the nucleophilic addition of asparagine with a carbonyl compound, preventing the formation of the Schiff's base, a critical intermediate in the formation of acrylamide (Mestdagh et al., 2008). Although this approach was successful at lowering acrylamide levels in fried potato products (Jackson & Al-Taher, 2005; Jung et al., 2003), treatments that lower the pH of foods may cause foods to have an undesirable taste (Pedreschi, Kack, & Granby, 2008). Another approach that reduces acrylamide by preventing Schiff's base formation includes the addition of mono- and divalent cations (Na^+ or Ca^{2+}) to foods (Gökmen & Senyuva, 2007; Lindsay & Jang, 2005; Park et al., 2005; Mestdagh et al., 2008; Sadd, Hamlet, & Liang, 2008). The addition of proteins or free amino acids other than asparagine (lysine, glutamine, glycine, cysteine) was studied as a method for reducing acrylamide formation by causing competitive reactions and/or covalently binding acrylamide via Michael addition reactions (Claeys et al., 2005; Hanley et al., 2005; Mestdagh et al., 2008; Sadd et al., 2008). These additions had low to moderate success at reducing acrylamide levels in both potato and cereal-based foods.

23.2.5.2 Treatments that Reduce the Levels of Acrylamide Precursors

Since reducing sugars and free asparagine are the major acrylamide precursors in food, removing either of these substrates is a strategy for reducing acrylamide formation (CAST, 2006). Procedures for reducing free asparagine and sugar levels in foods include rinsing and blanching treatments, use of asparaginase or microorganisms (fermentation), and control of storage conditions (potato products).

Rinsing, soaking and blanching treatments have been effective at reducing acrylamide formation in potato products (Jackson & Al-Taher, 2005; Grob et al., 2003; Pedreschi et al., 2008).

Soaking potato slices in room temperature water for at least 15 min before frying resulted in over 50% reduction in acrylamide (Grob *et al.*, 2003; Jackson & Al-Taher, 2005). Blanching slices in warm or hot water removed more glucose and asparagine from the potatoes than did water immersion (Pedreschi *et al.*, 2008). Soaking and blanching treatments reduce acrylamide formation by leaching out sugars and asparagine from the surface of the potato slice.

Use of asparaginase, an enzyme that hydrolyzes asparagine into aspartic acid and ammonia, has been successful at reducing acrylamide levels in potato and wheat-based bakery products (Amrein *et al.*, 2004; Ciesarova, Kiss, & Boegl, 2006; Pedreschi *et al.*, 2008; Vass *et al.*, 2004; Zyzak *et al.*, 2003). Amrein *et al.* (2004) reported that asparaginase treatment of gingerbread dough resulted in a 75% decrease in free asparagine and a 55% reduction in acrylamide levels in the baked product. At present, two commercial asparaginase preparations are available: Acrylaway® derived from *Aspergillus oryzae* (Novozymes, Denmark) and Preventase™ produced by *Aspergillus niger* (DSM Food Specialties, Denmark). The generally recognized as safe (GRAS) status from the FDA has now been obtained for asparaginase from *Aspergillus niger* (FDA, 2009).

Extensive fermentation with yeast is a way to reduce acrylamide content of bread by eliminating free asparagine (Konings *et al.*, 2007; Fredricksson, Tallving, Rosen, & Aman, 2004). Prolonged (2 hour) fermentation of whole wheat and rye dough caused an 87 and 77% reduction in acrylamide concentrations in whole grain and rye breads, respectively (Fredricksson *et al.*, 2004). Sourdough fermentation was less effective than yeast fermentation in reducing the asparagine content of the dough (Fredricksson *et al.*, 2004).

Several ingredients may increase acrylamide formation during baking of cereal-based products. A study by Amrein *et al.* (2004) showed that the baking agent, ammonium bicarbonate, enhanced acrylamide formation in bakery products by possibly creating more reactive carbonyl compounds. Use of sodium hydrogen carbonate as an alternative baking agent reduced acrylamide content by more than 60% (Amrein *et al.*, 2004). Similarly, use of sucrose rather than honey or inverted sugar syrup can reduce acrylamide formation in cookies, breads and cakes (Gökmen, Acar, Köksel, & Acar, 2007; Amrein *et al.*, 2004).

23.2.5.3 Changing Processing/Cooking Conditions

Acrylamide levels in foods can be reduced by reducing cooking times and temperatures. However, since the Maillard reaction which is responsible for acrylamide formation, also guarantees desirable flavor and color compounds in heated food, reducing the cooking time and temperature may compromise food color, flavor and texture. Conditions that minimize acrylamide in French fries involve frying or baking potato pieces as long as necessary to get the surface golden in color and the texture crispy (Grob *et al.*, 2003; Jackson & Al-Taher, 2005). Overall, the available information suggests that prolonged baking or excessive browning should be avoided to minimize acrylamide formation in baked cereal-based foods (Konings *et al.*, 2007). Since acrylamide formation increases linearly in the baking process, an important factor for minimizing acrylamide formation is to determine the proper cooking end-point. This indicates that the degree of surface browning could be used as a visual indicator of acrylamide formation during cooking.

23.2.5.4 Agronomic Factors

Selective breeding of potatoes or cereal grains is a potential method for controlling acrylamide levels by decreasing levels of acrylamide precursors (reducing sugars and asparagine, respectively) (CAST, 2006). Since 2002, several groups of researchers have demonstrated the importance of variety selection on formation of acrylamide in potato products (Foot *et al.*, 2007; Grob *et al.*, 2003; Rydberg *et al.*, 2003). Amrein *et al.* (2003) found a 50-fold variation in total reducing sugars in the different potato cultivars they studied. Cultivars with low reducing sugar content were found to be more suitable for potato products (French fries, potato chips) cooked or processed at high temperatures. In addition to cultivar selection, a reverse correlation between amount of fertilizer applied in potato cultivation and acrylamide content in foods was established (De Wilde *et al.*, 2006).

Asparagine is the major determinant of the acrylamide forming potential in cereal-based products. Studies by Claus *et al.* (2006) revealed a significant impact of cultivar and fertilizer application rate on acrylamide levels in bakery products due mainly to differences in the asparagine and crude protein contents of the raw material (Konings *et al.*, 2007). A study showed that nitrogen fertilization resulted in high amounts of amino acid and protein contents, causing increased acrylamide levels in breads, ranging from 10.6 to 55.6 µg/kg (Claus *et al.*, 2006). When wheat was grown with sulfate depletion, asparagine levels were 3600–5200 µg/kg compared to 600–900 µg/kg in wheat grown in soils with proper amounts of sulfate fertilizer (Friedman & Levin, 2008).

More research is needed to understand the factors affecting acrylamide formation in food. A better understanding of these factors will enable food manufacturers to minimize the acrylamide content of food without compromising food safety and quality.

23.2.6 Health Effects of Dietary Acrylamide

Experimental studies in animals have shown acrylamide to have neurotoxic, genotoxic and carcinogenic properties (CAST, 2006; Doerge *et al.*, 2008; Klaunig, 2008; Rice, 2005; LoPachin & Gavin, 2008). Chronic acrylamide exposure was shown to be carcinogenic in rats and mice, causing tumors at many organ sites when given in drinking water or by other means (Bull *et al.*, 1984; Johnson *et al.*, 1986; Friedman, Dulak, & Stedhman, 1995; Klaunig, 2008). In mice, acrylamide increased the incidence of lung and skin tumors (Bull *et al.*, 1984). In two bioassays in rats, acrylamide administered in drinking water consistently produced mesotheliomas of the testes, thyroid tumors, and mammary gland tumors (Friedman *et al.*, 1995; Johnson *et al.*, 1986). In one of the rat bioassays, acrylamide induced formation of pituitary tumors, pheochromocytomas, and uterine and brain tumors (Johnson *et al.*, 1986).

The mechanism by which acrylamide causes cancer in laboratory animals is not clear. Genotoxic and non-genotoxic mechanisms have been suggested (Hogervorst *et al.*, 2008). In animals, acrylamide is oxidized to the epoxide glycidamide (2,3-epoxypropionamide) by an enzymatic reaction involving cytochrome P450 2E1. Both acrylamide and glycidamide can form hemoglobin adducts with amino groups of DNA (Bagdonaite *et al.*, 2008). Possible non-genotoxic mechanisms by which acrylamide can induce cancer are that acrylamide reacts with glutathione and may influence the redox status of cells, or it may interfere with DNA repair (Hogervorst *et al.*, 2008). Based on the results of rodent carcinogenicity studies, IARC deemed acrylamide to be a likely human carcinogen through the formation of glycidamide (IARC, 1994).

The FDA National Center for Toxicological Research (NCTR) has completed a 2-year chronic rodent carcinogenicity bioassay in rats and mice under the auspices of the National Toxicology Program. This assay included study of dose-response relationships, histopathology, and correlation of adduct levels in target tissues with tumor incidence. This study addressed deficiencies in early carcinogenicity assays and will provide more reliable data on the potential carcinogenic risks of acrylamide exposure

(Robin, 2007). The results of this chronic study will soon be summarized and disseminated.

More than one-third of the calories consumed by the US and European populations are derived from food that contains acrylamide (Friedman & Levin, 2008). Human dietary exposure to acrylamide is not negligible and can amount to $100 \mu g/day$ (Galesa *et al.*, 2008; Mottram *et al.*, 2004). Studies have been done to determine whether the amount of acrylamide in the human diet is an important cancer risk factor. Most of the epidemiological studies examining the relationship between dietary intake of acrylamide and cancers of the colon, rectum, kidney, bladder, and breast have found no association between intake of acrylamide-containing foods and the risk of these cancers (Mucci *et al.*, 2003; Mucci, Lindblad, Steineck, & Adami, 2004; Mucci, Adami, & Wolk, 2006; Mucci & Wilson, 2008). However, epidemiological studies conducted by Hogervorst *et al.* (2008) and Olesen, Olsen, and Frandsen (2008) have shown that dietary exposure to acrylamide increased the risks of renal cancer and ovarian cancer, respectively. Clearly, more work is needed to determine the health consequence of acrylamide from dietary sources.

23.2.7 Regulatory Status/Risk Management

Owing to its carcinogenic potential and its low limits of exposure, acrylamide is considered a potential health hazard (JECFA, 2005). Therefore, food authorities in many countries have requested food manufacturers to take measures to limit acrylamide formation in their products (Amrein, Andres, Escher, & Amado, 2007). In 2002, the German minimization concept for acrylamide was established by the Federal Office of Consumer Protection and Food Safety (BVL). The concept was based on a voluntary agreement among the BVL, the Federal Ministry of Food, Agriculture and Consumer Protection (BMELV), the German

federal state authorities, and the stakeholders of the affected industry. The aim of the minimization concept is to achieve gradual reduction of acrylamide content of foods by avoiding formation. This requires the development of mitigation procedures that lower the acrylamide content of food without changing the characteristics of the food (Göbel & Kliemant, 2007).

Currently, the FDA and other regulatory agencies are still in the information gathering stages on acrylamide and have not instituted any regulatory action (Robin, 2007). Until expert scientific committees and regulatory agencies understand the mechanisms of formation and toxicology of acrylamide more clearly, it will be difficult to set the appropriate limits for acrylamide (Mills *et al.*, 2009; Robin, 2007). The results of long-term carcinogenicity assays will soon be announced. It is likely that the outcome of these studies will shape the future for acrylamide regulation and risk management (Mills *et al.*, 2009).

The issue of acrylamide in food has been an area of discussion for the Codex Alimentarius Commission (CAC), an international body established by the WHO and FAO for the purpose of protecting the health of consumers and ensuring fair food trade practices. CAC has written a discussion paper on the topic (CAC, 2006; Mills *et al.*, 2009). The Codex Committee on Food Additives and Contaminants (CCFAC) has produced a first draft of a Code of Practice for the Reduction of Acrylamide in Foods (CAC, 2008). The Code of Practice is being developed in the international arena as a means of disseminating information that will help reduce acrylamide levels in internationally traded foods and will assist governments that are unable to investigate the issue themselves (Mills *et al.*, 2009). It consists of methods that have been established in a commercial setting for minimizing acrylamide levels in foods. The Code of Practice was finalized and considered for adoption at the 32nd Session of the Codex Alimentarius Commission (Rome, 29 June–4 July 2009).

Several national regulatory agencies and research organizations have issued advice to consumers for reducing exposure to dietary acrylamide (FDA, 2008; Health Canada, 2009; HEATOX, 2007; Food Standards Agency, 2005). Overall, these groups suggest consumers not to make major dietary changes, but to eat a balanced diet, choosing a variety of foods that are low in *trans* fat and saturated fat, and rich in high-fiber grains, fruits and vegetables.

23.3 FURAN

23.3.1 Introduction

Furan is a volatile (boiling point = 31.4°C) cyclic ether found in cigarette smoke, and is used in the production of resins and lacquers, agrochemicals, and pharmaceuticals (Goldmann, Périsset, Scanlan, & Stadler, 2005). Furan and furan derivatives have long been known to occur in heated foods and contribute to the sensory properties of food (Maga, 1979; Zoller, Sager, & Reinhard, 2007). However, attention has been brought to the presence of furan in a wide variety of heated processed foods (coffee, juices, soups, and canned and jarred fruits and vegetables, including baby foods) by the FDA following the posting on its website in 2004 of data on the occurrence of the contaminant in food. The concerns over furan stem from its classification as a 'possible carcinogen to humans' (Group 2B) (IARC, 1995), and the finding that the compound causes cancer in rodents (National Toxicology Program, 1993).

Shortly after FDA published data on furan levels in food, there was interest by the scientific and regulatory community to determine occurrence of the contaminant in different food categories, determine exposure to furan, explore the mechanisms of formation of furan, and access methods for reducing furan levels in foods. The following sections summarize the current state of information on occurrence and levels of furan in food, mechanisms of formation, processing factors, health effects and regulatory status.

23.3.2 Occurrence and Levels of Furan in Food

Since furan has become a potential food safety issue, several international food agencies such as the FDA and the European Food Safety Authority (EFSA) have launched monitoring programs to survey the furan content of selected foods and beverages (Altaki, Santos, & Galceran, 2009). However, only limited data on furan concentration in various foods and dietary exposure to furan exist (Bolger, Tao, & Dinovi, 2009).

The majority of information on furan levels in food can be obtained from surveys conducted by the FDA in 2004–2006 on furan levels in thermally treated food commodities (FDA, 2007a). Table 23.3 summarizes the data from FDA's exploratory survey on furan levels in different food categories. FDA's exploratory survey included analysis of baby and infant foods (jarred foods, infant formulas), canned mixed foods (soups, sauces, broths, chili), canned fish and meat products, canned fruit, fruit juices and vegetables, breads, nut butters, beers, and other foods. Of the foods analyzed, high levels were found in jarred infant/toddler foods (sweet potatoes, 73–108 ppb), canned baked beans (56–122 ppb), brewed coffee (34–84 ppb), and canned soups containing meat and vegetables (50–125 ppb).

Limited data are available on furan levels in food commodities obtained in Europe, Africa and Asia. In a survey of food items purchased in Spain, Altaki *et al.* (2009) reported the highest levels (820 and 1100 ppb) in powdered instant coffees and in a jarred baby food entrée containing spaghetti and beef (40 ppb). A wide variety of food items purchased in Switzerland were analyzed for furan (Reinhard, Sager, Zimmermann, & Zoller, 2004; Zoller *et al.*, 2007). Furan levels were higher in jarred baby foods containing both meat and vegetables (21–153 ppb) than

TABLE 23.3   Summary of furan levels in various food categories[1]

Food category	Furan concentration (µg/kg)	Food product with highest level of furan
Infant and toddler foods	<0.8–108	Jarred sweet potatoes
Infant formula	ND–26.9	Milk-based infant formula concentrate
Mixtures (soups, sauces, broths, chili)	<5.0–125	Vegetable beef soup
Fish	<5.0–8.1	Canned sardines in tomato sauce
Canned fruit and vegetables	ND–122	Baked Beans with Pork
Fruit and vegetable juices, punches and drinks	ND–30.5	Prune juice
Bread	ND– < 2.0	Whole wheat bread
Breakfast cereals	9.2–47.5	Corn flakes
Crackers and crispbreads	4.2–18.6	Whole grain crispbread
Baked cereal products	ND–8.9	Graham crackers
Meats	ND–31.6	Potted meat food product
Nuts and nut butters	6.1–7.5	Peanut butter
Beer	ND–1.6	–
Nutrition drinks	ND–66.5	Strawberry shake
Dairy and eggs	10.9–15.3	Evaporated milk
Fats and oils	ND–5.4	Vegetable shortening
Jams, jellies and preserves	1.2–15.9	Apple butter spread
Gravies	13.3–173.6	Roast turkey gravy
Desserts	<0.8–13	Rice pudding
Snacks	<3.2–64.7	Pretzels
Candy bars	<0.8–1.7	Chocolate bar
Chocolate drink mixes, cocoa, chocolate syrups, and chocolate drinks	<0.4–3.3	Chocolate syrup
Miscellaneous	ND–88.3	Maple syrup

ND = Not Detected.
[1]Data from FDA (2007a).

baby foods containing solely meat, vegetables or fruit. Minimal amounts of furan were found in jarred baby foods containing solely meat (3–6 ppb) or fruit (1–16 ppb). Similar to FDA's survey, Zoller *et al*. (2007) found moderate amounts (17–80 ppb) of furan in jarred vegetable foods. Breads contained up to 30 ppb furan, and the majority of the furan was present in the crust (Zoller *et al*., 2007). Ground roasted coffee beans contained up to 5900 ppb furan while brews of

the coffees contained from 13–151 ppb (Zoller *et al*., 2007).

Dietary exposure assessments to furan were developed by FDA in 2004 and revised in 2007 (FDA, 2007). The FDA 2007 assessment reported a mean and 90th percentile of 0.26 and 0.61 µg furan/kg body weight/day for 2 + -year-olds, respectively, and 0.41 and 0.99 µg furan/kg body weight/day for 0 to 1-year-olds from the consumption of adult and infant foods, respectively

TABLE 23.4 Exposure to furan from adult food types[1]

Food category	Amount of furan contributed to diet (µg/kg body weight/day)
Brewed coffee	0.15
Chili	0.04
Cereals	0.01
Salty snacks	0.01
Soups containing meat	0.01
Pork and beans	0.004
Canned pasta	0.004
Canned pasta	0.004
Canned string beans	0.004
Pasta sauces	0.001
Juices	0.001
Canned tuna (water packed)	0.000008

[1]From FDA (2007b).

(Bolger et al., 2009). Based on an exposure assessment conducted by FDA (FDA, 2007b), brewed coffee contributes the greatest proportion of furan to the adult diet followed by chili, cereals, snack foods and soups containing meat (Table 23.4).

It is clear that more work is needed to expand the database on furan levels in foods, especially for regional and ethnic foods, to determine variability between and within brands, and the effects of home cooking on furan levels. EFSA has issued a call for data on furan levels in foods and beverages. This information which will be collated in 2009, will allow a more sound dietary exposure assessment for risk assessment purposes.

23.3.3 Mechanisms of Formation

Furan forms in a wide variety of foods of different compositions suggesting several pathways to formation. Precursors that have been found to form furan during thermal treatment include: ascorbic acid and its derivatives, Maillard reaction systems containing reducing sugars and amino acids, lipids containing unsaturated fatty acids, carotenoids, and organic acids (Becalski & Seaman, 2005; Fan, 2005; Fan, Huang, & Sokorai, 2008; Frankel, Neff, Selke, & Brooks, 1987; Limacher, Kerler, Conde-Petit, & Blank, 2007; Locas & Yaylayan, 2004; Maga, 1979; Mottram, 1991). An overview of the major routes of formation of furan from amino acids, carbohydrates and ascorbic acid and polyunsaturated fatty acid precursors is shown in Figure 23.2.

Mechanistic studies on furan formation were carried out by Locas and Yaylayan (2004) using model systems containing $^{13}C_3$-labeled sugars, amino acids and ascorbic acid heated at 250°C (pyrolysis conditions). Among the precursors studied, ascorbic acid had the highest potential to form furan, followed by glycolaldehyde/ alanine>erythrose>ribose/serine>sucrose/ serine>fructose/serine>glucose/cysteine. In similar experiments, Mark et al. (2006) found that ascorbic acid had the greatest potential to form furan in simple model systems than other precursors (glyceryl trilinolenate, linolenic acid, trilinolein, and erythrose).

Ascorbic acid and its derivatives (isoascorbic acid, dehydroascorbic acid) have been shown to be a major precursor of furan formed during different processing conditions (pyrolysis, thermal decomposition, roasting, retorting, γ-irradiation) of aqueous solutions and in food (Becalski & Seaman, 2005; Fan, 2005; Fan & Geveke, 2007). In experiments using simple model systems, levels of furan formed ranged from 0.1 µmol furan/mol ascorbic acid to about 1 mmol furan/ mol ascorbic acid (Limacher et al., 2008). In more complex systems such as food, Limacher et al. (2007, 2008) found that formation of furan from ascorbic acid is significantly reduced due to competing reactions. These results illustrate the difficulty in extrapolating results from simple model systems to foods.

Pyrolysis of sugars at extreme temperatures resulted in the formation of furan and alkylated derivatives. Hexoses, pentoses, tetroses and polysaccharides generated furan

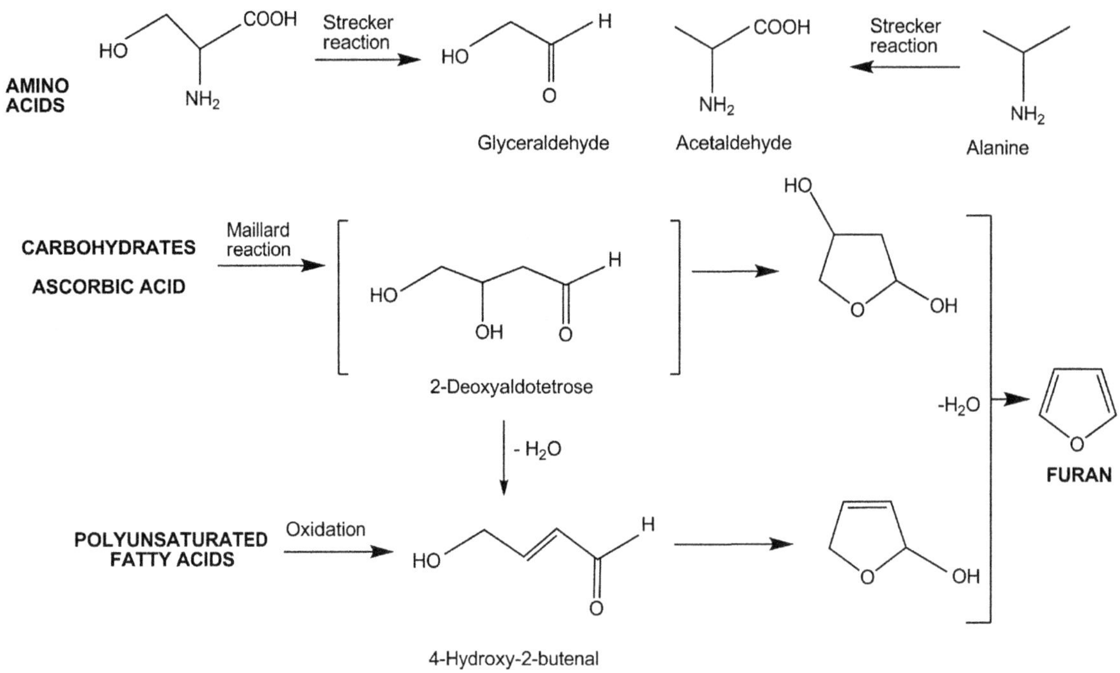

FIGURE 23.2   Mechanisms of formation of furan in heated foods from amino acids, carbohydrates, ascorbic acid and polyunsaturated fatty acid precursors. Adapted from Crews and Castle (2007), Mark *et al.* (2006) and Locas and Yaylayan (2004).

and its derivatives while glyceraldehyde, a triose, is less efficient (Locas & Yaylayan, 2004). Overall, sugars or amino acids when heated alone are not efficient at producing furans (Fan *et al.*, 2008; Locas & Yaylayan, 2004), but when heated in combination, are significant precursors of furan in heated food. Of the sugars studied, erythrose is efficient at producing furan, but only when heated at temperatures (i.e. >250°C) that do not represent typical food-processing conditions (Locas & Yaylayan, 2004; Mark *et al.*, 2006). In experiments using labeled sugars, Limacher *et al.* (2008) identified two major pathways of furan formation from sugars: 1) from the intact sugar skeleton; and 2) by recombination of reactive C2 and C3 fragments. Serine, threonine, and alanine promote furan formation by a recombination of C2 fragments such as acetaldehyde and glycolaldehyde (Vranova & Ciesarova, 2009).

Several amino acids alone, such as serine or cysteine, can undergo thermal degradation to produce furan; while others, such as alanine, threonine and aspartic acid, require the presence of reducing sugars, serine or cysteine to produce furan (Locas & Yaylayan, 2004). Reducing sugars in the presence of amino acids undergo the Maillard reaction and generate reactive intermediates that can ultimately form furan. The presence of amino acids such as threonine, serine or alanine, promotes furan formation from sugars (Limacher *et al.*, 2008). In simple model systems simulating roasting conditions, furan and methyl furan were formed at levels of up to 330μmol/ mol precursor from mixtures of sugars and selected amino acids (Limacher *et al.*, 2008).

Furan can be formed during thermal treatment of unsaturated fatty acids and the yield of furan increases with the degree of unsaturation (Becalski & Seaman, 2005; Crews &

Castle, 2007; Hasnip, Crews, & Castle, 2006). Becalski and Seaman (2005) found that furan can be formed by oxidation of polyunsaturated fatty acids at elevated temperatures and that formation is reduced by the addition of antioxidants such as tocopherol acetate. Overall, these results suggest that the formation of furan is linked with the process of free radical autoxidation (Crews & Castle, 2007; Locas & Yaylayan, 2004).

A considerable amount of information has been generated on formation of furan and its derivatives (2-methyl furan and further alkylated derivatives) in model systems containing a variety of precursors. Although these studies provide important information about possible mechanisms of formation of furan, they do not necessarily mimic furan formation in food since food systems tend to be more complex in nature and processing conditions are typically less severe.

23.3.4 Factors Affecting Furan Formation in Food

Many factors can affect the formation of furan, but those thought to have the greatest effect include food composition and processing or cooking conditions. However when the available information is examined, it is difficult to clearly define the effects of these factors on furan levels in food. This may be due to the inherent volatility of furan making quantitation difficult, and the fact that furan is formed by at least several mechanisms and with different classes of food precursors. When surveys (FDA, 2007a; Zoller et al., 2007) and experimental (Limacher et al., 2008) data are examined, it becomes apparent that furan levels tend to be greater in foods containing complex mixtures of carbohydrates, fatty acids and proteins than those of simple composition. As mentioned previously, furan can form from thermal processing of a variety of different food components. In food systems such as apple cider (containing mainly sugars with small amounts of ascorbic

acid and fatty acids), very low amounts of furan formed during heating at 120°C for 10 min. In contrast, more furan was produced by heating pumpkin puree, a food matrix that contains a mixture of starch, simple sugars, fatty acids, carotenoids and ascorbic acid (Limacher et al., 2008).

The presence of phosphate and the pH of a food may influence furan formation. In a model system consisting of ascorbic acid and fructose, phosphate increased furan formation (Fan et al., 2008). It was speculated that phosphates may increase furan production from sugars through the formation of reactive intermediate compounds from the Maillard reaction which can recombine to form furan (Fan et al., 2008). More furan was formed from heated ascorbic acid or sucrose solutions as the pH was reduced from 8 to 3 (Fan, 2005; Fan et al., 2008).

At present, there is no evidence of systematic studies on the effects of cooking/processing temperature and time on furan formation in food. Furan levels tend to be greater in foods that are heat processed in cans or jars since the furan that forms cannot escape from the closed container. Fan et al. (2008) reported that significant amounts of furan were produced in apple cider only at higher temperatures (>100°C) and prolonged times (>4 min). Similarly, Hasnip et al. (2006) reported greater levels of furan in bread toasted at 170–200°C than at 140–160°C.

The highest levels of furan are found in retorted canned and jarred foods (Roberts et al., 2008). Several reports (Goldmann et al., 2005; Hasnip & Castle, 2006; Roberts et al., 2008) have shown that furan in jarred or canned foods is lost during opening, cooking (at lower temperatures) and stirring/mixing. Of the cooking methods studied, heating canned and jarred foods in an open saucepan resulted in greater losses of furan than microwave-cooked foods (Roberts et al., 2008). Furan levels in cooked foods and beverages decreased upon sitting, and stirring foods before consumption also reduced furan levels (Goldmann et al., 2005; Roberts et al., 2008).

Heating jars of baby food by immersion in a hot water bath followed by stirring the contents of the jar, resulted in decreases in furan levels (Goldmann *et al.*, 2005; Roberts *et al.*, 2008).

Overall, the work to date indicates that furan in retail foods persists during the normal heating practices that precede consumption (Hasnip *et al.*, 2006). However, some treatments that may reduce consumer exposure to furan include heating, cooking in open containers, and stirring food before consuming. More work is needed on determining the effects of food preparation/processing procedures on furan level in food as they are consumed. Research is also needed to obtain a better understanding of the mechanisms by which furan is formed. This may enable the development of mitigation approaches for furan in food.

23.3.5 Health Effects of Dietary Furan

Furan is a hepatocarcinogen in both rats and mice and induces heptocellular carcinomas and cholangiocarcinomas (NTP, 1993). Furan has also been shown to cause a dose-dependent increase in mononuclear leukemia in male and female rats (NTP, 1993). The mechanism of carcinogenic activity of furan in rodents has not been elucidated but may be due to the activation of furan to the toxic metabolite, cis-2-butene-1,4-dial, by cytochrome P450 in the liver (Fransson-Steen, Goldsworthy, Kedderis, & Maronpot, 1997; Hamadeh *et al.*, 2004). There is some evidence that cis-2-butene-1,4-dial can react with DNA in target cells and induce the production of tumors (Wilson, Goldsworthy, Popp, & Butterworth, 1992; Chen, Hecht, & Peterson (1995)).

There is currently little information on the reproductive and developmental toxicities of furan and the toxicological effects of furan in humans from dietary sources (Heppner & Schlatter, 2007). Jun *et al.* (2008) measured urinary furan levels in healthy individuals consuming a normal diet and detected up to 3.14 ppb in over half (56%) of the subjects. In individuals with detectable urinary furan, the level of γ-glutamyltranspeptidase, a marker for liver disease, was strongly correlated with urinary furan concentration. This study points to the need to study the metabolic fate and potential toxicity of dietary furan in humans.

23.3.6 Regulatory Status

To date, the discovery of furan in food has generated less research interest than acrylamide. However, this situation may change when more information is available about dietary exposure to furan and the toxicity of the chemical (Robin, 2007). A the time of writing, FDA has not initiated any regulatory action on furan. EFSA has expressed the opinion that 'furan is clearly carcinogenic in rats and mice' and that 'the weight of evidence indicates that furan-induced carcinogenicity is probably attributable to a genotoxic mechanism (EFSA, 2004a). The EFSA Panel on Contaminants in the Food Chain elaborated a scientific report reviewing data on methods of analysis, occurrence, formation, and exposure toxicity (EFSA, 2004a). From the available data, it seems that there is a relatively small difference between possible human exposure and doses in experimental animals that produce carcinogenic effects, probably by a genotoxic mechanism. However, at present the limited availability of occurrence data in food does not allow a sound dietary exposure assessment. EFSA has issued a call for more information on the occurrence of furan in foods.

23.4 TRANS FATTY ACIDS

23.4.1 Introduction

Trans fatty acids (TFA) have received great attention over the past several years because of their effects on human health. There is an indication that unsaturated fats may cause more harm than saturated fats. *Trans* fatty acids, like saturated fatty acids, raise blood levels of low density lipoprotein (LDL) cholesterol, thereby increasing the risk of coronary heart disease. At equivalent dietary levels, TFA may also increase the risk of coronary heart disease more than saturated fats. This is because, unlike saturated fats, TFAs also reduce blood levels of high density lipoprotein (HDL) cholesterol and increase blood levels of triglycerides (Ascherio & Willett, 1997; EFSA, 2004b; Hu *et al.*, 1997; Judd *et al.*, 1994). A study estimated that between 30,000 and 100,000 cardiac deaths per year in the US are due to the consumption of *trans* fats (Mozaffarian *et al.*, 2006). In light of these findings, consumers are advised to limit their intake of *trans* fats.

Trans fats is the common name for a type of unsaturated fat with *trans*-isomer fatty acid(s). *Trans* fats may be monounsaturated or polyunsaturated. *Trans* fats occur naturally in trace amounts in some animal-based foods (i.e. dairy and beef fat) due to bacterial transformation of unsaturated fatty acids in the rumen of ruminant animals (Dijkstra, Hamilton, & Hamm, 2008; IFIC, 2003). *Trans* fatty acids can be present at trace levels in most vegetable oils and in variable amounts in a wide range of foods, including most foods made with partially hydrogenated oils, such as baked goods and fried foods, and some margarine products (Food Standards Australia New Zealand, 2005; Institute for International Research, 2006). Typically, ordinary vegetable oils, such as soybean, corn, cottonseed, sunflower, peanut, and olive, are moderately low in saturated acids, and the double bonds within unsaturated acids are in the *cis* configuration. Vegetable oils are sometimes hydrogenated in processed foods to improve their oxidative stability, extend their shelf-life, and give a more desirable texture (IFIC, 2003; List, 2004). For example, by using partially hydrogenated vegetable oil to make some margarine products, manufacturers can produce a spreadable topping that is lower in saturated fat than butter. Similarly, manufacturers can produce shortenings to make French fries, flaky piecrusts and crispy crackers (IFIC, 2003).

Trans fatty acids formed by hydrogenation are considered to be nutritionally undesirable. Hydrogenation is a process whereby hydrogen atoms are added to cis-unsaturated fats in the presence of a catalyst, breaking the double bond and making them more saturated. These saturated fats have a higher melting point, which makes them desirable for baking and extends their shelf-life. However, the process frequently turns some cis-isomers into *trans*-unsaturated fats instead of hydrogenating them completely (Dijkstra *et al.*, 2008; Institute for International Research, 2006). Concerns exist about the potential health effects of TFA, especially those that are derived from partial hydrogenation of vegetable oils. As a result, many countries including the United States, Canada and some European countries have either placed restrictions on the use of TFA in processed foods or more commonly, mandated labeling requirements for TFA in foods.

23.4.2 Regulatory Status/Risk Management

Some countries have acted to reduce consumption of *trans* fats. Denmark was the first country, in March 2003, to issue an order (Order no. 160), strictly regulating the content of *trans* fats in foods. The order does not apply to *trans* fatty acids in animal fats, but bans partially hydrogenated oils (Dijkstra *et al.*, 2008; List, 2004b). A limit of 2% TFA of fats and oils is allowed for human consumption and a *trans*-free claim can be made if the product has less than 1% TFA and includes all C_{14}-C_{22} *trans* isomers (Dijkstra *et al.*, 2008; List, 2004b). Switzerland followed Denmark's *trans* fats ban, and implemented the same regulation beginning in April 2008 (Anonymous, 2008). The

European Union (EU) favors voluntary labels except where nutrition claims are made. TFA are not included, but are declared on many packets of margarine. The EU is currently reviewing *trans* fat in the food industry (List, 2004b). Similarly, the Australia New Zealand Food Standards Code does not require manufacturers to label the *trans* fatty acid content of foods unless they make a nutritional claim about cholesterol, saturated, unsaturated or *trans* fatty acids. However, voluntary labeling is permitted and many edible oil spread manufacturers in Australia and New Zealand have chosen to voluntarily label their products (Food Standards Australia New Zealand, 2005).

On 11 July 2003, the FDA announced final rules requiring that *trans* fatty acids be stated in the nutrition label of conventional foods and dietary supplements (Dijkstra *et al.*, 2008; FDA, 2003). As of 1 January 2006, the TFA content of foods have been labeled as a separate line on the Nutrition Facts label. Products containing less than 0.5 grams per serving of TFA can be listed as 0 grams *trans* fat on the food label (Dijkstra *et al.*, 2008; FDA, 2003).

Since December 2005, Health Canada has required that food labels list the amount of *trans* fat in the nutrition section for most foods. Products containing less than 0.2 grams of *trans* fat per serving may be labeled as free of *trans* fats (Canadian Food Inspection Agency, 2005). In June 2006, a task force co-chaired by Health Canada and the Heart and Stroke Foundation of Canada recommended a limit of 5% *trans* fat (of total fat) in all products sold to consumers in Canada and 2% for tub margarines and spreads (Health Canada, 2006). On 20 June 2007, the Canadian Government agreed to regulate *trans* fats according to the 2006 recommendations (Health Canada, 2007). On 1 January 2008, Calgary became the first city in Canada to ban *trans* fats from restaurants and fast food chains. *Trans* fats present in cooking oil may not be greater than 2% of the total fat content (Anonymous, 2007).

23.4.3 Hydrogenation

Hydrogenation is important for two reasons in the fats and oils industry. It converts the liquid oils into semisolid or plastic fats for special applications, such as in shortenings and margarine, and it improves the oxidative stability of the oil (Dijkstra *et al.*, 2008; Nawar, 1996). Hydrogenation involves the reaction between unsaturated liquid oil and hydrogen adsorbed on a metal catalyst. The oil is mixed with a suitable catalyst (usually nickel), heated (140–225°C), then exposed, while stirred, to hydrogen at pressures up to 60 psi (Nawar, 1996). First, a carbon-metal complex is formed at either end of the olefinic bond. This intermediate complex then reacts with an atom of catalyst-adsorbed hydrogen to form an unstable half-hydrogenated state in which the olefin is attached to the catalyst by only one link and is thus free to rotate. The half-hydrogenated compound may either (a) react with another hydrogen atom and separate from the catalyst to generate the saturated product, or (b) lose a hydrogen atom to the nickel catalyst to restore the double bond. The regenerated double bond can be either in the same position (cis) as in the unhydrogenated compound, or a positional and/or geometric isomer (*trans*) of the original double bond (Dijkstra *et al.*, 2008; Nawar, 1996). The hydrogenation process is usually monitored by determining the change in refractive index, which is related to the degree of saturation of the oil. The hydrogenated oil is then cooled and the catalyst is removed by filtration (Nawar, 1996).

The rate of hydrogenation and the formation of *trans* acids depends on the processing conditions (hydrogen pressure, intensity of agitation, temperature, and kind and concentration of catalyst). For many years, manufacturers of fats have been trying to devise hydrogenation processes that minimize isomerization while avoiding the formation of high amounts of fully saturated material (Nawar, 1996; Patterson, 1994).

Temperature is the most important variable in *trans* isomer control. Lowering the temperature below the traditional levels of 140°C causes a significant *trans* isomer reduction, but an increase in saturate levels (Patterson, 1994). A TFA level of 6% can be achieved with a hydrogenation temperature of 40–60°C with a nickel catalyst, but this decreases the catalytic activity. It is, therefore, important to use a catalyst that can saturate the double bonds at these lower temperatures. Conventional hydrogenation plants are configured for typical initiation reaction temperatures in the 110–150°C range (Patterson, 1994).

23.4.4 Decreasing *Trans* Fatty Acids in Fats and Oils

Approximately 92 million tons of edible fats and oils were consumed worldwide between 2001 and 2002. Fifty-nine percent were soybean oil (29 million tons) and palm oil (25.4 million tons). Although soybean oil is low in saturated acids (15%), it is a significant source of TFA in the US diet because it requires partial hydrogenation for use in salad/cooking oils, spreads and shortenings. Salad oils and spreads typically contain 9–11% TFA and shortenings contain 12–25% TFA (List, 2004b). On the other hand, palm oil contains no *trans* fat, but it contains about 50% saturated acids. This makes it attractive for use in these products, especially when modified by interesterification and/or fractionation (List, 2004a).

In 1995, the International Margarine Association of the Countries of Europe (IMACE) recommended a level of less than 5% TFA in all products and that once implemented, the total of saturates plus *trans* fats would not be increased. In 2002, IMACE made a recommendation that European retail margarine and spreads not exceed 1% TFA, while products used in processed foods not exceed 5%, and the total saturate and TFA content does not increase (List, 2004b).

European processors have reduced the *trans* fat content by using several techniques. These include use of lauric oils (coconut, palm kernel), palm fractions, completely hardened vegetable oils (stearines), interesterification, lower-temperature deodorization to minimize thermal *trans* formation, and chemical refining rather than physical refining (List, 2004b). Methods that can be used to provide an oil blend with the required physical and chemical properties include the blending of different oils and fats, single- or multi-stage fractionation, interesterification and combination of these processes. A *trans*-free margarine fat blend can, for example, be produced by blending a lauric oil and a non-lauric oil; fully hydrogenating the mixture; randomizing the fully hydrogenated fat by interesterification; fractionating the interesterified product to eliminate high-melting triglycerides and/or low-melting triglycerides, and blending the olein or mid-fraction with a liquid oil. This oil can also be subjected to a direct interesterification process to reduce the saturated fatty acid content of the fat blend (Dijkstra *et al.*, 2008).

23.4.5 Interesterification

The process of random interesterification was used in Europe during the 1950s and 1960s. This process can change the original order of distribution of the fatty acids in the triglyceride-producing products. Chemical and enzymatic interesterification processes can affect physical properties by changing the melting properties and in some cases the crystal behavior of the original oil or fat. Commercially, interesterification is used for processing edible fats and oils to produce confectionery or coating fats, margarine oils, cooking oils, frying fats, shortenings, and other special application products (O'Brien, 2004). Unlike hydrogenation, interesterification does not affect the degree of saturation or cause isomerization of the fatty-acid double bond. In this process, fatty acids are removed from the glyceride molecules, these acids are shuffled, and replaced on the glyceride in random positions with the aid of a catalyst (List, 2004a; O'Brien, 2004).

Interesterification has not been extensively used in the US (O'Brien, 2004). Lard was the main interesterification product in the US. It could be randomized to improve its crystal habits and shortening properties by the addition of some fully hydrogenated fat (Patterson, 1994). However, chemical interesterification has disadvantages. It forms by-products such as soaps, methyl esters, and partial glycerides, thus requiring post-processing procedures to remove them (List, 2004b).

Enzymatic interesterification is currently being used commercially in Europe to formulate margarine and shortening oils. The major advantages of the enzymatic interesterification over the chemical processes are that the lipase catalysts are specific and the reaction can be better controlled (O'Brien, 2004). Oil modification by lipases is performed under anhydrous conditions at temperatures up to 160°F (70°C). Catalysts/enzymes are expensive, but there are no side-products and no post-processing (List, 2004b; O'Brien, 2004).

In 2003, Archer Daniels Midland introduced the Nova-Lipid™ line, which is based on enzymatic interesterification of soybean and hydrogenated soybean and cottonseed oils. These products include low *trans* fats in an 'all-purpose' baking shortening, cake shortening and a baking margarine. TFA contents of 9% allow nutritional labels to state '1 gram TFA/serving.' Other TFA products that ADM manufacture include all-purpose shortenings, pie shortenings, cake and icing shortenings, and all-purpose vegetable shortenings formulated from interesterified soybean and cottonseed oils with 4.5–5.5% TFA (List, 2004b).

Interesterification can be used to formulate products with less saturated or isomerized fatty acids for the production of products with low or no *trans*-acids (O'Brien, 2004). Interesterifying palm stearine with fully hydrogenated high-erucic-acid rapeseed oil can provide a hardstock that allows *trans*-free margarines to be made that also contain low saturated fatty acids (Patterson, 1994).

23.4.6 Fractionation

A *trans*-free margarine fat blend can also be produced by fractionating the interesterified product to remove high-melting triglycerides and/or low melting triglycerides and blending the olein or mid-fraction with a liquid oil (Patterson, 1994). Dry fractionation is the standard industry method (List, 2004a). Palm oil is the most popular oil used for fractionation. Palm oil (IV 51–53) is fractionated into olein (IV 56–59) and stearine (IV 32–36) fractions (List, 2004a). Fractionation produces products with different properties. A fat forms crystals by cooling and these crystals are then separated from the mother liquor by filtration. The crystals are isolated as a filter cake and are called the stearine fraction and the filtrate is referred to as the olein fraction (O'Brien, 2004).

Single-stage fractionation generates an olein fraction with a cloud point of <10°C. It is used as a substitute for soft oils in frying or cooking or it can be fractionated further (O'Brien, 2004). The olein (more liquid) fraction can then be fractionated into mid-fractions, super oleins and top oleins. The palm mid-fractions (IV 42–48) are further processed into harder fractions (IV 32–36). Fractionation of the stearine (more solid) (IV 32–36) gives softer and super stearines (IV 40–42 and 17–21, respectively). These fractions can be incorporated into margarines/shortenings and confectionery fats. However, replacing *trans* fat with highly saturated palm fractions will increase saturated acid content (List, 2004a).

Multi-stage fractionation of palm oil is applied to produce high-IV superoleins (IV >65) and soft-palm mid-fractions (S-PMF with IV 45–47). High-IV superoleins combine a low cloud point with good oxidative stability and are therefore used as frying oil and salad oil. S-PMF is increasingly used as *trans*-free hardstock in margarines and shortenings (O'Brien, 2004). Dry fractionation is also used for the modification of other vegetable oils (cottonseed oil, partially hydrogenated soybean oil, etc.) and animal fat (lard, fish, oil, etc.) (Dijkstra *et al.*, 2008).

23.4.7 Modified Fatty Acid Composition

Several transgenic and plant breeding techniques have been used to create oilseeds with altered fatty acid composition. These include low-linolenic soybean, high-oleic corn (maize) and soybean, high-oleic and mid-oleic sunflower and high-saturate lines (List, 2004b). The low-linolenic soybean and the high-oleic sunflower, soybean and corn oils can be used as frying oils and can reduce *trans* fatty acids in fried snack foods. High-oleic oils (i.e. palmitic acid or stearic acid) are used without hydrogenation for frying and in high-stability applications. High-saturate oils are used in margarines, spreads and shortenings. They may require blending with higher melting components (i.e. palm oil, cottonseed/soybean stearines) or interesterification of their glyceride structures for functionality (List, 2004b).

23.5 CONCLUSIONS

Processing plays an essential role in the modern world in providing a safe, palatable, nutritious and consistent food supply. Despite these benefits, processing can result in the formation of chemical hazards such as the heat-produced toxicants, acrylamide and furan, and *trans* fatty acids, a product of hydrogenation of oils. All three compounds have been found to have adverse physiological effects in laboratory animals, and possibly humans. Acrylamide and furan are produced by chemical reactions responsible for the desirable flavor, aroma and color of cooked foods. *Trans* fatty acids are generated during processes that improve the texture of oils and render them more stable to oxidative stresses. Changing processing conditions to minimize the formation of acrylamide, furan and *trans* fatty acids can result in undesirable effects on food safety and quality. Regulatory agencies in collaboration with the food industry and academia have placed an emphasis on gathering more information on the mechanisms by which they are formed and the health consequences resulting from dietary exposure to these compounds. This information will provide ways for managing these chemical hazards in food.

References

Altaki, M. S., Santos, F. J., & Galceran, M. T. (2009). Automated headspace solid-phase microextraction versus headspace for the analysis of furan in foods by gas chromatography-mass spectrometry. *Talanta*, 78, 1315–1320.

Amrein, T. M., Andres, L., Escher, F., & Amado, R. (2007). Occurrence of acrylamide in selected foods and mitigation options. *Food Additives and Contaminants*, 24(S1), 13–25.

Amrein, T. M., Schonbachler, B., Escher, F., & Amado, R. (2004). Acrylamide in gingerbread: Critical factors for formation and possible ways for reduction. *Journal of Agricultural and Food Chemistry*, 52, 4282–4288.

Amrein, T. M., Bachmann, S., Noti, A., et al. (2003). Potential of acrylamide formation, sugars, and free asparagine in potatoes: A comparison of cultivars and farming systems. *Journal of Agricultural and Food Chemistry*, 51, 5556–5560.

Anonymous. (2007). Calgary moves against trans fat. CBC News. 2007–12–29. http://www.cbc.ca/canada/story/2007/12/29/calgary-fats.html (accessed 9 February 2009).

Anonymous. (2008). Deadly fats: why are we still eating them? The Independent. http://www.independent.co.uk/life-style/health-and-wellbeing/healthy-living/deadly-fats-why-are-we-still-eating-them-843400.html (accessed 16 June 2008).

Ascherio, A., & Willett, W. C. (1997). Health effects of trans fatty acids. *The American Journal of Clinical Nutrition*, 66(suppl), 1006S–1010S.

Bagdonaite, K., Derler, K., & Murkovi, M. (2008). Determination of acrylamide during roasting of coffee. *Journal of Agricultural and Food Chemistry*, 56, 6081–6086.

Becalski, A., Lau, B. P.-Y., Lewis, D., et al. (2004). Acrylamide in French Fries: Influence of free amino acids and sugars. *Journal of Agricultural and Food Chemistry*, 52, 3801–3806.

Becalski, A., & Seaman, S. (2005). Furan precursors in food: A model study and development of a simple headspace method for determination of furan. *Journal of AOAC International*, 88, 102–106.

Biedermann, M., Noti, A., Biedermann-Brem, S., et al. (2002). Experiments on acrylamide formation and possibilities to decrease the potential of acrylamide formation in potatoes. *Mitteilungen Lebensmittel Hygiene*, 93, 668–687.

Blank, I., Robert, F., Goldmann, T., et al. (2005). Mechanism of acrylamide formation: Maillard-induced transformations of asparagine. In M. Friedman & D. Mottram (Eds.), *Chemistry and safety of acrylamide in food* (pp. 171–189). NY: Springer.

Bolger, P. M., Tao, S. S.-H., & Dinovi, M. (2009). Hazards of dietary furan. In R. H. Stadler & D. R. Lineback (Eds.), *Induced food toxicants: Occurrence, formation, mitigation and health risks* (pp. 117–134). Hoboken, NJ: John Wiley & Sons.

Boon, P. E., de Mul, A., van der Voet, H., et al. (2005). Calculations of dietary exposure to acrylamide. *Mutation Research, 580*, 143–155.

Bull, R. J., Robinson, M., Laurie, R. D., et al. (1984). Carcinogenic activity of acrylamide in the skin and lung of Swiss-ICR mice. *Cancer Letters, 24*, 209–212.

CAC. (2006). Discussion paper on acrylamide in food. ftp://ftp.fao.org/codex/ccfac38/fa38_35e.pdf (accessed 6 February 2009).

CAC. (2008). *Report of the 2nd Session of the CODEX Committee on Contaminants in Foods*, The Hague, The Netherlands, March 31–April 4, 2008, ftp://ftp.fao.org/codex/alinorm08/al31_41e.pdf (accessed 6 February 2009).

Canadian Food Inspection Agency. (2005). Information letter: Labelling of trans fatty acids. http://www.inspection.gc.ca/english/fssa/labeti/inform/20050914e.shtml.

CAST. (2006). Acrylamide in food. June 2006, Number 32 (available at: http://www.cast-science.org/websiteUploads/publicationPDFs/acrylamide_ip.pdf).

Chen, L. J., Hecht, S. S., & Peterson, L. A. (1995). Identification of cis–2-butene–1,4-dial as a microsomal metabolite of furan. *Chemical Research, 8*, 903–906.

CIAA. (2006). The CIAA acrylamide 'Toolbox', confederation of food and drink industries of the EU. http://www.ciaa.be/documents/brochures/CIAA_Acrylamide_Toolbox_Oct2006.pdf (accessed 23 September 2009).

Ciesarova, Z., Kiss, E., & Boegl, P. (2006). Impact of L-asparaginase on acrylamide content in potato products. *Journal of Food and Nutrition Research, 45*, 141–146.

Claeys, W. L., DeVleeschouwer, K., & Hendrickx, M. E. (2005). Kinetics of acrylamide formation and elimination during heating of an asparagine-sugar model system. *Journal of Agricultural and Food Chemistry, 53*, 9999–10005.

Claus, A., Weisz, G. M., Scieber, A., & Carle, R. (2006). Pyrolytic acrylamide formation from purified wheat gluten and gluten-supplemented wheat bread rolls. *Molecular Nutrition and Food Research, 50*, 87–93.

Crews, C., & Castle, L. (2007). A review of the occurrence, formation and analysis of furan in heat-processed foods. *Trends in Food Science and Technology, 18*, 365–372.

De Wilde, T., De Meulenaer, B., Mestdagh, F., et al. (2006). Influence of fertilization on acrylamide formation during frying of potatoes harvested in 2003. *Journal of Agricultural and Food Chemistry, 54*, 404–408.

Dijkstra, A. J., Hamilton, R. J., & Hamm, W. (Eds.), (2008). *Trans fatty acids*. Hoboken, NJ: Wiley-Blackwell.

Doerge, D. R., Young, J. F., Chen, J. J., et al. (2008). Using dietary exposure and physiologically based pharma-cokinetic/pharmacodynamic modeling in human risk extrapolations for acrylamide toxicity. *Journal of Agricultural and Food Chemistry, 56*, 6031–6038.

Dybing, E., Farmer, P. B., Andersen, M., et al. (2005). Human exposure and internal dose assessments of acrylamide in food. *Food and Chemical Toxicology, 43*, 271–278.

EFSA. (2004a). Report of the scientific panel on contaminants in the food chain on provisional findings of furan in food http://www.efsa.europa.int/science/contam/contam_documents/760/contam_furan_report7-11-05.pda. *EFSA Journal, 137*, 1–20.

EFSA. (2004b). European Commission Press Release. Trans fatty acids: EFSA Panel reviews dietary intakes and health effects. August 31, 2004. http://www.efsa.europa.eu/EFSA/efsa (accessed 30 January 2009).

European Commission. (2006). European Union Acrylamide Monitoring Database. http://irmm.jrc.be/html/activities/acrylamide/database.htm (accessed 3/14/09).

Fan, X. (2005). Formation of furan from carbohydrates and ascorbic acid following exposure to ionizing radiation and thermal processing. *Journal of Agricultural and Food Chemistry, 53*, 7826–7831.

Fan, X., & Geveke, D. J. (2007). Furan formation in sugar solution and apple cider upon ultraviolet treatment. *Journal of Agricultural and Food Chemistry, 55*, 7816–7821.

Fan, X., Huang, L., & Sokorai, K. J. B. (2008). Factors affecting thermally induced furan formation. *Journal of Agricultural and Food Chemistry, 56*, 9490–9494.

FDA. (2003). Food labeling: Trans fatty acids in nutrition labeling. *Federal Register, 68*, 41433–41506.

FDA. (2006a). Survey data on acrylamide in food: Individual food products. US Food and Drug Administration, Center for Food Safety and Applied Nutrition, 2006, http://www.cfsan.fda.gov/~dms/acrydata.html (accessed 4 February 2009).

FDA. (2006b). Survey data on acrylamide in food: Total diet survey results. US Food and Drug Administration, Center for Food Safety and Applied Nutrition, 2006, http://www.cfsan.fda.gov/~dms/acrydata2.html (accessed 4 February 2009).

FDA. (2006c). The 2006 exposure assessment for acrylamide. FDA/CFSAN. http://www.cfsan.fda.gov/~dms/acryexpo/acryex1.htm. (accessed 4 February 2009).

FDA. (2007a). Exploratory data on furan in food: Individual food products. U.S. Food and Drug Administration, Center for Food Safety and Applied Nutrition, October 2006. http://www.cfsan.fda.gov/~dms/furandat.html. (accessed 4 February 2009).

FDA. (2007b). An updated exposure assessment for furan from consumption of adult and baby foods. US Food and Drug Administration, Center for Food Safety and Applied Nutrition, April 2009. http://www.cfsan.fda.gov/~dms/furanexp/sld01.htm (accessed 5 February 2009).

FDA. (2008). Additional Information on Acrylamide, Diet, and Food Storage and Preparation. May 2008. http://

www.fda.gov/Food/FoodSafety/FoodContaminants Adulteration/ChemicalContaminants/Acrylamide/ucm151000.htm (accessed 5 February 2009).

FDA. (2009). Numerical listing of GRAS notices. US Food and Drug Administration, Center for Food Safety and Applied Nutrition, April 2009. http://www.foodsafety.gov/~rdb/opa-gras.html (accessed 4 April 2009).

Fohgelberg, P., Rosen, J., Hellenäs, K.-E., & Abramsson-Zetterberg, L. (2005). The acrylamide intake via some common baby food for children in Sweden during their first year of life—an improved method for analysis of acrylamide. *Food and Chemical Toxicology, 43*, 951–959.

Food Standards Agency. (2005). Acrylamide: Your Questions Answered. Jan. 2005. http://www.food.gov.uk/safereating/chemsafe/acrylamide_branch/acrylamide_study_faq/ (accessed 7 February 2009).

Food Standards Australia New Zealand. (2005). *Trans Fatty Acids.* 12 April 2005. Fact Sheets. http://www.foodstandards.gov.au/newsroom/factsheets/factsheets2005/ (accessed 9 January 2009).

Foot, R. J., Haase, N. U., Grob, K., & Gondé, P. (2007). Acrylamide in fried and roasted potato products: A review on progress in mitigation. *Food Additives and Contaminants, 24*(S1), 37–46.

Frankel, E. N., Neff, W. E., Selke, E., & Brooks, D. D. (1987). Thermal and metal-catalyzed decomposition of methyl linolenate hydroperoxides. *Lipids, 22*, 322–327.

Fransson-Steen, R., Goldsworthy, T. L., Kedderis, G. L., & Maronpot, R. R. (1997). Furan-induced liver cell proliferation and apoptosis in female B6C3F1 mice. *Toxicology, 118*, 195–204.

Fredricksson, H., Tallving, J., Rosen, J., & Aman, P. (2004). Fermentation reduces free asparagine in dough and acrylamide content in bread. *Cereal Chemistry, 81*, 650–653.

Friedman, M., & Levin, C. E. (2008). Review of methods for the reduction of dietary content and toxicity of acrylamide. *Journal of Agricultural and Food Chemistry, 56*, 6113–6140.

Friedman, M. A., Dulak, L. H., & Stedham, M. A. (1995). Lifetime oncogenicity study in rats with acrylamide. *Fundamental and Applied Toxicology, 27*, 95–105.

Göbel, A., & Kliemant, A. (2007). The German minimization concept for acrylamide. *Food Additives and Contaminants, 24*(S1), 82–90.

Gökmen, V., Acar, O., Köksel, H., & Acar, J. (2007). Effects of dough formula and baking conditions on acrylamide and hydroxymethylfurfural formation in cookies. *Food Chemistry, 104*, 1136–1142.

Gökmen, V., & Senyuva, H. Z. (2007). Acrylamide formation is prevented by divalent cations during the Maillard reaction. *Food Chemistry, 103*, 196–203.

Goldmann, T., Périsset, A., Scanlan, F., & Stadler, R. H. (2005). Rapid determination of furan in heated foodstuffs by isotope dilution solid phase micro-extraction-gas chromatography–mass spectrometry (SPME-GC-MS). *The Analyst, 130*, 878–883.

Granvogl, M., & Schieberle, P. (2006). Thermally generated 3-aminopropionamide as a transient intermediate in the formation of acrylamide. *Journal of Agricultural and Food Chemistry, 54*, 5933–5938.

Guenther, H., Anklam, E., Wenzl, T., & Stadler, R. H. (2007). Acrylamide in coffee: Review of progress in analysis, formation and level reduction. *Food Additives and Contaminants, 24*(S1), 60–70.

Haase, N. U. (2006). The formation of acrylamide in potato products. In K. Skog & J. Alexander (Eds.), *Acrylamide and other hazardous compounds in heat-treated foods* (pp. 41–59). England: Woodhead Publishing, Cambridge.

Hamadeh, H. K., Jayadev, S., Gaillard, E. T., et al. (2004). Integration of clinical and gene expression endpoints to explore furan-mediated hepatotoxicity. *Mutation Research, 549*, 169–183.

Hamlet, C. G., & Sadd, P. A. (2009). Chloropropanols and chloroesters. In R. H. Stadler & D. R. Lineback (Eds.), *Process-induced food toxicants* (pp. 175–214). Hoboken, NJ: Wiley.

Hanley, A. B., Offen, C., Clarke, M., et al. (2005). Acrylamide reduction in processed foods. In M. Friedman & D. Mottram (Eds.), *Chemistry and safety of acrylamide in food* (pp. 387–392). New York: Springer.

Hasnip, S., Crews, C., & Castle, L. (2006). Some factors affecting the formation of furan in heated foods. *Food Additives and Contaminants, 23*, 219–227.

Health Canada. (2006). TRANSforming the food supply. Trans Fat Task Force. http://www.hc-sc.gc.ca/fn-an/nutrition/gras-trans-fats/tf-gt-rep-rap-eng.php (accessed 4 February 2009).

Health Canada. (2007). Canada's new government calls on industry to adopt limits for trans fat. http://www.hc-sc.gc.ca/ahc-asc/media/nr-cp/2007/2007_74_e.html (accessed 8 January 2009).

Health Canada. (2009). Acrylamide. What you can do to reduce exposure. February 2009, http://www.hc-sc.gc.ca/fn-an/securit/chem-chim/food-aliment/acrylamide/acrylamide_rec-eng.php (accessed 5 March 2009).

HEATOX. (2007). Guidelines in home cooking and consumption. http://www.slv.se/upload/heatox/documents/D59_guidelines_to_authorities_and_consumer_organisations_on_home_cooking_and_consumption.pdf (accessed 12 January 2009).

Heppner, C. W., & Schlatter, J. R. (2007). Data requirements for risk assessment of furan in food. *Food Additives and Contaminants, 24*(S1), 114–121.

Hogervorst, J. G., Schouten, L. J., Konings, E. J., et al. (2008). Dietary acrylamide and the risk of renal cell, bladder and prostate cancer. *The American Journal of Clinical Nutrition, 87*, 1428–1438.

Hu, F. B., Stampfer, M. J., Manson, J. E., et al. (1997). Dietary fat intake and the risk of coronary heart disease in women. *The New England Journal of Medicine, 337,* 1491–1499.

Hunter, J. E. (2005). Dietary levels of *trans*-fatty acids: Basis for health concerns and industry efforts to limit their use. *Nutrition Research, 25,* 49–513.

IARC. (1994). Acrylamide. *Some Industrial Chemicals;* Monographs on the Evaluation of Carcinogenic Risks to Humans; International Agency for Research on Cancer, Lyon, France.

IARC. (1995). Furan. IARC Monographs on the Evaluation of Carcinogenic Risks to Humans, International Agency for Research on Cancer, Vol. 63, pp. 3194–3407, Lyon, France.

IFIC. (2003). Questions and Answers about Trans fats. International Food Information Council. http://www.ific. org/publications/qa/transqa.cfm. (accessed 30 January 2009).

Institute for International Research. (2006). Fats and Oils— Tapping into oil innovation. http://foodreview.ihs. com/news/2006/fatty-acids.htm (Accessed 30 January 2009).

Jackson, L., & Al-Taher, F. (2005). Effects of consumer food preparation on acrylamide formation. In M. Friedman & D. Mottram (Eds.), *Chemistry and safety of acrylamide in food: Vol. 561* (pp. 447–465). New York: Springer.

JECFA. (2005). Summary and Conclusions of the Sixty-fourth Meeting of the Joint FAO/WHO Expert Committee on Food Additives. Joint FAO/WHO Expert Committee on Food Additives JECFA/65/SC.

Johnson, K. A., Gorzinski, S. J., Bodner, K. M., et al. (1986). Chronic toxicity and oncogenicity study on acrylamide incorporated in the drinking water of Fischer 344 rats. *Toxicology and Applied Pharmacology, 85,* 154–168.

Judd, J. T., Clevidence, B. A., Muesing, R. A., et al. (1994). Dietary *trans* fatty acids: Effects on plasma lipids and lipoproteins of healthy men and women. *The American Journal of Clinical Nutrition, 59,* 861–868.

Jun, H.-J., Lee, K.-G., Lee, Y.-K., et al. (2008). Correlation of urinary furan with plasma γ-glutamyltranspeptidase levels in healthy men and women. *Food and Chemical Toxicology, 46,* 1753–1759.

Jung, M. Y., Choi, D. S., & Ju, J. W. (2003). A novel technique for limitation of acrylamide formation in fried and baked corn chips and in French fries. *Journal of Food Science, 68,* 1287–1290.

Klaunig, J. E. (2008). Acrylamide toxicity. *Journal of Agricultural and Food Chemistry, 56,* 5984–5988.

Konings, E. J. M., Ashby, P., Hamlet, C. G., & Thompson, G. A. K. (2007). Acrylamide in cereal and cereal products: A review on the progress in level reduction. *Food Additives and Contaminants, 24*(S1), 47–59.

Limacher, A., Kerler, J., Conde-Petit, B., & Blank, I. (2007). Formation of furan and methylfuran from ascorbic acid in model systems and food. *Food Additives and Contaminants, 24*(S1), 122–135.

Limacher, A., Kerler, J., Davidek, T., et al. (2008). Formation of furan and methylfuran by Maillard-type reactions in model systems and food. *Journal of Agricultural and Food Chemistry, 56,* 3639–3647.

Lindsay, R. C., & Jang, S. J. (2005). Chemical intervention strategies for substantial suppression of acrylamide formation in fried potato products. In M. Friedman & D. Mottram (Eds.), *Chemistry and safety of acrylamide in food* (pp. 393–404). New York: Springer.

List, G. R. (2004a). Decreasing *trans* and saturated fatty acid content in food oils. *Food Technology, 58,* 23–31.

List, G. R. (2004b). Processing and reformulation for nutrition labeling of *trans* fatty acids. *Lipid Technology, 16,* 173–177.

Locas, C. P., & Yaylayan, V. A. (2004). Origin and mechanistic pathways of formation of the parent furan—A food toxicant. *Journal of Agricultural and Food Chemistry, 42,* 6830–6836.

LoPachin, R. M., & Gavin, T. (2008). Acrylamide-induced nerve terminal damage: Relevance to neurotoxic and neurodegenerative mechanisms. *Journal of Agricultural and Food Chemistry, 56,* 5994–6003.

Maga, J. A. (1979). Furans in foods. *CRC Critical Reviews in Food Science and Nutrition, 11,* 355–400.

Mark, J., Pollien, P., Lindinger, C., et al. (2006). Quantitation of furan and methylfuran formed in different precursor systems by proton transfer reaction mass spectrometry. *Journal of Agricultural and Food Chemistry, 54,* 2786–2793.

Mestdagh, F., Maertens, J., Cucu, T., et al. (2008). Impact of additives to lower the formation of acrylamide in a potato model system through pH reduction and other mechanisms. *Food Chemistry, 107,* 26–31.

Mills, C., Mottram, D. S., & Wedzicha, B. L. (2009). Acrylamide. In R. H. Stadler & D. R. Lineback (Eds.), *Process-induced food toxicants* (pp. 23–50). Hoboken, NJ: Wiley.

Mottram, D. S. (1991). Meat. In H. Maarse (Ed.), *Volatile compounds in foods and beverages: Vol. 44* (pp. 107–177). New York: Marcel Dekker.

Mottram, D. S., Wedzicha, B. L., & Dodson, A. T. (2002). Acrylmide is formed in the Maillard reaction. *Nature, 419,* 448–449.

Mozaffarian, D., Katan, M. B., Ascherio, A., et al. (2006). Trans fatty acids and cardiovascular disease. *The New England Journal of Medicine, 354,* 1601–1613.

Mucci, L. A., Adami, H. O., & Wolk, A. (2006). Prospective study of dietary acrylamide and risk of colorectal cancer among women. *International Journal of Cancer, 118,* 169–173.

Mucci, L. A., Dickman, P. W., Steineck, G., et al. (2003). Dietary acrylamide and cancer of the large bowel, kidney and bladder: Absence of an association in a population study in Sweden. *British Journal of Cancer, 88,* 84–89.

Mucci, L. A., Lindblad, P., Steineck, G., & Adami, H. O. (2004). Dietary acrylamide and risk of renal cell cancer. *International Journal of Cancer, 109*, 774–776.

Mucci, L. A., & Wilson, K. M. (2008). Acrylamide intake through diet and human cancer risk. *Journal of Agricultural and Food Chemistry, 56*, 6013–6019.

Muttucumaru, N., Elmore, J. S., Curtis, T., et al. (2008). Reducing acrylamide precursors in raw materials derived from wheat and potato. *Journal of Agricultural and Food Chemistry, 56*, 6167–6172.

Nawar, W. (1996). Lipids. In O. R. Fennema (Ed.), *Food chemistry* (3rd ed) (pp. 225–319). New York: Marcel Dekker, Inc.

Noti, A., Biedermann-Brem, S., Biedermann, M., et al. (2003). Storage of potatoes at low temperatures should be avoided to prevent increased acrylamide formation during frying or roasting. *Mitteilungen Lebensmittel Hygiene, 94*, 167–180.

NTP. (1993). Toxicology and Carcinogenesis Studies of Furan in F–344/N Rats and B6C3F1 Mice. National Toxicology Program Technical Report 402. US Department of Health and Human Services, Public Health Service, National Institute of Health, Research Triangle Park, NC, USA.

O'Brien, R. D. (2004). *Fats and oils: Formulating and processing for applications* (2nd ed). Boca Raton, Fl: CRC Press.

Olesen, P. T., Olsen, A., & Frandsen, H. (2008). Acrylamide exposure and incidence of breast cancer among postmenopausan women in the Danish diet, cancer and health study. *International Journal of Cancer, 122*, 2094–2100.

Park, Y. W., Yang, H. W., Storkson, J. M., et al. (2005). Controlling acrylamide in French fry and potato chip models and a mathematical model of acrylamide formation—acrylamide: Acidulants, phytate and calcium. In M. Friedman & D. Mottram (Eds.), *Chemistry and safety of acrylamide in food* (pp. 343–356). New York: Springer.

Patterson, H. B. W. (1994). *Hydrogenation of fats and oils: Theory and practice*. Champaign, IL: AOCS Press.

Pedreschi, F., Kaack, K., & Granby, K. (2008). The effect of asparaginase on acrylamide formation in French fries. *Food Chemistry, 109*, 386–392.

Reinhard, H., Sager, F., Zimmermann, H., & Zoller, O. (2004). Furan in foods on the Swiss market- method and results 543–535. *Mitteilungen aus Lebensmitteluntersuchung und Hygiene, 95*.

Rice, J. M. (2005). The carcinogenicity of acrylamide. *Mutation Research, 580*, 3–20.

Roberts, D., Crews, C., Grundy, H., et al. (2008). Effect of consumer cooking on furan in convenience foods. *Food Additives and Contaminants, 25*, 25–31.

Robin, L. (2007). Regulatory Report. Acrylamide, furan and the FDA. *Food Safety Magazine*, June/July 2007, vol.13 (3), pp. 17–21. http://www.foodsafetymagazine.com/articlePF.asp?id=1967&sub=sub1. (accessed 6 August 2008).

Rupp, H. (2003). Chemical and physical hazards produced during food processing, storage and preparation. In R. H. Schmidt & G. E. Rodrick (Eds.), *Food Safety Handbook* (pp. 233–263). Hoboken, NJ: John Wiley & Sons.

Rydberg, P., Erikson, S., Tareke, E., et al. (2003). Investigations of factors that influence the acrylamide content of heated foodstuffs. *Journal of Agricultural and Food Chemistry, 51*, 7012–7018.

Sadd, P. A., Hamlet, C. G., & Liang, L. (2008). Effectiveness of methods for reducing acrylamide in bakery products. *Journal of Agricultural and Food Chemistry, 56*, 6154–6161.

Sikorski, Z. E. (2005). The effect of processing on the nutritional value and toxicity of foods. In W. M. Dabrowski & Z. E. Sikorski (Eds.), *Toxins in Food* (pp. 285–312). Boca Raton, FL: CRC Press.

Skog, K., & Alexander, J. (Eds.), (2006). *Acrylamide and other Hazardous Compounds in Heat-treated Foods*. Cambridge, England: Woodhead Publishing.

Stadler, R. H. (2006). The formation of acrylamide in cereal products and coffee. In K. Skog & J. Alexander (Eds.), *Acrylamide and other hazardous compounds in heat-treated foods* (pp. 23–40). Cambridge, England: Woodhead Publishing.

Stadler, R. H., Blank, I., Varga, N., et al. (2002). Acrylamide formed in the Maillard reaction. *Nature, 419*, 449.

Stadler, R. H., & Lineback, D. R. (Eds.), (2009). *Process-induced food toxicants*. Hoboken, NJ: Wiley & Sons.

Stadler, R. H., Robert, F., Riediker, S., et al. (2004). In-depth mechanistic study on the formation of acrylamide and other vinylogous compounds by the Maillard reaction. *Journal of Agricultural and Food Chemistry, 52*, 5550–5558.

Surdyk, N., Rosén, J., Andersson, R., & Aman, P. (2004). Effects of asparagine, fructose, and baking conditions on acrylamide content in yeast-leavened wheat bread. *Journal of Agricultural and Food Chemistry, 52*, 2047–2051.

Taeymans, D., Wood, J., Ashby, P., et al. (2004). A review of acrylamide: An industry perspective on research, analysis, formation, and control. *Critical Reviews in Food Science and Nutrition, 44*, 323–347.

Tareke, E., Rydberg, P., Karlsson, P., et al. (2002). Analysis of acrylamide, a carcinogen formed in heated foodstuffs. *Journal of Agricultural and Food Chemistry, 50*, 4998–5006.

Taubert, D., Harlfinger, S., Henkes, L., et al. (2004). Influence of processing parameters on acrylamide formation during frying of potatoes. *Journal of Agricultural and Food Chemistry, 52*, 2735–2739.

Vass, M., Amrein, T. M., Schönbächler, B., et al. (2004). Ways to reduce the acrylamide formation in cracker products. *Czech Journal of Food Science, 22*, 19–21.

Vranova, J., & Ciesarova, Z. (2009). Furan in food, A review. *Czech Journal of Food Science, 27*, 1–10.

Wenzl, T., & Anklam, E. (2007). European Union database of acrylamide levels in food: Update and critical review of data collection. *Food Additives and Contaminants, 24*(S1), 5–12.

Wenzl, T., Lachenmeier, D. W., & Gökmen, V. (2007). Analysis of heat-induced contaminants (acrylamide, chloropropanols and furan) in carbohydrate-rich foods. *Analytical and Bioanalytical Chemistry, 389*, 119–137.

Wilson, D. M., Goldsworthy, T. L., Popp, J. A., & Butterworth, B. E. (1992). Evaluation of genotoxicity, pathological lesions, and cell proliferation in livers of rats and mice treated with furan. *Environmental and Molecular Mutagenesis, 19*, 209–222.

Yaylayan, V. A., Locas, C. P., Wronowski, A., & O'Brien, J. (2005). Mechanistic pathways of formation of acrylamide from different amino acids. In M. Friedman & D. S. Mottram (Eds.), *Chemistry and safety of acrylamide in food* (pp. 191–204). NY: Springer.

Zoller, O., Sager, F., & Reinhard, H. (2007). Furan in food: Headspace method and product survey. *Food Additives and Contaminants, 24*(S1), 91–107.

Zyzak, D. V., Sanders, R. A., Stojanovic, M., et al. (2003). Acrylamide formation mechanism in heated foods. *Journal of Agricultural and Food Chemistry, 51*, 4782–4787.

CHAPTER

24

Responding to Incidents of Low Level Chemical Contamination in Food

Elizabeth A. Szabo[1], Edward Jansson[1], David Miles[1], Tracy Hambridge[2], Glenn Stanley[2], Janis Baines[2] and Paul Brent[2]

[1]The New South Wales Food Authority, Silverwater NSW, Australia
[2]Food Standards Australia New Zealand, Canberra BC ACT, Australia

OUTLINE

24.1 INTRODUCTION

There is a community expectation in Australia and New Zealand that food will be safe, and, in general, for most of the people most of the time, this expectation is met. The safety of food, however, is dependent on many factors, not all of which can be controlled through government legislation and regulations. Much of the shared responsibility for food safety lies within the agricultural sector and the processed food industry to ensure that reliable, preventative procedures are in place to produce consistently safe foods.

Food outlets and consumers also share responsibility to ensure food is handled and prepared in ways that do not introduce new risks.

Food risks can result from a broad range of microbiological, chemical or physical factors. In this chapter we will focus on the contamination of food by chemical hazards. Chemicals may be present in foods through the intentional and legitimate use of various chemicals, such as pesticides, veterinary medicines and other agricultural chemicals and via chemicals used in food production, such as food additives and processing aids. Chemical contamination may occur from environmental pollution by heavy metals; chemicals found naturally in foods such as some plant toxins; migration of chemicals from packaging materials; and as a result of food processing.

The potential human health effects, though infrequently manifested, of chemical contaminants found in food are as diverse as the variety of contaminants. These range from relatively modest changes such as effects on enzyme activity and body weight, to more significant changes such as birth defects and cancer (WHO, 2008a). The onset of health effects and association with a foodborne chemical contaminant might occur months to years after past or current exposure. Our knowledge of the potential health risks of chemicals has increased with developments in medical science and in the availability of analytical tools for discovering new chemicals or detecting them in increasingly minute amounts.

The intent of this chapter is to explore strategies for responding to low level chemical contamination of food. We use case studies of incidents involving environmental (dioxins in seafood), natural (cyanogenic glycosides in cassava-based snacks), and deliberate (melamine in dairy-based foods) chemical contamination of food to illustrate response approaches. Common to each issue is the use of a widely accepted method called risk analysis, which identifies, assesses and manages food-related health risks within a structured framework.

24.2 RISK ANALYSIS

Risk analysis can be used across a broad range of circumstances and can lead to effective management strategies even when the available data are limited. The framework used in Australia and New Zealand is based on the general framework endorsed by the Codex Alimentarius Commission (Codex, 2004). As discussed briefly below, the risk analysis framework is comprised of three distinct but interrelated components, namely risk assessment, risk management and risk communication.

Risk assessment involves a science-based approach that utilizes experimental and other available data to characterize the risk and arrive at a conclusion regarding the potential risk associated with a food or food ingredient.

Risk management assists in defining the risk assessment scope and questions to be addressed. It also considers options for managing identified food risks in the broader context, taking into account the potential benefits of the food as well as relevant policy, consumer behaviors and economic issues associated with use of the food.

Risk communication is the interactive exchange of information and opinions regarding risks, risk-related factors, and risk perceptions among all concerned parties, or stakeholders, throughout the entire risk analysis process. It is an ongoing process that engages stakeholders and the public in decision making to the maximum extent possible. Risk communication is also important in bridging the gap which sometimes exists between the scientific assessment and consumers' perception of the health risk.

Any risk analysis framework needs to be supported by guiding principles. These might include:

- *Use the best available data and methodologies.* Scientific, economic and other data and information come from both published and unpublished sources, but in both cases, data should be as reliable and as objective as possible. Critical evaluation of the available data is an essential element in establishing the basis for the safety of food and subsequent risk management decisions. Where possible, collaboration with other experts or organizations, both national and international should be sought.

- *Recognize uncertainty in risk analysis.* It is inevitable that decisions in relation to the safety of food will be made in the presence of scientific uncertainty. In deciding on the risk management options, it is appropriate to recognize, document and address scientific uncertainty. Depending on the level and nature of uncertainty, a cautious approach to risk management options, such as proposed changes to current food regulations, may be taken to ensure that the overall risk remains low. However, scientific uncertainty should not be a reason for inaction when there is reasonable evidence to indicate a potential health risk. Where high levels of uncertainty exist, further information or data may need to be collected, and a revised risk assessment conducted, before risk management options can be considered. As new evidence emerges over time, risk management options need to be revised and updated.
- *Tailor the risk management approach to the risk.* In managing food-related health risks, there are generally a number of options available, depending on the nature of the risk. Quantifying and comparing different risks is difficult, but qualitative comparisons are generally possible using criteria such as the severity of the outcome and the likelihood of the risk. In deciding on the risk management approach, consideration needs to be given to the level of potential risk; which in the case of food, will also depend on the importance of the food in the context of the total diet or for a particular population sub-group. Another factor influencing the level of protection in a particular case will be the level of risk which is acceptable to the community.

- *Involve interested and affected groups.* The involvement of groups that have an interest in the outcome of a risk analysis can enhance the process through the provision of scientific data; identifying relevant social, ethical and economic factors; and suggesting alternative management approaches. While the processes and rules for such involvement need to be clear, interested and affected groups can provide opportunities for building trust as well as contributing credibility to the successful implementation of the ultimate risk management decisions.
- *Communicate in an open and transparent manner.* Documents outlining risk management options in relation to food-related health risks should generally be publicly available and public submissions on these documents should be taken into account in the regulatory decisions. Confidential commercial information can be protected. Dialogue with industries, consumers and health professionals on food regulatory matters is integral to the risk analysis process. It is also facilitated by encouraging stakeholders to comment on documents outlining risk management options.
- *Review the regulatory response.* In some cases, it is not easy to predict with certainty the outcome of a regulatory decision regarding food. After a certain period, it is necessary to examine the impact of the regulation to ensure that the predicted outcome was achieved and/or that the assumptions used in the assessment were correct. Surveys of the food supply and key stakeholder groups affected by regulatory changes, such as the food industry, health professionals, enforcement officers or consumers, can generally provide information to evaluate the outcome and determine whether further regulatory action is required.

The general principles supporting the risk analysis framework are relevant in responding to rapidly emerging incidents, however, time constraints may impact on the sequence of steps within this framework, dictated on a case-by-case basis.

24.3 GENERAL CONTROL MEASURES FOR CHEMICALS

Many countries have established regulatory levels for the control of chemical contaminants in food. This can be either a maximum residue limit (MRL) in the case of an agricultural or veterinary chemical, or a maximum level (ML) for a contaminant or natural toxicant in the food supply. For example, the Australia New Zealand Food Standards Code (the Code) outlines the limits that relate to agricultural and veterinary residues or contaminants in food. Food containing chemicals at levels greater than the MRL or ML are viewed as breaching the Code and subject to regulatory enforcement action at the border and within the nation.

24.3.1 Maximum Residue Limits for Agricultural and Veterinary Residues in Food

The MRL is the highest concentration of a chemical residue that is legally permitted or accepted in a food. The MRL does not indicate the amount of chemical that is always present in a food but it does indicate the highest residue that could possibly result from the registered conditions of use. Testing for agricultural and veterinary residue levels in food assists in indicating whether an agricultural or veterinary chemical product has been used according to its registered use and if the MRL is exceeded then this indicates a likely misuse of the chemical product. In addition, MRLs, while not direct public health limits, act to protect public health and safety by minimizing residues in food while enabling the effective control of pests and diseases.

Standard 1.4.2 of the Code lists the limits for agricultural and veterinary chemical residues that may occur in foods. If a MRL is not listed for a particular agricultural or veterinary chemical-commodity combination, the default limit is that there must be no detectable residues of that chemical in that food. This general prohibition means that in the absence of the relevant MRL in Standard 1.4.2, legitimately treated produce may not be sold where there are detectable residues. In the current Australian regulatory system, there may be a time gap in the approval of MRLs for agricultural and veterinary chemical use on crops or animals, and the adoption of these MRLs into the Code that apply to saleable food.

In assessing the public health and safety implications of agricultural and veterinary residues, the dietary exposure to chemical residues from all potentially treated foods in the diet is compared to the relevant reference health standards such as the acceptable daily intake (ADI) and/or the acute reference dose (ARfD). The steps undertaken in conducting a dietary exposure assessment are:

- Determination of the residues of a chemical in a treated food; and
- Calculation of the dietary exposure to that food using food consumption data from national nutrition surveys and comparing this to the acceptable reference health standard.

24.3.2 Maximum Levels for Contaminants in Foods

Maximum Levels for contaminants and natural toxicants are listed in Standard 1.4.1 of the Code, where it has been established that a ML can serve an effective risk management function and only for those foods that provide a significant contribution to the total dietary exposure. Foods not listed in Standard 1.4.1 may contain low levels of contaminants or natural toxicants. As a general principle, regardless of whether or not a ML exists, the levels of contaminants and natural toxicants in all foods should be kept *as low as reasonably achievable* (the ALARA principle) (Abbott *et al.*, 2003).

In practice, MLs are set at a level that is slightly higher than the normal range of variation in levels in foods in order to avoid undue disruptions of food production and trade (ANZFA, 1998). However, MLs are not direct safety limits and cannot fulfill the purpose of being direct safety limits. This is because it is the exposure to a contaminant from the entire food supply that is most relevant to estimating public health implications, not exposure from a specific food.

Therefore, for many contaminant/food combinations, a ML has not been established or cannot be justified when a risk assessment indicates a low health risk. This does not mean that chemical contamination events for which there is no regulatory level are ignored and left unmanaged. In circumstances of chemical contamination where there are no established MLs, it is necessary to undertake an assessment of the risk for that particular situation, usually within a short timeframe. The first step in assessing the risk in relation to a chemical contaminant is understanding the nature of the potential adverse health effects associated with exposure to the contaminant and, if possible, to establish a safe level of dietary exposure. For many contaminants, there is a paucity of reliable data to identify and characterize the potential hazards, and thus to establish a safe level of human exposure.

Where data are available, it may be possible to establish a reference health standard or so-called 'tolerable intake', which can be calculated on a daily, weekly or longer basis. These reference values are usually established internationally by the Joint (FAO/WHO) Expert Committee on Food Additives (JECFA). The tolerable intake is also generally referred to as 'provisional' since there is often a lack of data on the consequences of human exposure at low levels, and new data may result in a change to the tolerable level.

For contaminants that accumulate in the body over time such as lead, cadmium, dioxin and mercury, the provisional tolerable weekly intake (PTWI) or monthly intake (PTMI) is used as a reference value in order to minimize the significance of daily variations in dietary exposures. For contaminants that do not accumulate in the body such as arsenic, the provisional tolerable daily intake (PTDI) is used. The PTDI, PTWI and PTMI apply to total exposure (i.e. food and non-food uses) and all sources of exposure need to be considered when comparing exposure to the reference health standard (WHO, 1987).

Many contaminants do not have an established reference health standard and data limitations might make it impossible to establish a provisional tolerable intake (PTI). In these cases, it might be possible to use a margin-of-exposure approach to determine the potential level of risk, by comparing the lowest level at which adverse effects occur (or the benchmark dose level) with the estimated level of exposure.

Estimation of dietary exposure to contaminants relies on concentration data for the contaminant in various foods together with data on the consumption level for each of these foods amongst various population groups; the more robust and extensive the input data, the more accurate the estimate of exposure. This information is then compared to the reference health standard (if available), or to a level known to cause adverse effects in animal or human studies resulting in a quantitative estimation of the level of risk from the diet. This input to risk management decision-making on the safety and suitability of food is equally applicable to the control of chemicals and during incident management.

24.3.3 National Food Incident Response Protocol

Ensuring food safety risks are understood and managed is a joint government and industry responsibility in Australia and New Zealand. The onus on industry is to produce food that is safe and suitable, and on governments to regulate on a risk basis to ensure industry has mechanisms in place to produce safe and suitable food.

The Australia New Zealand regulatory framework is discussed in more detail in Section 2.6 of Chapter 2 Development of Food Legislation around the World. In brief, the framework has four key elements: stakeholder input; policy development; standards setting; and implementation. One of the primary outputs of the framework is the Australia New Zealand Food Standards Code (the Code). The Code is implemented by food legislation in each Australian state and territory and in New Zealand. For example, in the state of New South Wales (NSW) this is achieved via the Food Act 2003. Competent authorities in states and territories have the responsibility for enforcing and policing the Code. All food offered for sale in Australia (imported or locally manufactured) must comply with the requirements of the Code. When food incidents occur, legislation enables competent authorities to take action.

Food incidents can not only result in public health and safety risks among consumers but can also cause widespread consumer concern and significant disruption to domestic and international trade. Whilst the majority of food incidents may be limited to a local area or jurisdiction, the modern nature of food distribution and retailing increases the possibility that a food incident will impact across a number of jurisdictions. Past experiences of Australian food regulatory agencies in responding to a national food incident have highlighted the importance of coordination between jurisdictions during a food incident and of gaining consensus on the appropriate response (e.g. level and extent of food recall). Inconsistencies in the response by jurisdictions on the same issue could render all jurisdictions vulnerable to criticism and scrutiny, and result in consumer confusion.

For these reasons, the National Food Incident Response Protocol (Australian Government, 2007) was developed and in 2007 endorsed by all members of the Food Regulation Standing Committee and the Australia New Zealand Food Regulation Ministerial Council. The Protocol formalized current arrangements between jurisdictions for responding to national food incidents.

The Protocol does not override the existing (emergency) response protocols of individual agencies or jurisdictions rather it provides a link between the protocols of Australian Government and State and Territory agencies responsible for food safety and food issues.

There are three main phases in responding to a national food incident:

1. Alert phase
2. Action phase
3. Stand-down phase.

An outline of the steps involved in responding to a national food incident is given in Figure 24.1. Not all incidents will trigger the Protocol. For example, the detection of a chemical contaminant in nationally distributed food at a level of public health concern would require a national response and triggering of the protocol. The detection of elevated levels of a chemical contaminant in a food made and distributed in a single jurisdiction would not trigger the protocol. Other mechanisms exist to enable information sharing with other jurisdictions when a national response is not required.

24.4 CASE STUDIES

Although risk analysis provides a structured framework for approaching issues of chemical contamination, users should not have the expectation that it will deliver the same response outcome time and time again. Rather, the framework offers flexibility in response determined on a case-by-case basis. This is best illustrated via the following case studies.

24.4.1 Environmental Contamination: *Dioxins*

24.4.1.1 *The Issue*

Sydney Harbour (meaning the harbor and its estuaries) has been a working harbor for over 100

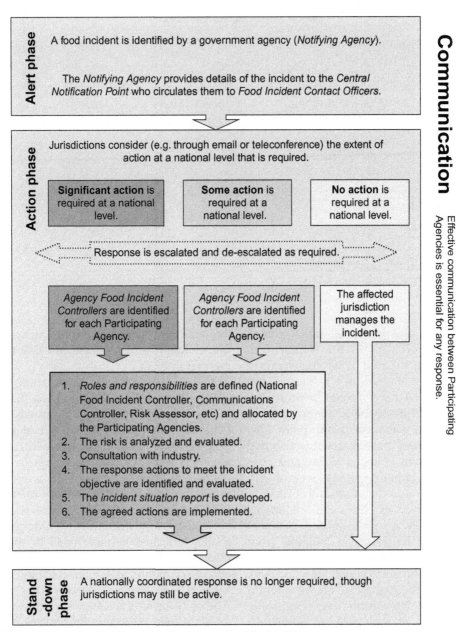

Alert phase

A food incident is identified by a government agency (*Notifying Agency*).

The *Notifying Agency* provides details of the incident to the *Central Notification Point* who circulates them to *Food Incident Contact Officers*.

Action phase

Jurisdictions consider (e.g. through email or teleconference) the extent of action at a national level that is required.

Significant action is required at a national level.

Some action is required at a national level.

No action is required at a national level.

Response is escalated and de-escalated as required.

Agency Food Incident Controllers are identified for each Participating Agency.

Agency Food Incident Controllers are identified for each Participating Agency.

The affected jurisdiction manages the incident.

1. *Roles and responsibilities* are defined (National Food Incident Controller, Communications Controller, Risk Assessor, etc) and allocated by the Participating Agencies.
2. The risk is analyzed and evaluated.
3. Consultation with industry.
4. The response actions to meet the incident objective are identified and evaluated.
5. The *incident situation report* is developed.
6. The agreed actions are implemented.

Stand-down phase

A nationally coordinated response is no longer required, though jurisdictions may still be active.

Communication

Effective communication between Participating Agencies is essential for any response.

FIGURE 24.1 The steps involved in responding to a national food incident.

years with many industries lining its foreshores. One such site was the Rhodes peninsula along Homebush Bay with several chemical plants situated in the area since 1928 (see Figure 24.2). Union Carbide was one of the plants producing chemicals containing dioxin, including the herbicide mixture called Agent Orange. Reclamation work, sometimes using contaminated material,

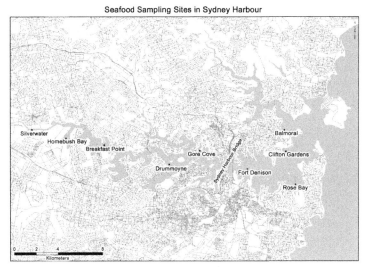

FIGURE 24.2   Seafood sampling sites in Sydney Harbour.

and runoff from the industrial sites created a contamination problem in the sediment of Homebush Bay. In the mid 1980s the chemical plants were closed. Subsequent testing of soil and sediment showed significant chemical contamination. From 1988 to 1993, initial remediation work on land was undertaken. From 1989 to 1991, when dioxins were detected in fish and prawn samples from Homebush Bay and elsewhere in Sydney Harbour, various levels of fishing bans were introduced and are still current.

A national survey of dioxins in sediments published in 2004 as part of the National Dioxins Program found levels ranging from 0.002 to 520 pg TEQ[1]/g dry weight across the Australian environment (Müller *et al.*, 2004). Not surprisingly, the highest levels were found in the vicinity of Homebush Bay: specifically the lower reaches at and west of Homebush Bay (100 and 520 pg TEQ/g) and in some areas east of Homebush Bay (78 and 130 pg TEQ/g).

Remediation work, including almost 10% of the sediment in the Homebush Bay area, commenced in 2006.

Prior to undertaking remediation work, the NSW Maritime Authority funded a study to look at levels of dioxins in fish and prawns in Sydney Harbour. The project was designed to provide baseline data for comparison with data taken after the remediation was completed to demonstrate the effectiveness of the work. The first results became available in November 2005 and included prawns sampled from five sites between Silverwater and Drummoyne (Figure 24.2). These results indicated similar levels to those found during previous testing, except that samples from outside prohibited commercial fishing zones also showed high levels of dioxins. The NSW Food Authority, being the competent authority for the safety of food for sale in the state of New South Wales, was informed and called upon to respond to the findings.

[1] The overall toxicity of a mixture of dioxins is expressed as a TEQ or Toxic Equivalent. This is the sum total of the amounts of each chemical detected when they are expressed as an equivalently toxic amount to the most toxic of the overall dioxin group, 2,3,7,8-tetrachloro-dibenzo-dioxin (TCDD).

24.4.1.2 *The Hazard*

'Dioxins' is a generic term for a group of 210 environmentally persistent chemicals. It includes 17 related polychlorinated dibenzodioxins (PCDDs) and dibenzofurans (PCDFs) considered by the World Health Organization to have significant toxicity to humans. Also included in the dioxin group are 12 compounds, called dioxin-like polychlorinated biphenyls (PCBs), out of a group of 209 PCBs (European Commission, 2000). The most dangerous chemical in the dioxin group is 2,3,7,8-tetrachlorodibenzo-para-dioxin (TCDD). In 1997, the International Agency for Research on Cancer (IARC)—part of the World Health Organization—nominated this compound as a Class 1 carcinogen, meaning a 'known human carcinogen' (IARC, 1997).

Dioxins are not manufactured intentionally. They are formed by natural processes such as volcanic activity and forest or grass fires. It is thought that bushfires contribute at least 20–30% of the total release of dioxin-like compounds to the Australian environment (Australian Government, 2004a). Humans and the environment have been exposed to and coping with low levels of dioxin-like compounds from combustion sources for hundreds of thousands of years. Dioxins are also produced as by-products of industrial processes such as waste incineration, pulp and paper bleaching, and the synthesis of certain chemicals. PCBs, on the other hand, were manufactured for approximately 50 years for use as components of insulating fluids in transformers and other electrical equipment, and are no longer manufactured.

Dioxins persist for a very long time in the environment. As they are fat soluble they can bioaccumulate along the food chain and have been found to be present in many foods such as dairy products, meat, fish and shellfish. International and Australian studies have concluded that around 95% of human exposure to dioxins occurs through the diet, with foods of animal origin such as meat, dairy products and fish being the main sources (Australian Government, 2004b).

Unborn children are exposed to dioxin-like compounds *in utero*, and nursing infants are exposed to these contaminants present in breast milk. People may also have some limited exposure through other routes such as breathing in air contaminated by dioxins (e.g. in smoke from bushfires or from incinerator emissions) but exposure to dioxins by such routes is not significant.

There have been some well publicized incidents of contamination of food supplies by dioxins:

- In 1999 dioxins were the cause of a food scare in Belgium affecting poultry and eggs; animal feed contaminated by PCB oil was the likely source;
- Also in 1999 dioxins were found in milk in Germany and traced back to Brazilian citrus pulp pellets contaminated by dioxin-containing lime, imported to Europe and used as a feed component for cattle;
- In 2008 a major recall of fresh and processed pig meat was instigated by Irish authorities after the detection of dioxin in the product destined for human consumption, again likely to be due to feed contamination.

Until 2005, Australian authorities had not encountered such an incident. Our knowledge of dioxins in the Australian environment came mainly from the National Dioxins Program, funded by the Australian Government and managed by the Department of the Environment and Heritage (DEH) during 2001–2004. The Department of the Environment and Heritage collected information on the levels of dioxin-like compounds in various environmental media in Australia, including air, soil, and sediments. It also collected data on concentrations of dioxins in the blood serum of different segments of the population.

In related projects, Food Standards Australia New Zealand (FSANZ) measured the levels of these compounds in various foods and estimated dietary exposures for different population subgroups, the Australian Department of Health and Ageing (DHA) measured dioxin-like compounds in breast milk, and the Australian Department of Agriculture, Fisheries and Forestry (DAFF) reported on levels in various agricultural commodities including meat, milk and fish. An overall risk assessment of exposure to dioxins in Australia (Australian Government, 2004b) concluded that:

- the Australian population can be confident that current background exposures to dioxin-like compounds are generally low compared with other similar countries;
- in the light of the environmental persistence and long biological half-lives for many of the dioxin-like compounds, it is prudent to take all reasonable steps to further reduce human exposure.

Although the exact impact of dioxins on human health is not fully understood, many governments take measures to keep dioxins in the food supply as low as possible. For example, the European Commission on 3 February 2006 adopted a maximum level for muscle meat of fish and fishery products of 4 pg TEQ/g fresh weight for PCDD/Fs and one of 8 pg/g fresh weight for the combined total of PCDD/Fs and dioxin-like PCB, which was enforced in November 2006 (European Commission, 2006). No such level has been set in Australia as it was determined by FSANZ that the level of exposure from food was well below the established reference health standard (the Australian Tolerable Monthly Intake for dioxins, TMI, is 70 pg TEQ dioxins/kg body weight per month).

With regard to Sydney Harbour, the dioxin results from prawns tested by the NSW Maritime Authority were compared to levels reported in the National Dioxins Program and to maximum levels used in the European Union (NSW Food Authority, 2006). A decision was made to conduct further testing of prawns (*Metapenaeus macleayi*) and extend the testing to bream (*Acanthopagrus australis*) as a representative of a bottom feeding finfish species likely to contain higher levels of dioxins. Overall, samples were taken from nine sites across Sydney Harbour and its tributaries as illustrated in Figure 24.2.

The National Measurement Institute analyzed prawn and bream samples for total dioxins using high resolution gas spectrometry/high resolution mass spectrometry. Amounts detected were translated using the World Health Organization toxic equivalency factors and expressed as pg TEQ/g fresh weight (WHO, 1998) for the 29 dioxin congeners determined by the WHO to be of concern.

Thirty-six composite prawn samples were taken across seven sites (Silverwater, Parramatta River near Homebush Bay, Breakfast Point, Drummoyne, Gore Cove, Fort Denison, and Clifton Gardens). The content of dioxins in the samples ranged from 3.1–22.9 pg TEQ/g fresh weight. The compound 2,3,7,8-TCDD (considered the most toxic dioxin) predominated. The mean across the sample sites was 11.3 pg TEQ/g fresh weight.

Forty composite bream samples were taken across eight sites (from Silverwater in the west to Balmoral in the east). The content of dioxins in the samples ranged from 6.6–141 pg TEQ/g fresh weight. The compound 2,3,7,8-TCDD predominated in all but one sample where a dioxin-like PCB compound predominated. The mean across the sample sites was 29.1 pg TEQ/g fresh weight. Excluding samples taken from the Homebush Bay area which was known to be highly contaminated, the adjusted mean level was 19.5 pg TEQ/g fresh weight.

Compared to European limits of dioxins in fish muscle meat (4 pg TEQ dioxins and furans/g fresh weight and 8 pg TEQ total dioxin/g fresh weight), results of dioxin testing of commercially important species taken from Sydney Harbour and its esturaries (2005/2006) were higher.

Because recreational fishing was also permitted in Sydney Harbour, testing of 14 other seafood species of particular interest to recreational fishing was undertaken. Species tested were crab, flounder, kingfish, luderick, sand whiting, sea mullet, silver biddy, silver trevally, tailor, trumpeter whiting, yellowtail scad, squid, dusky flathead, and fan-bellied leatherjacket. From March to September 2006, there were 243 samples of crustacea, fish and molluscs collected. The dioxin concentrations ranged significantly between the types of fish. For example, sea mullet, silver biddie, silver trevally and tailor had mean concentrations of 99, 41, 29 and 38 pg TEQ/g, respectively.

The mean dioxin concentration across the whole geographical sample area for crustacea was 11 pg TEQ/g, the mean concentration for fish was 25 pg TEQ/g and molluscs had a mean concentration of 17 pg TEQ/g. The Sydney Harbour Bridge was used as a reference point because it is a readily recognizable landmark. Seafood dioxin concentrations differed significantly from east to west of the bridge, and closer to the contaminated Homebush Bay site. The mean concentration in fish east of the bridge was 11 pg TEQ/g, while to the west, fish had a noticeably higher mean concentration of 37 pg TEQ/g. When separating crustacea samples between east and west of the bridge, the mean concentrations were 6 pg TEQ/g and 13 pg TEQ/g, respectively. Molluscs collected east of the bridge had a mean concentration of 6 pg TEQ/g with the mean concentration of samples west of the bridge at 24 pg TEQ/g.

24.4.1.3 *The Risks*

In December 2005, the NSW Food Authority formed an Expert Panel on Dioxins (NSW Food Authority, 2006) to provide advice on the public health risks posed by the levels of dioxins in seafood caught in Sydney Harbour. The panel was comprised of people with expertise in toxicology, marine biology, environmental science, analytical testing, medicine, risk management, food regulation, dietary exposure assessment, and risk communication.

The first dietary exposure assessment conducted for this issue was based on the test results from *commercially* important species from Sydney Harbour (predominantly prawns and bream) and was undertaken by FSANZ (2006). This showed that for seafood caught from Sydney Harbour, there was the potential for frequent eaters (for example, recreational or commercial

fishers who eat their own catch) to exceed the reference health standard for dioxins and relates to the 29 dioxin congeners determined by WHO to be of concern (the Australian TMI is 70 pg TEQ dioxins/kg body weight per month). People who very rarely consume seafood from Sydney Harbour (2 or 3 times per year, or less) were not likely to have dietary exposures to dioxins that exceeded the reference health standard.

Levels of dioxins in seafood caught in Sydney Harbour were higher than for seafood found in other areas of Australia. It was noted that previous surveys in other areas of Australia revealed dioxins in all other fish samples tested at less than 1 pg TEQ/g. Furthermore, it was calculated that on average more than one 150 gram serve per month of fish, or two 150 gram serves of prawns, from Sydney Harbour (excluding Homebush Bay itself where no fishing is allowed) could result in consumers exceeding the recommended TMI for dioxins.

The Dioxin Expert Panel noted that information presented to them suggested widespread contamination of dioxins in seafood caught in Sydney Harbour and the levels of dioxins in prawns and bream, used as 'indicator' species, were equivalent to or higher than levels found in some seafood caught from other highly contaminated areas in the world. The Panel advised that unless new empirical data is generated on a species-by-species basis, any risk management strategy applied to commercial fishing should be applied to all species.

Based on the data before them, the Panel concluded that seafood caught by commercial fishers in Sydney Harbour posed a possible public health risk and should not be consumed on a regular long-term basis until further data demonstrated the safety of the product. However, consumption patterns that fall within the restrictions outlined in the dietary exposure assessment should have no health implications. The Dioxin Expert Panel agreed that no more than one 150 gram serve per month of fish, or two 150 gram serves of prawns, should be consumed from Sydney Harbour.

The second dietary exposure assessment was based on the test results from *recreationally* important species from Sydney Harbour (Table 24.1) and was also undertaken by FSANZ (2007). Separate dietary modeling on data east and west of the Sydney Harbour Bridge was provided to the Dioxin Expert Panel. The Panel noted that on a species-by-species basis, the mean serves per month that an individual could consume before the reference health standard was exceeded varied greatly. In considering the dioxin levels in seafood sampled west of the bridge, the Panel noted the general trend for higher levels of dioxin in species in that area. The Panel considered it appropriate to revise the dietary advice for seafood caught in the harbor and advised that seafood caught west of the bridge should not be consumed. The key points in the Panel's advice were:

- Recreational fishers should avoid consuming seafood caught west of the bridge;
- Recreational fishers who eat a variety of seafood caught east of the bridge can consume 150 g of seafood from this source per week;
- Recreational fishers who frequently eat certain species of seafood caught east of the bridge require access to more detailed information on a species-by-species basis to ensure their intake remains within the reference health standard (Table 24.1); and
- In the absence of data on a particular species, the general advice noted above for east and west of the bridge should guide any risk management strategy.

TABLE 24.1   Estimates of the maximum number of 150 g serves before the tolerable monthly intake (TMI) is exceeded

		East of the Harbour Bridge		
Seafood	Number of samples[1]	Mean conc. of dioxins (pg TEQ/g)	Maximum grams before TMI exceeded	No. 150 gram serves before TMI exceeded
All Crustacea	**12**	**6**	**625–748**	**4 per month**
Prawns	6	6	625–748	4 per month
Crab	6	5	750–898	5 per month
All Fish	**146**	**11**	**341–408**	**2 per month**
Bream	15	18	208–249	1 per month
Flounder	9	2	1876–2245	12 per month
Kingfish	8	2	1876–2245	12 per month
Luderick	16	2	1876–2245	12 per month
Sand Whiting	23	3	1251–1496	8 per month
Sea Mullet	8	70	54–64	1 every 3 months
Silver Biddie	14	23	163–195	1 per month
Silver Trevally	6	5	750–898	5 per month
Tailor	6	24	156–187	1 per month
Trumpeter Whiting	21	2	1876–2245	12 per month
Yellowtail Scad	14	3	1251–1496	8 per month
Molluscs (Squid)	**15**	**6**	**625–748**	**4 per month**

[1]One sample represents a composite of up to ten individuals.

24.4.1.4 *The Response*

Australia is a signatory to the Stockholm Convention on Persistent Organic Pollutants (POPs) and so is committed to reducing and, where possible, eliminating production and release of POPs into the environment. Dioxins are one of the groups of chemicals covered by this Convention. Just prior to the emergence of the issue of dioxins in seafood from Sydney Harbour, the Australian government released a National Action Plan for addressing dioxins in October 2005. In relation to food, the Plan stated that the Australian food supply contained low levels of dioxins in comparison to the rest of the world and it committed Australia to resurvey the Australian food supply in 2010 to ensure that this was still the case, as resources allow (Australian Government, 2005).

Australia does not have a standard imposing a maximum level for dioxins in food. To assist with the management of the issue of dioxins in seafood from Sydney Harbour, a temporary action level was endorsed by the Dioxin Expert Panel. This is not an enforceable level but a level where appropriate counter-measures can be considered on a case-by-case basis. The aim of the temporary action level was to guide further investigation of the reasons for high levels of dioxins. Seafood exceeding the temporary action level triggered an investigation of consumption patterns in relation to risk.

The temporary action level was calculated for seafood using:

- average meal size for seafood of 150 g per week derived from 1998/99 Australian Bureau of Statistics data for average annual consumption (Australian Bureau of Statistics, 2000);
- average body weight of 70 kg;
- current background level of exposure to dioxins from food in Australia estimated at up to 22% of the TMI (FSANZ, 2004) leaving a further 54 pg TEQ/kg body weight/month before the recommended TMI of 70 pg TEQ/ kg body weight/month is exceeded. This 'additional' capacity of 54 pg TEQ/kg body weight/month translates to a weekly intake of around 13 pg TEQ/kg body weight.

The temporary action level was calculated as the acceptable weekly intake × average body-weight/average meal size. That calculation ($13 \times 70/150$) resulted in a temporary action level of 6 pg TEQ/g fresh weight for dioxins in seafood from Sydney Harbour.

The issue of dioxins in seafood from Sydney Harbour required a response on two fronts: 1) commercial fishing; and 2) recreational fishing.

Commercial fishing in Sydney Harbour was a small yet viable industry contributing less than 2% of finfish and less than 1% of prawns sold in markets around the State. Discussions on the future of commercial fishing in Sydney Harbour would affect the livelihoods of 44 commercial fishers. Several risk management options were considered and discussed with stakeholders (commercial fishers, seafood markets, government). The range of ways of protecting consumers were:

1. Seafood from Sydney Harbour should be labeled and marketed separately from seafood from other catchments together with consumption advice (stakeholders indicated that it was unlikely that consumers would purchase such seafood, industry were concerned of broader negative impacts);
2. Given that only high level consumers were at risk, co-mingling of seafood from Sydney Harbour with seafood from elsewhere would reduce the risk of a consumer exceeding the TMI for dioxins—this would need to be coupled with a consumer education campaign (stakeholders were concerned about consumer confusion and that this would result in consumers reducing the amount of seafood in their diet);
3. Provide consumption advice only (stakeholders were concerned about consumer confusion and consumers

reducing or excluding seafood from their diet); or

4. Close Sydney Harbour to commercial fishing (stakeholders agreed this was the best option available to protect the public and the broader industry).

A complete closure of Sydney Harbour and its estuaries to commercial fishing was implemented in 2006 and is effective until 2011.

Risk assessment results and the subsequent risk management approach was communicated to affected stakeholders via industry meetings, the media (print, radio, television), foreshore signage, websites, letters and brochures to commercial fishers. The New South Wales government announced a AU$5.8 million package that included a voluntary buy out of commercial fishing businesses, further testing for dioxins in the fish, and a public information campaign to advise recreational fishers and the community about the risks of eating seafood caught in the Harbour.

With regard to recreational fishing in Sydney Harbour, as the Dioxin Expert Panel advised that fish caught west of the bridge should not be consumed it was considered there were only two options available.

1. Prevent all fishing in Sydney Harbour (east and west of the bridge) by putting in place a fishing ban; or
2. Develop a communication strategy to ensure that recreational fishers are aware of the consumption advice.

Option 2 was preferred for the following reasons:

- A closure mandating 'catch and release' would be difficult to police and provide a false sense of security;
- A complete closure would unnecessarily prevent recreational fishing east of the bridge where dioxin levels in seafood were lower;
- An advisory option would allow a much more productive and positive interaction with fishers with an ability to disseminate

other information and build better rapport and trust, and hence compliance with the recommendations;

- Anecdotal information suggested that the advisory program put in place when the Harbour was closed for commercial fishing was working well.

The lower dioxin concentrations found in seafood caught east of the bridge had the potential to result in a relaxation to seafood consumption advice. However, it was generally agreed by risk managers that the existing advice of 150 g per month of mixed seafood should remain in force as a precaution. This is because anglers may lack the skill to differentiate species and effectively interpret the more detailed advice. An option for fishers to review the type of seafood they consumed and adjust consumption based on specific species advice was provided and communicated to recreational fishers via foreshore signage, brochures, and the NSW Food Authority's website (www.foodauthority. nsw.gov.au).

Table 24.2 provides an outline of the timeline of response to this issue.

24.4.2 Naturally Occurring Contamination: *Cyanogenic Glycosides*

24.4.2.1 The Issue

Adapting 'traditional' food from other countries to 'Western' style diets can lead to the inadvertent exposure of consumers to potentially harmful, naturally occurring chemicals. For example, cassava (Manihot esculenta Crantz) is a hardy plant grown in many tropical countries where it is an important food source. Cassava-based products have been available to Western consumers for many years and their profile has increased as manufacturers use the gluten-free nature of cassava to provide variety and choice for consumers with gluten intolerances, particularly in the snack food sector. Cassava contains,

TABLE 24.2 Timeline of key events in responding to dioxins contamination of seafood from Sydney Harbour

Focus	Date	Key event
Remediation work	Nov 2005	Monitoring shows prawns with elevated levels of dioxins, competent food safety authority notified
Dioxins and commercial fishing	Nov 2005	Testing program for prawns and bream commences
	Dec 2005	Temporary closure of Sydney Harbour to commercial prawning
		Formation of Dioxin expert panel
	Jan 2006	Test results reviewed by Dioxin expert panel and public risk identified
	Feb 2006	Closure of Sydney Harbour to all commercial fishing until 2011
	Feb 2006	NSW Government announces AU$5.8 M buy-out package for industry (includes funding for further testing and risk communication)
Dioxins and recreational fishing	Mar 2006	Testing of seafood species relevant to recreational fishing commences
	Nov 2006	Dioxin expert panel reviews new dietary advice for recreational fishing east and west of the Sydney Harbour Bridge and identifies higher risk of consuming seafood west of the Harbour Bridge
	Dec 2006	Risk management and communication strategies developed for recreational fishers east and west of the Harbour Bridge
		Public release of new advice east and west of the Harbour Bridge for recreational fishers
Remediation work	Jan 2007	Remediation work continues at Homebush Bay

in its natural state, compounds called cyanogenic glycosides. A problem can occur with cassava-based products under certain circumstances (Cardoso *et al.*, 2005). If insufficiently processed, the cassava can retain elevated levels of cyanogenic glycosides which bacteria in the human gut can break down to form hydrogen cyanide (or hydrocyanic acid, HCN) as an end product.

In January 2008, the NSW Food Authority received advice of the detection in Japan of higher than normal levels of HCN in cassava-based chips/crackers that were manufactured in New South Wales. Japanese authorities regarded the level (59 mg/kg or 59 parts per million, ppm) as 'a danger to damage human health' (translation). The cassava-based chips/crackers were derived from dried cassava pellets, which were made from a mixture of tapioca flour and fresh

cassava. The pellets were deep fried, flavored, packaged and distributed for retail sale.

24.4.2.2 The Hazard

Linamarin is the main (93%) cyanogenic glycoside present in cassava together with a small amount of lotaustralin (7%) (FSANZ, 2008a). The formation of HCN is a two-step process that is performed by endogenous enzymes as shown in Figure 24.3. Initially, a β-glucosidase enzyme (linamarase) hydrolyzes the glycosidic bond linking the glucose to the α-hydroxynitrile (cyanohydrin); then hydrogen cyanide (or hydrocyanic acid) is dissociated from acetone cyanohydrin (or from butanone cyanohydrin for lotaustralin) either non-enzymatically or through action of another enzyme, a hydroxynitrile lyase.

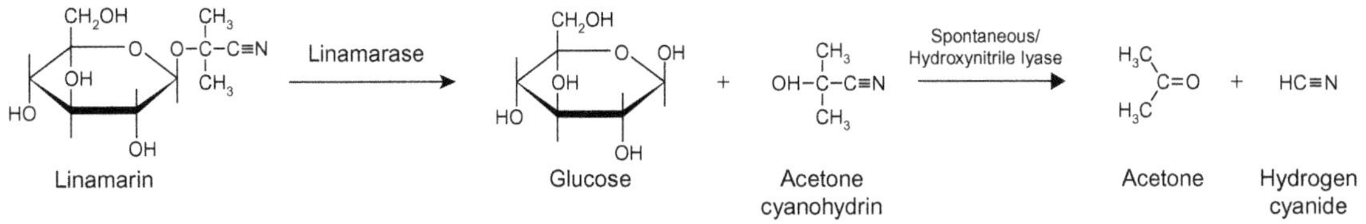

FIGURE 24.3   Chemical reaction for the formation of hydrocyanic acid from linamarin.

The non-enzymatic pathway is pH-dependent. At pH >6, high rates of dissociation occur; but at pH 5, the yield of hydrocyanic acid is much lower (Cooke, 1978). In spite of this, cyanohydrin co-exists with intact glucoside and hydrocyanic acid in differently processed cassava products. Therefore, cyanide in cassava products may exist in three forms: (i) the glucosides (linamarin and lotaustralin); (ii) the cyanohydrin; and (iii) free hydrogen cyanide.

It is essential that the linamarin content of raw cassava is reduced before human consumption and there are established processing methods to enable this to occur (Bradbury, 2006; Cumbana, Mirone, Cliff & Bradbury, 2007; FAO, 1977). HCN inhibits mitochondrial oxidation. If the level of exposure to HCN exceeds the capacity of normal physiological detoxification mechanisms, death can result. Clinical manifestations of acute cyanide poisoning, especially non-lethal doses are often non-specific and typically include headaches, dizziness, stomach pain, or mental confusion.

These symptoms closely resemble that of overindulgence or mild gastro-intestinal tract disturbance. Because the dose–response curve is steep, and symptoms occur some hours after ingestion, individuals exposed to dangerous levels of HCN may not recognize warning symptoms before consuming a lethal dose. Death in humans has been reported from HCN doses as low as 0.58 mg/kg body weight.

In some developing countries where cassava is the primary source of carbohydrate for the population, long-term exposure to sub-lethal concentrations of cyanogenic glycosides present ongoing health issues, such as Konzo, an irreversible motor neuron disease; clinical signs include the inability to walk, limited arm movement, and speech difficulties (Ernesto et al., 2002; Oluwole, 2008). Cassava products are not consumed to these levels in developed countries such as Australia and this situation is not expected to occur there. Sub-lethal exposure to cassava leading to mild clinical signs of intoxication would not be expected to lead to presentation at hospital emergency departments or general practitioners, and therefore would not be reported in most instances.

The correct processing of raw cassava ensures that the linamarin content in a processed product will be within an acceptable range. The processing methods use varying combinations of peeling, grating, soaking in water, and mild heat for the primary purpose of allowing the natural conversion of linamarin to HCN. The hydrogen cyanide formed is volatile and is released in the air rather than remaining in the food. To determine the risks associated with linamarin remaining in food, FSANZ considered toxicity studies conducted directly on linamarin and established an acute reference dose (ARfD) of 0.7 mg/kg body weight on the basis of death in hamsters at doses greater than 70 mg/kg body weight and applying a 100-fold uncertainty factor to account for intra-species variability and inter-species extrapolation (FSANZ, 2008). The available data suggested that there is sufficient enzymatic capacity in the microflora of the cecum to completely hydrolyze large amounts of linamarin as no unchanged linamarin was excreted in the feces following oral ingestion.

As total HCN levels are more readily determined than linamarin levels, the linamarin ARfD was converted to an ARfD for total HCN measured in cassava, for analytical convenience. One mole of linamarin can release one mole of hydrocyanic acid if hydrolysis is complete and on this basis the linamarin ARfD equates to an ARfD for HCN in cassava of 0.08 mg/kg body weight. As the lowest reported fatal absorbed dose for HCN is 0.58 mg/kg body weight, the ARfD for hydrocyanic acid provided a margin of exposure of seven which, given the steep dose–response curve for HCN toxicity, was considered to be appropriate.

Cassava-based products have been available to Western consumers for many years and are eaten in a variety of ways ranging from flour to vegetable dishes and desserts. Their profile has increased as manufacturers use the gluten-free property of cassava to provide variety and choice for consumers with gluten intolerances, particularly in the snack food sector. These products also are marketed as an alternative or substitute to potato crisps. While cassava products are not consumed in Western countries to the same levels as in some developing countries, industry and government still need to assess any potential health impact and manage it accordingly.

In the Code the following HCN limits apply: 25 mg/kg in confectionery; 5 mg/kg in stone fruit juices; 50 mg/kg in marzipan; 1 mg/kg per 1% alcohol in alcoholic beverages. Sweet cassava is defined in the Code, *Standard 1.1.2—Supplementary Definitions for Foods,* as containing less than 50 mg/kg hydrogen cyanide (hydrocyanic acid) on a fresh weight basis. Bitter varieties of cassava (listed in the Code in *Standard 1.4.4—Prohibited and Restricted Plants and Fungi* as a banned plant material) require extensive processing to remove the cyanogenic glycosides as they tend to be more evenly distributed throughout the root. When the issue emerged, a product standard for cassava-based snack foods was not available in Australia.

In the EU, the maximum permitted levels of HCN are as follows; 1 mg/kg in foodstuffs, 1 mg/kg in beverages, with the exception of 50 mg/kg in nougat, marzipan or its substitutes or similar products, 1 mg per percent of alcohol in alcoholic beverages and 5 mg/kg in canned stone fruit. An acceptable level in food and water referred to in the US is 25 mg/kg.

As a follow-up to the Australian-made product rejected by Japan, further testing of both domestic and imported cassava cracker/chip products was undertaken. Equally high levels of total HCN were found, when analyzed by a method developed by Bradbury, Egan, and Bradbury (1999). A total of 300 samples of ready-to-eat cassava chips were analyzed (Table 24.3), with the results showing significant variation in levels of total HCN.

Testing also included 12 samples of chip pellets (prior to deep frying to form the chip). These too showed significant variability, with levels of total HCN ranging from <10 to 237 mg/kg (mean value 96.7 mg/kg). It is unclear whether these levels resulted from inadequate processing of the sweet cassava prior to pellet formation, use of a cassava cultivar with inherently higher levels of cyanogenic glycosides, or the use of bitter cassava.

24.4.2.3 The Risks

A significant difficulty in determining levels of total HCN in cassava chip products, that is the sum of hydrogen cyanide evolved during enzymatic hydrolysis (see Figure 24.3), is the absence of a standard or reference analytical method. For a more general discussion on analytical methods, see Chapter 5 (Global Harmonization of Analytical Methods). It appeared that some laboratories were adapting methods for HCN in water and as a consequence were only determining the 'free' HCN content of the product, which resulted in a substantial under-reporting of the total hydrocyanic acid content of the food.

It was not possible to replicate the method used by Japanese authorities, which was a combined thermal and enzymatic method. Independent expert advice identified the Bradbury method

TABLE 24.3   Levels of total hydrocyanic acid found in local and imported cassava-based crackers

| Country of Origin | Brand | Level of total hydrocyanic acid expressed as mg/kg | | | |
		Number of samples	Mean Level (Std dev)	Minimum	Maximum
Australia	Brand 1	193	66.6 (27.7)	<10	145
Australia	Brand 2	10	10.1 (0.8)	<10	12
Australia	Brand 3	68	45.8 (14.4)	24	86
Australia	Brand 4	5	<10	<10	<10
China		3	<10	<10	<10
Indonesia	Brand 1	5	77.0 (6.9)	71	85
Indonesia	Brand 2	2	<10	<10	<10
Indonesia	Brand 3	3	38.3 (22.0)	13	53
Indonesia	Brand 4	1	<10	<10	<10
Korea		5	<10	<10	<10
Malaysia		5	<10	<10	<10
TOTAL		**300**	**55.8 (29.6)**	**<10**	**145**

(Bradbury *et al.*, 1999), as the most appropriate test available. Test results from 300 samples of ready-to-eat cassava chips on the Australian market were used by FSANZ to conduct a dietary exposure assessment for HCN in cassava chips. The assessment needed to take two key, variable parameters into consideration; the range of levels of total HCN likely to be found in these chips, and the range of exposures likely for a single sitting for various age groups.

Dietary exposure assessment used consumption data reported in the 1995 Australian National Nutrition Survey (Australian Bureau of Statistics, 1999) and the 1997 New Zealand National Nutrition Survey (New Zealand Government, 1999). Consumption of ready-to-eat cassava chips was not reported separately and was considered as captured under the 'extruded snacks' or 'other snacks' categories. Throughout the dietary exposure assessment, the combined consumption of equivalent salty snacks (crisps, extruded and other salty snacks) was used to estimate the amount

of ready-to-eat cassava chips that might be consumed in 1 day, on the assumption that consumers may substitute any similar salty snack with ready-to-eat cassava chips. Two dietary exposure assessment approaches were used; deterministic and probabilistic.

The deterministic assessment was based on acute dietary exposures to total HCN from ready-to-eat cassava chips and was estimated for the Australian and New Zealand populations, and for age and gender population sub-groups. The results showed that the mean concentration of total hydrocyanic acid of 63 mg/kg in cassava chips available for sale in January 2008 (sampled from domestic and imported cassava chips and a variety of products of the major suppliers of these products), could result in dietary exposures above the ARfD for all groups assessed. The assessment identified 2–4-year-old children as having the highest risk of exceeding the ARfD, with adults being less at risk. At a concentration of 25 mg/kg, most groups, particularly children, still exceeded the ARfD. At concentrations of 10 mg/kg, the lowest considered in the report, 2–4-year-old children remained at risk. However, such exposure would most likely only occur if a young child consumed more than 100 g of cassava chips in a single sitting. The risk is increased by the irregular eating patterns and low body-weight of this age group.

Exposure was also assessed using a probabilistic approach, which better accounted for the interplay of the parameters impinging on the risks to the key age group of 2–4-year-olds. A distribution of possible dietary exposures in the target age group and a calculation of the probability of exceeding the ARfD, were achieved through a simulation carried out by randomly multiplying each point of the distribution of salty snacks consumption with each point of the actual and simulated distributions of HCN concentration. The likelihood of 2–4-year-old Australian children exceeding the ARfD from consuming cassava chips with a mean concentration of 63 mg/kg was estimated at 56%; i.e. approximately one out of two occasions of eating cassava chips with this level of HCN may result in exposure above the ARfD.

The probability of exceeding the ARfD decreased to 17–22% at a mean concentration of 25 mg/kg, and 2–4% at a mean concentration of 10 mg/kg and a standard deviation of 5 or 10 mg/kg. Because of the short half-life of HCN, however, the consequences of exceeding the ARfD will depend on the time over which the exposure occurs, one sitting or across a day. Consequently, the probability of exceeding the ARfD is not necessarily equivalent to the probability of being at risk of an adverse event (illness). Available food consumption data does not distinguish between that eaten in a single sitting and that eaten across the day so refinement of the calculations was not possible. However, the 97.5th percentile consumption for salty snacks is approximately 100 g (male and female combined) for 2–4-year-olds and this quantity of snack is readily consumable in a single sitting.

For children aged 2–4 years, reducing the mean concentration of HCN in cassava chips to 10 mg/kg would reduce the potential incidence of exposures above the ARfD by 93–97%. Reducing the concentration to 25 mg/kg would lead to a lesser reduction of 61–70%.

Toxicologists from academia and government departments reviewed the dietary exposure assessment and concluded that inadequate processing of raw cassava that resulted in appreciable residual quantities of total HCN as detected in products on the Australian market might represent a public health risk. Children clearly were most at risk. The conclusions of the assessment were subsequently supported by the peer review of international experts.

24.4.2.4 The Response

Within 24 hours of the notification of the detection in Japan, the National Food Incident Response Protocol was activated and expert independent toxicological advice was sought. Preliminary expert advice was that if eaten in excess (between 100–200 g), the levels detected might manifest as mild symptoms such as vomiting, abdominal pain, anxiety, constriction of the throat, dizziness and weakness. Children were the most vulnerable group in this regard. The manufacturer was contacted, informed of the results and the health concern. In response, the company voluntarily recalled all their gluten-free product range. Jurisdictions across Australia issued media releases advising consumers to be cautious; namely, to avoid eating large quantities or overindulge in the consumption of cassava-based vegetable chip/cracker products—particularly children.

The extent of the problem was assessed by testing the product available on the Australian market. To support this activity, a preliminary risk assessment undertaken by FSANZ provided a guidance level of 25 mg/kg total HCN in cassava chips, considered a safe level to consume (FSANZ, 2008a). Cassava chips containing total hydrogen cyanide above this level presented a potential health risk (NB: the risk assessment was subsequently revised as described above). The manufacturers and importers of cassava chip products where testing detected levels above 25 mg/kg, were given notice that the product contained higher than acceptable levels of HCN. Businesses were asked to indicate what actions they intended to take to meet the guidance level of 25 mg/kg. The action taken by most companies was to voluntarily withdraw the product from the market.

The issuing of advisory notices warning consumers to limit their consumption of cassava-based chip products to an appropriate level gained good media coverage. However, the long-term effectiveness of these messages is not considered appropriate as a basis for a long-term risk management strategy. In addition, testing showed significant variability in levels of total HCN in cassava-based chip products.

Initial risk communication messages to the public were predicated on test results available at that stage of the incident. The average level detected was 80 mg/kg in the finished product and it was estimated that a 'safe' consumption level was around 200 g of chips for a 20 kg child. However, levels as high as 145 mg/kg were detected in some ready-to-eat cassava chip products, meaning that the 'safe' amount to consume would almost be halved. Batch to batch variability of total HCN in the product was observed, which tended to undermine the communication to the public regarding safe consumption levels. This also indicated that manufacturers needed to assert stronger control over the ingredients being used to make the cassava chips (and other ready-to-eat foods containing cassava) such that the total HCN acid in their products would consistently be as low as reasonably achievable. Production approaches to achieving this are well-documented (Cardoso *et al.*, 2005).

For these reasons, FSANZ prepared Proposal P1002 to assess the public health risks associated

with hydrocyanic acid (hydrogen cyanide) in ready-to-eat cassava chips. This was released for public consultation on 6 March 2008 and gazetted on 30 April 2009. The Code now includes a maximum level of 10 mg/kg for hydrocyanic acid in ready-to-eat cassava chips. This is in-line with a Codex standard for cassava flour.

Table 24.4 provides an outline of the timeline of response to this issue.

24.4.3 Deliberate Contamination: Melamine

24.4.3.1 The Issue

In September 2008, FSANZ became aware of media reports, which indicated that more than 50,000 infants and young children in China had sought treatment for renal tube blockages and kidney stones following consumption of infant formula adulterated with melamine. The addition of melamine to food or infant formula is not approved anywhere in the world. By the end of November 2008, the Chinese Ministry of Health reported that 294,000 infants were affected and six children died from melamine-contaminated infant formula. It is understood that melamine, a source of nitrogen, was added to milk to boost its apparent protein content, when tested by measuring nitrogen content. The adulterated milk was subsequently used as an ingredient in the manufacture of infant formula.

The Australian Quarantine and Inspection Service (AQIS) and the Infant Formula Manufacturers' Association of Australia very quickly confirmed that Australia does not import infant formula from China. However, laboratory findings from Singapore emerged, which indicated that the contaminated milk was used as an ingredient in other products such as soft confectionery. The first of these products to come to international attention was White Rabbit creamy candy from China. AQIS confirmed that this product and others with a dairy-base were imported into Australia.

TABLE 24.4 Timeline of key events in responding to cyanogenic glycosides in cassava-based crackers/chips

Focus	Date	Key event
Notification	Jan 2008	NSW Food Authority notified of the detection of hydrogen cyanide in cassava-based crackers by Japanese authorities
		Expert toxicological advice sought and National food incident response protocol activated
		Product voluntarily recalled from the market
		Laboratory established a method to test for total hydrogen cyanide, testing commences
Monitoring	Feb 2008	Consumer advisories issued
		Preliminary risk assessment completed with guidance level of 25 mg/kg
		Test results lead to additional voluntary product withdrawals
		NSW Food Authority request Food Standards Australia New Zealand to urgently consider appropriate standards for these products
Standards	Mar 2008	Proposed standard for hydrocyanic acid (hydrogen cyanide) of 10 mg/kg in ready-to-eat cassava chips released for public comment
	Sept 2008	Final approval report (including revised risk assessment) released for public comments
	Dec 2008	Ministerial Council review of proposed standard requested
	April 2009	Food Standards Code amended

24.4.3.2 *The Hazard*

Melamine resins are used for kitchenware, plastic resins, flame retardant fibers and components of paper and cardboard. It is possible for such resins to come into contact with food during food production. This might result in the presence of trace quantities of melamine in food that does not pose any risk to human health.

In 2007, a similar food adulteration event involving melamine was detected by authorities in the US. An adulterated pet food ingredient (gluten) imported from China resulted in renal failure and death in cats and dogs. Analysis of some adulterated pet food scraps detected melamine and a number of melamine-related compounds (e.g. cyanuric acid, ammelide, and ammeline).

The US Food and Drug Administration (FDA) responded to this event by preparing an interim risk assessment for melamine and related compounds (US FDA, 2007). The risk assessment established a tolerable daily intake (TDI) of 0.63 mg/kg body weight/day that included a 100-fold safety factor and considered the likely risk to humans arising from consumption of meat and eggs derived from animals that had eaten feed contaminated with melamine compounds. The risk assessment concluded that the dietary risk to humans from this source was very low.

Investigations into the nature of the kidney stones that were present in the pets that died in the 2007 incident revealed that they were composed of melamine-cyanurate. Furthermore, subsequent experimental tests confirmed that cats fed pet food adulterated with melamine and cyanuric acid (in combination) died because of kidney failure through intratubular obstruction caused by the presence of melamine-cyanurate kidney stones (US FDA, 2007). In contrast, cats did not die if fed either melamine or cyanuric acid separately at the equivalent concentration.

Evidence showing that the synergistic action of melamine and cyanuric acid could produce an effect that was greater than each compound separately caused reconsideration about the adequacy of the melamine TDI for human health risk assessment purposes. To address this, the FDA proposed to apply an additional 10-fold uncertainty factor to its risk assessment for exposure to melamine and its analogs in food (US FDA, 2008). Based on its worst case exposure scenario the FDA concluded that if 50% of the diet was contaminated with melamine and its analogs at a level of 2.5 mg melamine/kg of food a person's daily exposure would be 0.063 mg/kg body weight/day. Hence there is a 1000-fold difference between the estimated dietary exposure and the level of melamine that does not cause any toxicity in animals. Other countries also undertook similar dietary exposure determinations. For Europe this was based on a TDI of 0.5 mg/kg body weight/day (EFSA, 2008) and in Canada this was based on a toxicological reference dose for melamine of 0.35 mg/kg body weight/day (Canadian Government, 2008).

The World Health Organization convened an expert panel in December 2008 to consider toxicological risks posed by melamine (WHO, 2008b). The outcome of that meeting was the establishment of a TDI at 0.2 mg/kg bodyweight for melamine. Based on this, it leads a 50 kg person to a tolerable amount of 10 mg melamine per day. The TDI applies to melamine alone. The TDI for cyanuric acid alone remains at 1.5 mg/kg body weight as data were not available at the meeting to evaluate the TDI. While co-occurrence of melamine with cyanuric acid seems to be more toxic, the available data do not allow the calculation of a health-based guidance value for this co-exposure.

24.4.3.3 The Risks

Trace quantities of melamine and related compounds that are of no toxicological importance may legitimately be present in food. This might arise during processing through leaching from food-grade melamine contact material. Although there are no published reports on the likely leached levels of melamine in foods, some studies report levels of melamine that can be leached from melamine kitchenware under very severe conditions. Melamine may be detected in beverages at levels of 0.5, 0.7, 1.4 and 2.2 mg/kg in coffee, orange juice, fermented milk and lemon juice respectively (Ishiwata, Inoue, Yamazaki, & Yoshihira, 1987). These levels originate from migration of melamine from the cup, made of melamine-formaldehyde resin, into the beverage under experimental hot and acidic conditions (95°C for 30 min). Given the extreme use conditions used to generate these data, it is considered that a level of 2.5 mg melamine/kg food would represent the upper levels likely to be legitimately found in foods. Therefore, melamine levels in food exceeding 2.5 mg/kg would be indicative of food adulteration.

In October 2008, FSANZ undertook a preliminary dietary exposure assessment on melamine in soft confectionery for the whole population (Australians aged 2 years and above and New Zealanders aged 15 years and above) and the Australian population sub-groups of children aged 2–3 years and 4–8 years. Based on levels of melamine detected in White Rabbit creamy candy (imported from China into New Zealand, see next section), a concentration of melamine of 180 mg/kg was assigned to foods similar to White Rabbit Candy (e.g. soft, chewy textured confectionery). In order to determine if the level of potential exposure to melamine could be a public health and safety concern, the estimated dietary exposures were compared to the TDI of 0.63 mg/kg body weight/day (FDA value). For all adults and children 4–8 years, dietary exposure was estimated to be below the TDI. For 2–3-year-old children, dietary exposure was 115% TDI at the 90th percentile of melamine exposure. For a child weighing 30 kg, about 105 g of these sweets would have to be consumed before the TDI was exceeded. However, in general, Chinese-made sweets are likely to be consumed infrequently and in small amounts so they are not considered to be a high-risk food for ongoing dietary exposure to melamine.

The overall conclusions of the risk assessment were:

- A maximum level of 1 mg/kg for melamine in infant formula is considered appropriate;
- A maximum level of 2.5 mg/kg for melamine in dairy-based foods and foods containing dairy-based ingredients is appropriate and acceptable;
- A level of melamine above 2.5 mg/kg is indicative of food adulteration;
- For infant formula, even at relatively low levels of adulteration an infant will quickly exceed the Tolerable Daily Intake for melamine, if consuming formula only;
- Foods with low levels of dairy-based ingredients, such as candies and biscuits, are likely to be infrequently consumed and in small amounts so they are not considered to be a high-risk food for potential dietary exposure to melamine even if the dairy ingredient has been adulterated.

24.4.3.4 *The Response*

The National Food Incident Response Protocol was activated within 24 hours upon learning of media reports from the Chinese and international press. New Zealand authorities were participants in the response protocol. In the first instance, regulatory authorities in Australia and New Zealand deployed officers to inspect premises, predominantly in areas with a high Asian demographic, and focused on the country of origin labeling of infant formula offered for sale. No infant formula products from China were found during these inspections, reinforcing the import information supplied by border control authorities that infant formula products were not permitted to be imported into Australia from China.

A number of dairy-based products were purchased from Asian retail outlets and importers, and were submitted to laboratories for melamine testing. This included; soft confectionaries, drinks, soups, ice cream, sweetened condensed milk, biscuits, and sweeteners. New Zealand authorities received their results first. In certain batches of White Rabbit creamy candy, the level of melamine detected was 180 mg/kg. As a result, the risk management strategy adopted in New Zealand was to put out a consumer advisory statement and approach importers to voluntarily withdraw the products, which subsequently occurred.

In Australia, a two-pronged approach was agreed for national action in response to the findings in New Zealand. First, FSANZ issued an advisory to the media about the detection of melamine in White Rabbit creamy candy in New Zealand. Second, all known importers of these products were informed of the FSANZ advisory and were requested to voluntarily withdraw their products from the market until further testing and investigation were completed. Importers willingly complied with this request.

The first round of test results in Australia also showed positive levels of melamine in certain batches of White Rabbit creamy candies ranging from 35 to 168 mg/kg. As these had already been voluntarily removed from the market as a proactive step by importers, no further action was required.

A nationally coordinated monitoring program of products containing ingredients from China that might have been adulterated by melamine began in October 2008. Generally, immediate attention from Australian or overseas authorities was given to products that tested positive in overseas surveys; imported products that were dairy-based; and food with dairy-based ingredients which were at high risk of adulteration. This was then extended to products imported from China into Australia where price was determined partially by protein content as tested by nitrogen content; for example, with gluten, corn, soy, ingredients that have potential for addition of melamine to boost nitrogen content.

With test results expected on a broad range of products from coordinated efforts, a national risk management strategy was developed. This was represented as a decision tree (Figure 24.4) for the purpose of providing guidance and a consistent approach to managing the presence of melamine in food. The decision tree applied to final food, not ingredients for use in foods and also did not apply to infant formula. The decision tree was used in conjunction with the risk assessment and referral levels for dairy foods and foods containing dairy-based ingredients adulterated with melamine (FSANZ, 2008b).

Either as a result of testing of products in Australia or manufacturers taking a precautionary approach because of test results elsewhere, at the time of writing, the following products have been withdrawn from the Australian market: White Rabbit cream candy, Lotte biscuits, Kirin Milk Tea, Orion Tiramisu Italian cake, Dali Yuan brand First Milk vanilla flavored drink, Boxer Lovers Body Pen Set (body paint), Munchy's Mini crackers, Four Seas Premium cake (three flavors), Danco Waffles and Mengniu Monmilk.

While there was international agreement on the level of melamine contamination that indicated adulterated products, the risk management response varied from country to country. Australia made assessments on a case-by-case basis as did New Zealand. Authorities in the US and Hong Kong indicated that food, other than infant formula, containing in excess of 2.5 mg melamine/kg would not be permitted. The EU, Canada and China set a level of 2.5 mg melamine/kg for dairy-based foods. For infant formula a level of 1 mg melamine/kg applied in Hong Kong, China and the US. In Canada the 1 mg melamine/kg maximum level applied to infant formula and sole nutrition products including meal replacement

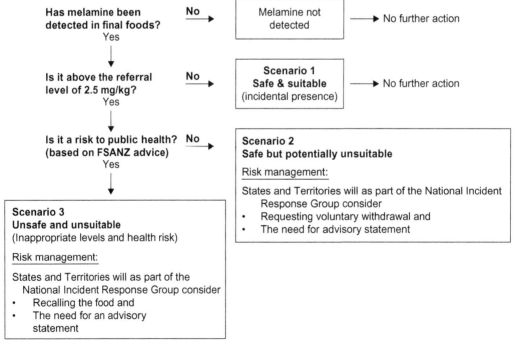

FIGURE 24.4 A risk management decision tree for melamine in food containing dairy ingredients (excluding infant formula).

products until December 2008. Canada revised the level for infant formula following the WHO Expert Meeting held in December 2008 such that a level of 0.5 mg/kg applies to ready-made formula and other infant formula products. The EU and Australia are currently not permitting any importation of infant formula from China.

Table 24.5 provides an outline of the timeline of response to this issue.

24.5 CONCLUSION

The need to respond to low-level chemical contaminants is often prompted by an emerging food incident that requires a response at local, national or international levels within a short time-frame. The case studies presented illustrate how risk analysis offers a structured and flexible framework in considering the risks associated with food. Incorporating the key components of risk assessment, risk management and risk communication, risk analysis provides a systematic and disciplined approach to establishing and implementing risk management options applicable to the severity of risk and local circumstances.

Illustrated within each case study was the need for risk managers to recognize that, in all cases, risk assessment results contained a degree of uncertainty depending on the quality of the available data. Advances in scientific knowledge will have an impact on these risk management decisions. Subsequently, review of risk management decisions is essential in determining whether advance knowledge has made an impact on scientific advice previously used to make decisions resulting in policy, regulation or action.

ACKNOWLEDGEMENTS

The authors praise the professionalism, dedication and commitment of national and international regulatory colleagues and scientific experts involved in responding to the issues presented as case studies. Some of the material featured in this chapter appears in the public domain on government websites: the New South Wales

TABLE 24.5 Timeline of key events in responding to melamine adulteration of dairy-based foods

Focus	Date	Key event
Notification	Sept 2008	Media reports of illness associated with infant formula adulterated with melamine in China. High levels of melamine detected in confectionary product in Singapore
		Confirmation from AQIS that no Chinese infant formula imported into Australia
		Consumer advisories issued and importers of confectionary contacted
		Products voluntarily withdrawn from the market
		Expert toxicological advice sought
		Laboratory adapts test method to range of food products
Monitoring	Oct 2008	Risk assessment completed and risk management decision tree developed
		Monitoring program designed and implemented
		Test results lead to additional product withdrawals
	Nov 2008	Test results lead to additional product withdrawals
	Dec 2008	Monitoring of high risk products (completed in March 2009)

Food Authority (www.foodauthority.nsw.gov.au) and the Food Standards Australia New Zealand (www.foodstandards.gov.au). Full links to the material is provided in the reference section.

References

Abbott, P., Baines, J., Fox, P., et al. (2003). Review of the regulations for contaminants and natural toxicants. *Food Control, 14*, 383–389.

ANZFA. (1998). *The regulation of contaminants and other restricted substances in food: Policy paper.* Canberra: Australia New Zealand Food Authority.

Australian Bureau of Statistics (1999). 4804.0—National Nutrition Survey: Foods Eaten, Australia, 1995 (available at: http://www.abs.gov.au/AUSSTATS/abs@.nsf/ProductsbyCatalogue/9A125034802F94CECA2568A9001393CE?OpenDocument).

Australian Bureau of Statistics (2000). 4306.0— Apparent Consumption of Foodstuffs, Australia, 1997–98 and 1998–99 (available at: http://www.abs.gov.au/AUSSTATS/abs@.nsf/0/123FCDBF086C4DAACA2568A90013939A?OpenDocument).

Australian Government (2004a). Department of the Environment and Heritage, *Dioxins in Australia: A Summary of the Finding of Studies Conducted from 2001 to 2004, National Dioxin Program.* Australian Government Department of the Environment and Heritage, Canberra, Australia.

Australian Government (2004b). Department of Health and Ageing, Office of Chemical Safety, *Human Health Risk Assessment of Dioxins in Australian, National Dioxin Program, Technical Report No. 12.* Australian Government Department of the Environment and Heritage, Canberra, Australia.

Australian Government (2005). Environment Protection & Heritage Council. National Dioxins Program. National Action Plan for Addressing Dioxins in Australia. Environment Protection & Heritage Council, Canberra, Australia.

Australian Government (2007). Department of Health and Aging *National Food Incident Response Protocol* (available at: http://www.health.gov.au/internet/main/publishing.nsf/Content/CDA339ACBEE60CF8CA25709600193198/$File/response.pdf).

Bradbury, J. H. (2006). Simple wetting method to reduce cyanogen content of cassava flour. *Journal of Food Composition and Analysis, 19*, 388–393.

Bradbury, M. G., Egan, S. V., & Bradbury, J. H. (1999). Picrate paper kits for determination of total cyanogens in cassava roots and all forms of cyanogens in cassava products. *Journal of the Science of Food and Agriculture, 79*, 593–601.

Canadian Government (2008). Health Canada's Human Health Risk Assessment Supporting Standard Development for Melamine in Foods (available at: http://www.hc-sc.gc.ca/fn-an/pubs/melamine_hra-ers-eng.php).

Cardoso, A. P., Mirione, E., Ernesto, M., et al. (2005). Processing of cassava roots to remove cyanogens. *Journal of Food Composition and Analysis, 18*, 451–460.

Codex (2004). Working Principles for Risk Analysis for Application in the Framework of the Codex Alimentarius. In: *Codex Alimentarius Commission Procedural Manual Ed. 14.* Joint FAO/WHO Food Standards Programme, Rome.

Cooke, R. D. 1978. An enzymatic assay for the total cyanide content of cassava (*manihot esculenta crantz*). *Journal of the Science of Food and Agriculture, 29*(4), 345–352.

Cumbana, A., Mirione, E., Cliff, J., & Bradbury, J. H. (2007). Reduction of cyanide content of cassava flour in Mozambique by the wetting method. *Food Chemistry, 101*, 894–897.

Ernesto, M., Cardoso, A. P., Nicala, D., et al. (2002). Persistent konzo and cyanogen toxicity from cassava in Northern Mozambique. *Acta Tropica, 82*, 357–362.

European Commission (2000). Health and Consumer Protection Directorate-General Opinion of the Scientific Committee on Food on the Risk Assessment of Dioxins and Dioxin-like PCBs in Food. Document SCF/CS/CNTM/DIOXIN/8 Final, 23 November 2000. Brussels, Belgium: European Commission.

European Commission (2006), Commission Regulation (EC) No 199/2006 of 3 February 2006 amending Regulation (EC) No 466/2001 setting maximum levels for certain contaminants in foodstuffs as regards dioxins and dioxin-like PCBs (available at: http://europa.eu.int/eur-lex/lex/LexUriServ/site/en/oj/2006/l_032/l_03220060204en00340038.pdf).

EFSA. (2008). Statement of EFSA on risks for public health due to the presences of melamine in infant milk and other milk products in China (available at: http://www.efsa.europa.eu/cs/BlobServer/Statement/contam_ej_807_melamine,0.pdf?ssbinary = true). *The EFSA Journal, 807*, 1–10.

FAO. (1977). Cassava processing. *FAO Plant Production and Protection Series No 3.* Food and Agriculture Organization (available at: http://www.fao.org/docrep/X5032E/x5032E00.htm).

FSANZ. (2004). *Dioxins in food: Dietary Exposure Assessment and Risk Characterisation, Technical Report Series No. 27.* Food Standards Australia New Zealand (available at: http://www.foodstandards.gov.au/technicalreportseries/index.cfm).

FSANZ. (2006). *Dioxins in Prawns and Fish from Sydney Harbour: An Assessment of the Public Health and Safety Risk, Technical Report Series No. 43.* Food Standards

Australia New Zealand (available at: http://www.food-standards.gov.au/technicalreportseries/index.cfm).

FSANZ. (2007). *Dioxins in Seafood from Sydney Harbour. A Revised Assessment of the Public Health and Safety Risk* (updated), *Technical Report Series No. 44*. Food Standards Australia New Zealand (available at: http://www.food-standards.gov.au/technicalreportseries/index.cfm).

FSANZ. (2008a). *Proposal P1002 Hydrocyanic acid (hydrogen cyanide) in ready-to-eat cassava chips: Assessment report*. Food Standards Australia New Zealand (available at: http://www.foodstandards.gov.au/_srcfiles/P1002_Cassava_in_Vege_chips_AR.pdf).

FSANZ. (2008b). *Risk assessment and referral levels for dairy foods and foods containing dairy-based ingredients adulterated with melamine*. Food Standards Australia New Zealand (available at: http://www.foodstandards.gov.au/news-room/factsheets/factsheets2008/melamineinfoods-fromchina/riskassessmentandref4064.cfm).

IARC. (1997). IARC Monographs on the Evaluation of Carcinogen Risks to Humans. Vol 69. *Polychlorinated Dibenzo-para-dioxins and Polychlorinated Bibenzofurans*. Lyon, France: International Agency for Research on Cancer.

Ishiwata, H., Inoue, T., Yamazaki, T., & Yoshihira, K. (1987). Liquid chromatographic determination of melamine in beverages. *Journal - Association of Official Analytical Chemists, 70*, 457–460.

Müller, J., Muller, R., Goudkamp, K. et al. (2004). *Dioxins in the Aquatic Environments in Australia, National Dioxin Program, Technical Report No. 6*. Canberra, Australia: Australian Government Department of the Environment and Heritage.

New Zealand Government (1999) Ministry of Health: 1997 National Nutrition Survey (available at: http://www.moh.govt.nz/moh.nsf/0/8F1DBEB1E0E1C70C4C2567D80009B770).

NSW Food Authority (2006). Dioxins in Seafood in Port Jackson and its Tributaries: Report of the Expert Panel (available at: http://www.foodauthority.nsw.gov.au/consumer/pdf/Report_of_the_Expert_Panel_on_Dioxins_in_Seafood.pdf).

Oluwole, O. S. A. (2008). Cyanogenicity of cassava varieties and risk of exposure to cyanide from cassava food in Nigerian communities. *Journal of the science of Food and Agriculture, 88*, 962–969.

US FDA. (2007). *Interim Melamine and Analogues Safety/Risk Assessment*. United States of America Food and Drug Administration (available at: http://www.cfsan.fda.gov/~dms/melamra.html).

US FDA. (2008). *Interim Safety and Risk Assessment of Melamine and Melamine-related Compounds in Food*. United States of America Food and Drug Administration (available at: http://www.fda.gov/bbs/topics/NEWS/2008/NEW01895.html).

WHO. (1987). *Principles for the safety assessment of food additives and contaminants in food*. International Programme on Chemical Safety. Geneva, Switzerland: World Health Organisation.

WHO. (1998). *Assessment of the Health Risks of Dioxins: Re-Evaluation of the Tolerable Daily Intake (TDI)*. Executive Summary of the WHO Consultation, 25–29 May 1998, Geneva, Switzerland.

WHO. (2008a). *Chemical risks in food* (available at: http://www.who.int/foodsafety/chem/en/).

WHO. (2008b). Expert meeting to review toxicological aspects of melamine and cyanuric acid (available at: http://www.who.int/foodsafety/fs_management/infosan_events/en/index.html).

1

Integrating Risk Assessment and Cost Benefit Analysis: An Economics Perspective on International Trade and Food Safety

Cristina McLaughlin, Peter Vardon, and Clark Nardinelli

US Food and Drug Administration, Center for Food Safety and Applied Nutrition, MD, USA

ABSTRACT

The World Trade Organization (WTO) was created to promote international trade liberalization without discrimination. The WTO's Sanitary and Phytosanitary (SPS) Agreement was added to protect human, animal and plant life and health from transmissible risks in accordance with science-based risk assessments, equivalence and harmonization, while still promoting trade (Roberts, D. & Unnevehr, L., 2005, Resolving trade disputes arising from trends in food safety regulation: the role of the multilateral governance framework. *World Trade Rev, 4*, 469–497). Some research shows that WTO rules have not been consistently successful at promoting trade liberalization (Rose, A. K., 2002, *Do WTO members have a more liberal trade policy? NBER Working Paper*, No. 9347, Cambridge, MA: NBER; Subramanian, A. & Wei, S. J., 2006, *The WTO promotes trade, strongly but unevenly.* NBER Working Paper, No. 10024, Cambridge, MA: NBER, and IMF Working Paper). The SPS Agreement risk analysis process may not have been successful at promoting trade with the parts of the world that are riskiest—the developing world. Risk analysis is the framework for decision makers and regulators to use risk assessment, risk management, and risk communication in order to reduce the public impact of risks, especially, health and safety risks. The agreement allows nations to establish a self-selected appropriate level of (risk) protection (ALOP) including zero-levels of risk, which can amount to an import ban (Gruszczynski, L., 2008, Risk management policies under the WTO Agreement on the application of sanitary and phytosanitary measures. *AJWH*, Vol. 3, March 2008, No. 1).

The purpose of this perspective is to show that integrating risk assessment and cost–benefit analysis (CBA) into the SPS risk analysis framework could better help member nations to identify cost-effective levels of risk protection—options less likely to include unwarranted import bans based on zero-risk levels. Resulting import policies could in turn be more transparent and more likely to promote trade. Although many risk assessments are used in conjunction with economic analysis, both types of analyses are seldom explicitly combined. One of the difficulties caused by separate analyses is that results may have differing starting or end points or both. This lack of a common metric can lead to confusion and extensive lag times from onset of the analyses to policy making. Without integrating risk assessments and economic analyses, finite resources may be allocated to reducing an already low risk, while higher risks may continue to be tolerated (Williams, R. A. & Thompson, K. M., 2004, Integrated analysis: combining risk and economic assessments while preserving the separation of powers. *Risk Analysis*, 24(6), 1613–1623).

ABSTRACT

2

Food Additives and Other Substances Added to Human Foods

Larry Keener

International Product Safety Consultants, Seattle, WA, USA

ABSTRACT

Great disparities exist globally with regard to regulations and standards relating to the control of substances allowed for addition, directly or indirectly, to human food. A number of countries have adopted strict criteria for both defining and classifying the various types of substances that are permitted for inclusion in foods and food ingredients. Likewise, there are nations that have promulgated legislation regulating the precise manner in which the various classes of approved substances might be added to human food. By contrast, the food additive standards and regulations of other nations that participate in the global trade in food and food ingredients are far less refined and robust.

In general substances found in human food can be assigned as one of the six following classifications: 1) Residues; 2) Unavoidable Contaminants; 3) Prohibited Substances; 4) Supplements; 5) Food Additives; or 6) Cosmetic Additives. Included in these various classifications are color and flavor agents, as well as pesticide residues, vitamins, veterinary compounds and environmental contaminants (Schultz, H. W., 1981, *Food law handbook*, Westport CT: AVI Publishing).

According to the Extension Services of Iowa, Kansas, and Nebraska (report by Redlinger & Nelson, 1993) there are presently upwards of 2800 additives approved for use in the United States. In the US there are greater than 400 million pounds of additives used annually in processed meats (Food Product Development, 1980). The average US citizen is reported to consume between 140 and 150 pounds of additives per year (Redlinger & Nelson, 1993). Worldwide, approximately 98% of the additive compounds consumed are sugar, corn sweeteners, salt, citric acid, pepper, vegetable color, mustard, yeast and baking powder (Redlinger & Nelson, 1993). Safety testing in the US is conducted on all additives, except those that are prior-sanctioned and generally recognized as safe (GRAS) substances. During the period from 1978 to 2008, the US food additives business grew from about $1billion to nearly $13.0 billion in annual sales.

According to Codex, a 'food additive' is 'any substance not normally consumed as a food by itself and not normally used as a typical ingredient of the food, whether or not it has nutritive value, the intentional addition of which to food for a technological (including organoleptic) purpose in the manufacture, processing, preparation, treatment, packing, packaging, transport or holding of such food results, or may be reasonably expected to result, (directly or indirectly) in it or its by-products becoming a component of or otherwise affecting the characteristics of such foods.' The definition goes on to state that the term *does not include* 'contaminants, or substances added to food for maintaining or improving nutritional qualities, or sodium chloride' (The Codex General Standard for the Labeling of Prepackaged Foods, CODEX STAN 1-1985). It is easily conceived that confusion could rapidly ensue using this definition as to what is and what is not a food additive. The issue is further complicated when one considers the implications associated with the multitude of national definitions and norms related to food additives. The US Food and Drug Administration, for example, accepts that food additives 'promote health and wellness,' 'improve nutritional value,' and 'flavor development and stabilization.' Clearly these functional characteristics are in conflict with Codex's food additive definition. Salt, for example, is used for both flavor development and preservation. Which begs the question, is salt a food additive or not?

Processing aids and carry-over compounds, sub-classifications of food additives, are also an exceedingly confusing subject. According to Codex, processing aids are *'a "chaotic subject" where member states have disparate views due to their own individual experiences and long histories of regulatory development'* (Codex Alimentarius Commission, Guidelines and Principles on the use of Processing Aids; Codex discussion paper CCFAC; New Zealand Delegation.). The subject may even be chaotic *within* national regulatory frameworks. Consider that in the US, regulations of the Federal Food, Drug and Cosmetic Act allow for the definition and use of Processing Aid (US

Food and Drug Administration, 1986, US Code of Federal Regulations, 21CFR101.100(a)(3) in the production of food that is intended for human use. By contrast, however, the US Department of Agriculture's Food Safety and Inspection Service regulations are mute on the subject. Likewise, the Canadian Food Inspection Agency does not have specific regulations governing this class of food additive compounds called processing aids (Salminen, 2005, Chemical Health Hazard Assessment Division, Health Products and Food Branch, Health Canada, Personal Communication).

Japan defines processing aids as 'substances that are added to a food during the processing of such food but are removed from the food before it is prepared in its finished form, <substances> that are added to a food during processing that are converted into components ubiquitously present in the food, and do not significantly increase the level of the constituents naturally found in food, or < substances> that are added to a food for their technical or functional effect in the processing but are present in the finished food at an insignificant level and do not have any technical or functional effect in the food' (Codex Alimentarius Commission, Guidelines and Principles on the use of Processing Aids, Codex discussion paper CX/FAC 02/0905).

Codex's definition takes a somewhat different view of processing aids and it has defined this class of additives accordingly: *'Processing aid—* any substance or material not including apparatus or utensils, and not consumed as a food ingredient by itself, intentionally used in the processing of raw materials, foods or its ingredients to fulfill a certain technological purpose during treatment or processing and which may result in the non-intentional but unavoidable presence of residues or derivatives in the final product' (The Codex General Standard for the Labeling of Prepackaged Foods, CODEX STAN 1-1985).

Processing aids are an important but complex class of food additives. They play a role in facilitating the stabilization and preservation of many food products. Hydrogen peroxide, for example, is used in processing liquid eggs and allows the egg to be pasteurized using mild thermal processing conditions that will not result in protein denaturation. Utilizing this heat and hydrogen peroxide process requires the use of yet another processing aid, the enzyme Catalase. Catalase is added to the process for the removal of residual hydrogen peroxide and thereby enables compliance with the aspect of the US regulation requiring that the processing aid is removed and not present in the final food. Chemicals in this grouping are used to promote separation, clarification, mixing, blending, and foam suppression, as well as for management of material flow characteristics. Included in this classification is a very broad array of both chemical and biological agents. Processing aids may be derived from biotechnology, from other natural foods

sources, or they may result from synthesis in a chemical manufacturing facility.

In terms of substances that are allowed for addition to human foods, processing aids hold a unique status in that many countries have elected to exempt them from labeling requirements. This exemption frequently raises questions and concerns for both regulatory officials and consumers about the public health status and safety of foods to which these substances have been added. The vagaries and nuances in this area are enormous and also frequently an impediment to international trade.

This chapter explores both the opportunities and impediments to harmonization of the definitions, permissible usage and labeling of the substances permitted for inclusion in the production of foods that are intended for human consumption.

ABSTRACT

3

Global Harmonization of Food Regulations: Benefits and Risks of Organic Food

Alain Maquet

European Commission, DG Joint Research Centre, Institute for Reference Materials and
Measurements, Geel, Belgium

ABSTRACT

The state-of-the-art of organic food is investigated with respect to regulations; to the harmonization of standards; to the ongoing debate over whether organically grown produce is safer and/or healthier than conventionally grown produce; and to the research currently underway and proposed to sustain the development of the organic market.

Food quality and food safety aspects related to organic food commodities are depicted within the framework of the European food law. Some specific issues of organic food safety (e.g. pesticide residues, nitrates, pathogenic microorganisms, mycotoxins) and potential nutritional benefits (e.g. polyphenols, antioxidant capacity, proteins) are detailed on the basis of recent scientific evidence. Few studies have attempted to directly measure the impact of diets comprising organic or conventional foods on animal and human health. However, their overview does not yet provide clear evidence on whether or not the food production method affects any aspect of human health.

Research activities based on organic food and farming systems can contribute greatly towards the overall sustainability of agriculture and food production. The ideas proposed by scientists are intended to promote, among other priority areas, high quality foods. Research concerning claims on the authenticity, safety and nutritional values of organic food is also still relevant today despite increased scientific efforts in this last decade.

Index

Printed in the United States
By Bookmasters